This book is to be re~
the last d~~

Drugs in Anaesthesia:
mechanisms of action

Edited by

Stanley A. Feldman
BSc, MB BS, FFARCS, DA

Consultant Anaesthetist
Westminster Hospital
Charing Cross and Westminster Medical School
University of London

Cyril F. Scurr
CBE, LVO, FRCS, FFARCS,Hon FFARCS (I)

Honorary Consulting Anaesthetist
Westminster Hospital
London

Sir William Paton
CBE, FRS, MA, DM, FRCP, FFARCS

Emeritus Professor of Pharmacology
University of Oxford

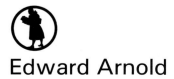

Edward Arnold

© Edward Arnold (Publishers) Ltd 1987

First published in Great Britain 1987 by
Edward Arnold (Publishers) Ltd, 41 Bedford Square, London WC1B 3DQ

Edward Arnold (Australia) Pty Ltd, 80 Waverley Road, Caulfield East,
    Victoria 3145, Australia

Edward Arnold, 3 East Read Street, Baltimore, Maryland 21202, U.S.A.

ISBN 0 7131 4515 3

Erratum:

Figs A4.1, A4.2 and A4.3 on pp. 432 and 433 are
taken from Hull, C.J. (1984) Opioid Infusions.
In: *Acute Pain* (International Medical Reviews
Vol. 1) (Eds. Smith, G. and Covino, B.G.),
Butterworth & Co (Publishers) Ltd: Sevenoaks,
Kent. (Reproduced with permission.)

Whilst the advice and information in this book is believed to be true and accurate at
the date of going to press, neither the authors nor the publisher can accept any legal
responsibility or liability for any errors or omissions that may be made.

Text set in 10/11pt Times
by Tek-Art Ltd, Croydon, Surrey
Printed in Great Britain
by Butler & Tanner Ltd, London and Frome

List of Contributors

Editors

Stanley A. Feldman BSc, MB BS, FFARCS, DA
Consultant Anaesthetist
Westminster Hospital
Charing Cross and Westminster Medical School
University of London, UK

Cyril F. Scurr CBE, LVO, FRCS, FFARCS, Hon FFARCS(I)
Honorary Consulting Anaesthetist
Westminster Hospital
London, UK

Sir William Paton CBE, FRS, MA, DM, FRCP, FFARCS
13 Staverton Road
Oxford, UK

Contributors

Jeffrey M. Baden MB BS, FFARCS, MRCP (UK)
Associate Professor of Anesthesia
Stanford University School of Medicine
        and
Assistant Chief, Anesthesiology Service
Veterans Administration Medical Center
Palo Alto, California 94304, USA

P.K. Barnes MB BS, MRCS, LRCP, FFARCS
Consultant Anaesthetist
Magill Department of Anaesthetics
Westminster Hospital
London, UK

D.J. Chapple BSc
Pharmacologist
Department of Pharmacology I
Wellcome Research Laboratories
Beckenham, Kent, UK

Benjamin G. Covino PhD, MD
Chairman of Anesthesia
Brigham and Women's Hospital
    and
Professor of Anesthesia
Harvard Medical School
Boston, Massachusetts, USA

David J.R. Duthie MB ChB, FFARCS
Lecturer in Anaesthesia
University of Sheffield, UK

P. Foëx, DM(Geneva), DPhil, FFARCS
Clinical Reader and Honorary Consultant in Clinical Physiology
University of Oxford
Radcliffe Infirmary, UK

Valerie A. Goat MB ChB, FFARCS
Consultant Anaesthetist
Radcliffe Infirmary
Oxford, UK

C.J. Hull MB BS, MRCS, LRCP, FFARCS, DA
Professor of Anaesthesia and Honorary Consultant Anaesthetist
University of Newcastle upon Tyne
Royal Victoria Infirmary, UK

D.H. Jenkinson PhD
Professor of Pharmacology
University College London, UK

Vincent Marks MA, BM BCh, DM, FRCP, FRCPath
Professor of Clinical Biochemistry
University of Surrey
Guildford, UK

Laurence E. Mather PhD, FFA RACS
Reader in Anaesthesia and Intensive Care
Flinders University of South Australia
School of Medicine
Adelaide SA 5042
Australia

H. Mattie MD, PhD
Clinical Pharmacologist
Department of Infectious Diseases and Internal Medicine
University Hospital
Leiden, Netherlands

Keith W. Miller MS, DPhil, AM
Edward Mallinckrodt, Jr
Professor of Pharmacology
Harvard Medical School
      and
Department of Anesthesia
Massachusetts General Hospital
Boston, MA 02114, USA

Walter S. Nimmo BSc, MB ChB, MD, FRCP, FFARCS
Professor of Anaesthesia
University of Sheffield, UK

Felicity Reynolds MD, MB BS, FFARCS
Reader in Pharmacology (applied to Anaesthesia)
St Thomas' Hospital
London, UK

W.B. Runciman BSc (Med), MB BCh, FFA RACS, FFA RACS(Intens), PhD
Senior Specialist, Intensive Care Unit
Flinders Medical Centre
      and
Senior Lecturer
Flinders University
South Australia

T.W. Smith MSc, PhD
Section Leader
Department of Pharmacology I
Wellcome Research Laboratories
Beckenham, Kent, UK

Neil Soni FFA RACS
Senior Lecturer in Anaesthesia
Westminster and Charing Cross Medical School
London, UK

T.W. Stone DSc
Professor of Neurosciences
St. George's Hospital Medical School
University of London, UK

Preface

Arguably in the last twenty-five years the greatest contribution to anaesthetic advancement has come not from the development of new drugs but from a better appreciation of how to use safely and effectively those agents already available.

It was our conviction that the safe and effective use of potent drugs required an understanding of the science of pharmacology that provided the motivation for this book. With the assistance of an international panel of pharmacologists and anaesthetists we have compiled a book to cover the basis of the pharmacology of most of those groups of drugs used in anaesthesia and intensive care. In Part One we have considered the mechanisms by which drugs react with receptors, the factors that determine their distribution, metabolism and excretion, and how these may be affected by anaesthesia. Part Two covers the fundamental mechanism of action of the various drugs commonly used by anaesthetists, whilst Part Three, the appendices, presents the mechanisms by which drug interactions, side effects and toxicity occur, together with methods of drug analysis and delivery.

This book is not intended as a textbook of pharmacology listing all drugs, their doses, side effects and interactions. This purpose is already served by standard textbooks and by pharmacopoeias. It has been our intention to produce a framework of basic scientific data and principles upon which detailed information about specific drugs can be built and which will allow an enlightened assessment and critique of the specific attributes of the ever increasing numbers of new drugs being produced.

It became evident whilst compiling this book that the depth of knowledge of the mechanisms of drug action varies greatly from one group of drugs to another. Whilst the cellular and sub-cellular mechanisms may be well understood for one group of agents they are often less well known and more speculative for others.

In those instances where the cellular reactions producing the observed effects are only known in general and non-specific terms it has been necessary to describe the physiological changes observed and the clinical response in patients to appreciate the possible mechanisms of action that might be involved.

Inevitably when producing a book for a speciality such as anaesthesia one has to make arbitrary decisions as to which groups of drugs one should include and which should be omitted in order to keep the book within the bounds of a readily readable textbook. Our selection of topics reflects the extent of contemporary interest and the areas of major new research. To have tried hard to be all embracing would have diluted the basic objective of producing a book dedicated to scientific method.

1986   SAF
                                                                                               CFS
                                                                                               WP

Contents

viii   Contents

Part one
General Principles

1

An introduction to receptors and their actions

D.H. Jenkinson

The aims of this chapter are to outline what is known about receptors and their function, to describe the main methods that can be used to study both, and to draw attention to some gaps that remain in our knowledge. Whenever practicable, these matters are discussed and illustrated in relation to the actions of drugs used in the practice of anaesthesia.

Definition, general characteristics and localization of receptors

Receptors are commonly defined as those cellular structures with which neurotransmitters, hormones and drugs combine to produce their action. This encompasses two concepts: that of *recognition* (because of the ability of the receptors to combine with considerable selectivity with specific molecules), and that of *transmission* (because combination of the receptor with such a molecule leads to a change in the functioning of the cell on, or in, which the receptor is located).

The definition does not specify how much of the structure is to be regarded as the receptor. Is it just the binding site for the neurotransmitter or hormone, or the entire macromolecule which carries the site (or sites)? In practice, the term is used in both senses. This can be illustrated in relation to a remarkable recent achievement, the isolation of the acetylcholine receptor of the kind found in skeletal muscle, and the determination of its complete amino acid composition and sequence (for reviews, see Stroud and Finer-Moore, 1985; and McCarthy *et al.*, 1986). Here 'receptor' refers to the whole macromolecule, made up of five subunits, of four different kinds, and with a total relative molecular mass of about 250 000. However, in a statement such as 'tubocurarine competes with acetylcholine for its receptors', the term now means the immediate binding site, comprising only a few of the hundreds of amino acids which, together with carbohydrate moieties, make up the macromolecule.

The lack of an exact definition bears on the vexed question of the molecular mechanism of action of general anaesthetics. Although this is discussed in more appropriate detail in Chapter 6, we may note here that there is increasing evidence to suggest that at least some general anaesthetics may become associated with specific hydrophobic regions of certain membrane proteins, whose function is thereby altered. Should these regions then be regarded as receptors? To form a view, we need to consider the definition and characteristics of receptors a little further.

As already stated, receptors *recognize* and *transmit*. Recognition is by virtue of the ability of the receptor to combine with specific molecules. Hence the receptor has the property of discriminating between the many small molecules to which it will be exposed *in situ*. Evidently, this is possible because the structure of the binding site is to some degree complementary to that of the neurotransmitter or hormone. The complementarity applies not only to shape (the small molecule must 'fit') but also to the distribution of electrical charge. Thus at physiological pH many neurotransmitters carry a net charge which may be positive (e.g. acetylcholine, noradrenaline, 5-hydroxytryptamine) or negative (e.g. glutamate, ATP), and which interacts with a site of opposite charge on the receptor. One or more polar groups are generally also present so that each molecule has a characteristic electron distribution which cannot, however, be regarded as invariant. Indeed, the study of the complementarity of drugs and their binding sites is made particularly difficult, and challenging, by the certainty that both the shape and the charge distribution not only of the drug molecule but also of its receptor will alter as 'docking' occurs (see Dean and Wakelin, 1979; Dean, 1981a, b; Weinstein, 1986).

The importance of shape is underlined by the large differences which generally exist between the affinities of receptors for the stereoisomers of hormones or drug molecules (for an excellent general account, see Ariëns, Soudijn and Timmermans, 1983). Thus, (−)-hyoscyamine (atropine is racemic hyoscyamine) has an approximately 320-fold greater affinity for the muscarinic receptors of the ileum than that of the (+)-isomer. Another striking example is provided by the steroidal anaesthetic alphaxalone. Here anaesthetic activity is completely dependent on the correct stereochemistry at one of the 19 carbon atoms in the molecule. Further, the 'wrong' conformation at another nearby carbon results in an agent which causes paraesthesia as well as anaesthesia (for references, see Phillips, 1974).

Thus, those disposed to regard the site of action of at least some general anaesthetics as a form of receptor will be concerned to demonstrate a dependence of activity on the size, shape and charge distribution of the anaesthetic molecule (see Franks and Lieb, 1984, 1985). The dependence on shape is certainly very striking for the steroidal anaesthetics, although scarcely evident for smaller molecules such as halothane and ether.

Localization of receptors
In keeping with their function of enabling cells to respond to neurotransmitters and/or hormones, receptors are often located on the cell membrane. In specialized cells such as skeletal muscle and some neurons, they may be largely restricted to those regions of the membrane which are exposed to neurotransmitter. For example, in skeletal muscle the receptors are packed at a density of over $15\,000/\mu m^2$ in the junctional membrane, as compared with less than $30/\mu m^2$ in the extrajunctional region. There is a corresponding gradient of messenger RNA for acetylcholine (ACh) receptor synthesis (Merlie and Sanes, 1985). Further details of the spatial distribution of the ACh

receptors in skeletal muscle can be found in Chapter 7, and all that need be added here is that receptors are concentrated in the immediate vicinity of the nerve endings in other kinds of cells (e.g. the soma of postganglionic neurons in the parasympathetic system (Harris, Kuffler and Dennis, 1971)) and on the dendrites of CNS neurons (for references, see the review by Poo, 1985).

A striking change in the localization of ACh receptors occurs when a skeletal muscle is chronically denervated or damaged. The extrajunctional receptors (i.e. those away from the end-plate region) then increase greatly in number, to the extent that the entire surface of the muscle fibre becomes highly, although not uniformly, responsive to ACh. There can be as much as a 30-fold rise in the total number of receptors (albeit of a slightly different kind – see, for example, Fambrough, 1979). The tissue accordingly becomes more sensitive to diffusely applied ACh and other cholinergic agonists ('denervation supersensitivity'). One consequence is that the effects of depolarizing neuromuscular blocking agents are no longer restricted to the motor end-plate region: the increase in sodium and potassium permeability, and the ensuing depolarization, which these agents cause now occurs along the length of the muscle fibres. This may well underlie the hyperkalaemia which can result when suxamethonium is administered to patients with denervated or otherwise damaged skeletal muscle (see the accounts by Smith, 1976; and Feldman, 1984).

An increase in receptor number is not, however, the only factor involved in denervation supersensitivity and indeed may not occur at all in some tissues. Adrenergically innervated smooth muscle provides an example. Here the increase in responsiveness to noradrenaline which is seen following chronic denervation is due partly to loss of the neuronal uptake mechanism present in the nerve endings (and which is capable of greatly reducing the local concentration of externally applied noradrenaline – see, for example, Guimaraes and Trendelenburg, 1985) and partly to complex changes in the smooth muscle cells (Fleming, 1980, 1984).

Finally, it should be mentioned that the receptors for some hormones are located within the cell rather than exclusively on the cell membrane. Examples include the receptors for all the steroidal hormones and for those of the thyroid gland.

Methods for the study of receptors

Methods based on the measurement of tissue responses

For many years receptors could be studied only indirectly, by careful observation of tissue responses either *in vivo* or *in vitro*. Although this approach has now been supplemented by the more direct methods to be described, it has provided a great deal of useful information, and is still the mainstay both of pharmacological analysis and of new drug development. Isolated tissues are generally preferred for such work because there is less uncertainty about the concentration of applied drugs, although even then it certainly cannot be assumed that the concentration attained at the receptors is the same as that in the fluid bathing the tissue. Comparable experiments *in vivo* have the added complications that (1) it is often difficult to maintain a steady concentration of the drug in the plasma, (2) the drug may be bound to plasma proteins (so that the concentration 'free' to equilibrate with the receptor may be much reduced) and (3) the drug may be metabolized to compounds of uncertain activity. Evidently, the interpretation of such measurements needs particular care.

A variety of responses may be measured in work with isolated tissues, and the traditional pharmacological preparations (e.g. the resting or transmurally stimulated guinea-pig ileum; the right and left atria of the guinea-pig; the field-stimulated rat vas deferens) continue to play a central part in studies of the classification and action of receptors (see also the later sections on dose–response relations and competitive antagonism). A comprehensive list of these preparations, together with comments on the experimental conditions needed for success with them, can be found in the excellent review by Kenakin (1984).

Some important problems are not, however, amenable to such methods, and require the measurement of the response of individual cells, or even limited regions of a cell. The development of intracellular recording using fine-tipped microelectrodes has made the study of single cell responses relatively straightforward. It is now also practicable to work with isolated cells (e.g. a single muscle fibre or a neuron in a cell culture) which can then be exposed to known concentrations of drugs with relatively little delay due to diffusion. Furthermore, those agonist molecules (the majority) which carry a net electrical charge can be applied by ionophoresis from a fine-tipped micropipette so that the response of a limited area of the cell membrane may easily be studied. The remarkable spatial and time resolution which can be achieved with this method is illustrated in Fig. 1.1.

Further advances have followed the more recent development of the 'patch electrode' technique which enables the opening and closing of single ion channels to be recorded (Neher and Sakmann, 1976). A flat-tipped micropipette is pressed against a cell membrane in such a way as to allow the study of the electrical properties and responses of the minute area (often only a few square micrometres) of membrane under the pipette tip. Agonists such as ACh can be included in the patch pipette, and this has allowed the responses to the activation of single receptors to be observed for the first time. Results obtained using this technique are illustrated in Fig. 1.2. Ingenious and powerful variants of the method have since been devised and it is now possible, for example, to excise from the cell the patch of membrane under the pipette. Drugs or other agents can then be applied to either face of the membrane with little delay due to diffusion. Full accounts can be found in the books edited by Sakmann and Neher (1983) and by Eisenberg, Frank and Stevens (1984).

Despite these remarkable advances, some aspects of receptor function remain difficult to investigate by studies of drug response alone. For example, it is still not straightforward, and often impossible, to deduce from the response of a tissue what is the proportion of receptors occupied by an agonist. There are several reasons, of which two merit mention here. The first is, as discussed later, that occupied receptors may exist in several interconvertible states, only one of which gives rise to the response which is observed. Second, the concentration–response relationships for the action of agonists on single cells often have a sigmoidal form which suggests that full activation of the receptor

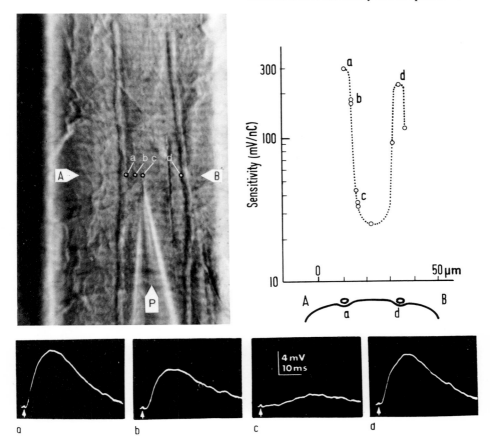

Fig. 1.1   Differences in acetylcholine sensitivity across the surface of a frog muscle fibre with closely spaced nerve terminals. *Photomicrograph:* Cutaneous pectoris muscle fibre viewed under Nomarski optics. Acetylcholine was applied ionophoretically from a micropipette at a series of points along a line running perpendicularly to two parallel terminals about 22 μm apart. P = acetylcholine pipette. *Records:* Acetylcholine depolarizations elicited at each of the spots marked with a white dot on the photomicrograph. Moving the pipette as little as 3 μm from the edge of the terminal caused a 34 per cent drop in sensitivity. *Graph:* Profile of sensitivity between the two terminals. (Reproduced, with permission, from Peper and McMahan (1972).)

occurs only when two or more binding sites on the receptor macromolecule are occupied by agonist molecules. This was first noted for the ACh receptor of skeletal muscle (Katz and Thesleff, 1957; Jenkinson, 1960) and the same is seen for responses mediated by the receptors for GABA (Takeuchi and Takeuchi, 1975; Kaneko and Tachibana, 1986) and glutamate (Dekin and Edwards, 1983; see also Werman, 1969). The interactions between these sites (and their possible non-equivalence, for which there is direct structural evidence in the case of the ACh receptor) greatly increase the difficulty of analysing the relationship between agonist concentration and response.

ACH. 100 nmol/l

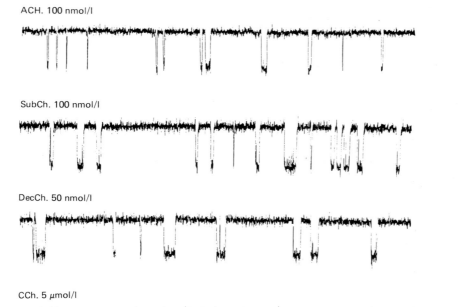

SubCh. 100 nmol/l

DecCh. 50 nmol/l

CCh. 5 μmol/l

4 pA

100 ms

Fig. 1.2   Records showing the minute electrical currents (downward deflections) flowing through single ion channels in the postjunctional membrane of frog skeletal muscle fibres. These currents result from brief transitions of individual receptors to an active state, in response to various agonists (ACh = acetylcholine; SubCh = suberyldicholine; DecCh = the dicholine ester of decan-1,10-dicarboxylic acid; CCh=carbamylcholine). (Reproduced, with permission, from Colquhoun and Sakmann (1985), where further details may be found.)

Direct measurement of the binding of drugs to receptors

Reversible ligands

In 1965, Paton and Rang introduced a method which allowed the binding of a drug to membrane receptors to be studied directly. The technique is simple in principle: an isolated tissue is exposed to a known concentration of a radiolabelled drug for long enough for equilibrium to be reached, and the amount of drug bound to the receptors is then determined from the radioactivity of the tissue, after allowing for the quantity of labelled drug in the extracellular spaces. A variety of difficulties may be encountered in practice. Perhaps the most important is that the tissue often has a number of other binding sites for the labelled drug, each with a characteristic affinity. One way of allowing for this is to repeat the binding experiments, but now in the presence of an appropriate concentration of an unlabelled agent that is known

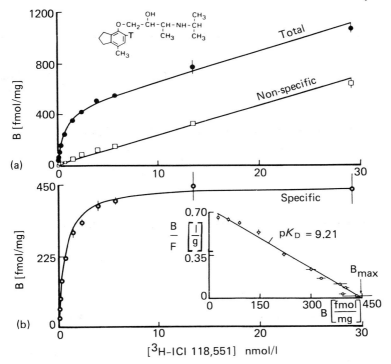

Fig. 1.3 The radiolabelled ligand-binding technqiue. In this example, the ligand is a tritiated β_2-adrenoceptor antagonist, ICI 118,551 (for structure, see top: T indicates the position of the label). The tissue being studied is guinea-pig lung, and (a) shows the amounts of the ligand binding to membrane particles at various ligand concentrations. 'Total' and 'non-specific' refer to the binding (B) observed in the absence and presence respectively of 0.2 mmol/l $(-)$-isoprenaline which was used to determine what proportion of the binding is non-specific – i.e. not to the receptors (see text). (b) A plot of the specific binding, again as a function of the free (i.e. unbound) concentration (F) of [3H]-ICI 118,551. *Inset* A means of analysing the binding data in order to obtain estimates of the affinity constant for binding, and of the maximum binding capacity (B_{max}). For further details, and an account of the exacting statistical analysis which was applied (the lines show the theoretical fit), see Lemoine, Ehle and Kaumann (1985). (Reproduced, with permission, from Lemoine, Ehle and Kaumann (1985).)

from other evidence to combine with the receptors under study. The reduction in binding which this agent causes should then correspond to the amount of the labelled drug bound to the receptors, and is generally (if sometimes rather optimistically) referred to as the specific binding. Better terms are *displaceable* or *inhibitable* binding. Although the procedure carries the potential risk of circularity, it has been enormously useful in practice (see, for example, Furchgott, 1978; and the general account by Yamamura, Enna and Kuhar, 1985). An example of its application to the study of β-adrenoceptors is illustrated in Fig. 1.3.

One of the most valuable features of the radioligand-binding technique is that it provides an estimate not only of the affinity constant for binding but also of the number of binding sites. The latter is quite unobtainable from classical pharmacological methods alone. Also, once a suitable radiolabelled ligand is available, and has been characterized, the ability of other unlabelled drugs to compete with it for the receptors can be studied, so that estimates of the affinity constants of these drugs too can be obtained.

Binding experiments can be done with intact tissues (as in the original study by Paton and Rang), with isolated cells or with broken cell preparations (e.g. of cell membranes). The last approach avoids certain problems which can be met when intact cells are used. One such complication is that the labelled drug may be taken into the cell by specific membrane transport systems such as that for monoamines in some nerve endings. The use of membrane preparations does, however, carry the risk that the properties of the receptor may change as the cell is disrupted. The choice of an appropriate bathing fluid can also be a problem. Nevertheless, the agreement between the affinity constants for competitive antagonists as determined by ligand binding to cell fragments and by the classical pharmacological techniques to be described is often excellent. An example is shown in Fig. 1.4.

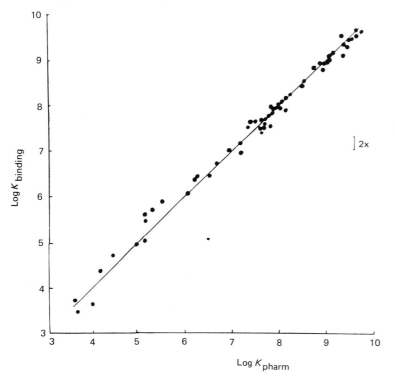

Fig. 1.4 Comparison of affinity constants for muscarinic antagonists as determined by the radiolabelled ligand-binding technique (ordinate) and by the classic pharmacological method using isolated tissue (guinea-pig ileum) in an organ bath (abscissa). Each point represents a single muscarinic antagonist. The binding experiments were done by measuring the ability of the compounds to inhibit the binding of the labelled muscarinic receptor antagonist [^{3}H]propylbenzilyl choline to membrane fragments prepared from rat cerebral cortex. (Reproduced, with permission, from Birdsall (1986).)

The ligand-binding method has been applied to many human tissues obtained either during operative procedures (e.g. cardiac surgery, allowing β-adrenoceptors in the heart to be studied: Gille *et al.*, 1985) or by biopsy (as when the presence of oestrogen receptors is assessed in planning the treatment of breast cancer – see, for example, Seibert and Lippman, 1982). The formed elements of blood have also been widely used (e.g. platelet α-adrenoceptors: Motulsky and Insel, 1982; Swart and Barnett, 1985; β-adrenoceptors in lymphocytes: Molinoff and Aarons, 1983; for a general review, see Insel, 1985). Such measurements have been used to examine changes in the number of β-adrenoceptors during drug treatment (e.g. Aarons *et al.*, 1980; Molinoff and Aarons, 1983) and in response to physical training programmes (Butler *et al.*, 1982).

A recent development is based on the use of drug molecules labelled with positron-emitting isotopes such as ^{18}F. Computer-assisted tomography can then be deployed to study the distribution of certain receptors in conscious man (Mintun *et al.*, 1984; Baron *et al.*, 1985). Recent advances in this and other methods for receptor mapping have been reviewed by Kuhar, De Souza and Unnerstall (1986).

Irreversible ligands

A related approach is to use labelled ligands which bind irreversibly, or nearly so, to receptors. α-bungarotoxin, found in a snake venom, provides an excellent example. This peptide, with a relative molecular mass of approximately 8000, binds to the nicotinic receptor of the motor end-plate with remarkably high affinity and selectivity. It can be labelled either radioisotopically or with a fluorescent group, so allowing (respectively) the receptors to be counted (e.g. using quantitative autoradiography – see Fertuk and Salpeter, 1976) or 'seen' by means of fluorescence microscopy (e.g. Anderson and Cohen, 1974; Colquhoun and Sakmann, 1985). The receptor deficit in myasthenia gravis was detected in this way (Fambrough, Drachman and Satyamurti, 1973; see also the reviews by Fambrough, 1979; Vincent, 1980; Lindstrom, 1985).

Receptor isolation

This was first achieved for the nicotinic receptor of the kind found at the neuromuscular junction, and also as it happens at a higher density in the electric organs of certain fish, including *Electrophorus* and *Torpedo*, which therefore provided excellent starting material. The initial successes were attained by labelling *Torpedo* receptors either with a compound such as TDF (*p*-(trimethylammonium) benzene diazonium fluoroborate) which is capable of forming a covalent bond with the receptor, or with radioiodinated α-bungarotoxin, and then applying protein separation methods to isolate the material carrying the label (for references, and an excellent review, see Changeux, 1981). However, the technique of affinity chromatography is now more often employed. Here a suitable ligand (often a cobra venom toxin related to α-bungarotoxin, but less irreversible in its action) is chemically attached to an inert material which can be placed in a chromatographic column. When a mixture of detergent-solubilized membrane proteins, including the receptors, is applied to the column, the receptors bind to the immobilized ligand and so their passage is much delayed in relation to the other material. Hence the receptors can be separated, and subsequently eluted from the column by using a high concentration of a competing ligand such as carbachol or ACh itself. When a receptor molecule dissociates from the material in the column, it is likely to combine with the eluting ligand, and is no longer trappable by the immobilized toxin. Similar procedures, but using immobilized adrenoceptor antagonists, have been used to isolate α- and β-adrenoceptors (for references, see Caron *et al.*, 1985; and Dixon *et al.*, 1986).

How can the success of the isolation be assessed? Clearly, the material must show the appropriate binding (i.e. recognition) characteristics. There are two other commonly applied tests. One is to raise antibodies against the receptor preparation in another species, and to see if there is cross-reaction with receptors *in situ*. This was first done with the nicotinic receptor purified from *Torpedo*, and administered to rabbits. Antibodies were formed, and this was observed to be associated with the development of a use-dependent fatigue of neuromuscular transmission strikingly similar to that seen in myasthenia gravis. Indeed these experiments (Patrick and Lindstrom, 1973; for reviews, see Vincent, 1980; Lindstrom, 1985) provided the first direct evidence to support the proposal (Simpson, 1960) that myasthenia gravis is an autoimmune disease.

The second and more stringent test (again pioneered with the nicotinic ACh receptor) is to incorporate the putative receptor into an artificial lipid membrane, and then show that the application of agonist will elicit its characteristic actions (in the case of acetylcholine receptor, the opening of ion channels with the same properties as those in intact tissues). This, too, has been convincingly demonstrated (Schindler and Quast, 1980; see also Latorre *et al.*, 1985; and Miller, 1986).

Reconstitution experiments can also be done with β-adrenoceptors (see, for example, Asano *et al.*, 1984; Hekman *et al.*, 1984; and the review by Birnbaumer *et al.*, 1985). In this instance, three components (the receptor macromolecule itself, a guanine nucleotide regulatory protein and the enzyme adenylate cyclase) are needed (see p. 23) for the expression of one of this receptor's primary actions, the activation of adenylate cyclase.

The study of receptor synthesis and structure

The discovery that either chronic denervation or damage to skeletal muscle leads to the appearance of ACh receptors over the entire fibre surface (see earlier) raised the question of whether the increase in receptors is a consequence of the unmasking of previously existing, but 'latent', receptors, or of either an increase in synthesis or a reduction in degradation. These possibilities were distinguished by testing the effects of protein synthesis inhibitors and by using labelled precursors. The results showed clearly that the change is in receptor synthesis. The nature of the signal for this increased synthesis is still unclear, although an important clue is that electrical stimulation, via implanted electrodes, of denervated muscles causes both the number and the localization of receptors to return towards (Lømo and Rosenthal, 1972; Purves and Sakmann, 1974), although not always attain, the situation in normal muscle (for a review, see Fambrough, 1979).

A powerful method which allows the step-by-step synthesis of receptors to be studied is based on the experimental 'subversion' of another cell's protein synthetic machinery. Amphibian oocytes are often chosen for this purpose, because of their large size and synthetic capabilities. Perhaps not altogether surprisingly, these cells do not normally make nicotinic receptors. However, they can be forced to do so by injecting into their cytoplasm messenger RNA from another cell type which expresses these receptors (Sumikawa *et al.*, 1981; Barnard, Miledi and Sumikawa, 1982; Miledi, Parker and Sumikawa, 1982). The method can be used to examine the synthesis of the subunits of receptors, the assembly of the subunits into the receptor macromolecule, and the post-translational modification of receptors, for example, by the attachment of glycoside residues to that part of the structure which projects from the outer face of the membrane when the receptor is in position. The synthesis of other kinds of receptor, and of receptor-controlled ion channels, is equally readily studied, and the method has already been applied to receptors for 5-hydroxytryptamine, glycine, GABA and glutamate (e.g. Gundersen, Miledi and Parker, 1984; Houamed *et al.*, 1984).

Further advances have been made possible by developments in gene cloning. This technique has already been applied to determine the complete amino acid sequence of each of the subunits of the nicotinic receptor (see Momoi and Lennon, 1986, and the reviews by Stroud and Finer-Moore, 1985, and McCarthy *et al.*, 1986). Site-directed mutagenesis, whereby amino acids at a known part of the sequence can be deleted or replaced by others, has also become possible, and studies of the resulting changes in the function of the modified receptor have already provided useful information about the molecular events which underlie receptor activation (see Sakmann *et al.*, 1985, and earlier references therein).

Gene cloning has also been applied to determine the amino acid sequence of other receptors; for example, for epidermal growth factor (Staros, Cohen and Russo, 1985), for oestrogen (Green *et al.*, 1986) and for the β actions of catecholamines (Dixon *et al.*, 1986). An exciting (though still not fully understood) outcome of such studies is the discovery that the sequences often show unexpected common features with other, at first sight unrelated, proteins. For example, there is considerable homology between the β-adrenoceptor and rhodopsin, and between oestrogen receptors and certain proteins associated with oncogenic activity.

Dose–response curves and the characterization of drug receptor interactions

Agonists and partial agonists

Figure 1.5 shows concentration–response relationships for three hypothetical agonists (*A*, *B* and *C*) which act through the same receptors. *C* evidently cannot elicit as large a response as *A* and *B*, and is described as a partial agonist. The ratio of the maximum response which it can produce to that observed with a 'full' agonist (e.g. *A* and *B*) of the same pharmacological class

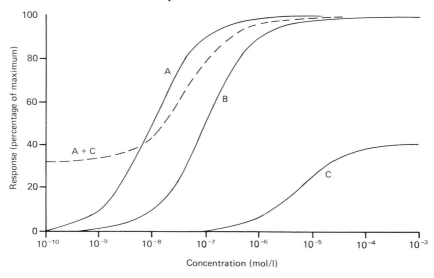

Fig. 1.5 Concentration–response curves for three hypothetical agonists, A, B and C, of which C is a partial agonist (see text). The broken line shows the relationship to be expected for varying concentrations of A applied in the presence of a constant submaximal concentration of C. At low concentrations of A, the simultaneous action of C increases the response. However, when [A] is large, C now causes a reduction (because the additional contribution to the response by receptors occupied by C is more than offset by the reduction in receptor occupancy by the full agonist, A).

is now generally described as the *intrinsic activity*. In principle, and often in practice, it is possible to have a complete range of substances from full agonists, through partial agonists with varying intrinsic activities, to agents which combine with the receptors but do not activate them to any appreciable extent, and so are competitive antagonists (see later).

Two other aspects of partial agonism deserve comment. The fact is that the maximum response to a partial agonist may vary not only between tissues in the same species but also in the same tissue under different experimental conditions. These points are illustrated in Figs. 1.6 and 1.7 respectively. The second point is that even though the agonists *A* and *B* in Fig. 1.5 are both able to cause a maximum response, and hence by definition have the same intrinsic activity (unity), it cannot be concluded that they are equally effective in activating the receptors. This is because many tissue responses (both *in vivo* and *in vitro*) are elicited, and may even be maximal, when only a small proportion of the receptors are activated. Hence *A* in Fig. 1.5 might need to occupy only 1 per cent of the receptors in order to produce a maximum response, as compared with 20 per cent for *B*. *A* is clearly more effective than *B*. It was the need to encompass this possibility that led to the introduction by Stephenson (1956) of the concept of *efficacy* as a measure of the ability of agonists to activate receptors. According to the convention suggested by Stephenson a partial agonist which can produce at most a half-maximal response has an efficacy of unity. It scarcely needs saying that the term

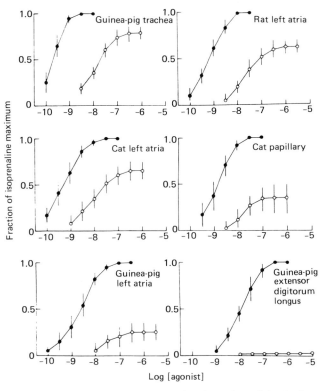

Fig. 1.6 Concentration–response relationships for the action of the β-adrenoceptor agonists isoprenaline (●) and prenalterol (○) on a range of isolated tissues from cat, guinea-pig and rat. Note that the maximum response to the partial agonist prenalterol varies considerably from tissue to tissue even though prenalterol has little β_1/β_2-adrenoceptor selectivity. (Reproduced, with permission, from Kenakin and Beek (1980).)

'efficacy' is here being used in a specifically pharmacological sense. Fuller accounts of the definition of efficacy and of the methods that can be used to measure and compare efficacies can be found elsewhere (e.g. Mackay, 1977; Jenkinson, 1979; Kenakin, 1984, 1985). Before leaving the topic it is worth noting an important extension of the concept by Furchgott (1966) who, recognizing that the magnitude of the 'message' communicated to a cell by its receptors must be a function of the total number of receptors as well as the nature of the drug that activates them, introduced the term *intrinsic efficacy*, ε. Here ε is the notional efficacy associated with a single receptor. The product of ε and the number (or notional concentration) of receptors is equivalent to efficacy as defined by Stephenson (see also the review by Kenakin, 1984, and the critique by Colquhoun, 1986b).

The phenomenon of partial agonism is potentially important in the use of drugs. For example, some β-adrenoceptor blockers have intrinsic activity; that is, they activate the β-adrenoceptors, albeit weakly (hence they are said to possess 'intrinsic sympathomimetic activity'). This could confer therapeutic

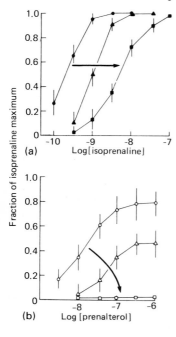

Fig. 1.7 Concentration–response curves for the relaxant effect of (a) isoprenaline and (b) prenalterol on guinea-pig tracheal smooth muscle. The measurements were made both in the absence (circles) and presence (triangles and squares) of carbachol at either 1 μmol/l or 10 μmol/l respectively. Carbachol tends to cause contraction, so greater concentrations of the β-agonists are needed for a given relaxation. Because the maximum activation of the β-adrenoceptors that prenalterol can cause is limited, and much less than that of isoprenaline, carbachol also reduces the maximum relaxation attainable with prenalterol but not isoprenaline (see arrows). (Reproduced, with permission, from Kenakin and Beek (1980).)

advantages, although whether this is important in practice is debated (see, for example, McDevitt, 1983; Gerber and Nies, 1985). In principle at least, the fact that the dose–response curves for partial agonists are less steep than those for full agonists (see Figs. 1.5–1.7) could be useful under some circumstances, as when the newer inotropic agents (e.g. dobutamine, prenalterol) are employed. The ability of a partial agonist to add to the response to a low concentration of a full agonist (such as a circulating hormone) but to reduce that to a high concentration (see Fig. 1.5, broken line) could also be important.

How can the existence and properties of partial agonists be explained in terms of molecular events at the receptor? There is now much evidence to suggest that receptor activation occurs in at least two steps. The first is the formation of a drug–receptor complex. This may then isomerize to a form in which the receptor is active (i.e. capable of altering cell function).

$$A + R \underset{}{\overset{K_1}{\rightleftharpoons}} AR \underset{}{\overset{K_2}{\rightleftharpoons}} AR^*$$

If the concentration of A is high enough, and if equilibrium is reached, all the receptors will be either in the AR (inactive) or AR* (active) form (provided that desensitization has not occurred – see later). The position of the equilibrium $AR \rightleftharpoons AR^*$ then determines the maximum response to the agonist in question. For an effective agonist, AR* will predominate, whereas for a weak partial agonist the value of the equilibrium constant K_2 is such that there will be more AR than AR*. The relationship between K_2 and efficacy (in the sense introduced by Stephenson, 1956) has been discussed by Colquhoun (1986b).

Some of the most compelling evidence for such an explanation comes from 'patch clamp' experiments of the kind already mentioned. It is found (Gardner, Ogden and Colquhoun, 1984; see also Fig. 1.2) that the single ion channels opened by a variety of nicotinic agonists have almost exactly the same electrical conductance, as though receptor function is all-or-none. The implication is that the effectiveness of AR* does not depend on the nature of A. What differs between agonists is the proportion of time for which the receptors are in the active state (determined in turn by the rates of the transitions between R, AR and AR*).

Whilst such a scheme can account for much that is known about receptor function, it should be kept in mind that a substance may be a partial agonist because, in addition to activating receptors, it may also interfere with some subsequent step or steps. For example, decamethonium not only activates ACh receptors (hence causing the relatively maintained depolarization that is the primary cause of the neuromuscular block which it initiates) but also blocks the ion channels that open in response to its presence (Adams and Sakmann, 1978). Acetylcholine itself, and carbachol, can block the channels (Colquhoun and Sakmann, 1985; Ogden and Colquhoun, 1985), as can tubocurarine, although the effect is not large at normal membrane potentials (Colquhoun, Dreyer and Sheridan, 1979; Waud and Waud, 1985; see also Colquhoun, 1986a).

Receptor desensitization

To conclude this section on agonists, we may note that the response of a tissue often declines spontaneously despite the continued presence of the agonist. Several factors may contribute. One is receptor desensitization, a process which may contribute to depolarization block of the kind caused by suxamethonium, although the matter is controversial (see the discussions by Zaimis (1976), Bowman (1980), Colquhoun (1986a) and by Feldman in Chapter 7 of this volume). Although desensitization is only partly understood a contributory factor is a change in the receptor to an inactive (desensitized) form (R_D), so an extra step has to be added to the scheme already discussed:

$$A + R \rightleftharpoons AR \rightleftharpoons AR^* \rightleftharpoons AR_D$$

Perhaps surprisingly at first sight, R_D may have a higher affinity for the agonist than has the R form of the receptor (Katz and Thesleff, 1957; Sine and Taylor, 1979, 1982). Further discussion, and other references, can be found in the articles by Adams (1981) and Carmeliet and Mubagwa (1986).

Prolonged application of agonists may cause the response to decline through yet other mechanisms (see, for example, Hollenberg, 1985). The β-adrenoceptors have been studied in particular detail (for a review, see Sibley and Lefkowitz, 1985; also Helmreich and Pfeuffer, 1985), and here at least three processes can contribute to the fall in response.

1. A change in the receptor to a form that has a reduced capacity to combine with guanine nucleotide regulatory proteins (see later). Phosphorylation by an intracellular protein kinase may be involved.
2. Sequestration of the receptor, which may enter the cell where it is no longer available for activation. Many other kinds of receptor (e.g. for epidermal growth factor and insulin) are internalized by endocytosis, and this plays a part in the control of receptor number (see Goldstein et al., 1985).
3. Over a much longer period (several hours or days rather than minutes or seconds), the total number of receptors may diminish (down-regulation). This has been shown to occur in man; for example, in response to β-adrenoceptor agonists (e.g. Molinoff and Aarons, 1983). The administration of antagonists can have the opposite effect (e.g. Aarons et al., 1980) although the therapeutic importance of this is uncertain (e.g. Gerber and Nies, 1985).

Finally, we may note that desensitization produced by one agonist may under some circumstances reduce the response to another, acting through a different receptor (heterologous as compared with homologous desensitization). This can arise when the response is limited by some common step which is either involved in receptor activation (e.g. the availability of a guanine nucleotide regulatory protein) or occurs subsequent to receptor activation (e.g. the release of calcium from intracellular stores).

Competitive antagonism

It is first worth observing that the term 'competitive' is used in two slightly different senses in pharmacology. One is to imply that the antagonist combines with the same binding site as the agonist being blocked, so that their binding is mutually exclusive. If this is so, and if the combination with the receptors is freely reversible, certain predictions follow. Perhaps the most important is that the antagonism should be surmountable; that is, it should always be possible to elicit a response by sufficiently raising the concentration of agonist. This is because, provided that enough time is allowed (and only a few seconds may be needed), the agonist and antagonist will come into equilibrium with the receptors so that the relative proportion occupied by each is determined only by the respective concentrations and affinities for the receptor.

The second usage of 'competitive' is to convey that the inhibitory effect of an antagonist can be overcome by increasing the dose of the agonist, and that this can be done over a wide range of concentrations. This second meaning is included in the first, provided that the antagonist–receptor complexes are readily dissociable. If, however, the antagonist (e.g. α-bungarotoxin, phenoxybenzamine) combines irreversibly with the same binding site as the agonist then the antagonism is competitive in the first sense discussed, but not the second. One consequence of this ambiguity in usage is that some authors describe such antagonists as *irreversible competitive*, whereas others (with the second meaning in mind) classify them as *non-competitive*. No confusion need arise if the terms are used consistently (see also the discussions by Ginsborg and Jenkinson, 1976; and Colquhoun, 1986a).

Reversible antagonists

The characteristics of reversible competitive antagonism have been well established by the work of Clark, Gaddum and Schild, and need be summarized only briefly here. First, the competitive antagonist displaces the log concentration–response curve for the agonist to the right, and in a parallel fashion. Secondly, the extent of the displacement, as assessed by the dose ratio (i.e. the factor, x, by which the agonist concentration must be raised in order to restore a given submaximal response elicited in the presence of the antagonist), should be related to the antagonist concentration, [B], by the simple relationship.

$$x - 1 = K_B [B]$$

where K_B is the affinity constant for the combination of the antagonist with the receptor. This expression is known as the Schild equation (Schild, 1949; Arunlakshana and Schild, 1959; see also the reviews by Kenakin, 1982, 1984), and it has been shown to apply over a wide range of concentrations of competitive antagonists of many pharmacological classes. The results of such measurements are often displayed as a *Schild plot*, as illustrated in Fig. 1.8, and from them estimates of K_B are readily obtained. This offers a powerful and versatile means not only of characterizing antagonists but also of classifying receptors, since if the receptors in two tissues are the same, the K_B values obtained for an antagonist known to act on these receptors should be identical. The assumptions involved, and other approaches to receptor classification, are discussed in the volume edited by Black, Gerskowitch and Jenkinson (1986). An excellent example of their application can be found in a series of papers, on the muscarinic receptors concerned in the vagal control of gastric secretion, by Black, Leff and Shankley (1985a, b) and Black and Shankley (1985a, b).

The action of competitive antagonists on synaptic transmission

The classical analysis of competitive antagonism as outlined above is based on the assumption that enough time is available for the applied steady concentrations of agonist and antagonist to come into dynamic equilibrium with the receptors (or nearly so: see the analysis by Rang, 1966). The problem of quantifying the action of a competitive antagonist on synaptic transmission in an intact tissue such as skeletal muscle is more difficult, not least because the transmitter may be present for only a millisecond or so after each nerve impulse. It is unlikely (though still uncertain) that this is long enough for the proportion of receptors occupied by an antagonist such as tubocurarine to fall appreciably. Hence the presence of tubocurarine may simply reduce the number of receptors available to the transmitter (though the antagonism is still competitive in the first of the senses already discussed). This has been studied in much detail: see the papers by Paton and Waud (1967) and Pennefather and

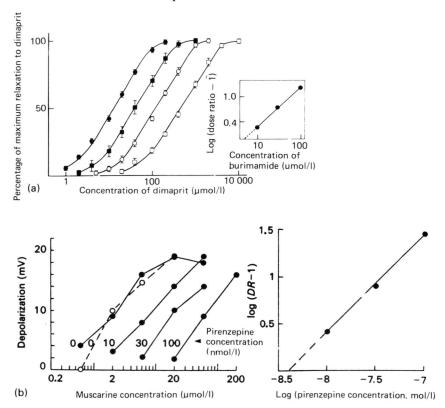

Fig. 1.8 Competitive antagonism. (a) The effect of three concentrations (10 μmol/l, ■; 30 μmol/l, ○; 100 μmol/l, □) of the H_2-receptor antagonist burimamide on the concentration–response relations for the relaxant action of the histamine H_2-receptor agonist dimaprit on a strip of guinea-pig lung. Pyridylethylamine (100 μmol/l) was present throughout, to induce tone. *Right*: Schild plot (see text) based on these observations. (b) Another example, showing the influence of the muscarinic antagonist pirenzepine on the action of muscarine. In this instance, all the observations were made on a single cell, a neuron in the submucous plexus of the guinea-pig small intestine. It was also possible to demonstrate the recovery of the response (membrane depolarization) on washing out pirenzepine (○). (Reproduced, with permission, from: (a) Foreman, Rising and Webber (1985); and (b) North, Slack, and Suprenant (1985).)

Quastel (1981, 1982) as well as the reviews by Ginsborg and Jenkinson (1976) and Colquhoun (1986a) and the volume by Bowman (1980). In addition, the cleft between the motor nerve ending and the postsynaptic membrane is very narrow, so that if some antagonist does dissociate from the receptors during the presence of the transmitter, the concentration in the cleft will rise, hence tending to counteract the reduction in binding. Thus the binding is to some extent buffered (see Armstrong and Lester, 1979; and Colquhoun, 1986a).

These factors make it difficult to measure the rates of association and dissociation of agonists and antagonists with receptors in intact tissues (for a general introduction to the study of the kinetics of drug–receptor interaction, see Colquhoun, 1981, 1986a). Indeed, it can be surprisingly hard to distinguish between reaction rates on the one hand, and the time required for diffusion on the other, as limiting factors in the kinetics of drug action; furthermore, diffusion in a restricted space may be greatly slowed by binding (see, for example, Colquhoun, Henderson and Ritchie, 1972). To complete this account of the problems likely to be faced when kinetics are to be studied in intact tissues, it may be mentioned again that it is difficult to deduce receptor occupancy from the response of a tissue, especially if the response measured is an indirect one (as when the reduction in the twitch of a skeletal muscle is used as an index of receptor blockade by, say, tubocurarine). In this situation, more than 80 per cent of the receptors may have to be occupied before there is an appreciable decline in the twitch (see Paton and Waud, 1967; Waud and Waud, 1975; and Chapter 7). Moreover, this safety margin may itself alter with the conditions of the measurement. For example, it could be expected to change during or following anoxia, and it will also be affected by local changes in ion concentration (particularly of potassium and calcium; see Waud, Mookerjee and Waud 1982). This is not of course to deny the value of such studies which indeed are essential for a full understanding of the action of skeletal muscle relaxants – see also Chapter 7.

This account of competitive antagonism, and its analysis, can be concluded by observing that a more complex model is required for those receptor macromolecules (such as that for ACh) which possess more than one binding site for the agonist. If these sites are non-equivalent, as the asymmetry of the nicotinic receptor macromolecule suggests, the single 'affinity constant' determined for an antagonist such as tubocurarine must be a function of the individual affinities for the site on each of the two subunits. This has been analysed by Sine and Taylor (1981, 1984; see also Waud and Waud, 1985; Colquhoun, 1986a).

Irreversible antagonists

These agents are exemplified by α-bungarotoxin, benzilylcholine mustard and phenoxybenzamine which block (respectively) skeletal muscle nicotinic receptors, muscarinic receptors and α-adrenoceptors. Figure 1.9 illustrates their characteristic influence on the concentration–response relationship. The parallel shift which is seen following a relatively limited application of the antagonist in this example occurs because not all of the receptors have to be activated even for a maximal response: although many receptors have been irreversibly blocked, enough are left to allow a full response on applying a higher concentration of agonist. Only when the proportion of receptors available to the agonist has been reduced even further does the maximum response become smaller, so that the antagonism is then insurmountable.

How receptors alter cell function

'Fast' receptors
Although receptors are usually, and best, classified in terms of the substances which activate or block them, an alternative classification, based on their

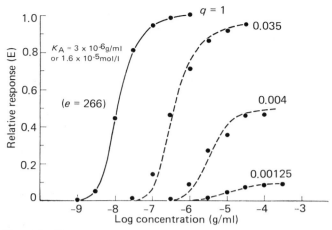

Fig. 1.9 The effect of progressive blockade of receptors by an irreversible antagonist, dibenamine, on the contractile response to carbachol of a strip of smooth muscle from rabbit stomach. The muscle was subjected to three 20-minute exposures to dibenamine. Following each exposure and washout, the concentration–response relationship for carbachol was redetermined. The numbers given for each curve are the estimated proportions (q) of receptors left unblocked. Note that the maximum response that carbachol can cause is little reduced even when q is as small as 0.035. The broken lines are theoretical curves based on (1) the dose–response curve before blockade (solid curve), (2) the estimated equilibrium constant, K_A, for the combination of carbachol with the receptors, and (3) the q values shown. Further details can be found in the review by Furchgott (1966). (Reproduced, with permission, from Furchgott (1966).)

rapidity of action, can also be helpful. The nicotinic receptor for ACh is the most fully understood *fast* receptor, and it responds to the presence of ACh within microseconds. The response is triggered by the combination of ACh with its binding sites on the two α-subunits of the pentameric macromolecule, which then changes shape in an all-or-none way (see p. 17 and Fig. 1.2), so creating a channel which allows the passage of sodium, potassium and calcium ions across the cell membrane (see the reviews by Stroud and Finer-Moore, 1985; and McCarthy *et al.*, 1986). If enough channels are opened the outcome is that the membrane potential falls to the point at which an action potential is set up in the postsynaptic cell. This is discussed in more detail in Chapter 7, and all that need be added here is that it seems likely that other fast receptors (e.g. those for amino acid neurotransmitters such as glutamate, glycine and γ-aminobutyric acid (GABA)) act in a broadly similar way, although in the case of glycine and GABA (more precisely, the $GABA_A$ receptor subtype) the permeability increase is to small anions rather than cations.

Receptors with an intermediate speed of response

A second, larger group of receptors respond on a slower time scale (from some tens of milliseconds to a few seconds). Examples include the muscarinic receptors for ACh, α- and β-adrenoceptors, and the H_1- and H_2-receptors for histamine. It is now clear that these act quite differently from the 'fast' variety. Perhaps most important, they are not in themselves able to form ion channels, although their activation can cause changes (which may be in either direction) in the ion permeability of the cell membrane. The underlying mechanism has only recently begun to be understood. Combination of such a receptor with an agonist causes an increase in the activity of a membrane-bound enzyme. For some receptors (e.g. α_1-adrenoceptors) this is a phosphodiesterase (similar in its action to phospholipase C), which acts on a specific membrane phospholipid, phosphatidylinositol bisphosphate. As a result, inositol 1,4,5-trisphosphate and diacylglycerol are formed. These two substances (possibly in conjunction with others yet to be identified) then initiate the still incompletely understood cellular events, such as an increase in cytosolic calcium and activation of protein kinases, which lead to the final response (e.g. contraction of vascular smooth muscle, or glycogenolysis and a change in membrane permeability in a liver cell). This mechanism has been reviewed by Downes and Michell (1985) and Hirasawa and Nishizuka (1985).

Other receptors in this general class (e.g. β-adrenoceptors; those for glucagon and corticotrophin) influence the activity of another membrane-bound enzyme, adenylate cyclase. This catalyses the formation of cyclic adenosine monophosphate (cAMP) from adenosine triphosphate (ATP). The cAMP then acts as an intracellular 'second messenger' which, by in turn activating specific protein kinases, initiates the characteristic cell response (e.g. the initiation of steroid synthesis in the adrenal cortex; accelerated glycogenolysis in most types of cell; an increase in the proportion of calcium channels opening during the action potential in cardiac muscle cells). A further important group of receptors (e.g. α_2-adrenoceptors, opioid receptors) can *inhibit* adenylate cyclase. This enzyme is thus the target for a wide range of receptors, and it has been studied in great detail. One of the most fruitful discoveries has been the essential role of at least two kinds of guanine

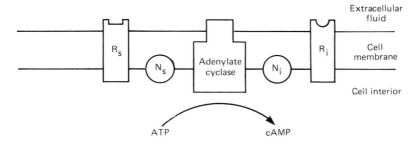

Fig. 1.10 Diagrammatic representation of the action of receptors (R_s, R_i) which stimulate (R_s) or inhibit (R_i) the activity of adenylate cyclase, an enzyme which catalyses the formation of the 'second messenger' cyclic AMP. R_s receptors include those for glucagon, corticotrophin and adrenaline (β-adrenoceptors). R_i receptors are activated, for example, by opioids and by noradrenaline (α_2-adrenoceptors). Combination of a hormone with a receptor of either class causes the latter to become associated with, and activate, a regulatory protein (N_s or N_i) which has a binding site for the guanine nucleotide GDP. The result of the activation is that GDP is replaced by GTP, with the consequence that N_s now becomes capable of increasing the activity of adenylate cyclase (whereas N_i can inhibit it). Both of the N proteins can also hydrolyse the bound GTP, and when this happens the influence on adenylate cyclase is terminated. The hydrolysis can be inhibited by the action of cholera toxin on the N_s protein. Complex as it may seem, the scheme is still an oversimplification (e.g. there may be interactions between N_s and N_i, each of which is made up of three subunits which dissociate during activity). A fuller account can be found in the reviews by Caron *et al.* (1985), Helmreich and Pfeuffer (1985) and Levitzki (1986).

nucleotide-binding regulatory proteins which are intermediates in the sequence of events through which the combination of a hormone or neurotransmitter with its receptor changes the rate of action of adenylate cyclase, in either direction. This new information has been summarized in Fig. 1.10. The importance of the guanine nucleotide regulatory units is underlined by the more recent findings that they are the target for cholera and pertussis toxins, and that when activated by receptors they may open or close ion channels without the involvement of adenylate cyclase (for references, see Stevens, 1986).

Yet other receptors, exemplified by those for insulin and epidermal growth factor, are now known to possess an enzymic activity which is intrinsic to at least some of their functions. The receptors are in fact tyrosine protein kinases, catalysing the transfer of phosphate groups from ATP to tyrosine residues in target proteins, which can include the receptors themselves (Houslay, 1985; Kahn, 1985). This phosphorylation may be the first step in the diverse and incompletely understood actions which follow.

Slow receptors
This brief account of receptor action can be completed by turning to a third broad class of receptors whose effects are seen over a time scale of minutes or hours. Examples are the receptors for thyroid and steroidal hormones. These receptors are mainly located within the cell, either in the cytosol or in the nucleus (recent evidence favours the latter; for references, see the review by Ringold, 1985). Following combination with an agonist, they change in conformation to the extent that they are now able to alter the transcription of DNA, resulting in the first instance in the production of messenger RNA molecules coding for one or more specific proteins. These proteins then modify cellular function in a way characteristic for the cell in question (see Ringold, 1985). For example, it is likely that the anti-inflammatory action of the adrenocortical hormones is a consequence of the formation of a specific protein, lipocortin, which in turn inhibits phospholipase A_2, thus decreasing the production of arachidonic acid, and so of all the inflammatory mediators derived therefrom. This has been reviewed by Schleimer (1985) – see also Flower (1986).

Epilogue

If at all successful, this summary of the study and properties of receptors will have conveyed the impression of an exciting area of research, although one in which remarkably detailed information (such as the complete amino acid sequence of a receptor) coexists with large gaps in knowledge (e.g. of the proportion of receptors which are in an active form when a tissue responds; or of the values of the association and dissociation rate constants for the combination of agonists and antagonists with receptors in situ). It will also have become clear from this chapter that many of the drugs most useful in the practice of anaesthesia have long had an additional role as tools in the study of receptors, and their importance in this regard is likely to continue.

References

Aarons, R.D., Nies, A.S., Gal, J., Hegstrand, L.R. and Molinoff, P.B. (1980) Elevation of beta-adrenergic receptor density in human lymphocytes after propranolol treatment. *Journal of Clinical Investigation* **65**, 949–957

Adams, P.R. (1981) Acetylcholine receptor kinetics. *Journal of Membrane Biology* **58**, 161–174

Adams, P.R. and Sakmann, B. (1978) Decamethonium both opens and blocks endplate channels. *Proceedings of the National Academy of Sciences, USA* **75**, 2994–2998

Anderson, C.R. and Cohen, M.W. (1974) Fluorescent staining of acetylcholine receptors on vertebrate skeletal muscle. *Journal of Physiology* **237**, 385–400

Ariëns, E.J., Soudijn, W. and Timmermans, P.B.M.W.M. (Eds.) (1983) *Stereochemistry and Biological Activity of Drugs*. Blackwell Scientific: Oxford

Armstrong, D.L. and Lester, H.A. (1979) The kinetics of tubocurarine action and restricted diffusion within the synaptic cleft. *Journal of Physiology* **294**, 365–386

Arunlakshana, O. and Schild, H.O. (1959) Some quantitative uses of drug antagonists. *British Journal of Pharmacology* **14**, 48–58

Asano, T., Katada, T., Gilman, A.G. and Ross, E.M. (1984) Activation of the inhibitory GTP-binding protein of adenylate cyclase, G_i, by beta-adrenergic receptors in reconstituted phospholipid vesicles. *Journal of Biological Chemistry* **259**, 9351–9354

Barnard, E.A., Miledi, R. and Sumikawa, K. (1982) Translation of exogenous messenger RNA coding for nicotinic acetylcholine receptors produces functional receptors in *Xenopus* oocytes. *Proceedings of the Royal Society, B* **215**, 241–246

Baron, J.C., Maziere, B., Loc'h, C., Sgouropoulos, P., Bonnet, A.M. and Agid, Y. (1985) Progressive supranuclear palsy: loss of striatal dopamine receptors demonstrated *in vivo* by positron tomography. *Lancet* **1**, 1163–1164

Birdsall, N.J.M. (1986) Can complex binding phenomena be resolved to provide a safe basis for classification? In: *Towards the Classification of 'Hormone' Receptors* (Eds. Black, J.W., Gerskowitch, P. and Jenkinson, D.H.). Liss: New York (In press)

Birnbaumer, L., Codina, J., Mattera, R. *et al.* (1985) Structural basis of adenylate cyclase stimulation and inhibition by distinct guanine nucleotide regulatory proteins. In: *Molecular Mechanisms of Transmembrane Signalling* (Eds. Cohen, P. and Houslay, M.D.), pp. 131–182. Elsevier: Amsterdam

Black, J.W. and Shankley, N.P. (1985a) Pharmacological analysis of muscarinic receptors coupled to oxyntic cell secretion in the mouse stomach. *British Journal of Pharmacology* **86**, 601–607

Black, J.W. and Shankley, N.P. (1985b) Pharmacological analysis of the muscarinic receptors involved when McN-A 343 stimulates acid secretion in the mouse isolated stomach. *British Journal of Pharmacology* **86**, 609–617

Black, J.W., Gerskowitch, P. and Jenkinson, D.H. (Eds.) (1986) *Towards the Classification of 'Hormone' Receptors*. Liss: New York.

Black, J.W., Leff, P. and Shankley, N.P. (1985a) Further analysis of anomalous pK_B values for histamine H_2-receptor antagonists on the mouse isolated stomach assay. *British Journal of Pharmacology* **86**, 581–587

Black, J.W., Leff, P. and Shankley, N.P. (1985b) Pharmacological analysis of the pentagastrin–tiotidine interaction in the mouse isolated stomach. *British Journal of Pharmacology* **86**, 589–599

Bowman, W.C. (1980) *Pharmacology of Neuromuscular Function*, pp. 71–85. John Wright: Bristol

Butler, J., O'Brien, M., O'Malley, K. and Kelly, J.G. (1982) Relationship of β-adrenoceptor density to fitness in athletics. *Nature* **298**, 60–62

Carmeliet, E. and Mubagwa, K. (1986) Desensitization of the acetylcholine-induced increase of potassium conductance in rabbit cardiac Purkinje fibres. *Journal of Physiology* **371**, 239–255

Caron, M.G., Benovic, J.L., Stiles, G.L. *et al.* (1985) Biochemical properties of the adrenergic receptors delineated by purification and photoaffinity labelling. In: *Adrenergic Receptors: Molecular Properties and Therapeutic Implications* (Eds. Lefkowitz, R.J. and Lindenlaub, E.), pp. 7–27. Schattauer: Stuttgart, New York

Changeux, J.-P. (1981) The acetylcholine receptor: an 'allosteric' membrane protein. *Harvey Lectures* **75**, 85–254

Colquhoun, D. (1981) How fast do drugs work? *Trends in Pharmacological Sciences* **2**, 212–217

Colquhoun, D. (1986a) On the principles of postsynaptic action of neuromuscular blocking agents. In: *New Neuromuscular Blocking Agents*, Handbook of Experimental Pharmacology, vol. 79 (Ed. Kharkevich, D.A.), pp. 59–113. Springer-Verlag: Berlin

Colquhoun, D. (1986b) Affinity, efficacy and receptor classification. Is the classical theory still useful? In: *Towards the Classification of 'Hormone' Receptors* (Eds. Black, J.W., Gerskowitch, P. and Jenkinson, D.H.). Liss: New York (In press)

Colquhoun, D. and Sakmann, B. (1985) Fast events in single-channel currents activated by acetylcholine and its analogues at the frog muscle end-plate. *Journal of Physiology* **369**, 501–557

Colquhoun, D., Dreyer, F. and Sheridan, R.E. (1979) The action of tubocurarine at the frog neuromuscular junction. *Journal of Physiology* **293**, 247–284

Colquhoun, D., Henderson, R. and Ritchie, J.M. (1972) The binding of labelled tetrodotoxin to non-myelinated nerve fibres. *Journal of Physiology* **227**, 95–126

Dean, P.M. (1981a) Drug-receptor recognition: electrostatic field lines at the receptor and dielectric effects. *British Journal of Pharmacology* **74**, 39–46

Dean, P.M. (1981b) Drug-receptor recognition: molecular orientation and dielectric effects. *British Journal of Pharmacology* **74**, 47–60

Dean, P.M. and Wakelin, L.P.G. (1979) The docking manoeuvre at a drug receptor: a quantum mechanical study of intercalative attack of ethidium and its carboxylated derivative on a DNA fragment. *Philosophical Transactions of the Royal Society, B* **287**, 571–604

Dekin, M.S. and Edwards, C. (1983) Voltage-dependent drug blockade of L-glutamate activated channels of the crayfish. *Journal of Physiology* **341**, 127–138

Dixon, R.A.F., Kobilka, B.K., Strader, D.J. *et al.* (1986) Cloning of the gene and cDNA for mammalian β-adrenergic receptor and homology with rhodopsin. *Nature* **321**, 75–79

Downes, C.P. and Michell, R.H. (1985) Inositol phospholipid breakdown as a receptor controlled generator of second messengers. In: *Molecular Mechanisms of Transmembrane Signalling* (Eds. Cohen, P. and Houslay, M.D.), pp. 3–56. Elsevier: Amsterdam

Eisenberg, R.S., Frank, M. and Stevens, C.F. (Eds.) (1984) *Membranes, Channels, and Noise*. Plenum: New York and London

Fambrough, D.M. (1979) Control of acetylcholine receptors in skeletal muscle. *Physiological Reviews* **59**, 165–216

Fambrough, D.M., Drachman, D.B. and Satyamurti, S. (1973) Neuromuscular junction in myasthenia gravis: decreased acetylcholine receptors. *Science* **182**, 293–295

Feldman, S. (1984) Neuromuscular blocking drugs. In: *A Practice of Anaesthesia* (Ed. Churchill-Davidson, H.C.), pp. 676–707. Lloyd–Luke: London

Fertuk, H.C. and Salpeter, M.M. (1976) Quantitation of junctional and extrajunctional acetylcholine receptors by electron microscope autoradiography after ^{125}I-α-bungarotoxin binding at mouse neuromuscular junctions. *Journal of Cell Biology* **69**, 144–158

Fleming, W.W. (1980) The electrogenic Na^+,K^+-pump in smooth muscle: physiologic and pharmacologic significance. *Annual Review of Pharmacology and Toxicology* **20**, 129–149

Fleming, W.W. (1984) A review of postjunctional supersensitivity in cardiac muscle. In: *Neuronal and Extraneuronal Events in Autonomic Pharmacology* (Eds. Fleming, W.W., Graefe, K.-H., Langer, S.Z. and Weiner, N.), pp. 205–219. Raven Press: New York

Flower, R.J. (1986) The mediators of steroid action. *Nature* **320**, 20

Foreman, J.C., Rising, T.J. and Webber, S.E. (1985) A study of the histamine H_2-receptor mediating relaxation of the parenchymal lung strip preparation of the guinea-pig. *British Journal of Pharmacology* **86**, 465–473

Franks, N.P. and Lieb, W.R. (1984) Do general anaesthetics act by competitive binding to specific receptors? *Nature* **310**, 599–601

Franks, N.P. and Lieb, W.R. (1985) Mapping of general anaesthetic target sites provides a molecular basis for cutoff effects. *Nature* **316**, 349–351

Furchgott, R.F. (1966) The use of β-haloalkylamines in the differentiation of receptors and in the determination of dissociation constants of receptor–agonist complexes. In: *Advances in Drug Research*, vol. 3 (Eds. Harper, N.J. and Simmonds, A.B.), pp. 21–55. Academic Press: London

Furchgott, R.F. (1978) Pharmacological characterization of receptors: its relation to radioligand-binding studies. *Federation Proceedings* **37**, 115–120

Gardner, P., Ogden, D.C. and Colquhoun, D. (1984) Conductances of single ion channels opened by nicotinic agonists are indistinguishable. *Nature* **309**, 160–162

Gerber, J.G. and Nies, A.S. (1985) Beta-adrenergic blocking drugs. *Annual Review of Medicine* **36**, 145–164

Gille, E., Lemoine, H., Ehle, B. and Kaumann, A.J. (1985) The affinity of (−)-propranolol for β₁- and β₂-adrenoceptors of human heart. *Naunyn-Schmiedeberg's Archives of Pharmacology* **331**, 60–70

Ginsborg, B.L. and Jenkinson, D.H. (1976) Transmission of impulses from nerve to muscle. In: *Neuromuscular Junction*, Handbook of Experimental Pharmacology, vol. 42 (Ed. Zaimis, E.), pp. 229–364. Springer-Verlag: Berlin

Goldstein, J.L., Brown, M.S., Anderson, R.G.W., Russell, D.W. and Schneider, W.J. (1985) Receptor-mediated endocytosis. *Annual Review of Cell Biology* **1**, 1–39

Green, S., Walter, P., Kumar, V. *et al.* (1986) Human oestrogen receptor cDNA: sequence expression and homology to υ-*erb*-A. *Nature* **320**, 134–139

Guimaraes, S. and Trendelenburg, U. (1985) Deviation supersensitivity and inhibition of saturable sites of loss. *Trends in Pharmacological Sciences* **6**, 371–374

Gundersen, C.B., Miledi, R. and Parker, I. (1984) Messenger RNA from human brain induces drug- and voltage-operated channels in *Xenopus* oocytes. *Nature* **308**, 421–424

Harris, A.J., Kuffler, S.W. and Dennis, M.J. (1971) Differential chemosensitivity of synaptic and extrasynaptic areas of the neuronal surface membrane in parasympathetic neurons of the frog, tested by microapplication of acetylcholine. *Proceedings of the Royal Society of London, B* **177**, 541–554

Hekman, M., Feder, D., Gal, A. *et al.* (1984) Reconstitution of β-adrenergic receptor with components of adenylate cyclase. *EMBO Journal* **3**, 3339–3345

Helmreich, E.J.M. and Pfeuffer, T. (1985) Regulation of signal transduction by β-adrenergic hormone receptors. *Trends in Pharmacological Sciences* **6**, 438–443

Hirasawa, K. and Nishizuka, Y. (1985) Phosphatidylinositol turnover in receptor mechanism and signal transduction. *Annual Review of Pharmacology and Toxicology* **25**, 147–170

Hollenberg, M.D. (1985) Pathophysiological and therapeutic implications of receptor regulation. *Trends in Pharmacological Sciences* **6**, 334–337

Houamed, K.M., Bilbe, G., Smart, T.G. *et al.* (1984) Expression of functional GABA, glycine and glutamate receptors in *Xenopus* oocytes injected with rat brain mRNA. *Nature* **310**, 318–321

Houslay, M.D. (1985) The insulin receptor and signal generation at the plasma membrane. In: *Molecular Mechanisms of Transmembrane Signalling* (Eds. Cohen, P. and Houslay, M.D.), pp. 279–334. Elsevier: Amsterdam

Insel, P.A. (1985) Adrenergic receptors on human blood cells. In: *Pharmacology of Adrenoceptors* (Eds. Szabadi, E., Bradshaw, C.M. and Nahorski, S.R.), pp. 215–224. Macmillan: London

Jenkinson, D.H. (1960) The antagonism between tubocurarine and substances which depolarize the motor end-plate. *Journal of Physiology* **152**, 309–324

Jenkinson, D.H. (1979) Partial agonists in receptor classification. In: *Proceedings of the VI International Symposium on Medicinal Chemistry* (Ed. Simpkins, M.A.), pp. 373–383. Cotswold Press: Oxford

Kahn, C.R. (1985) The molecular mechanism of insulin action. *Annual Review of Medicine* **36**, 429–451

Kaneko, A. and Tachibana, M. (1986) Effect of γ-aminobutyric acid on isolated cone photoreceptors of the turtle retina. *Journal of Physiology* **373**, 443–461

Katz, B. and Thesleff, S. (1957) A study of the 'desensitization' produced by acetylcholine at the motor end-plate. *Journal of Physiology* **138**, 63–80

Kenakin, T.P. (1982) The Schild regression in the process of receptor classification. *Canadian Journal of Physiology and Pharmacology* **60**, 249–265

Kenakin, T.P. (1984) The classification of drugs and drug receptors in isolated tissues. *Pharmacological Reviews* **36**, 165–222

Kenakin, T.P. (1985) The quantification of relative efficacy of agonists. *Journal of Pharmacological Methods* **13**, 281–308

Kenakin, T.P. and Beek, D. (1980) Is prenalterol (H133/80) really a selective beta-1 adrenoceptor agonist? Tissue selectivity resulting from differences in stimulus–response relationships. *Journal of Pharmacology and Experimental Therapeutics* **213**, 406–413

Kuhar, M.J., De Souza, E.B. and Unnerstall, J.R. (1986) Neurotransmitter receptor mapping by autoradiography and other methods. *Annual Review of Neuroscience* **9**, 27–59

Latorre, R., Alvarez, O., Cecchi, X. and Vergara, C. (1985) Properties of reconstituted ion channels. *Annual Review of Biophysics and Biophysical Chemistry* **14**, 79–111

Lemoine, H., Ehle, B. and Kaumann, A.J. (1985) Direct labelling of β_2-adrenoceptors. Comparison of binding potency of ^{3}H-ICI 118,551 and blocking potency of ICI 118,551. *Naunyn-Schmiedeberg's Archives of Pharmacology* **331**, 40–51

Levitzki, A. (1986) Coupling of β-adrenoceptors to adenylate cyclase and the role of the GTP binding protein in signal transduction. In: *Towards the Classification of 'Hormone' Receptors* (Eds. Black, J.W., Gerskowitch, P. and Jenkinson, D.H.). Liss: New York (In press)

Lindstrom, J. (1985) Immunobiology of myasthenia gravis, experimental autoimmune myasthenia gravis and Lambert–Eaton syndrome. *Annual Review of Immunology* **3**, 109–131

Lømo, T. and Rosenthal, J. (1972) Control of acetylcholine sensitivity by muscle activity in the rat. *Journal of Physiology* **221**, 493–513

McCarthy, M.P., Earnest, J.P., Young, E.F., Choe, S. and Stroud, R.M. (1986) The molecular neurobiology of the acetylcholine receptor. *Annual Review of Neuroscience* **9**, 383–413

McDevitt, D.G. (1983) Beta-adrenergic blocking drugs and partial agonist activity: is it clinically relevant? *Drugs* **25**, 331–338

Mackay, D. (1977) A critical survey of receptor theories of drug action. In: *Kinetics of Drug Action*, vol. 47 (Ed. van Rossum, J.M.), pp. 255–322. Springer-Verlag: Berlin

Merlie, J.P. and Sanes, J.R. (1985) Concentration of acetylcholine receptor mRNA in synaptic regions of adult muscle fibres. *Nature* **317**, 66–68

Miledi, R., Parker, I. and Sumikawa, K. (1982) Properties of acetylcholine receptors translated by cat muscle mRNA in *Xenopus* oocytes. *EMBO Journal* **1**, 1307–1312

Miller, C. (1986) *Ion Channel Reconstitition*. Plenum: New York and London

Mintun, M.A., Raichle, M.E., Kilbourn, M.R., Wooten, G.F. and Welch, M.J. (1984) A quantitative model for the *in vivo* assessment of drug binding sites with positron emission tomography. *Annals of Neurology* **15**, 217–227

Molinoff, P.B. and Aarons, R.D. (1983) Effects of drugs on β-adrenergic receptors on human lymphocytes. *Journal of Cardiovascular Pharmacology* **5**, S63–S67

Momoi, M.Y. and Lennon, V.A. (1986) Evidence for structural dissimilarity in the neurotransmitter binding region of purified acetylcholine receptors from human muscle and *Torpedo* electric organ. *Journal of Neurochemistry* **46**, 76–81

Motulsky, J.H. and Insel, P.A. (1982) [^{3}H] – Dihydroergocryptine binding to alpha-adrenergic receptors of human platelets. *Biochemical Pharmacology* **31**, 2591–2597

Neher, E. and Sakmann, B. (1976) Single-channel currents recorded from membrane of denervated frog muscle fibres. *Nature* **260**, 799–802

North, R.A., Slack, B.E. and Suprenant, A. (1985) Muscarinic M_1 and M_2 receptors mediate depolarization and presynaptic inhibition in guinea-pig enteric nervous system. *Journal of Physiology* **368**, 435–452

Ogden, D.C. and Colquhoun, D. (1985) Ion channel block by acetylcholine, carbachol and suberyldicholine at the frog neuromuscular junction. *Proceedings of the Royal Society, B* **255**, 329–355

Paton, W.D.M. and Rang, H.P. (1965) The uptake of atropine and related drugs by intestinal smooth muscle of the guinea-pig in relation to acetylcholine receptors. *Proceedings of the Royal Society of London, B* **163**, 1–44

Paton, W.D.M. and Waud, D.R. (1967) The margin of safety of neuromuscular transmission. *Journal of Physiology* **191**, 59–90

Patrick, J. and Lindstrom, J. (1973) Autoimmune response to acetylcholine receptor. *Science* **180**, 871–872

Pennefather, P. and Quastel, D.M.J. (1981) Relation between subsynaptic receptor blockade and response to quantal transmitter at the mouse neuromuscular junction. *Journal of General Physiology* **78**, 313–344

Pennefather, P. and Quastel, D.M.J. (1982) Modification of dose-response curves by effector blockade and uncompetitive antagonism. *Molecular Pharmacology* **22**, 369–380

Peper, K. and McMahan, U.J. (1972) Distribution of acetylcholine receptors in the vicinity of nerve terminals on skeletal muscle of the frog. *Proceedings of the Royal Society of London, B* **181**, 431–440

Phillips, G.H. (1974) Structure–activity relationships in steroidal anaesthetics. In: *Molecular Mechanisms in General Anaesthesia* (Eds. Halsey, M.J., Millar, R.A. and Sutton, J.A.), pp. 32–46. Churchill: Edinburgh

Poo, M.-m. (1985) Mobility and localization of proteins in excitable membranes. *Annual Review of Neuroscience* **8**, 369–406

Purves, D. and Sakmann, B. (1974) The effect of contractile activity on fibrillation and extrajunctional acetylcholine-sensitivity in rat muscle maintained in organ culture. *Journal of Physiology* **237**, 157–182

Rang, H.P. (1966) The kinetics of action of acetylcholine antagonists in smooth muscle. *Proceedings of the Royal Society, B* **164**, 488–510

Ringold, G.M. (1985) Steroid hormone regulation of gene expression. *Annual Review of Pharmacology and Toxicology* **25**, 529–566

Sakmann, B. and Neher, E. (1983) (Eds.) *Single Channel Recording*. Plenum: New York and London

Sakmann, B., Methfessel, C. Mishina, M. *et al*, (1985) Role of acetylcholine receptor subunits in gating of the channel. *Nature* **318**, 538–543

Schild, H.O. (1949) pA$_x$ and competitive drug antagonism. *British Journal of Pharmacology* **4**, 277–280

Schindler, H. and Quast, U. (1980) Functional acetylcholine receptor from *Torpedo marmorata* in planar membranes. *Proceedings of the National Academy of Sciences, USA* **77**, 3052–3056

Schleimer, R.P. (1985) The mechanisms of antiinflammatory steroid action in allergic diseases. *Annual Review of Pharmacology and Toxicology* **25**, 381–412

Seibert, K. and Lippman, M.E. (1982) Hormone receptors in breast cancer. *Clinical Oncology* **1**, 735–793

Sibley, D.R. and Lefkowitz, R.J. (1985) Molecular mechanism of receptor desensitization using the β-adrenergic receptor-coupled adenylate cyclase system as a model. *Nature* **317**, 124–129

Simpson, J.A. (1960) Myasthenia gravis – a new hypothesis. *Scottish Medical Journal* **5**, 419–436

Sine, S.M. and Taylor, P. (1979) Functional consequences of agonist-mediated state transitions in the cholinergic receptor. *Journal of Biological Chemistry* **254**, 3315–3325

Sine, S.M. and Taylor, P. (1981) Relationship between reversible antagonist occupancy and the functional capacity of the acetylcholine receptor. *Journal of Biological Chemistry* **256**, 6692–6699

Sine, S.M. and Taylor, P. (1982) Local anesthetics and histrionicotoxin are allosteric inhibitors of the acetylcholine receptor. *Journal of Biological Chemistry* **257**, 8106–8114

Sine, S.M. and Taylor, P. (1984) Examination of ligand occupation and the permeability response of the nicotinic acetylcholine receptor on intact cells. In: *Investigation of Membrane-located Receptors* (Eds. Reid, E., Cook, G.M.W. and Morré, D.), pp. 369–380. Plenum: New York and London

Smith, S.E. (1976) Neuromuscular blocking drugs in man. In: *Neuromuscular Junction*, Handbook of Experimental Pharmacology, vol. 42 (Ed. Zaimis, E.), pp. 593–660. Springer-Verlag: Berlin

Staros, J.V., Cohen, S. and Russo, M.W. (1985) Epidermal growth factor receptor: characterization of its protein kinase activity. In: *Molecular Mechanisms of Transmembrane Signalling* (Eds. Cohen, P. and Houslay, M.D.), pp. 253–277. Elsevier: Amsterdam

Stephenson, R.P. (1956) A modification of receptor theory. *British Journal of Pharmacology* **11**, 379–393

Stevens, C.F. (1986) Modifying channel function. *Nature* **319**, 622

Stroud, R.M. and Finer-Moore, J. (1985) Acetylcholine receptor structure, function and evolution. *Annual Review of Cell Biology* **1**, 317–351

Sumikawa, K., Houghton, M., Emtage, J.S., Richards, B.M. and Barnard, E.A. (1981) Active multi-subunit ACh receptor assembled by translation of heterologous mRNA in *Xenopus* oocytes. *Nature* **292**, 862–864

Swart, S.S. and Barnett, D.B. (1985) Adrenoceptors and abnormal platelet function. In: *Pharmacology of Adrenoceptors* (Eds. Szabadi, E., Bradshaw, C.M. and Nahorski, S.R.), pp. 225–233. Macmillan: London

Takeuchi, A. and Takeuchi, N. (1975) The structure–activity relationship for GABA and related compounds in the crayfish muscle. *Neuropharmacology* **14**, 627–634

Vincent, A. (1980) Immunology of acetylcholine receptors in relation to myasthenia gravis. *Physiological Reviews* **60**, 756–824

Waud, B.E. and Waud, D.R. (1985) Interaction among agents that block end-plate depolarization competitively. *Anesthesiology* **63**, 4–15

Waud, B.E., Mookerjee, A. and Waud, D.R. (1982) Chronic potassium depletion and sensitivity to tubocurarine. *Anesthesiology* **57**, 111–115

Waud, D.R. and Waud, B.E. (1975) *In vitro* measurement of margin of safety of neuromuscular transmission. *American Journal of Physiology* **229**, 1632–1634

Weinstein, H. (1986) Classification based on ligand binding: on the chemical meaning of ligand affinity in studies of drug receptor interactions. In: *Towards the Classification of 'Hormone' Receptors*. (Eds. Black, J.W., Gerskowitch, P. and Jenkinson, D.H.). Liss: New York (In press)

Werman, R. (1969) An electrophysiological approach to drug–receptor mechanisms. *Comparative Biochemistry and Physiology*, **30**, 997–1017.

Yamamura, H.I., Enna, S.J. and Kuhar, M.J. (1985) *Neurotransmitter Receptor Binding*. 2nd Edit. Raven: New York

Zaimis, E. (1976) The neuromuscular junction: areas of uncertainty. In: *Neuromuscular Junction*, Handbook of Experimental Pharmacology, vol. 42. (Ed. Zaimis, E.), pp. 1–21. Springer-Verlag: Berlin

2

Principles of pharmacokinetics

C.J. Hull

This chapter presents a systematic outline of pharmacokinetic principles, with a minimum of jargon, mathematics and model-dependent concepts. In order that an account of *pharmacokinetics* is not interrupted by explanations of principles familiar to most readers, an elementary understanding of several basic concepts (such as exponential mathematics) will be assumed. The reader wishing to refresh these topics may find the appendices to this chapter useful. Symbols follow the convention adopted by the *British Journal of Anaesthesia* (Hull, 1979).

When a drug is administered, it is subject to a number of *pharmacokinetic* influences. For example, some fraction of the dose will reach the systemic circulation by *uptake* processes. In the case of intravenous injection, uptake may be regarded as both instantaneous and complete. Upon reaching the circulation, most drugs are *partitioned* between different blood components. Then the drug will be *distributed* to organs and tissue zones, in one or more of which it may exert pharmacological effects. These effects may be regarded as 'useful' or 'adverse', depending upon the prescriber's intentions! The microenvironment in which drug molecules come into intimate association with their sites of action is often referred to as the *biophase*, which may be anatomically definable but more often must be regarded as a widely dispersed set of 'microzones' with similar functional characteristics. From the outset, the drug may be subject to one or more *eliminational* processes, which may involve direct excretion or transformation to more excretable products.

On reaching the biophase, the drug will cause an *effect*, often by occupancy of one or more receptor types. The relationship between drug in biophase and the magnitude and time-course of the consequent effect is governed by *pharmacodynamic* factors.

Holford made an elegant distinction between the two processes: '*Pharmacokinetics* is what the body does to the drug, whereas *pharmacodynamics* is what the drug does to the body'.

Uptake and availability

Oral administration

Many drugs are administered by the oral route. This may be simply for convenience, since the agent can be non-sterile, and administration does not usually require skilled help or supervision. However, since this route also allows the pharmacist considerable control over the rate at which the drug becomes available for absorption (see below), it may be actively preferred under some circumstances.

Disintegration

Before the drug can be absorbed, it must enter solution. If the preparation is taken in solid tablet form, then disintegration is an essential preliminary stage. The tablet may be formulated so as to disintegrate or even effervesce in water, thus facilitating dissolution by breaking the active drug into fine particles. On the other hand, close compaction with binding agents may result in much slower disintegration and therefore slower absorption.

Capsules may also be used as drug vehicles, with a variety of characteristics. In the simplest form the envelope is simply gelatin; this protects the patient from unpleasant taste, but dissolves rapidly to release the drug in the stomach. Enteric-coated capsules will resist the acid medium of the stomach and release the drug in the lower regions of the tract. This may protect the stomach from irritants, but may also protect drugs such as penicillin from destruction by a strongly acid environment.

Sustained-release formulations may be non-homogenous, with some parts disintegrating rapidly, others more slowly. More complex vehicles are designed to sustain their physical integrity throughout, releasing drug at controlled rates throughout the gastrointestinal transit.

Dissolution

The rate at which a drug is absorbed depends upon its solubility, since passive transfer depends upon the concentration gradient of *diffusible* drug. Thus if a drug is very poorly water soluble, uptake will be slow because only the minute proportion in solution can actually diffuse across cell membranes. Moreover, only a fraction of the dissolved drug is able to cross the hydrophobic layer of cell membranes lining the gastrointestinal tract. This is because many drugs are partially ionized in aqueous solution, and only the non-ionized fraction can penetrate lipid structures. The un-ionized drug in solution should be regarded as the *absorbable fraction*.

Absorption (see Orme, 1984)

The rate at which diffusible drug is absorbed depends upon its lipid solubility; thus methadone is absorbed more rapidly than morphine. Many drugs (e.g. pethidine) are almost entirely ionized at gastric pH; soluble but unavailable. Only on entering the more alkaline milieu of the small bowel does a significant fraction become free base and thus absorbable. The opposite may also apply, as with aspirin, which, being poorly ionized in the acid medium of the stomach, undergoes rapid absorption after oral dosing. The behaviour of individual drugs depends upon whether they are acids or bases, and upon their pK_a values. The principles involved are considered in Appendix A of this chapter.

When uptake does not commence until drug is released by the stomach (as with any opioid), the process may be both complex and unpredictable, due to great variation in the rate of gastric emptying. This may be caused by food, drugs or disease processes.

By influencing both gastric secretion and emptying, food may either enhance or impede the absorption of drugs depending upon the preferential sites of absorption and the effect of pH on the drug structure. The drug may also be adsorbed by food particles, thus reducing the dose available for absorption.

Other drugs may influence uptake in a variety of ways. They may modify the intragastric pH (e.g. H_2 antagonists). They may promote or delay gastric emptying (e.g. metoclopramide and morphine). Finally they may interact in the gastrointestinal tract itself; antacids may form stable complexes with drugs such as digoxin, and thereby make them 'unavailable'.

First-pass metabolism

Generally, drugs administered by the oral route enter the portal circulation and therefore must pass through the liver. Consequently, some fraction of the dose will be metabolized before reaching the systemic circulation (see later definition of extraction ratio). This process is known as *first-pass metabolism*. If a large fraction is eliminated in this way, the effective dose (so far as the target tissue is concerned) is greatly diminished. Thus drugs such as propranolol must be given in much larger doses when administered orally.

Presystemic metabolism may also take place in the gut wall; this mechanism contributes to the first-pass elimination of both morphine and chlorpromazine.

Bioavailability

All the above effects influence the effective dose which enters the systemic circulation and has the opportunity to perfuse the target tissue. *Bioavailability* may be defined as the ratio of *effective dose* to the *administered dose*. This ratio permits calculation of an equivalent oral dose from a known systemic dose, and vice versa. Bioavailability can be estimated by giving the same dose both orally and intravenously (on different occasions), followed by measurement of plasma concentrations throughout the elimination phase. Then, following estimation of the area under each concentration–time curve (AUC_o and AUC_{iv} respectively), bioavailability can be calculated as AUC_o/AUC_{iv}.

Sublingual and rectal administration

First-pass effects can be avoided if the drug is absorbed from a surface whose circulation does not drain into the portal circulation. This can be achieved if the agent is rapidly absorbed from a sublingual tablet or from the rectal mucosa.

In the former case, the route is limited to potent, rapidly absorbed drugs (such as glyceryl trinitrate, isosorbide dinitrate and buprenorphine), so that an effective mass of drug can be absorbed during a limited period of retention. Drugs with high lipid solubility have the greatest permeability, but it is also important that the agent is sufficiently water soluble to reach high concentration in saliva. Drugs with high lipid solubility (such as buprenorphine) may be stored at the site of absorption, thus delaying (and prolonging) systemic uptake.

Rectal administration is popular in some countries, but has the disadvantage that evacuation may precede absorption or, conversely, local inflammatory disease may greatly accelerate absorption with consequent excessive plasma concentrations.

Transdermal administration

If a drug is sufficiently potent, therapeutic quantities may be absorbed directly through the skin. In the case of a drug whose dosage is not critical (e.g. glyceryl trinitrate), a simple ointment may approximate to a *zero-order* input (see Appendix B of this chapter). The rate of uptake is related to the area and perfusion of the skin surface, and may therefore be regulated (to some extent) by choice of site and prescribing the drug 'by the inch'. In more critical applications, truly zero-order devices have been developed which release drug at a constant rate. Here, a drug depot is separated from the skin by a diffusion-limiting membrane, and secured by means of an adhesive 'patch'. So long as the depot drug mass is large compared to the delivered dose, the diffusion-limiting membrane will release drug at an almost constant rate for extended periods.

This technique has been notably effective in the treatment of motion sickness using hyoscine, and the management of angina with glyceryl trinitrate. In both cases, predictable administration rates can be sustained for at least 24 hours. The administration of potent opioids is an obvious application for this technique, and a 'patch' device for delivering fentanyl is undergoing clinical trials.

As with sublingual administration, lipid-soluble drugs accumulate in the dermis, so uptake continues for some time after removal of the transdermal patch.

Administration by inhalation

Gases and vapours

The respiratory tract can be used in a variety of modes. The inhalation of gases and vapours is perhaps the most fundamental of all anaesthetic routes, and follows simple but often misunderstood principles. The great majority of uptake takes place from the alveoli, and is dependent upon the partial pressure gradient between alveolus and plasma. At the commencement of inhalation successive tidal volumes mix with the functional residual capacity (FRC) and the alveolar concentration begins to rise towards that in fresh gas. Then, uptake from each alveolus depends upon the capillary blood flow (with which a continuous equilibrium is maintained), the vapour partial pressure of the agent in plasma (initially zero), and the blood/gas partition coefficient. The uptake of drug from the alveoli limits the rate at which alveolar drug tension rises towards that in inspired air. Thus the alveolar tension of an agent with high blood solubility (e.g. trichlorethylene) rises much more slowly than that of one with low solubility (e.g. nitrous oxide), and more drug is required to achieve an anaesthetic tension. These differences can be demonstrated graphically by plotting the ratio of alveolar to inspired concentrations against time (Fig. 2.1).

Since the intensity of pharmacological effect is determined by the drug

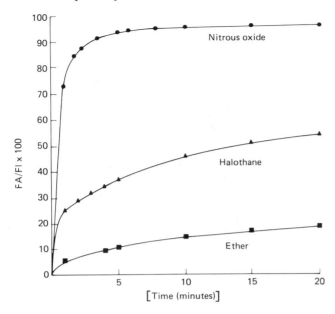

Fig. 2.1   The concentrations of some anaesthetic agents in alveolar gas during inhalation of a constant mixture, expressed as a fraction of the inspired concentration. This enables agents of widely varying potency to be compared directly. (After Eger, 1980; reproduced with permission.)

tension in blood perfusing the brain, and this follows closely behind alveolar tension, Fig. 2.1 also indicates a physical basis for the very different rates of onset for a range of agents.

The rate of uptake of a gas is dependent upon the partial pressure gradient. Thus it follows that eventually the alveolar tension will reach that of inspired gas. Then the net uptake will be zero, unless some gas is eliminated by other routes. Under these conditions, the alveolar partial pressure of the anaesthetic agent approaches that in the inspired mixture. Then if the solubility in plasma is known, the plasma concentration can be calculated with some precision. Elimination depends upon the same processes operating in reverse.

Administration by inhalation has a fundamental advantage over all other techniques. After dosing by any other route, elimination must follow some quite separate pathway whose characteristics are determined by a different set of parameters. Thus it is not possible to relate plasma concentration to the rate of administration with the same certainty.

The close relationship between inspired concentration and plasma partial pressure (and thus to intensity of effect) is fundamental to the intelligent practice of inhalational anaesthesia. Equally, it is important to appreciate why this does *not* apply to a drug given by intravenous infusion.

Aerosols
Many drugs are rapidly absorbed from both alveoli and bronchial mucosa. If the agent is water soluble, a solution can be finely divided as an aqueous

aerosol. Many years ago asthmatic patients self-administered adrenaline as a spray, but the large droplet size caused rapid rain-out before reaching the terminal bronchioles and alveoli. In fact, some drugs delivered as large droplets may be swallowed and act through gastrointestinal absorption. Modern aerosols can be made to deliver controlled droplet sizes in the micron range, so that a high proportion of the dose reaches the alveoli with consequently very rapid uptake. Pressurized aerosols in which the drug is dispensed directly into a propellant such as Freon are more convenient for day-to-day use.

In many cases (e.g. glyceryl trinitrate) aerosol administration is simply a non-invasive means of giving a small intravenous dose. However, some drugs (such as salbutamol) are more effective if given by this route, since direct diffusion to bronchial β_2-adrenoceptors results in higher intensity of effect without increasing the administered dose.

A number of 'social' drugs are administered by aerosols. Nicotine is the best example in our culture, but others such as cannabis and opium are highly effective when 'smoked'.

It must be remembered that the respiratory tract is an extremely efficient means of administration. Thus when local anaesthetic agents are applied to the trachea and bronchi for endoscopic procedures, an appreciable fraction of the dose will be absorbed *very rapidly indeed*.

Intramuscular and subcutaneous administration

If the variation associated with the oral route is to be avoided and a sustained effect is required, in many cases there is no alternative to administration by injection. In principle, a depot of drug is placed in a tissue in which it is not pharmacologically active, and gradual absorption into the systemic circulation follows. Uptake will usually be first-order (see Appendix C of this chapter).

The rate of uptake depends upon the following.

1. *Bioavailability*. This is often 100 per cent, but should not be assumed to be so.
2. *Local tissue solubility and binding*. High solubility or binding at the injection site may greatly diminish immediate availability (especially when lipid-soluble drugs are injected into subcutaneous fat). Since the processes are reversible, this should not be seen as diminished bioavailability, but as partitioning which diminishes the diffusible concentration.
3. *Water solubility*. Drug cannot diffuse to capillaries except in aqueous solution. As the drug solution pH shifts from that of the preparation to that of the tissue, a reduction in ionized fraction may result in lowered solubility so that some drug may come out of solution.
4. *Permeability*. The drug's ability to diffuse through tissues is enhanced by small molecular weight and lipid solubility. Thus uptake is favoured by low ionization as long as the drug can remain in aqueous solution.
5. *Perfusion*. This factor is responsible for much of the observed variation in uptake rate. Blood flow in different muscle sites may differ considerably, especially when the subject is physically active. Perfusion of subcutaneous sites may be very poor, resulting in slow uptake. Accidental subcutaneous

injection is a frequent cause of apparently ineffective intramuscular injections.

Spinal and epidural administration

Some drugs such as local anaesthetic agents have long been administered both intrathecally and by extradural injection but it is only recently that opioids have been given by this route.

The term *uptake* is difficult to define in this context because two quite separate processes are at work. While drug is undergoing systemic uptake in the conventional sense it is also diffusing directly to neural tissues where (presumably) the pharmacological action occurs. Thus the biophase is reached without first entering the systemic circulation.

In the case of intrathecal injection, these two uptake mechanisms occur simultaneously (with heavy emphasis on neural uptake) while the drug disperses through the CSF under the influence of the specific gravity of the administered solution and the patient's posture.

However, disposition after extradural administration is more complex, since the drug disperses through the space primarily by displacement while undergoing systemic uptake (much more rapidly than from the CSF) and diffusion both through the dura and into the nerves traversing the epidural space. Whilst neural and systemic uptake are favoured by high lipid solubility, the dura acts as a simple diffusion barrier where molecular weight is the determining factor: small molecules diffuse faster than big ones.

Modification of local capillary blood flow, either by direct effects of the drug itself or by the action of some added vasopressor, may greatly modify the balance between systemic and neural uptake. By this means it is possible to limit systemic side effects and intensify the neural blockade.

Drug disposition in blood

Ionization

When drug enters the blood stream, it cannot be assumed to form a simple homogenous solution. Many drugs exist in both ionized and un-ionized forms, the relative proportions of the two species depending upon the pK_a of the drug and the pH (see Appendix A of this chapter). Thus at pH 7.4 thiopentone is 40 per cent ionized, whilst diazepam is only 0.01 per cent ionized (Fig. 2.2).

Since the ionized form is generally poorly lipid soluble and crosses lipid membranes (such as the blood–brain barrier) with great difficulty, non-ionized drug should be regarded as the 'diffusible fraction'. This certainly applies so far as the brain (and, to a lesser extent, the placenta) is concerned. However, many capillary membranes are fenestrated, with less tightly applied junctions between cells so that ionized molecules of moderate size can pass. Were it not so, pancuronium would not be a neuromuscular blocking agent.

The ionized and non-ionized forms are readily interchangeable, and maintain a dynamic equilibrium at all times according to the local pH. Thus fentanyl crosses the blood–brain barrier as free base, but in brain CSF

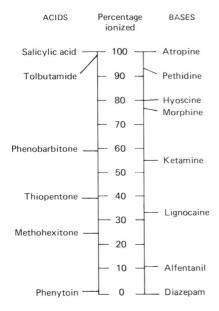

ACIDS   Percentage   BASES
               ionized

Salicylic acid ─── 100 ─── Atropine

Tolbutamide ── 90 ── Pethidine

── 80 ── Hyoscine
── Morphine

── 70 ──

Phenobarbitone ── 60 ──
── Ketamine
── 50 ──

Thiopentone ── 40 ──
── Lignocaine
── 30 ──

Methohexitone ── 20 ──

── 10 ── Alfentanil

Phenytoin ─── 0 ─── Diazepam

Fig. 2.2   The percentage ionization at pH 7.4 of some commonly used drugs.

(assuming pH 7.3) some 93 per cent becomes protonated. Indeed, this repartitioning process is essential since it is the protonated form which actually 'recognizes' and associates with the μ-receptor.

Protein binding

Many drugs bind reversibly to plasma proteins, and also to proteins in extravascular components. Since protein binding may be very extensive, the relative proportions of bound drug in various body spaces can have a profound effect upon overall drug disposition.

Generally, acidic drugs bind to albumin, but basic drugs may bind to gammaglobulins, lipoproteins and glycoproteins. It is of particular interest that drugs such as lignocaine, bupivacaine, propranolol and alfentanil bind extensively to α_1-acid glycoprotein. This has been called the 'stress protein', and increased concentrations may be found in chronic inflammatory disease, in malignancy and after myocardial infarction or major surgery.

Drugs may bind to more than one site on an individual protein structure, and may 'compete' with other drugs for the same site.

Taking the simplest possible situation where a drug binds reversibly to a single protein-binding site in a well-stirred medium, the relation between bound and unbound drug is governed by the mass action equation:

$$K_d = [\text{free}].[\text{vacant sites}]/[\text{bound}]$$

where K_d is the equilibrium dissociation constant and expresses the drug concentration at which 50 per cent of sites are occupied. As the drug concentration rises, [bound] increases and [vacant sites] diminishes as the equilibrium:

$$[free] + [vacant sites] \rightleftharpoons [bound]$$

shifts progressively to the right. If [vacant sites] is very large in proportion to [free] (i.e. drug concentration is much less than K_d), then the ratio [bound]:[free] remains almost constant. Thus it has been shown that approximately 85 per cent of fentanyl in plasma is protein bound over the entire therapeutic concentration range.

Saturation of binding sites
Less potent drugs such as salicylates which must achieve much greater plasma concentrations may occupy a significant proportion of all available sites. As [vacant sites] diminishes, [bound] no longer keeps pace with [free] and the binding ratio diminishes. Clearly, it is under these conditions that binding interactions with other drugs are most likely. For instance, salicylates may decrease the bound fraction of warfarin, and thereby cause a considerable increase of effect. It should be appreciated that the effect is caused by the *unbound* drug fraction; thus a small change in percentage binding from, say, 98 per cent to 90 per cent results in a fivefold increase in free drug.

Protein-bound drug is not immediately available for diffusion out of the vascular compartment. Outward diffusion of unbound drug is immediately followed by restoration of the binding equilibrium, making more unbound drug available. By this means all protein-bound drug may diffuse out of the plasma as it passes (for instance) through a hepatic capillary. However, the *rate* of diffusion is dependent on the concentration of unbound diffusible drug. Thus protein binding may have a considerable effect upon the *rate* at which drug diffuses out of the circulation. When taking ionization into consideration also, it becomes evident that the diffusible concentration of some drugs may be quite a small proportion of that measurable in plasma (i.e. only some 0.35 per cent of buprenorphine).

Uptake by red cells

Any lipophilic drug will diffuse into red cells, to reach a similar concentration as the unbound concentration in plasma. However, some drugs may bind to red cell proteins and thus reach a much higher concentration. For instance, the red cell concentration of fentanyl is very similar to that in plasma.

It is important to consider the whole-blood drug concentration when determining the capacity of the liver to remove drug from the body. For instance, if a drug is eliminated faster than the capacity of the *plasma* to deliver it to the liver, it might be concluded quite erroneously that elimination must occur at other sites.

Distribution of drug in the body

Physical characteristics

As drug enters the blood, it is very rapidly mixed with the circulating volume. Some drugs (e.g. dicoumarol) are so tightly bound to plasma proteins that virtually none leaves the circulation. Ionized drugs such as pancuronium can distribute to much of the extracellular space by passing through capillary endothelial pores, but cannot cross the non-fenestrated capillary membranes constituting the blood–brain barrier. The placental barrier is somewhat less selective for ionized molecules, and allows slow transfer of these agents.

By contrast, the un–ionized fraction of many weak acids and bases *can* cross the blood–brain barrier and thus reach all parts of the central nervous system. Many of these drugs enter the cellular space and become distributed throughout the body water.

Water/lipid partition

Lipid-soluble agents may enter lipid tissues, and over a period may reach high concentrations. When a drug is dissolved in two adjacent but different phases (i.e. water and lipid), it does not reach equilibrium with equal concentrations in each phase. In fact, equilibrium is reached with equal *chemical potential* in each phase, this being the thermodynamic energy of *solute* molecules interacting with those of the *solvent*. In the case of dissolved gases, this can be expressed directly as the *tension* or *partial pressure*. The chemical potential, which ranges from 0 to 1, can be expressed as the ratio of drug concentration (expressed as a fraction of total mass) to its solubility coefficient in the solvent concerned. Thus lipid-soluble drugs can achieve diffusional equilibrium with much higher concentrations in brain lipids than in plasma.

Variation in distribution rates

Distribution to different tissue zones may occur at grossly different rates, depending upon tissue perfusion, the nature of any cell membranes through which drug must diffuse, and the tissue/plasma partition coefficients. Drug binding to tissue proteins is also important, since this has the effect of increasing the apparent partition coefficient.

Thus thiopentone diffuses rapidly into the brain as a result of good perfusion and high lipid solubility. However, despite its lipid solubility this agent appears only very gradually in body fat. This is due to the poor perfusion of fat tissue, which limits drug access. Furthermore, since very little thiopentone can enter lipids during the brief period of high concentration after an intravenous bolus, the process must continue when concentrations have fallen to a much lower level. Thus distribution to storage lipid is very slow due to both perfusion limitation and initial distribution to better perfused tissues.

Morphine rapidly leaves the circulation for well-perfused tissues, as evidenced by a very rapid and profound fall in plasma concentration after an intravenous bolus dose. However, it apppears much more gradually in the brain, since here the poor lipid solubility is a limiting factor.

Non-depolarizing neuromuscular blocking agents leave the circulation relatively slowly due to slow transcapillary diffusion. As a result biophase concentrations rise slowly also, and maximal receptor occupancy does not develop for several minutes.

As a result of these widely differing rates of distribution, it may be difficult to identify sharply defined distributive and eliminational phases in the declining plasma concentration curve. Only too often, drug continues to distribute to very 'slow' tissues throughout the period of measurement; this can lead to gross overestimates of the rate of drug elimination.

Volume of distribution

If the plasma concentrations of a drug are measured after a single intravenous dose, it should be possible to estimate the volume of the space into which it distributes; i.e.

volume = dose/concentration

This is not as straightforward as it might appear, since the plasma concentrations do not equilibrate to a distributional steady state which can be measured. This is because the distributive process includes the organs of elimination (predominantly liver and kidney), so that elimination takes place from the outset. As a result, the plasma concentration curve (Fig. 2.3) commonly shows a very rapid initial decline due to rapid distribution *and* elimination. This is followed by a slower phase in which distributive processes play only a minor role and the rate of concentration decline is due principally to elimination. It must be stressed that although these phases are often

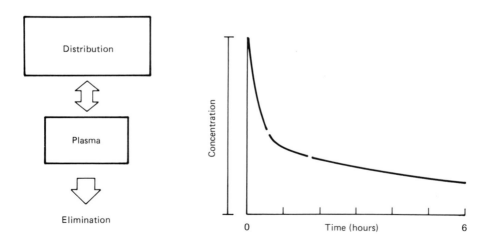

Fig. 2.3 When a drug is administered by the intravenous route, the plasma concentration is likely to decline rapidly at first as a result of simultaneous elimination and distribution. Later, the rate of fall diminishes as distributive processes become less significant.

described as 'distributive' and 'eliminational', the terms refer to the *dominant* process.

Determination of distribution volume

The simplest method is to assume that after the initial distributive phase the body behaves like a single well-stirred compartment, from which drug is eliminated along one or more first-order pathways. The first step is to fit an exponential function to the terminal phase data. This can be done with greatest precision by using a curve-fitting computer program, but an approximation may be made by plotting the data on semilogarithmic co-ordinates (see Appendix B of this chapter) and then drawing a straight line along the terminal phase points. The rate constant β is simply the gradient.

Now there are two alternatives. The first is to calculate the area under the concentration–time plot (AUC), and then calculate the apparent volume of distribution $Vd_{(area)}$ as:

$$Vd_{(area)} = \text{dose}/(AUC \times \beta)$$

Alternatively, the function fitted to the terminal phase data can be solved (by extrapolation) for B, the concentration at time zero (Fig. 2.4). Then the apparent volume $Vd_{(extrap)}$ can be calculated:

$$Vd_{(extrap)} = \text{dose}/B$$

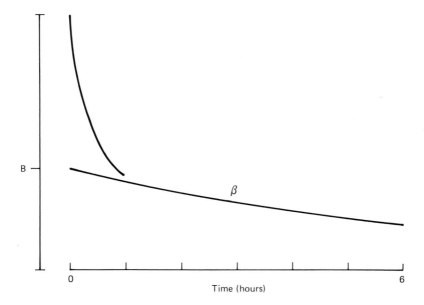

Fig. 2.4   If the terminal phase of concentration decline is extrapolated back to $t = 0$, the intercept B can be determined. This can be used to estimate the apparent volume of distribution (see text).

Although both methods present no difficulty, and can be calculated from single-dose data, they tend to overestimate the volume. During the elimination phase, drug is *returning* from a variety of tissues to the plasma, whence it is removed by the organs of elimination. Thus there are chemical potential *gradients* from tissue to plasma. Since the calculations above assume that the whole body behaves as a single well-stirred compartment (which it is not), the lower concentration in plasma leads to an overestimation of volume.

This limitation can be overcome by estimating the apparent distribution volume at steady state, where intercompartmental gradients will be minimized. This can be achieved only by giving a constant infusion of drug until steady state is achieved. Since this must continue for at least five times $T_{\frac{1}{2}}$, the procedure will be somewhat protracted. From serial plasma concentrations the following quantities are determined:

C^{ss}, the concentration at steady state.
AUC^{t}, the area under the curve until the infusion ceased at time t.
$AUC^{t \to \infty}$, the area under the curve from time t to infinity.

Then the steady state volume of distribution can be calculated:

$$V^{ss} = \mathrm{dose}/C^{ss}.\,(1 - \{AUC^{t} - AUC^{t \to \infty}\})$$

There are also model-dependent methods of calculation (Appendix D of this chapter) which require less work but more assumptions.

The apparent volumes of distribution for a range of drugs (Fig. 2.5) show wide variation, ranging from 4 to 700 litres in a 70 kg adult. Clearly if the apparent volumes are in excess of *body* volume, the reader may be tempted to doubt their validity. Not so; these are *apparent* litres, and simply reflect the relationship between the mass of drug in the body and the measured plasma

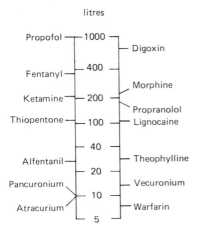

Fig. 2.5   The apparent volumes of distribution for some drugs used in anaesthesia. (Data partly from Rowland, 1978; reproduced with permission).

concentrations. Large volumes reflect the solubility or binding of drug outside the plasma, and express this as the volume of *plasma* which would be necessary to account for the observed concentrations. The value of the estimation is that although Vd is not a real volume, it does permit calculation of the dose required to yield a specified plasma concentration. Data for the plasma concentrations required to mediate the effects of individual drugs are becoming available, and an appreciation of distribution volume is essential if this is to be put to practical use.

Elimination of drugs from the body

The biochemical mechanisms of drug elimination are considered elsewhere; here the discussion will be limited to general principles and pharmacokinetic aspects of organ-specific elimination.

If serial plasma concentrations are measured during the late elimination phase after an intravenous bolus, it is often found that they decline exponentially. When this is the case, it is reasonable to conclude that one or more first-order processes are responsible. Then it can be stated that at any time the rate of elimination must be proportional to the plasma concentration at that time. This allows us to develop the concept of whole-body clearance.

Whole-body clearance

The term *clearance* describes not the rate but the *efficiency* of elimination. The efficiency of a first-order pathway cannot be determined by measuring the rate of elimination (i.e. mass/time), since this will vary according to the plasma concentration; nor is it indicated by the rate at which the plasma concentration declines (as evidenced by a rate constant or half-time), since this reflects also the *mass* of drug which must be eliminated to yield each unit decline in concentration. However, it can be expressed by the ratio of *elimination rate* to the *plasma concentration at which that rate occurs* (i.e. rate of elimination per unit concentration).

The dimensions of clearance can be derived from those of the contributing variables. Thus 'rate of elimination' is *mass/time*, whilst plasma concentration has the dimension *mass/volume*. Therefore, clearance must be *mass/time* × *volume/mass*. The mass terms cancel, leaving *volume/time*. It follows that clearance must be expressed in units such as 'litres per hour', 'millilitres per minute' etc.

Now it will not be surprising to learn that although high clearance may often be associated with a short plasma concentration half-time (as in the case of atracurium), there are many exceptions. For instance (Table 2.1), in common with many lipophilic drugs, fentanyl has a high clearance but a long terminal half-time. This is because after an intravenous bolus dose the plasma concentration declines rapidly as drug is dispersed into a very large apparent volume of distribution. Thus after the initial distributive phase plasma concentrations are very low, and although a high proportion of any drug entering the liver will be eliminated, this is only a very small proportion of the drug remaining in the body.

Table 2.1   Elimination half-time ($T_{1/2}$), clearance and apparent volume (V^β) of distribution of some drugs used in anaesthetic practice (approximate values for a 70-kg adult)

	Clearance (ml/min)	$T_{1/2}$ (min)	V^β (litre)
Thiopentone	224	600	120
Propofol	1900	380	1000
Morphine	1400	170	220
Fentanyl	900	360	330
Alfentanil	140	100	27
Pancuronium	70	100	10
Vecuronium	230	80	12
Atracurium	350	20	10
Diazepam	21	1800	85
Midazolam	490	140	95

Conversely, alfentanil has a lower clearance (probably due to less efficient hepatic biotransformation) but a much shorter half-time. In this case, a small distribution volume ensures that, despite lower eliminational efficiency, the much higher concentrations perfusing the liver result in a more rapid decline in plasma concentration.

Estimation of whole-body clearance

Clearance can be estimated following a single bolus dose of drug. The principle is based on the statement that clearance is the concentration divided by the rate of elimination. Thus over the lifetime of drug in the body, clearance must be the *mean* concentration divided by the *mean* rate of elimination.

Referring to Fig. 2.6, it will be evident that if t is the time taken to eliminate the drug, the mean concentration must be the area (AUC) under a plot of concentration vs time divided by t. Similarly, the mean elimination rate must be the dose given divided by the time t taken to eliminate it. Then,

$$Cl = (\text{dose}/t)/(AUC/t)$$
$$= (\text{dose}/t) \times (t/AUC)$$
$$= \text{dose}/AUC$$

Plasma concentrations are measured throughout the elimination period, plotted against time, and the 'area under the curve' is determined. Then clearance can be calculated easily. Many errors can occur; most are due to the estimation of AUC from a series of plasma concentrations, with inevitable assumptions regarding the changing concentration between samples, and an extrapolation from the last measured concentration to account for elimination beyond that time.

Clearance is best determined by a 'steady state' method. At steady state the rate of drug elimination must equate with the (constant) rate of drug infusion.

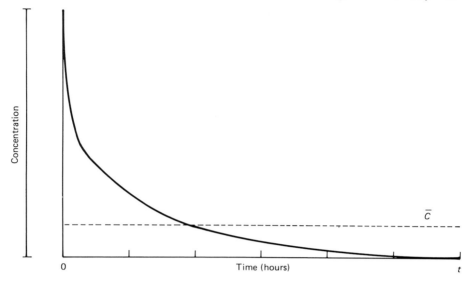

Fig. 2.6 Following a single dose of drug, the area (AUC) under the concentration–time curve (solid line) equals that under a rectangle of width t and height $\bar{c}$, where $\bar{c}$ is the mean concentration. Thus the mean concentration can be calculated as AUC/t. The mean rate of elimination must be dose/t.

Thus if the plasma concentration at steady state is given the symbol C^{ss}:

$$Cl = \text{infusion rate}/C^{ss}$$

The only limitation of this method is the long period which must be allowed for the plasma concentration to reach C^{ss}.

Whole body clearance is the sum of all individual clearances, including hepatic, renal and organ-independent mechanisms. These will be considered in terms of pharmacokinetic principles; actual biochemical pathways and the influences of age, gender, disease and other drugs are described in a later chapter.

Hepatic clearance

In the case of an organ which removes drug from the blood perfusing it, clearance has exactly the same definition as before; that is, the rate of elimination by the liver per unit concentration, with the result expressed in *millilitres per minute* (or similar).

The question now arises: millilitres of what? If clearance is calculated from concentration of drug in plasma, the answer is *plasma*. If it had been blood, then millilitres of *blood*.

Clearance by an organ can also be considered according to the Fick principle, by which organ plasma flow equals the rate at which a substance is added to or subtracted from the plasma by that organ, divided by the concentration difference in plasma entering and leaving the organ.

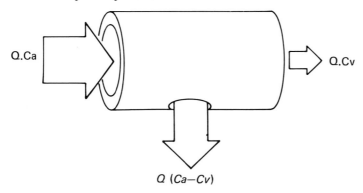

Q.Ca

Q.Cv

Q (Ca−Cv)

Fig. 2.7 A perfusion diagram of drug extraction by the liver, showing the relationship between perfusion, blood concentration and the rate of drug elimination. Q = hepatic blood flow; Ca and Cv = drug concentrations in blood entering and leaving the liver. (After Rowland, 1978; reproduced with permission.)

Thus (Fig. 2.7) if Q is the liver plasma flow, and Ca and Cv are the drug concentrations entering and leaving the liver:

$$Q = \text{rate of elimination}/(Ca - Cv)$$

Equally:

$$\text{Rate of elimination} = Q \times (Ca - Cv)$$

It is also possible to determine the fraction of drug in the incoming plasma which is removed or extracted by the liver. This is expressed as the *extraction ratio*:

$$ER = (Ca - Cv)/Ca$$

Drugs used in anaesthesia differ greatly in extraction ratio: thiopentone, diazepam and pancuronium have low ratios, whilst fentanyl, propofol, lignocaine and propranolol all have high ratios.

Clearance can be expressed by substituting $Q \cdot (Ca - Cv)$ for 'rate of elimination', and Ca for concentration:

$$Cl_h = Q \times (Ca - Cv)/Ca$$

However, since $(Ca - Cv)/Ca$ has been defined above as the extraction ratio (ER), this simplifies further to:

$$Cl_h = Q \times ER$$

Thus clearance and extraction ratio both express the efficiency of drug elimination by the liver.

The equation above leads to a further concept of clearance. Since extraction ratio can be expressed alternatively as the fraction of perfusing plasma which appears to be stripped entirely of drug, so clearance can be regarded as the volume of plasma apparently stripped of drug per unit time.

Drugs with high extraction ratios may exhibit clearances in excess of hepatic plasma flow. This may simply reflect the presence of drug in red corpuscles, extracted as blood passes through hepatic capillaries. If the concentration of drug in red cells is known, then clearance can be expressed in terms of whole blood. Too often, however, plasma clearance is simply scaled up according to the haematocrit. If the concentration in red cells differs from that in plasma (as is often the case), this will lead to serious error.

Intrinsic clearance

Hepatic clearance depends upon the hepatic blood flow, the proportion of drug bound to plasma and red cell proteins, the ease with which drug dissociates from those proteins, and the rate of diffusion out of red cells. The efficiency with which the liver tissue eliminates drug is often disguised by these factors, and should be assessed by a parameter which expresses the clearance of an unrestricted supply of free drug in plasma. This is *intrinsic clearance*.

Estimation of intrinsic clearance

Intrinsic clearance (Cl_{int}) can be regarded as the clearance which would be possible if perfusion were so great as to reduce the extraction ratio to zero. Under these conditions, clearance would reflect the capacity of hepatic enzyme systems to remove drug from plasma. Thus Cl_{int} can be calculated by correcting hepatic clearance (Cl_h) for the effect of extraction (Fig. 2.8):

$$Cl_{int} = Cl_h/(1 - ER)$$

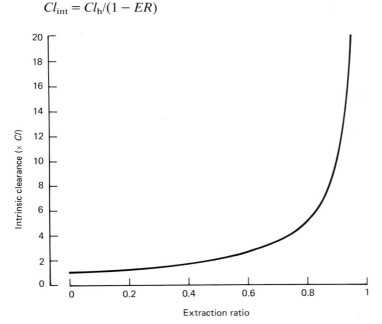

Fig. 2.8   The relationship between observed plasma clearance (Cl_p) and intrinsic clearance (Cl_{int}) depends upon the extraction ratio (ER). The vertical axis shows Cl_{int} expressed as a multiple of Cl_p. When ER is very low, Cl_{int} is very close to Cl_p. However, when ER approaches unity, plasma clearance is limited by perfusion, and therefore Cl_{int} is many times greater.

It is constructive to define Cl_h in terms of intrinsic clearance. The equation above can be rearranged to solve for Cl_h, and clearly demonstrates the interaction between intrinsic clearance and drug extraction:

$$Cl_h = Cl_{int} - (Cl_{int} \cdot ER)$$

Intrinsic clearance, extraction ratio, protein binding and perfusion

All the above factors influence the ultimate rate of drug elimination. As may be expected, each may have a limiting or modulating effect upon the others, resulting in a complex interaction. However, some basic principles can be stated without creating further confusion. These should be considered with reference to Figs. 2.9 and 2.10.

1. If intrinsic clearance is *high*, the plasma in each hepatic capillary is rapidly stripped of free (unbound) drug. Following disturbance of the equilibrium between free and bound drug, some dissociation occurs, thus restoring the [free]/[bound] ratio. More free drug diffuses into the hepatic cell, and the cycle is repeated until no bound drug remains. Thus binding is not a limiting factor.

The rate of elimination is dependent upon the hepatic blood flow and the drug concentration (see Fig. 2.9). This is referred to as *perfusion-limited clearance*. Thus drugs such as lignocaine are very dependent upon hepatic blood flow, and the situation is complicated even further by the haemodynamic effects of lignocaine itself, which may lead to changes in hepatic blood flow.

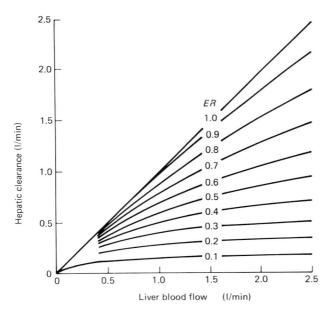

Fig. 2.9   The influence of extraction ratio upon the relationship between hepatic perfusion and plasma clearance. (From Wilkinson and Shand, 1975; reproduced with permission).

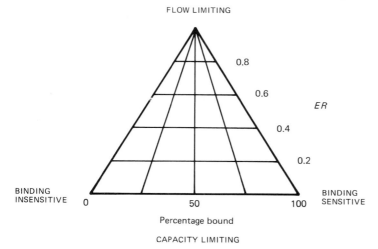

FLOW LIMITING

CAPACITY LIMITING

Fig. 2.10 Diagrammatic representation of the sensitivity of drug clearance to variation in perfusion and plasma protein binding. Drugs with high *ER* are sensitive to changes in perfusion, whilst those with low *ER* and high protein binding are sensitive to changes in binding. (After Blaschke, 1977; reproduced with permission.)

2. If intrinsic clearance is *low*, drug binding becomes important (Fig. 2.10). In this case, intracellular enzymes consume much less drug, and the rate becomes dependent upon the free drug concentration in plasma. This is reduced by high binding, so that drug uptake is low. Since only a small fraction of free drug is removed with each pass through the hepatic capillary, a correspondingly small fraction of bound drug will dissociate to restore the [bound]/[free] ratio. Therefore much of the bound drug remains bound. Under these conditions, changes in perfusion have little effect since the capillary retains a plentiful supply of drug. However, changes in binding may have dramatic effects. These must be seen in terms of *free* drug in plasma.

If the drug is highly bound the free fraction must be very small; in the case of diazepam (98 per cent bound) this will not normally exceed 2 per cent. Now if the bound fraction decreases to 90 per cent the free fraction rises to 10 per cent, a fivefold increase. Since the velocity of the enzyme reaction is proportional to the free drug concentration, there will be a dramatic increase in both extraction ratio and clearance.

In the case of drugs such as pancuronium (<50 per cent bound) or phenobarbitone (70 per cent bound) changes in binding will influence clearance, but without a multiplicative effect upon free fraction the change will be relatively small.

Drugs with low intrinsic clearance are said to be *capacity limited*. Those which are poorly protein bound (e.g. phenytoin) are unaffected by variation in binding. However, those (e.g. warfarin) which are also highly protein bound are said to be *binding sensitive*.

Non-linear hepatic clearance

Since hepatic elimination depends largely upon the activity of enzyme–substrate interactions, it follows that the velocities of these processes are determined by the Michaelis–Menten equation (Appendix C of this chapter). All such interactions are *saturable*, so if drug delivery to the liver cell raises the cytoplasmic drug concentration towards K_m the rate of reaction will no longer rise in linear proportion to the concentration. As the concentration rises further, the reaction may indeed reach saturation, under which conditions the rate of elimination will become constant, with no further increase in rate, regardless of concentration.

Only drugs with *capacity-limited* clearance are affected in this way. Obviously, a drug (such as propranolol) with an intrinsic clearance greatly in excess of actual clearance could not possibly be presented to the liver sufficiently rapidly to approach saturation. Phenytoin, theophylline and salicylates are good examples of drugs which may reach zero-order elimination in the clinical dose range, as may thiopentone in high dosage (Fig. 2.11).

Drugs with saturable excretion must be clearly distinguished from those with low intrinsic clearance. A low value of Cl_{int} with first-order drug excretion may be regarded as due to a relatively small *number* of enzymatic sites, with a K_m value well in excess of the clinically attainable concentration range. By contrast, an enzyme system having a K_m within the clinical concentration range will show non-linear or even zero-order excretion, regardless of the number of available sites.

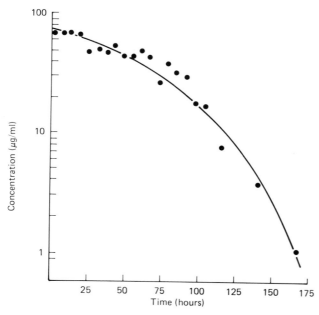

Fig. 2.11 Plasma concentrations of thiopentone (semilogarithmic scale) following very high dosage (502 mg/kg over 42 hours). Elimination is zero-order at very high concentrations, becoming first-order at lower levels. (From Stanski *et al.*, 1980; reproduced with permission.)

Renal elimination

Renal blood flow amounts to some 700 ml per minute in an average adult, and this represents the maximum possible blood clearance by the kidneys.

This may be achieved as the sum of two separate mechanisms: *glomerular filtration* and *tubular secretion* (Fig. 2.12).

Elimination by glomerular filtration

Approximately 18 per cent of renal plasma flow appears as glomerular filtrate (127 ml per minute), and will contain the same drug concentration as the non-protein-bound fraction in plasma. Of course, any drug carried in red cells is unaffected by passage through the glomerular capillary. However, lipid-soluble drugs will diffuse back into the peritubular capillaries; thus despite glomerular filtration the renal clearance of thiopentone is zero. Only the non-ionized drug fraction is reabsorbed, and therefore the *rate* of reabsorption depends upon the relative proportions of ionized and un-ionized species. In some cases a change in urinary pH may modify the un-ionized fraction enough to alter renal clearance. Thus acidification of urine increases the ionization of pethidine in glomerular filtrate, and may thereby cause a significant increase in renal clearance.

A number of drugs (e.g. penicillin, cimetidine and neostigmine) are actively secreted into the renal tubule, thus raising the possibility that renal clearance may reach (or even exceed) renal plasma flow. Like hepatic clearance, these transport mechanisms are active processes, and are therefore both saturable

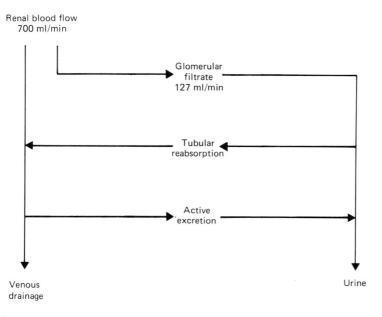

Fig. 2.12 Factors influencing renal clearance. Unless drug is actively excreted, the renal extraction ratio cannot normally exceed 0.18, this being the fraction of drug entering the kidneys which undergoes glomerulor filtration.

by very high concentrations and susceptible to substrate competition by other drugs.

As with the liver, the clearance of drugs with high renal extraction ratios (such as neostigmine) are very susceptible to changes in renal blood flow.

Organ-independent elimination

Some drugs are eliminated by mechanisms which do not depend upon perfusion of any organ of elimination. For instance, atracurium is degraded by the pH- and temperature-dependent Hofmann reaction, by which the drug molecule cleaves spontaneously to yield the inactive (at least at the neuromuscular junction) substance laudanosine. Since this reaction occurs in all sites to which the drug may distribute, drug does not need to return to the plasma prior to elimination. The apparent plasma clearance is high (380 ml per minute) in comparison with other non-depolarizing neuromuscular blocking agents such as pancuronium (125 ml per minute), but the distribution volume is also small, so the elimination half-life is very short indeed for a muscle relaxant (20 minutes). Hofmann elimination is not saturable since there is no enzyme–substrate interaction involved.

By contrast, a number of drugs are hydrolysed by plasma cholinesterase. Suxamethonium is the best-known example (also hydrolysed by acetylcholinesterase at the neuromuscular junction), but procaine, 2-chloroprocaine and propanidid also depend upon this route of elimination and interactions may occur when any two (or more) are used simultaneously.

Pharmacokinetic analysis

A number of important pharmacokinetic concepts have been introduced in the course of the foregoing sections.

The most important is that when a drug diffuses out of the plasma to some tissue in which it is more soluble, the ensuing plasma concentrations will behave as if the drug is dispersed throughout a much larger volume than the physically demonstrable space. In many cases the apparent volume of a tissue is simply the product of actual volume and the partition coefficient with plasma. Thus *distribution volume* does not require physical existence to be both valid and useful.

Second, *clearance* is of fundamental importance, and has much greater depth of meaning than the traditional 'litres of blood cleared per unit time'. Furthermore, it is a perfectly valid concept even when much of the 'clearing' takes place out of the vascular compartment.

Quite apart from their descriptive value, these pharmacokinetic parameters have practical application. For instance, if the clinician wishes to estimate the dose of a drug needed to 'load' a patient to a specified concentration, he need only solve the simple equation:

$$\text{Dose} = \text{concentration} \times Vd$$

Similarly, he can calculate the rate at which a constant drug infusion must run in order to achieve and then maintain a constant plasma concentration

(C^{ss}). This can be calculated by application of the basic concept of clearance: that *clearance equals the rate of elimination per unit concentration*. Thus if C^{ss} and Cl are known, the rate of elimination at steady state can be determined easily. Now at steady state, the rate of administration *must* equal the rate of elimination, so:

$$\text{Infusion rate} = Cl \cdot C^{ss}$$

Unfortunately, these very simple concepts have some limitations, since it is assumed that the body behaves as if it were a single well-stirred compartment. Figure 2.3 showed that an intravenous bolus of drug will often result in a decaying plasma concentration curve which initially falls too steeply to be consistent with first-order elimination. If the curve is replotted on semilogarithmic axes (Fig. 2.13) it can be seen that whilst the terminal section is now a straight line and therefore an exponential process (see Appendix B of this chapter), the initial section has a steeper and non-linear gradient.

In fact, if the exponential process accounting for the terminal section is identified, the *differences* between this function and the actual curve can be calculated. If now these differences are plotted against time on the same semilogarithmic plot, they are seen to fall in a straight line and therefore represent a second exponential function. Thus the drug decay curve usually can be identified (but by no means always) with a function consisting of the *sum* of two exponential terms. The process of curve fitting can be performed at various levels of sophistication from judicious use of eyeball, ruler and pencil to non-linear regression analysis programs (such as ELSFIT) which can be run on small digital computers. The process is deceptively easy but beset with pitfalls for the unwary.

When the decay curve *can* be identified with a 'biexponential' function,

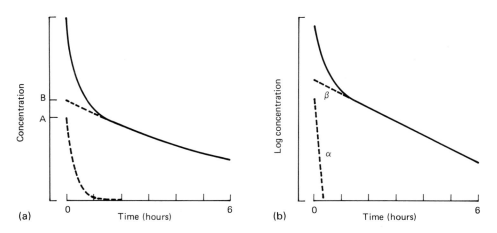

Fig. 2.13   The function $C = A \cdot e^{-\alpha t} + B \cdot e^{-\beta t}$ (solid line) is the sum of two simple exponential terms (broken lines) having zero-time intercepts and rate constants A, α and B, β. Drawn on (a) linear and (b) semilogarithmic ordinates.

derivation of pharmacokinetic parameters becomes very straight-forward. For instance, the area under the curve (AUC) can be determined using:

$$AUC = A/\alpha + B/\beta$$

which is very much simpler than planimetry or application of the trapezoidal rule.

The two-compartment model

It is possible, however, to go further without making many more assumptions. Any biexponential function (see Fig. 2.10) can be shown to characterize a set of feasible two-compartment models. All have drug added to the *central* compartment, which must include the plasma volume.

If it is accepted that drug may be eliminated from both compartments, there are innumerable feasible solutions. However, if (as is often very reasonable) it is assumed that drug is eliminated only from the central compartment, then only *one* model (Fig. 2.14) will behave according to the equation.

This model makes no assumptions regarding the distribution of drug to individual tissues; indeed, all temptations to assign physiological or anatomical significance to central and deep volumes should be resisted firmly.

The great advantage of this over the one-compartment model is that it accounts for *distribution*, which so clearly plays a vital role in drug disposition.

The value for V_1 represents the volume into which the drug appears to distribute initially, i.e before distributive processes begin. If a loading dose is based (as suggested above) on the total apparent volume ($V^{ss} = V_1 + V_2$), the initial concentration will be much higher than intended due to the initial volume being much smaller. Clearly this may not only be therapeutically unnecessary, but also result in unwanted side effects.

If, however, the loading dose is calculated on the basis of V_1, then the initial concentration will be in the desired range. Of course, distribution will cause an immediate reduction, but in practice this can be avoided by the use of more sophisticated methods outside the scope of this text.

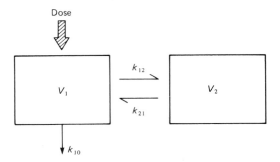

Fig. 2.14 The two-compartment open pharmacokinetic model. Rate constant notation indicates the direction of drug movement.

Clearance from a compartmental model can be derived easily. First, since clearance describes the *efficiency* of an elimination pathway, and it is (usually) assumed that drug is eliminated only from the central compartment, clearance can be determined by considering that compartment only.

Second, it has been shown (Appendix B of this chapter) that in a simple first-order system the rate constant k is (at any time) the rate of concentration decline expressed as a fraction of the concentration. Thus at any time:

k = rate of concentration decline/concentration

This expression can be expanded to reflect the changing mass of drug in the system. Since the *mass* of drug corresponding to a particular concentration must be the product of drug *concentration* and the *volume* into which it appears to be dispersed, it follows that:

$k \cdot V$ = rate of concentration decline $\times$ volume/concentration
= rate of drug elimination/concentration

Therefore it follows that:

$$Cl = k \cdot Vd$$

In two-compartment terminology, and remembering that we need only consider the central compartment:

$$Cl = k_{10} \cdot V_1$$

Not only does clearance define the rate of elimination per unit concentration; it also indicates the rate at which drug must be administered in order to maintain that unit concentration (since at equilibrium input must equal output). Thus for any desired plasma concentration C^{ss}, the required infusion rate k'_{01} is simply:

$$k'_{01} = C^{ss} \cdot Cl$$

The value of compartmental models
Models of this type are most useful for estimating the optimal dosing regimen, but also help in conceptualizing the differences between drugs. For instance, the apparently similar drugs vecuronium and atracurium have quite different pharmacokinetic profiles, and the compartmental approach enables the clinician to use these agents with both insight and intelligence.

Compartmental models are *not* predictors of drug behaviour in individual cases. They are derived from grouped data, and therefore have only very general predictive capacity. In individual cases the simple model can do no more than make broad indications, albeit more precisely than is likely by other means. A detailed account of the mathematics involved may be found elsewhere (Hull, 1983).

More complex kinetic models

In some cases, examination of decaying drug concentrations shows that a two-compartment model is not satisfactory but that the inclusion of a third compartment permits a good fit. Such a model requires a third term in the equation, and the regression must be made with less degrees of freedom. Three-compartment models should be proposed only after the most rigorous statistical analysis (Boxenbaum, Reigelman and Elashoff, 1974).

Some workers (i.e. Mather's group in Australia) have proposed more *physiological* models of drug action, which can, for instance, account for changes in cardiac output and tissue perfusion. Such models require vast amounts of data, relating plasma concentrations to individual organ blood flow data and the effects of physiological perturbations. Mapleson and his colleagues have developed valid human models for some anaesthetic gases and vapours (Chilcoat, Lunn and Mapleson, 1984), but systems of this complexity can be realized only with the aid of powerful computers.

Appendix A   Acids, bases and pK_a

An acid is a proton donor, a base a proton acceptor. Many drugs are weak acids or weak bases, and therefore are partially ionized in aqueous solution. The equilibrium between a weak acid and its salt with a strong base is expressed by the Henderson–Hasselbalch equation:

$$pH = pK_a + \log([\text{salt}]/[\text{acid}])$$

where K_a is the dissociation constant and pK_a its negative logarithm. pK_a is equal to the pH at which the drug is 50 per cent ionized. Thus:

$$pH = pK_a + [\text{ionized}]/[\text{non-ionized}]$$

Now if

$$s = \text{antilog}(pH - pK_a)$$

the ionized fraction Fi can be calculated:

$$Fi = 1/(1 + s)$$

Naturally, the ionization equation for a weak base must be:

$$pH = pK_a + [\text{non-ionized}]/[\text{ionized}]$$

and the ionized fraction will be:

$$Fi = s/(1 + s)$$

Thus, given the drug pK_a and the solution pH, the ionized fraction can be calculated easily.

Some drugs (e.g. nitrazepam) are *amphoteric*; that is, they can behave as either acids or bases. Thus an ampholyte reacts as an acid at pH values above its isoelectric pH to form anions, but acts as a base below the isoelectric pH to form cations. As might be expected, it will have two values of pK_a, and the above calculations can be applied to the relevant value, according to the pH.

Appendix B   Zero and first-order processes

Many biological processes can be characterized by the general equation:

$$dC/dt = -k \cdot C^n$$

where dC/dt is the rate at which some quantity (such as drug concentration) declines with time, k is the rate constant and n an exponent with value 1 or zero.

The exponent n determines the *order* of the equation. In the case of a *zero-order* process, $n = 0$ and the equation reduces to:

$$dC/dt = -k$$

The rate of change in C is constant throughout, and therefore C decrements by the same amount in every time period.

In a *first-order* process, $n = 1$. Here the rate of change is $-k \cdot C$, and therefore is a function of C itself.

Integration yields the familiar exponential function:

$$C = C^0 \cdot e^{-kt}$$

where C^0 is the value for C at time zero, and e is the base of the natural logarithm (2.7182...).

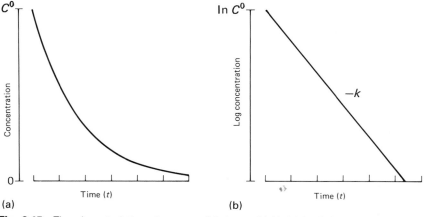

(a)   (b)

Fig. 2.15   The characteristics of exponential decay. (a) Variable C decays according to the function $C = C^0 \cdot e^{-kt}$, where C^0 is the value of C when $t = 0$. (b) The function in (a) is transformed by taking natural logarithms so that: $\ln C = \ln C^0 - kt$. $\ln C$ is plotted against time t, yielding a straight line of gradient $-k$.

If C is plotted against time (Fig. 2.15a) it can be seen that the function declines at a rate proportional to the current magnitude of C itself. At all times, the ratio of gradient to magnitude remains constant; thus slope/$C = k$. Since in this case the gradient is negative, it can be expressed as slope $= -k \cdot C$

It is often useful to express exponential functions in terms of the time taken for a certain change to take place. Now at time zero, $C = C^0$. Since the gradient expresses the ratio of C to t at any time, and at time zero equals $k \cdot C^0$, it follows that τ, the time taken for the initial gradient to reach zero, must be $1/k$. The *time constant* τ expresses the time taken for C to decline by a factor of e. In one time constant C will decline to 37 per cent of the initial value; in two time constants to 37 per cent of 37 per cent (14 per cent), and so on.

The time constant is mathematically convenient, but conceptually somewhat difficult. Many feel more comfortable with the *half-time*, which is the time taken for C to decline by a half. Half-time can be calculated using the expression:

$$T_{1/2} = \tau \cdot \ln 2$$

where ln 2 denotes the natural logarithm of 2 (0.693). The logic of this relationship can be readily verified by taking $C/C^0 = 0.5$ in the equation: $C/C^0 = e^{-kt}$, and then solving for t. Thus:

$$0.5 = e^{-kt}$$

Then take natural logarithms:

$$\ln 0.5 = -kt$$

Rearranging:

$$t = -\ln 0.5/k$$

Now ln 0.5 $= -0.693$. It is convenient to make use of the relationship $-\ln 0.5 = \ln 2$, thus eliminating the minus signs and yielding:

$$t = \ln 2/k$$

Of course it follows that:

$$t = \ln 2 \cdot \tau$$

Half-time is denoted by the SI symbol $T_{1/2}$, and often is followed by a further identifier (usually a Greek letter) to denote which of several exponential terms it describes.

It may be noted from the procedure above that taking logarithms transformed the exponential expression into linear form. Similarly, taking natural logarithms to the original exponential equation:

$$C = C^0 \cdot e^{-kt}$$

yields:

$$\ln C = \ln C^0 - kt$$

This can be confirmed (Fig. 2.15b) by plotting $\ln C$ against t. The semilogarithmic plot is a useful indicator of exponential properties; linearity implies that the variable is changing in proportion to its own magnitude, and therefore a half-time and rate constant can be calculated. However it does *not* legitimize extrapolation.

Appendix C   The Michaelis–Menten equation

The velocity of an enzymatic reaction (in which one enzyme molecule reacts with one of substrate) is governed by the Michaelis–Menten equation:

$$V = V_{max} \cdot C/(K_m + C)$$

where V_{max} is the maximum attainable velocity of the reaction (i.e. with unlimited substrate availability), C is the actual molar substrate concentration, and K_m the Michaelis constant (Fig. 2.16).

From examination of the equation it will be evident that when the reaction proceeds at 50 per cent of V_{max}, K_m must equal C. Thus K_m equals the substrate concentration at which the reaction velocity is $V_{max}/2$. Also, it will be clear that V is a hyperbolic function of C. However, when C is very small compared with

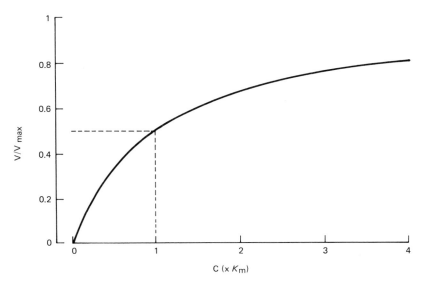

Fig. 2.16   Graphical representation of the Michaelis–Menten equation (see text).

K_m, the term $(K_m + C)$ can be simplified to K_m. Under these conditions the equation becomes linear:

$$V = V_{max} \cdot C/K_m$$

and so reaction velocity rises in proportion to the substrate concentration. However, it must be remembered that as the concentration rises towards K_m the relationship becomes markedly non-linear. When C is large compared with K_m, the term $(K_m + C)$ reduces to C; as a result the equation simplifies to:

$$V = V_{max}$$

Now the reaction proceeds at V_{max} and can go no faster whatever concentration is reached. When elimination of a drug is governed by a reaction of this type, the process will be first-order at low concentrations (i.e. rate of elimination is proportional to the concentration), becoming zero-order as the enzymatic reaction saturates.

References

Blaschke, T.F. (1977) Protein binding and kinetics of drugs in liver diseases. *Clinical Pharmacokinetics* 2, 35

Boxenbaum, H.G., Reigelman, S. and Elashoff, R.M. (1974) Statistical estimations in pharmacokinetics. *Journal of Pharmacokinetics and Biopharmaceutics* 2, 123

Chilcoat, R.T., Lunn, J.N. and Mapleson, W.W. (1984) Computer assistance in the control of anaesthesia. *British Journal of Anaesthesia* 56, 1417

Eger, E.I. (1980) Inhalational anaesthesia: pharmacokinetics. In: *General Anaesthesia*, vol. 1, 4th edn. (Eds. Gray, T.C., Nunn, J.F. and Utting, J.E.). Butterworths: London

Hull, C.J. (1979) Symbols for compartmental models (Editorial). *British Journal of Anaesthesia* 51, 815

Hull, C.J. (1983) General principles of pharmacokinetics. In: *The Pharmacokinetics of Anaesthesia*. (Eds. Prys-Roberts, C. and Hug, C.C.). Blackwell Scientific: Oxford

Orme, M. (1984) Drug absorption in the gut. *British Journal of Anaesthesia* 56, 59

Rowland, M. (1978) Drug administration and regimens. In: *Clinical Pharmacology: basic principles in therapeutics* (Eds. Melmon, K.L. and Morelli, H.F.). Macmillan: New York

Stanski, D.R., Mihm, F.G., Rosenthal, M.H. *et al.* (1980) Pharmacokinetics of high-dose thiopental used for cerebral resuscitation. *Anesthesiology* 53, 169

Wilkinson, G.R. and Shand, D.G. (1975) A physiological approach to hepatic drug clearance. *Clinical Pharmacology and Therapeutics* 18, 377

Further reading

Gibaldi, M. and Perrier, D. (1975) *Pharmacokinetics*. New York: Marcel Dekker

Prys-Roberts, C. and Hug, C.C. (1983) *The Pharmacokinetics of Anaesthesia*. Blackwell Scientific: Oxford

Stanski, D.R. and Watkins, W.D. (1982) *Drug Disposition in Anesthesia*. Grune & Stratton: New York

3
Transfer across membranes

Felicity Reynolds

The rate and extent of drug transfer across biological membranes depend on the nature of the membrane and also on the nature of the environment on either side of the membrane, as well as on the properties of the drug itself. There are three components to drug transfer:

1. The actual speed of passage of the drug across the membrane.
2. The ratio of the concentrations on either side of the membrane at equilibrium (which depends upon the relative affinity of the two environments for the drug).
3. The time taken to attain that equilibrium (this is determined by (1) and (2) and also by flow rates and compartment volumes on the two sides).

The nature of membranes

Most biological membranes are complex and consist of sheets of cells together with their basement membrane. The latter forms a microskeleton consisting of a network of mucopolysaccharides with some collagen fibres, and is generally freely permeable to water and solutes, although some types inhibit macromolecular passage. Since both intracellular and extracellular fluid are aqueous environments through which molecules can pass freely, the essence of any membranous barrier must reside in the cell membrane itself.

The cell membrane

A plasma membrane surrounds each cell and controls its internal environment. The membrane consists principally of phospholipid and protein. The lipid is arranged in two layers, with the long axes of the triglyceride molecules at right angles to the plane of the membrane. The phosphated glycerol end of each molecule is more hydrophilic and lies towards the inner (cytoplasmic) and outer surfaces, whilst the fatty acid chain which is lipophilic lies towards the centre of the membrane. Interspersed among the lipid are large coiled protein molecules, many of which extend right through the membrane from one surface to the other.

A lipid-soluble substance can diffuse across such a lipid membrane provided its molecular weight is less than 600–1000. Above 600, transfer is retarded, and above 1000 it virtually ceases. Molecular weights of most commonly used drugs fall well below this cut-off point. A hydrophilic molecule is always surrounded by a watery envelope, and its hydrated or hydrodynamic radius is considerably larger than the radius of the molecule itself. Water-soluble compounds which are non-ionized (uncharged) can cross lipid membranes, provided they are of molecular weight below 100. Larger water-soluble molecules, and all charged particles, cross lipid membranes extremely slowly, if at all, unless they can make use of special transport processes (see below, 'Modes of transfer'). Such transport processes are presumably mediated via the protein component of the cell membrane, which, it is assumed, also provides the small aqueous pores for the passage of uncharged hydrophilic particles. Certain membranes possess brush borders, and may carry out pinocytosis (see below), a means whereby macromolecules enter cells.

Complex membranes

Capillary endothelium
Certain complex membranes are functionally more porous than the plasma membrane, which never of itself contains gaps to allow macromolecules to pass passively into the cytoplasm. Thus the endothelium of certain capillaries contains fenestrae, which allow free passage of water and solutes up to a molecular weight of 10 000–70 000 (depending on shape and charge) or a hydrodynamic radius of about 3.5 nm, *through* the endothelium, rather than *into* the cells. Other capillaries appear to allow passage of such particles by a form of transendothelial pinocytosis. Sinusoidal capillaries possess gaps *between* endothelial cells, large enough to allow passage of the· formed elements of the blood.

Lipid membranes
Most familiar membrane systems function as lipid membranes (often incorrectly termed lipid *barriers*; they function as barriers only to *non*-lipids). They include: the blood–brain barrier, which is embodied in the non-porous capillaries supplying the central nervous system, mucous membranes and the gastrointestinal tract, the renal tubule, and the placenta.

The environment

The various environments that a drug may encounter during its sojourn in the body differ in their affinity for certain chemicals. Thus at equilibrium concentrations of drugs in different body compartments are not necessarily equal. Sources of variations in affinity derive from differences in pH and in lipid and protein content between compartments. These factors are considered below under 'Principles governing transfer'.

Gas-filled compartments: A volatile agent diffuses into any gaseous environment (the alveolus, the intestinal lumen, a pneumothorax, the middle ear, etc.) until it reaches equilibrium according to its blood/gas partition coefficient. This is of importance for nitrous oxide because of its high volatility

Table 3.1   Molecular weights

Lipophilic		Hydrophilic	
Bupivacaine	288	Alcuronium	666
Thiopentone	264	Suxamethonium	290
Halothane	197	Mannitol	182
Diamorphine	369	Morphine	285
Physostigmine	275	Neostigmine	223

and low blood solubility, and because it is given in high concentration.

Differences in affinity that various tissues may have for drugs affect the final equilibrium concentration ratio, a somewhat theoretical concept. The time taken to attain such an equilibrium will, of course, also depend upon the blood flow to the individual tissue. Resultant inequalities in drug concentration in two adjacent compartments can be misinterpreted as being due to a diffusion barrier or an active transport process.

Chemistry of drugs

Drugs that may be encountered by anaesthetists have various important chemical attributes. First, they have molecular weights usually in the hundreds (Table 3.1), allowing for easy lipid diffusion but not for aqueous diffusion (see above, under 'The cell membrane').

Lipid-soluble, non-polar compounds

Inhalational anaesthetics are all relatively small lipid-soluble molecules which diffuse rapidly across biological membranes. Because of their volatility they can be given by inhalation – the parenteral administration of *non*-volatile non-polar compounds presents problems precisely because of their non-solubility in water: Althesin and propanidid have both caused problems because they were solubilized with Cremophor, which has proved unsafe.

Nitrous oxide, the least lipophilic of the inhalational anaesthetics, possesses a molecule so small (mol. wt 44) that diffusion presents no problems.

Weak electrolytes

Many agents are weak acids or weak bases which are partially ionized in aqueous solution. The ionized form is solely water soluble (ions can only *exist* in an aqueous medium), whilst the non-ionized form is variably lipid soluble and can therefore diffuse across lipid membranes.

Acid

Barbiturates are weak acids that are all around 50 per cent ionized at physiological pH, and of course become more ionized and water soluble in an alkaline medium. Hence their sodium salts are water soluble. The non-ionized forms vary in lipid solubility from the hydrophilic phenobarbitone on one hand, to the highly lipophilic thiopentone on the other. *Penicillins* and *salicylates* are examples of stronger (more highly ionized) acids with pK_a values of 2.5 and 3, respectively. Most penicillins diffuse only slowly across lipid membranes, whilst salicylates diffuse more readily, even though only a small proportion is non-ionized.

Bases

Weak bases in organic chemistry commonly take the form of amines, or piperidine or piperazine derivatives; this very large group includes opioid analgesics, local anaesthetics, phenothiazine derivatives, antimuscarinics, antihistamines and antidepressants. Such compounds are soluble in an acidic medium and are therefore commonly administered as acid salts (hydrochloride, sulphate, etc.) but at body pH are able to diffuse across lipid membranes in the non-ionized state. Although benzodiazepines are also bases, some, such as diazepam, are so weakly basic (pK_a 3) that they are insoluble in water at a pH which could safely be administered, and therefore require solubilization.

Polar compounds

Some compounds are lipid insoluble even though non-ionized; for example, peptide hormones (oxytocin, vasopressin, insulin, ACTH, etc.), mannitol (an alcohol), sugars and dextrans. The molecular weights of these substances are too high for simple aqueous diffusion across lipid membranes. Others, such as quaternary ammonium compounds, are fully ionized irrespective of the pH of the medium. All these compounds are completely hydrophilic, and can therefore cross lipid membranes only very slowly, if at all, unless a special transport process is available. With the exception of the higher molecular weight dextrans, they can, however, pass through capillary pores, and therefore the distribution of such polar foreign compounds tends to be limited to the *extracellular space*.

Modes of transfer

Most drugs cross most membranes by diffusion, and much of this chapter concerns drug diffusion. However, there are other modes of transfer which must be considered.

Filtration

A semipermeable membrane allows passage of solute depending on pore size and particle diameter. The rate of transfer of solute depends in part on hydrostatic pressure and also in part on concentration gradient. Fenestrated capillaries allow filtration of solute in this way.

The glomerulus filters huge volumes of water together with all the solutes in plasma up to a molecular weight close to that of albumin, at a rate very largely dependent upon hydrostatic pressure.

Bulk flow

Bulk flow permits passage of water and solutes, quite irrespective of concentration gradient and molecular size. Arachnoid villi contain valves which open under hydrostatic pressure to allow passage of unmodified cerebrospinal fluid into the venous sinuses. Sinusoids in liver, spleen and bone marrow possess no basement membrane, and have intercellular gaps which allow bulk flow of fluid, solutes and cellular elements. Lymphatic channels and venules do the same. Thus all types of drugs in aqueous solution *enter* the circulation easily if administered parenterally.

Facilitated diffusion

This is a system whereby water-soluble molecules such as sugars are selectively transported across lipid membranes down a concentration gradient, but at a rate more rapid than simple diffusion would allow. The process is selective for biologically desirable optical isomers such as D-glucose, and is presumed to involve a carrier mechanism, but consumes no energy.

Active transport

This type of process consumes energy and enables the transfer across membranes against a concentration gradient of essential requirements and waste products. Examples in nature are the transport of essential amino acids across the blood–brain barrier (Davson, 1976) and the placenta (Young, 1979), iodine uptake in the thyroid, catecholamine uptake, and the secretion of H^+ and urate in the renal tubule. Some drugs may 'hitch a lift' on active transport mechanisms; for example, adrenergic neurone-blocking drugs use the noradrenaline uptake process, and penicillins and other acidic drugs use the urate secretory mechanism.

Vesicular transport

Certain membranes possess brush borders which can engulf droplets and macromolecules. This they do by forming invaginations which become vesicles within the cell cytoplasm. This is termed *pinocytosis*. It is not an arbitrary process, as it involves the initial concentration of desirable material such as protein on the cell surface, which is then engulfed to form a vesicle. This is similar to the means whereby the amoeba obtains its nutrition, forming a vacuole which gradually shrinks within the cytoplasm as the material within it is assimilated (*endocytosis*).

In capillary endothelium, however, such vesicles may be visible which do not appear to shrink, but rather provide a vehicle for transport of material across the thickness of the flattened cell.

Exocytosis, the reverse of pinocytosis, is the process by which the contents of storage vesicles are extruded from cells, the vesicular membrane first becoming fused with the cell membrane and then continuous with it. By this means neurotransmitters and histamine are released.

Diffusion

Diffusion is far the most important means whereby drugs cross membranes. It is a passive process taking place only down a concentration gradient and consuming no energy.

Principles governing transfer

Diffusion rate

The term 'diffusion' means a spreading abroad, and implies the spreading out of a substance in all directions until the concentrations are equal throughout the environment. Diffusion across membranes implies transfer down a concentration gradient, or, in the case of a gas, down a pressure gradient.

Rate of diffusion, physically speaking, should really refer to the speed of passage through a medium in terms of velocity, or *distance* over *time*. In practice, however, passage across a membrane, whose thickness is small in relation to area, is more usefully considered in terms of *mass transferred per unit area*, over *time*.

Classically, the rate of diffusion of drugs across membranes has been expressed in the following equation:

$$\text{Rate of diffusion} = \frac{KA\,(C_1 - C_2)}{X}$$

where C_1 and C_2 are the concentrations on either side of the membrane, A is the area and X the thickness of the membrane, and K is the diffusion constant of the drug, which is said to be related to its molecular diameter, degree of ionization and lipid solubility. This classic equation requires modification before it can be applied to biological situations, for the following reasons.

1. Taking total concentrations on either side of the membrane ignores the effect of protein binding and other factors which may affect the partition coefficient of the drug across the membrane and the size of the *diffusible* fraction.
2. The equation yields an expression involving the product of *area* and *gradient* per unit of membrane thickness. Hence the concentration must be taken as that per unit volume of membrane, in which case the equation can be further simplified to $K \times$ mass per unit area. Although this is near our original concept, time is completely missing from the right-hand side of the equation. Molecular size and lipid solubility do not affect diffusion in a linearly related manner, as is explained below.
3. The degree of ionization is far from constant, but is dependent upon whether the agent is an acid or a base, and, if so, how strong, and upon the pH of the aqueous media on either side of the membrane.

In practice, area available for transfer will certainly affect the initial rate of transfer of drug across membrane, while for a freely diffusible substance the effect of membrane thickness will be principally to delay arrival rather than to retard transfer. For such a drug it is the *flow* (in other words, blood supply) which is the more important determinant of diffusion rate. This, too, is missing from the equation. Thus the equation above would be inappropriate to apply to drugs.

Molecular size

Graded permeability is apparent only over a comparatively narrow range of molecular weights, and hence molecular size essentially operates a cut-off point in membrane transfer.

Among *hydrophilic* non-ionized compounds, urea, of molecular weight 60, diffuses slowly across lipid membranes, while compounds of molecular weight greater than 100, such as mannitol (see Table 3.1) diffuse not at all (see also the sections 'The central nervous system' and 'The kidney'). No ionized particles can diffuse passively across lipid membranes.

Among *lipophilic* compounds the cut-off for transfer across lipid membranes is at molecular weights between 600 and 1000. Most drugs possess molecular weights below 1000 (see Table 3.1). Digoxin is an example of a drug which, having a molecular weight of 781, is somewhat slow in its membrane transfer.

Porous membranes present no barrier to transfer of drugs, whether hydrophilic or lipophilic, as they permit filtration and even bulk flow as well as diffusion; therefore a cut-off point exists only for macromolecules. Across a capillary membrane such as the glomerulus, dextrans are filtered freely up to a molecular radius of 1.8–2.0 nm whilst above 4.0 nm they are virtually barred (Bohrer *et al.*, 1978). This range coincides with molecular weights of 10 000–30 000. Ionization affects permeability of these molecules over a similar range of molecular sizes (see later, under 'The kidney').

Proteins behave in a similar manner. Thus inulin, on the one hand, is freely permeable and is cleared at the glomerular filtration rate, while plasma proteins are at or beyond the filtrable size. Albumin, for example, has a molecular radius of about 3.5 nm.

The protein-bound fraction of a drug cannot diffuse across membranes, but acts as a readily available store with which to replenish the free fraction as that diffuses away.

Lipid solubility

The term 'lipid solubility' is used here, according to popular though incorrect practice, to mean lipid/buffer partition coefficient.

Like molecular weight, lipophilicity exerts a largely all-or-none effect, and, so far as drug diffusion is concerned, is the much more important factor. Thus in Table 3.1 the drugs in the left-hand column, though (with the exception of halothane) partly ionized, are all of sufficient lipid solubility to equilibrate readily across lipid membranes. Suxamethonium and alcuronium, chosen as possessing the smallest and the largest molecules among neuromuscular blocking drugs in current use, are both barred from lipid diffusion, being quaternary ammonium compounds. Mannitol, though non-ionized and small, is still non-diffusible because of its lipid insolubility.

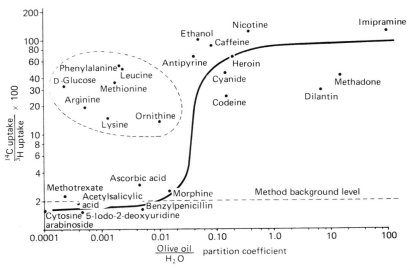

Fig. 3.1 Relationship between percentage clearance of radiolabelled drug (compared with that of water) and oil/buffer partition coefficient. The encircled points which do not show the expected relationship between lipid solubility and penetration, relate to amino acids for which active transport is available, and D-glucose for which there is a carrier mechanism. (Reproduced from Oldendorf, 1974a, by kind permission of the author and publishers.)

Diamorphine, though possessing a larger molecule than morphine (Table 3.1), is much more diffusible because of its enhanced lipid solubility. It can therefore equilibrate across the blood–brain barrier in a single circulation, whereas morphine cannot (Fig. 3.1).

Morphine, being a piperidine derivative, is a base, which should not therefore be compulsorily hydrophilic. However, it also possesses two hydroxyl groups, which are weakly *acidic*. It is therefore difficult to find, among an average population of morphine molecules, any that are wholly non-ionized. It is these two hydroxyl groups which are acetylated in the diamorphine molecule (Fig. 3.2), thereby negating their ionizing tendencies and enhancing its lipophilicity.

Physostigmine, although a larger molecule than neostigmine (see Table 3.1) is a tertiary amine and therefore lipid soluble and diffusible while neostigmine, a quaternary ammonium compound, is poorly absorbed by mouth and does not enter the central nervous system.

The all-or-none effect of lipid solubility is well shown in studies by Oldendorf (1974a) (see Fig. 3.1), and is exemplified in the behaviour of barbiturates. The *bolus effect* of thiopentone (i.e. the ability to produce sleep in one arm–brain circulation time which is rapidly reversed by drug redistribution) is familiar to anaesthetists. The same phenomenon is not seen with the less lipophilic barbiturates, which induce sleep rapidly only if given in massive doses, whose duration of action would be prolonged. This contrast was well demonstrated in rats by Goldstein and Aronow (1960) (Fig. 3.3).

Drugs which can equilibrate across a membrane in a single passage can be

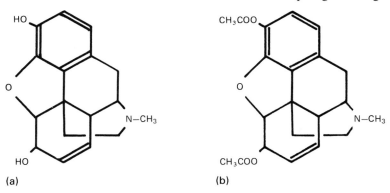

Fig. 3.2 Structural formulae of (a) morphine and (b) diamorphine.

expected to be flow-dependent in their transfer rates. Thus uptake of anaesthetics across the alveolar membrane is dependent upon ventilation and blood flow; transfer of pethidine across the placenta is dependent upon umbilical blood flow. Such circulation preserves the gradient for diffusion.

Lipid solubility not only affects the ability of a drug to cross a membrane by lipid diffusion; it also influences the equilibrium distribution. Intracellular and membrane lipid components concentrate highly lipid-soluble substances such as halothane. Highly lipophilic local anaesthetics tend to have a prolonged local effect because they are taken up into axonal membrane lipid, rather than remaining in the aqueous phase to be absorbed systemically via capillaries and lymphatics.

Gradient

Diffusible gradient differs from concentration gradient because of ionization and protein binding. Gradient is also affected by supply (usually flow) on the

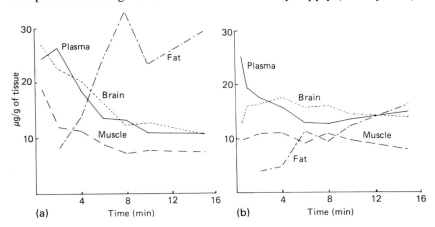

Fig. 3.3 Tissue concentration of (a) thiopentone and (b) pentobarbitone after intravenous injection of 15 mg/kg to male rats. Each point represents the mean value for four rats. (Data of Goldstein and Aronow, 1960, by kind permission of the authors.)

up side of the membrane, and compartment size or flow rate on the down side. In a closed system a gradient is time dependent and will ultimately disappear.

Ionization

Weak acids become more ionized the more alkaline the medium in which they find themselves, while weak bases are more ionized in an acid medium (both behave as buffers). Only the non-ionized portion is readily diffusible across lipid membranes. It is therefore this portion which exerts a gradient for diffusion, which ceases once the non-ionized fraction is equal on the two sides of a membrane.

The degree of ionization of a particular drug is a function of its pK and the pH of the environment. While this may have a small effect on the rate of membrane transfer, it has a much more important effect on the final distribution of that agent. For example, it is often supposed that the more ionized a drug, the less it will enter cells; while this may be so for acidic drugs, the reverse is true for bases. According to the principle of non-ionic diffusion, using the Henderson–Hasselbalch equation, one may calculate the relative concentrations of a basic drug in solution in intracellular and extracellular water. For this purpose one needs to know not only their pH values but also the pK_a of the drug – that is, the logarithm$_{10}$ of the reciprocal of its acid dissociation constant. Thus, for an intracellular environment at a pH of 7.2, and a weak base with a pK_a of 7.6 (e.g. diamorphine):

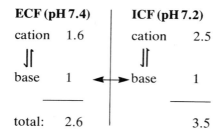

ECF (pH 7.4)		**ICF (pH 7.2)**	
cation	1.6	cation	2.5
base	1	base	1
total:	2.6		3.5

∴ ICF/ECF ratio = 1.35

Now for a *stronger* base, that is one with a higher pK_a, (say chlorpromazine, 9.3), this concentration ratio is a little higher.

ECF (pH 7.4)		**ICF (pH 7.2)**	
cation	79	cation	126
base	1	base	1
total:	80		127

∴ ICF/ECF ratio = 1.6

This ratio also becomes higher the greater the pH disparity. Thus bases, even when given parenterally, are concentrated in the intragastric lumen. Take fentanyl, pK_a 8.4:

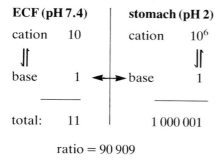

ECF (pH 7.4)		stomach (pH 2)	
cation	10	cation	10^6
base	1	base	1
total:	11		1 000 001

ratio = 90 909

Thus, were the entire cardiac output to be shunted through the gastric mucosa, basic drugs would all finish up in the stomach. This is known as the ion-trapping effect.

By contrast, acidic drugs in free solution tend to be more concentrated in the plasma than in cells, although the difference is less for weak acids such as barbiturates (e.g. thiopentone, pK_a 7.6):

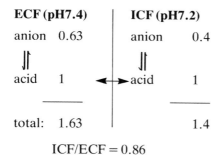

ECF (pH7.4)		ICF (pH7.2)	
anion	0.63	anion	0.4
acid	1	acid	1
total:	1.63		1.4

ICF/ECF = 0.86

that it is for stronger acids such as phenylbutazone (pK_a 4.5):

anion	795	anion	501
acid	1	acid	1
total:	796		502

ICF/ECF = 0.63

Again, for a small pH gradient the disparity in free concentration is not great. But taking the example of the stomach, acidic drugs will not be secreted into the stomach as will basic drugs, whereas they can be absorbed from it (see later, 'Gastrointestinal tract').

The pH of the renal tubular fluid is usually low, although variable, and will therefore strongly influence the excretion of weak acids and bases (see later, 'The kidney').

Protein binding

Plasma protein binding not only reduces the diffusible gradient of a strongly bound drug; it also alters the equilibrium distribution ratio.

Acidic drugs are bound to plasma albumin, which is of high capacity but variable affinity. Phenylbutazone, which possesses high affinity binding, tends to replace other acidic drugs by competition. This interaction is not usually of great clinical importance for drugs used chronically since the result is normally an increased tissue uptake and clearance of the raised free fraction. It is important, however, with warfarin, whose tissue uptake is not great, and may also be important with thiopentone, whose effect *depends* upon the transient uptake by the brain of the free fraction.

Many basic drugs (pethidine, local anaesthetics) are bound to α_1-acid glycoprotein, at much higher affinity than to albumin. The total binding capacity of the former small fraction is less than that of albumin but it is still the more important within the therapeutic range of drug concentration. The disparity in concentrations of these two protein fractions in mother and in baby is the principal cause of distributional inequalities across the placenta (see later, 'Placental transfer').

Open and closed systems: flow rates and compartment volumes

In an *open* system, so-called 'sink conditions' may pertain, and a gradient persists until the drug has completely disappeared from the up side.

Sink conditions are found in the kidney, in which the tubular fluid ultimately becomes urine and is voided to the exterior. They also operate across the blood–CSF barrier for hydrophilic drugs (see below, 'The central nervous system'), and virtually also into the stomach for basic drugs because of the ion-trapping effect (see above, 'Ionization').

In a *closed* system, a compartment of finite size gradually becomes saturated with drug, until the gradient is obliterated. Equilibration-time depends upon the relationship between the capacity of the compartment (the product of volume and affinity for the drug) and its blood supply. Thus inhalational anaesthetics, for example, equilibrate quickly into the vessel-rich group of tissues, for which their affinity is similar to that for blood, but they only slowly saturate adipose tissue, since its affinity is high but its blood supply poor. The same phenomenon is apparent for lipophilic non-volatile agents such as thiopentone (Fig. 3.3).

When a drug is administered chronically at a steady rate, the time taken for the plasma concentration to plateau is dependent upon the elimination rate of the drug, and is 93 per cent complete at four half-lives and 99 per cent at seven half-lives.

Table 3.2   Distribution volumes (V_D) of a range of drugs

	V_D (l/kg)
Nortriptyline	22.1
Lignocaine	1.5
Thiopentone	1.2
Tubocurarine	0.14

Tissue distribution

Ultimate tissue distribution at equilibrium is the resultant of all the factors which produce distributional inequalities: ion trapping, protein binding and lipid solubility. Thus thiopentone, for example, is a protein-bound acidic drug; one would therefore expect its plasma concentration to be higher than intracellular concentration, and consequently the distribution volume to be small. Yet because it is taken up in lipid and probably bound to tissue protein as well, the tissue concentration is higher than the plasma and its distribution volume is greater than total body water (Table 3.2). Highly lipid-soluble *basic* drugs such as chlorpromazine and tricyclic antidepressants, however, have distribution volumes considerably larger than those of acidic compounds whereas a less lipid-soluble base such as lignocaine is intermediate. Lipid-insoluble compounds are limited in their distribution to the extracellular fluid, hence their distribution volumes are proportionally small (Table 3.2).

The penetration of drugs to individual tissues depends upon the type of capillary supplying each tissue. A description of capillary histology and permeability, and how these may determine drug penetration, has been given elsewhere (Reynolds, 1980).

The lung

The lung presents an enormous surface area for the uptake and elimination of volatile agents. The alveolar membrane and capillary endothelium together present a very thin membranous diffusion barrier, which is freely permeable to respiratory gases and inhalational anaesthetics. Lung capillary endothelium possesses tight junctions (the borders of the cells are continuously welded together) and no fenestrae, while pinocytotic vesicles are rare. It is therefore ready-made for rapid diffusion of gases and lipid-soluble drugs, but proteins, other macromolecules and copious amounts of water do not, in normal circumstances, pass out into the interstitial fluid or alveolar spaces.

Despite the relatively small amount of solid tissue it contains, the lung does, of course, possess a massive blood supply (the cardiac output), and is an important repository for many lipid-soluble drugs. For example, an initial bolus of lignocaine is much attenuated after passage through the pulmonary circulation. This step is therefore of value in reducing the acute toxicity of an intravenous injection.

Mucous membranes

Mucous membranes of the upper air passages and gastrointestinal tract behave as lipid membranes across which lipid-soluble drugs pass readily. Mucous membranes of nose and mouth can provide access for such drugs to the systemic circulation, bypassing the portal system.

Drugs are usually applied to the nose for their local effects (nasal decongestants, local anaesthetics, etc.), but vasopressin, for example, may be taken as snuff and, being a lipid-insoluble peptide hormone, it is absorbed only very slowly. Were it to be swallowed, however, it would be broken down by peptidases in the gastrointestinal tract.

Certain drugs are taken sublingually or in the buccal cavity. Glyceryl trinitrate has been used by this route for many decades. Its rapid onset of action may be further accelerated by prior chewing. If swallowed, high first-pass clearance renders it useless. Buprenorphine, on the other hand, achieves a sustained effect of slow onset when taken sublingually, but if swallowed it, too, is prey to high first-pass clearance. Oxytocin, another hydrophilic peptide hormone, has also been given bucally for a slow sustained effect.

Local anaesthetics with adequate lipid solubility (all except procaine) produce good analgesia when applied to mucous surfaces, but they are also, with the exception of cocaine, rapidly absorbed into the circulation by this route. Cocaine is only slowly absorbed because it is a powerful vasoconstrictor.

Gastrointestinal tract

Drugs that are swallowed may be destroyed by gastric acid (penicillin), broken down enzymatically (peptide hormones), conjugated in the gut wall (morphine), or broken down in the liver (almost everything). Lipid-insoluble drugs such as quaternary ammonium compounds, aminoglycoside antibiotics, etc. are not absorbed passively, although some such as the orally active penicillins, amino acids such as levodopa, antimetabolites and so on may be actively transported. Some poorly absorbed drugs are therefore used for their local effects – for example, morphine in the management of diarrhoea, aminoglycosides to sterilize the bowel and antacids for dyspepsia. Equally, flesh from animals killed by curare is perfectly safe to eat (else the use of poisoned arrows would never have caught on!)

Weak bases become highly ionized in the acid gastric lumen, and cannot therefore be absorbed until they pass into the higher pH of the small intestine. Their onset of action is therefore very slow when stomach emptying is delayed. Moreover, when administered parenterally they are secreted into the stomach (see p. 73). Gastric lavage is therefore useful following overdose of basic drugs even if taken parenterally or swallowed many hours previously.

Weak acids are poorly ionized in the stomach. Thus aspirin, for example, which is a fairly strong acid, is highly ionized everywhere throughout the body *except* in the stomach. It *can* be absorbed in the stomach, although when it encounters the higher pH in the mucosal cells, it becomes highly ionized and therefore trapped. This is a factor in the production of gastric erosion by aspirin and all the non-steroidal anti-inflammatory drugs (NSAIDs). Because of the increase in surface area of the small intestine, acids as well as bases are absorbed more rapidly here than in the stomach.

Skeletal muscle

Muscle capillaries, histologically, are continuous capillaries with tight junctions and cytoplasmic vesicles although, functionally, they appear to possess large and small pores. Thus larger dextrans and albumin diffuse slowly out of limb vessels, whilst small hydrophilic solutes such as sucrose (Renkin and Garlick, 1970) and neuromuscular blocking drugs apparently pass rapidly into the muscle extracellular fluid. This may be through cytoplasmic vesicles, which, though they could theoretically constitute large pores, do not often appear to reach the contraluminal surface of capillary endothelium, and might not be very speedy. Intercellular clefts are hard to visualize histologically but might constitute small pores.

Hydrophilic drugs given by intramuscular injection gain ready access to the systemic circulation from the aqueous extracellular environment. This they do by way of either venules or lymphatic channels, both of which are sinusoidal, with large intercellular clefts. Thus any agent which is freely water soluble is well absorbed following intramuscular or indeed any form of parenteral injection. This applies to both weak acids and bases and to quaternary fully ionized compounds. Lipid-soluble compounds which are water *in*soluble are, by contrast, very *un*reliably absorbed following intramuscular injection. Diazepam, for example, is never given by this route; the anticonvulsant phenytoin is very poorly absorbed and actually precipitates out in muscle. Various agents may be administered intramuscularly in an oily base to prolong their effects; for example, hormone replacements such as vasopressin which cannot be taken by mouth.

The central nervous system (Davson, 1976; Oldendorf, 1974a, b, 1976)

Contrary to earlier belief, the brain *does* contain extracellular fluid, although after death it may be largely taken up by swelling brain cells. The extracellular fluid is in free communication with the cerebrospinal fluid, which acts as the lymphatic drainage of the brain.

The blood–brain barrier is, like any lipid membrane, a barrier to non-lipids. This barrier resides in the endothelium of the capillaries supplying the brain, and is therefore between the blood and the extracellular fluid. Brain capillaries are continuous, with tight junctions, no fenestrae and few if any pinocytotic vesicles, and are therefore impenetrable to macromolecules and lipid-insoluble drugs, everywhere except the area postrema, the median eminence and the pineal body. Metastases of solid tumours also acquire an abnormal vasculature with freely permeable capillaries.

The blood–CSF barrier, although structurally and functionally different from the blood–brain barrier, also shows the selective permeability characteristic of a lipid membrane. Capillaries of the choroid are fenestrated, for filtration of fluid into the space between capillary endothelium and the ependymal epithelium lining the ventricles, in the first step in CSF production. The ependymal cells which cover the choroid surface are sealed laterally by tight junctions; they restrict filtration and perform active transport, in the final modification of the CSF. Thus protein and hydrophilic molecules pass readily out of choroid capillaries into the perivascular connective tissue, but enter the

CSF only slowly. From here they are actively taken up again by the choroid plexus, thus giving an impression of greater barrier impermeability than actually exists.

Elsewhere the pia and ependyma are more permeable because adjacent epithelial cells do not possess occlusive tight junctions, but allow free communication between brain extracellular fluid and CSF, even for macromolecules. The CSF drains into venous sinuses via arachnoid granulations which possess valves opening under pressure and having a pore size greater than 10 nm. Water and all solutes irrespective of molecular size and charge can therefore pass out of the CSF into the venous system. This system provides a sink for hydrophilic substances, which pass slowly into brain and CSF but quickly out. Equilibrium between plasma and brain is therefore never attained for water-soluble molecules or ions. Similarly, metabolites may be rapidly cleared from brain via CSF.

Although drugs which diffuse slowly from blood to brain and CSF gain ready access to the brain if injected into the CSF, in the normal course of events any solute in plasma will tend to pass into brain and CSF at similar rates rather than passing first to one then to the other.

Drug transfer across the blood–brain barrier has generally been studied using the single-shot technique of Oldendorf. In this method the uptake of radiolabelled drug is compared with that of tritiated water. This examines rate of transfer but ignores steady state distribution ratios, which, if far from unity, can distort the results of rate studies.

Rate of transfer is principally dependent upon lipid solubility. Oldendorf and colleagues (1972) found that whereas uptake of morphine by brain was undetectable in a single circulation, that of diamorphine was 68 per cent (Fig. 3.1), and codeine and methadone were intermediate. Uptake by brain of ethanol, nicotine, caffeine and antipyrine was virtually complete, whilst that of many cytotoxic drugs was negligible (Oldendorf, 1974a, b, 1976) (see Fig. 3.1). Thus cerebral extension of leukaemias must be prevented by intrathecal administration of methotrexate, for example. Among barbiturates, thiopentone equilibrates between blood and brain in a single circulation, whereas less soluble members do not (Fig. 3.3).

Mannitol cannot pass from blood into brain extracellular fluid; it can therefore reduce intracranial pressure by exerting an osmotic effect across the blood–brain barrier. This is in contrast to other tissues where it can pass into the extracellular space, and serves to expand this at the expense of intracellular water. Neurotransmitters do not cross cerebral capillaries and, moreover, tend to be broken down by the endothelial cells. The management of Parkinsonism by levodopa makes use of the selective permeability of the blood–brain barrier. Dopamine, which is deficient, does not cross the blood–brain barrier, whereas its amino acid precursor, L-dopa, is actively transported, and taken up by dopaminergic neurones. The peripheral side effects of levodopa are treated by preventing its conversion to dopamine in the periphery, using a dopa-decarboxylase inhibitor which does not cross the blood–brain barrier. The side effects of nausea and vomiting are also reduced by the decarboxylase inhibitor because it can gain access to the chemoreceptor trigger zone in the area postrema whose capillaries possess increased permeability.

Increased blood–brain barrier permeability has been reported in a number of situations; for example, hypertension, seizures (Bolwig, Hertz and Westergard, 1977) (possibly because of associated hypertension), vasodilatation accompanying halothane anaesthesia (Forster *et al.*, 1977) and hyperosmolarity (Rapoport, Hori and Klatzo, 1971). It has been suggested that a common mechanism for increasing permeability in these conditions might be the splitting open of tight junctions. However, an increase in pinocytosis has been observed in such circumstances, and is a more plausible explanation.

Plasma protein binding
This affects steady state concentrations, and CSF/plasma ratios are generally equivalent to the plasma free fraction, as is the case with the highly bound anticonvulsant phenytoin. Uptake by lipids and tissue protein in brain, however, tends to counteract the effect of plasma protein binding at equilibrium (Houghton *et al.*, 1975).

Protein binding also alters the gradient for diffusion; hence the more marked effect of thiopentone in individuals in whom albumin binding is reduced. Drug binding interactions can also affect brain/plasma ratios (Green and Kitchen, 1975).

Plasma protein binding of certain basic drugs may be low in the neonate, in whom the binding protein α_1-acid glycoprotein is deficient (Krauer, Dayer and Anner, 1984). Brain/plasma concentration ratios for such drugs would therefore be expected to be higher in the neonate than in the adult, as has been found for methadone (Peters, 1975), although such findings are commonly attributed to a deficiency in the blood–brain barrier in the newborn. There is no blood–brain barrier, in neonate *or* adult, for such lipid-soluble drugs.

pH changes
Changes in pH in the arterial blood are much attenuated in brain ECF and CSF by efficient buffering. Thus a decrease in ionization of weak bases, such as narcotics, in alkalosis (Kaufman, Kofki and Benson, 1977; Schulman *et al.*, 1984) and of weak acids such as barbiturates or salicylates, in hypoventilation, will result in an increased brain/plasma ratio, and vice versa. Changes in $P\text{CO}_2$ alter the uptake and clearance of all drugs which equilibrate rapidly between blood and brain, not only because of acid–base changes, but also because of the effect of carbon dioxide on cerebral *blood flow*. Thus in the days of ether anaesthesia, carbon dioxide was administered during induction, not only to stimulate respiration but also because the resulting cerebral vasodilation accelerated brain uptake of ether. By contrast, hyperventilation, causing cerebral vasoconstriction, will slow equilibrium of readily diffusible agents.

The kidney

The glomerular capillaries are fenestrated but possess a dense basement membrane. They allow passage by filtration and bulk flow of water and all solutes up to a molecular radius of 2.0–4.0 nm (Fig. 3.4). This range coincides with a molecular weight for *dextrans* of 10 000–30 000, but for proteins the relationship is not the same. Thus albumin, molecular weight 68 000, has an effective radius of 3.5 nm. This impermeability to macromolecules would

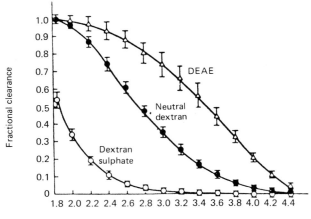

Fig. 3.4 Clearance of neutral dextran, polyanionic dextran (dextran sulphate) and polycationic dextran (DEAE) in rats, plotted as a function of effective molecular radius. Clearance is expressed as a percentage of inulin clearance. (Reproduced from Bohrer *et al.* (1978) by kind permision of Professor Channing R. Robertson and of the publishers.)

appear to derive from the basement membrane, since fenestrae have a diameter far in excess of this cut-off point, and the epithelium covering the glomerular tuft is equally permeable (Renkin, 1970). Small amounts of albumin *are* filtered in the glomerulus, but are actively taken up again by the cells of the proximal tubule.

All drugs, therefore, are filtered in the glomerulus, except for that portion which is protein bound. Protein binding, however, has less effect on renal clearance than might be supposed, since binding is freely reversible and because of the prolonged contact between blood and tubular fluid along the length of the nephron. Thus any free drug which passes from plasma to tubular lumen can be replaced from the bound store.

Following glomerular filtration, more than 99 per cent of the filtered water is reabsorbed in the course of urine production. Tubular cells are bound laterally by tight junctions, and therefore, apart from their active functions, behave as a lipid membrane for diffusion purposes. Peritubular capillaries are fenestrated and highly permeable, for the reabsorption of large volumes of water and solute (Schnermann, 1975). Any drug that is lipid soluble is therefore reabsorbed along with the water. The reabsorption of weak acids such as barbiturates or salicylate may be inhibited by rendering the tubular fluid alkaline and so increasing the ionization of the drug. The administration of sodium bicarbonate therefore not only reverses the metabolic acidosis encountered in salicylate overdose, it also accelerates excretion (Fig. 3.5). To promote the excretion of basic drugs, ammonium chloride can be used to acidify the urine, but this is rarely indicated. Most basic drugs, being extensively taken up in tissues, are excreted unchanged only to a minute degree. They are in the main converted into more polar compounds to reduce their distribution volume and enhance renal excretion. Examples of exceptions

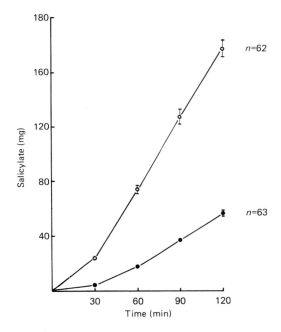

Fig. 3.5 Cumulative excretion of salicylate in 125 medical students after 856 mg orally (1 g of sodium salicylate). One group (○) received sodium bicarbonate, 10 g at −60 minutes, and the other (●) ammonium chloride 7 g. Vertical bars represent standard errors. (Republished from Reynolds, 1980, by kind permission of the publishers.)

to this general rule are amphetamine, and also procainamide, of which about 50 per cent may be excreted unchanged.

Polar compounds are filtered in the glomerulus and not reabsorbed in the renal tubule. Thus creatinine, inulin and mannitol are cleared by the kidney at the glomerular filtration rate. Mannitol alone acts as an osmotic diuretic because its molecule is so small (mol. wt 182), yet sufficiently above the 100 cut-off point to prevent any back-diffusion. Fully ionized drugs such as quaternary ammonium compounds are excreted equally rapidly.

Certain drugs, particularly acids, are actively secreted in the tubule, hitching a lift on the uric acid transport process. Thus penicillins are excreted at a rate approaching renal plasma flow. Thiazide and loop diuretics also compete for the uric acid secretory process, and in doing so tend to inhibit uric acid excretion. Aspirin may do the same, though in larger doses it also inhibits the much larger but less sensitive component, the uric acid reabsorption process, so acting as a uricosuric.

Placental transfer

The placenta in late gestation in the human is classified as haemomonochorial – that is, maternal blood is in direct contact with a single layer of fetal chorion, the syncytiotrophoblast. The layer beneath, the cytotrophoblast, exists at term only as isolated cells rather than a continuum. The placenta possesses numerous branching villi, each with a core of chorionic connective tissue in which lie fetal capillaries. As term approaches, the connective tissue becomes increasingly sparse, and fetal blood vessels tend to fill the villi. Syncytiotrophoblast overlying fetal capillaries becomes very thin and the two layers fuse to form vasculoyncytial membranes, areas well suited for rapid transfer of diffusible particles such as respiratory gases. The membrane which separates maternal from fetal blood is therefore thin at term and consists only of syncytiotrophoblast and fetal endothelium. Because of the syncytial nature of the chorion it is covered by a continuous lipid cell membrane, as is the case in all species. This therefore implies that lipid-soluble drugs will diffuse rapidly across the placenta, and purely water-soluble drugs will cross only slowly, following the rules for all lipid membranes. It is thus apparent that drugs which act quickly on the brain cross the placenta rapidly, whilst those which are confined in the body to the extracellular space cross the placenta only slowly.

The rate at which drugs cross the placenta is dependent upon both placental factors and drug characteristics. Placental factors are area available for maternal–fetal exchange and blood flow on either side of the placenta. Drug transfer across a given area of placenta is dependent upon its penetrative power and its *diffusible* concentration gradient. Drug characteristics which determine this are protein binding, lipid solubility and, to a small extent, ionization. All these factors interact, and time may also affect the gradient since it allows equilibration. The placenta offers no bar to diffusion of lipid-soluble drugs, which are therefore commonly said to be flow dependent in their transfer rate. The rate, however, is further modified by the equilibrium distribution, which is largely determined by protein binding, and also by ionization.

Protein binding
Since only unbound drug penetrates the placental membrane, high protein binding greatly reduces the diffusible gradient of drug. As there is often disparity in protein binding between fetus and mother, protein binding also affects equilibrium distribution. At term, albumin concentration may be higher in the fetus than in the mother, whilst α_1-acid glycoprotein is normally lower (Krauer, Dayer and Anner, 1984). Thus binding of acidic compounds and of diazepam is greater in fetus than mother, whereas that of basic drugs such as local anaesthetics and pethidine is higher in mother. The effect is that a highly bound drug such as bupivacaine not only crosses the placenta slowly but also never attains such a high concentration in fetal as in maternal plasma. The ultimate equilibrium ratio is dependent upon the glycoprotein gradient (Petersen *et al.*, 1981; Hamshaw-Thomas and Reynolds, 1985). The relationship between fetal/maternal ratio and protein binding is illustrated in Table 3.3. By contrast, diazepam, which is highly lipid soluble, poorly ionized and highly albumin bound (Nau *et al.*, 1983), rapidly attains higher concentrations in fetus than mother.

Ionization
Fetal plasma pH is lower than maternal, normally by about 0.1 of a pH unit. Thus ionization of free bases at equilibrium will be higher in fetus than mother, whilst the reverse is true of free acids. This effect is normally swamped with

Table 3.3   Factors affecting the placental transfer of some basic drugs

	F/M ratio	Maternal protein binding	Oleyl alcohol/ buffer partition coefficient
Bupivacaine	0.3	90	250
Lignocaine	0.55	75	29
Pethidine	1.0	50	18
Antipyrine	1.0	0	1.7

highly protein-bound drug by the effect of binding inequalities across the placenta. However, it has been shown that in the presence of fetal acidosis the fetal/maternal ratios of basic drugs such as lignocaine (O'Brien *et al.*, 1982) and bupivacaine (Kennedy *et al.*, 1979) are increased because of the ion-trapping effect (see p. 73). As one may assume that fetal acidosis is associated with a reduction in fetal flow, these findings emphasize the greater importance of equilibrium ratio than flow-dependent transfer rate in determining fetal dose.

Lipid solubility
This is of limited importance in that a drug of even the modest lipid solubility of pethidine penetrates the placenta so easily that it is largely flow dependent in its transfer rate (Hamshaw-Thomas, Rogerson and Reynolds, 1984). Thus greater lipophilicity can confer no greater penetrative powers (Table 3.3).

Purely *hydrophilic drugs* cross the placenta exceedingly slowly; thus fetal/maternal plasma concentration ratios of quaternary ammonium compounds and mannitol, for example, are low. Water-soluble drugs are, of course, rapidly excreted in the urine in the fetus as in the adult; thus sink conditions apply (see p. 74) and it is unlikely that materno–fetal equilibrium is ever attained. Although detectable levels of neuromuscular blocking drugs have been measured in umbilical venous blood, this is directly downstream of the placenta, and concentrations in fetal arterial blood do not rise sufficiently high to cause neuromuscular blockade following usual maternal doses. Paralysis has been detected in the neonate only following a maternal dose of tubocurarine of ten times normal (Older and Harris, 1968).

Placental factors
When considering the transfer of respiratory gases, the area available for materno–fetal exchange is all important, as the fetus is constantly consuming oxygen and manufacturing carbon dioxide. Such is not the case, however, with drugs, the more lipid soluble of which will ultimately tend to equilibrate across the placenta, and the efficiency of the placenta is therefore less crucial to drug than to respiratory gas exchange. However, the initial rate of transfer of freely diffusible drugs is dependent upon placental blood flow. In this respect umbilical flow is much more important than maternal or intervillous, flow, as umbilical flow is generally about half the intervillous flow, and maternal blood is normally very incompletely cleared of drug. An increase of umbilical relative to intervillous flow is therefore likely to be associated with an increase in the proportion of the intervillous flow that is cleared of drug (Hamshaw-Thomas, Rogerson and Reynolds, 1984; Vella, Knott and Reynolds, 1986). Highly lipid-

soluble drugs such as bupivacaine are therefore fetal-flow dependent in their transfer rates. By contrast, the less-lipid-soluble antipyrine (which is commonly used as a marker for the efficiency of materno–fetal exchange), not being bound to plasma protein, crosses the placenta more rapidly than bupivacaine in normal circumstances but is dependent on the adequacy of flow on both sides of the placenta (Wilkening *et al.*, 1982).

Materno–fetal equilibration

While umbilical venous drug concentration is an index of placental transfer, umbilical arterial concentration, taken in conjunction with umbilical venous or maternal levels, can give a measure of the extent of fetal equilibration. Thus while *lipid-soluble drugs* can probably approach equilibration across the placenta in a single circulation, they are, following transfer, taken up in fetal tissues and thus full equilibrium may take from about 40 minutes to a few hours. (Actual equilibrium fetal/maternal concentration ratios will be largely dependent upon protein binding either side of the membrane.) A drug such as thiopentone, which is given in a bolus to the mother, equilibrates across the placenta but does not put the baby to sleep because he represents a much deeper compartment than the maternal brain, and his brain is much more remote from maternal blood. With continuous administration, however, any lipid-soluble drugs will achieve active concentrations in the fetus. When maternal administration stops, lipid-soluble drugs and even slightly lipid-soluble metabolites cross the placenta back to the mother. The fetus, appropriately, does not produce more polar metabolites such as conjugates, in vast amounts, as they would be trapped in the fetal environment. Thus chloramphenicol, for example, which depends for its detoxification on conjugation, may be lethal to the neonate although the fetus *in utero* can survive an equivalent dose administered, and eliminated, transplacentally.

Purely *water-soluble drugs*, by contrast, cross the placenta slowly but are eliminated in fetal urine relatively rapidly; thus full materno–fetal equilibration is never achieved. Accumulation occurs in amniotic fluid, which the fetus drinks, but lipid-insoluble drugs are poorly absorbed from the gut and therefore may also accumulate in the gut lumen. This is commonly of little importance, though the prolonged maternal administration of the quaternary ammonium ganglion blocker hexamethonium as an antihypertensive has been associated with neonatal ileus.

A more detailed account of drug distribution into amniotic fluid may be found in Reynolds (1981), and of the principles of placental drug transfer in Reynolds (1986); individual drug transfer has been reviewed in Reynolds (1984).

References

Bohrer, M.P. Baylis, G., Humes, H.D. *et al.* (1978) Permselectivity of the glomerular capillary wall. Facilitated filtration of circulating polycations. *Journal of Clinical Investigation* **61**, 72

Bolwig, T.G., Hertz, M.M. and Westergaard, E. (1977) Acute hypertension causing blood–brain barrier breakdown during epileptic seizures. *Acta Neurologica Scandinavica* **56**, 335

Davson, H. (1976) The blood–brain barrier (Review Lecture). *Journal of Physiology* **255**, 1.

Forster, A., van Horn, K., Marshall, L.F. and Shapiro, H.M. (1977) Influence of anesthetic agents on blood–brain barrier function during acute hypertension. *Acta Neurologica Scandinavica* **56**, suppl., 60

Goldstein, A. and Aronow, L. (1960). The durations of action of thiopental and pentobarbital. *Journal of Pharmacology and Experimental Therapeutics* **128**, 1

Green, P.G. and Kitchen, I. (1985) Different effects of di-isopropylfluorophosphate on the entry of opioids into mouse brain. *British Journal of Pharmacology* **84**, 657

Hamshaw-Thomas, A. and Reynolds, F. (1985) Placental transfer of bupivacaine, pethidine and lignocaine in the rabbit. Effect of umbilical flow rate and protein content. *British Journal of Obstetrics and Gynaecology* **92**, 706

Hamshaw-Thomas, A., Rogerson, N. and Reynolds, F. (1984) Transfer of bupivacaine, lignocaine and pethidine across the rabbit placenta – influence of maternal protein binding and fetal flow. *Placenta* **5**, 61

Houghton, G.W., Richens, A., Toseland, P.A., Davidson, S. and Falconer, M.A. (1975) Brain concentrations of phenytoin, phenobarbitone and primidone in epileptic patients. *European Journal of Clinical Pharmacology* **9**, 73

Kaufman, J.J., Koski, W.S. and Benson, D.W. (1977) Temperature and pH sensitivity of the partition coefficient as related to the blood–brain barrier to drugs. *Experimental Eye Research* **25**, 201

Kennedy, R.L., Erenberg, A., Robillard, J.E., Merkow, A. and Turner, T. (1979) Effects of changes in maternal–fetal pH on the transplacental equilibrium of bupivacaine. *Anesthesiology* **51**, 50

Krauer, B., Dayer, P. and Anner, R. (1984) Changes in serum albumin and α_1-acid glycoprotein concentrations during pregnancy: an analysis of feto-maternal pairs. *British Journal of Obstetrics and Gynaecology* **91**, 875

Nau, H., Luck, W., Kuhnz, W. and Wegener, S. (1983) Serum protein binding of diazepam, desmethyldiazepam, furosemide, indomethacin, warfarin and phenobarbital in human fetus, mother and newborn infant. *Pediatric Pharmacology* **3**, 219

O'Brien, W.F., Cefalo, R.C., Grissom, M.P. *et al.* (1982) The influence of asphyxia on fetal lidocaine toxicity. *American Journal of Obstetrics and Gynecology* **142**, 205

Oldendorf, W.H. (1974a) Lipid solubility and drug penetration of the blood–brain barrier. *Proceedings of the Society for Experimental Biology and Medicine* **147**, 813

Oldendorf, W.H. (1974b) Blood–brain barrier permeability to drugs. *Annual Review of Pharmacology* **14**, 239

Oldendorf, W.H. (1976) Certain aspects of drug distribution to brain. *Advances in Experimental Medicine and Biology* **69**, 103

Oldendorf, W.H., Hyman, S., Braun, L. and Oldendorf, S.Z. (1972) Blood–brain barrier: penetration of morphine, codeine, heroin and methadone after carotid injection. *Science* **178**, 984

Older, P.O. and Harris, J.M. (1968) Placental transfer of tubocurarine. *British Journal of Anaesthesia* **40**, 459

Peters, M.A. (1975) Development of a 'blood–brain barrier' to methadone in the newborn rat. *Journal of Pharmacology and Experimental Therapeutics* **192**, 513

Petersen, M.C., Moore, R.G., Nation, R.L. and McMeniman, W. (1981) Relationship between the transplacental gradients of bupivacaine and α_1-acid glycoprotein. *British Journal of Clinical Pharmacology* **12**, 859

Rapoport, S.I., Hori, M. and Klatzo, I. (1972) Testing of a hypothesis for osmotic opening of the blood–brain barrier. *American Journal of Physiology* **223**, 323

Renkin, E.M. (1970) Permeability and molecular size in peripheral and glomerular capillaries. In: *Capillary Permeability* (Eds. Crone, C. and Lassen, N.A.), pp. 544–547. Munksgaard: Copenhagen

Renkin, E.M. and Garlick, D.G. (1970) Transcapillary exchange of large molecules between plasma and lymph. In: *Capillary Permeability* (Eds. Crone, C. and Lassen, N.A.), pp. 553–559. Munksgaard: Copenhagen

Reynolds, F. (1979) Drug transfer across the placenta. In: *Placental Transfer* (Eds. Chamberlain, G. and Wilkinson, A.) pp. 166–181. Pitman Medical: Tunbridge Wells

Reynolds, F. (1980) Transfer of drugs across membranes. In: *Topical Reviews in Anaesthesia–1* (Eds. Norman, J. and Whitwam, J.), pp. 135–178. John Wright: Bristol

Reynolds, F. (1981) Distribution of drugs in amniotic fluid. In: *Amniotic Fluid and its Clinical Significance* (Ed. Sandler, M.), pp. 261–275. Marcel Dekker: New York

Reynolds, F. (1984) The fetus and placenta. In: *Wylie and Churchill-Davidson's A Practice of Anaesthesia*, 5th edn. (Ed. Churchill-Davidson, H.C.), pp. 1069–1089. London: Lloyd-Luke

Reynolds, F. (1986) Placental transfer of respiratory gases and drugs. In: *Essentials of Obstetric Anaesthesia* (Ed. Morgan, B.M). Farrand Press: London

Schnermann, J. (1975) Transcapillary fluid flow in the peritubular microvasculature of the kidney. *Bibliotheca Anatomica* **13**, 36

Schulman, D.S., Kaufman, J.J., Eisenstein, M.M. and Rapoport, S.I. (1984) Blood pH and brain uptake of ^{14}C-morphine. *Anesthesiology* **61**, 540

Vella, L.M., Knott, C. and Reynolds, F. (1986) Transfer of fentanyl across the rabbit placenta – effect of umbilical flow and concurrent drug administration. *British Journal of Anaesthesia* **58**, 49

Wilkening, R.B., Anderson, S., Martensson, L. and Meschia, G. (1982) Placental transfer as a function of uterine blood flow. *American Journal of Physiology* **242**, H429

Young, M. (1979) Transfer of amino acids. In: *Placental Transfer* (Eds. Chamberlain, G.V.P. and Wilkinson, A.W.), pp. 142–158. Pitman Medical: Tunbridge Wells

4

Effects of anaesthesia on drug disposition

W.B. Runciman and L.E. Mather*

The average patient presenting for surgery will receive five to ten drugs in the perioperative period (Cullen and Miller, 1979). A large number of factors may influence the pharmacokinetics and pharmacodynamics of drugs given in this period, some of which have the potential for altering the therapeutic and/or toxic effects of the drugs given. Some of these factors have been the subjects of detailed reviews, such as the effects of anaesthesia and surgery on the cardiovascular system (Prys-Roberts, 1980) or on intermediary metabolism (Kehlet, 1984). However, the effects of anaesthesia *per se* on drug disposition have not been considered in any detail, even in recent texts on the pharmacology of drugs relevant to the anaesthetist (e.g. Wood and Wood, 1982b; Mazze, 1983; Sear, 1984) or on pharmacokinetics (Stanski and Watkins, 1982; Benet, Massoud and Gambertoglio, 1984; Prys-Roberts and Hug, 1984).

There have been many reports on the effects of anaesthesia or of various anaesthetic agents on drug disposition. However, a number of problems arise in reviewing the literature. Many of these reports were not intended to be of particular interest to the clinical anaesthetist (e.g. a comparison of the effects of ether and urethane anaesthesia in the rat), but have relevance to those using anaesthesia to facilitate surgical procedures in experimental animals or to those interested in drug metabolism. In this review, reports on anaesthetic agents and on drugs not used clinically have been included because they add to the body of evidence that there may be widespread effects on drug disposition involving many anaesthetic agents, many drugs and many metabolic pathways, and because they may help to shed some light on the possible mechanisms involved.

A further problem in reviewing the literature is that a wide range of experimental approaches has been used, including *in vivo* pharmacodynamic studies (using end-points such as loss of righting reflex), *in vivo* pharmacokinetic studies (using blood or urine drug concentrations), *in vivo* studies with the subsequent sacrifice of groups of animals for analysis of tissue drug and enzyme concentrations, and a full range of *in vitro* approaches (including the use of isolated perfused organs, tissue slices, cell and organelle

*The authors acknowledge the support of the National Health and Medical Research Council of Australia.

preparations). These studies are complicated because of variations in the routes, rates and timing of the administration of both the anaesthetic agents and the drugs in question, and by the fact that different parameters were often studied by different workers. Another problem is that the experimental design or method used rarely allowed discrimination between effects on blood flow and those on clearance or metabolism. In some cases it was possible, by examining the data, the experimental design and the drugs used, to form an opinion as to the likelihood of one or other of these effects operating. Because of the number of studies which have been performed, reports on the effects of anaesthesia and of anaesthetic agents on drug disposition have been tabulated and assigned a number for identification, so that they may conveniently be referred to in the text (see Tables 4.1 – 4.4).

Patients presenting for surgery may have pre-existing cardiovascular, hepatic or renal disease and may already be receiving treatment. Logistic and administrative problems frequently disrupt this treatment and, with drugs taken orally, inability to swallow, nausea and alterations in gastric emptying may further contribute to altered drug availability. Agents used for premedication, induction and maintenance of anaesthesia may each alter drug disposition. and further perturbations may be caused by the effects of surgery, of blood loss, of the patient's responses to noxious stimuli, and of alterations in hydrogen ion status and body temperature. Particular emphasis will be placed on the effects of anaesthetic agents themselves on drug distribution and clearance. As there have been recent reviews on the effects of hepatic, cardiac and renal disease on drug disposition (Benowitz and Meister, 1983; Blaschke, 1983; Fabre and Balant, 1983), on interactions between drugs commonly used in the perioperative period (Cullen and Miller, 1979) and on the effects of alterations in hydrogen ion status and body temperature (Bax and Woods, 1985), these topics will not be discussed any further.

Drug availability

Drug administration problems

A number of patients require long-term drug treatment which should be continued through the perioperative period; examples are those needing antihypertensive agents, anti-anginal agents or anticonvulsants. Even when these are correctly prescribed up to the time of the operation, they may not actually be given in the immediate postoperative period. In a recent study, only 40 per cent of such prescribed drugs were actually administered to the patients (Nimmo, 1985, personal communication).

Drugs given orally

Drugs prescribed for oral administration may not be taken by this route because of nausea or an inability to swallow or, if taken, may be vomited up before gastric emptying takes place. This is particularly important in the immediate postoperative period. For example, for these reasons, low and even undetectable   blood   propranolol   concentrations   were   found   after thyroidectomy, whereas normal blood concentrations could be achieved if the propranolol was given via a nasogastric tube (Feely *et al.*, 1980).

Alterations in gastric emptying are also important in the perioperative period; the effects of drugs and diseases on gastric emptying have been reviewed recently by Nimmo (1983). Absorption of orally administered drugs is largely dependent on gastric emptying, even for weakly acidic drugs such as aspirin and barbiturates which are highly lipid soluble at gastric pH. Delayed gastric emptying can lead to therapeutic failure with a large number of drugs. Although a wide range of drugs may influence gastric emptying – anticholinergics, phenothiazines, neurolepts, hypnotics, sedatives, anaesthetic agents and antacids – there have been few studies in man to demonstrate the magnitude or significance of this effect. However, a number of drug interaction studies in man have shown indirectly that anticholinergics, ganglion blockers, opioid analgesics and antacids produce effects which may be attributed to altered gastric motility, and some more specific direct studies have been done. For example, it has been shown that the time to empty 50 per cent of an ingested solution from the stomach is increased eight- to tenfold after pethidine, diamorphine or pentazocine and that this was not reversible by metoclopramide (Nimmo, 1983).

In another study it was shown that the mean time to peak blood lignocaine concentration after oral administration was increased from 45 minutes in healthy volunteers to 3 hours in patients undergoing laparoscopy and tubal diathermy under general anaesthesia after atropine premedication (Adjepon-Yamoah, Scott and Prescott, 1973). However, studies such as this, involving patients, are more difficult to interpret, as it is not possible to determine the relative importance of the several factors which may influence gastric emptying and drug absorption.

Many conditions encountered in surgical patients, such as peritoneal irritation, trauma or severe pain, are also thought to reduce gastric emptying (Elfstrom, 1979). However, there is a need for more well-controlled studies in this area as, in a recent study, anxiety and moderate pain before premedication were shown, in fact, not to reduce gastric emptying or drug absorption (Marsh, Spencer and Nimmo, 1984). In his review, Nimmo (1983) has emphasized that problems arising from delayed gastric emptying may remain unrecognized or be 'swept under the carpet' because therapeutic failure is less spectacular than drug toxicity. It would seem reasonable, therefore, to suggest that the intravenous route should be used whenever possible in the perioperative period, at least after premedication, especially when therapeutic failure may lead to life-threatening complications (e.g. with long-term β-blocker treatment, see Chapter 16).

Drugs given by intramuscular injection

As dose-dependent reductions in cardiac output are caused by halothane, enflurane and methoxyflurane (Hickey and Eger, 1980) and by barbiturates (Roberts, 1980), a reduction would be expected in the rate of absorption of drugs administered by intramuscular injection during anaesthesia with these agents, with a concomitant delay in, and a reduction of, peak tissue concentration. This has been shown to occur for ketamine with halothane

Table 4.1 Reports documenting reduction of drug clearance or metabolism by diethyl ether (ether)

	Author(s), year	Anaesthetic agent(s)/test drug(s)	Species	Experimental method used	Conclusions*
1	Aune, Olsen and Morland, 1981	Ether/antipyrine, paracetamol, sulphanilamide	Rat	Metabolism study in vitro on suspensions of isolated rat liver parenchymal cells	A dose-related ether inhibition of antipyrine and paracetamol metabolism was found, but there was no inhibition by ether of sulphanilamide metabolism
2	Baekeland and Greene, 1958	Ether/pentobarbitone	Rat	Pharmacokinetic study on the effects of ether in vivo. Enzymatic oxidation of pentobarbitone studied in rat liver homogenates in vitro	Significant increases in liver and plasma pentobarbitone levels were found in ether-treated rats in vivo. 45–96% inhibition of pentobarbitone metabolism was found in the presence of ether in vitro
3	Bombeck et al., 1969	Ether/N,N-dimethylaniline	Calf	Metabolism study on biopsies taken from isolated perfused calves' livers	Ether produced proliferative lesions of the smooth endoplasmic reticulum, but did not uncouple oxidative N-demethylation in hepatic microsomal fractions
4	Cooke and Cooke, 1983	Ether, pentobarbitone, urethane/iopanoate	Rat	Pharmacokinetics and metabolism of each iopanoate enantiomer studied with each anaesthetic agent in vivo	Ether and pentobarbitone significantly depressed the biliary secretion of each enantiomer as compared with urethane.
5	Hanew et al., 1984	Ether/aminopyrine; ethanol/aminopyrine; ether and ethanol/ aminopyrine	Rat	Pharmacokinetic study of effects of ether, ethanol, and ether and ethanol on aminopyrine kinetics in vivo	A 60% reduction in aminopyrine clearance was shown with ether, a 40% reduction with alcohol, and an 85% reduction with alcohol and ether. Probably reflects inhibition of metabolism, as aminopyrine clearance is generally recognized to be capacity limited*
6	Higashi et al., 1982	Ether/gentamicin, tobramycin	Rat	Pharmacokinetic study in rats on effects of ether or pentobarbitone on test drug disposition both during and after anaesthesia	Ether significantly reduced the clearance of both gentamicin and tobramycin; the effects persisted for at least 2 hours after anaesthesia. See Table 4.3 for studies on pentobarbitone.

7	Johannessen, Gadeholt and Aarbakke, 1981	Ether/antipyrine, paracetamol	Rat	Pharmacokinetic study of antipyrine and paracetamol both after a 5-minute exposure to ether and during continuous ether anaesthesia	A 5-minute exposure to ether reduced hepatic conjugation of paracetamol by 40%, but had no effect on antipyrine kinetics. Continuous ether anaesthesia interfered with both hepatic conjugation of paracetamol and hepatic oxidation of antipyrine
8	Lockwood and Houston 1982	Ether, cold stress/aminopyrine	Rat	Rats were exposed to 'cold stress' or to 'ether stress' (subanaesthetic ether concentrations) for 24 hours, and aminopyrine kinetics were then determined	'Cold stress' resulted in an enhanced rate of aminopyrine demethylation, whereas ether had no consistent effect in subanaesthetic concentrations
9	Umeda and Inaba, 1978	Ether, urethane/phenytoin	Rat	Study on the pharmacokinetics of phenytoin and on the biliary excretion of phenytoin metabolites with ether and with urethane anaesthesia	Phenytoin kinetics under urethane were similar to literature values for awake animals. However, ether anaesthesia produced a tenfold increase in phenytoin half-life and a threefold reduction in biliary excretion of phenytoin metabolites
10	Vermeulen et al., 1983	Ether/hexobarbitone	Rat	Pharmacokinetic study of hexobarbitone with and without ether anaesthesia	Ether anaesthesia resulted in a significant inhibition of the hepatic metabolism of hexobarbitone.

*A statement followed by an asterisk indicates further comment in interpretation of the data by the authors of this chapter.

anaesthesia in an elegant study by White *et al.* (1976). In control rats after an intramuscular ketamine injection, the plasma, brain, kidney and liver ketamine concentrations peaked at 5 minutes, and muscle concentrations peaked at 15 minutes. In rats under 0.8% halothane anaesthesia, the peak plasma, brain, kidney and liver concentrations were reduced to about 60 per cent of those in control animals and occurred at 15 minutes, while muscle concentration peaked only at 30 minutes. Significantly delayed and significantly lower peak concentrations of the two major metabolites of ketamine were also found in the plasma and tissues of the halothane-anaesthetized rats.

Drug distribution

Theoretically, anaesthetic agents may cause changes in the rate, pattern and apparent volume of drug distribution by producing changes in the rate and distribution of blood flow and changes in drug binding and uptake processes. However, very few studies of adequate experimental design have been carried out specifically to determine the extent to which such changes influence drug distribution.

Changes in rate and distribution of blood flow

All inhalational anaesthetic agents produce a dose-dependent depression of myocardial function *in vitro*. This also occurs in intact man, with cardiac output being reduced to about 75 per cent of control values at 1 MAC (minimal alveolar concentration) for halothane, methoxyflurane and enflurane; the reductions for nitrous oxide and isoflurane are insignificant at the doses used clinically in man (Hickey and Eger, 1980).

Kidney blood flow is reduced to an even greater extent than cardiac output, with reductions from about 30 per cent for the nitrous oxide–relaxant technique to greater than 60 per cent for some of the inhalational anaesthetic agents (Cousins, Skowronski and Plummer, 1983). Interpretation of the many studies which have been carried out is complicated by a host of uncontrolled variables. However, it seems that, with adequate hydration, reductions of about 40 per cent are usually produced during general anaesthesia with the halogenated hydrocarbons (Bastron, 1980).

Changes in intrarenal distribution of blood flow, depressed autoregulation and alterations in renal tubular function are probably of more importance, but have not been studied systematically. Functional reserve for oxygen delivery to the kidneys may also be reduced, as a significant reduction in renal vein oxygen tension has been noted to accompany these flow changes in the sheep (Runciman *et al.*, 1984a–c).

General anaesthesia also produces reductions of between 20 and 50 per cent in hepatosplanchnic blood flow, with slightly smaller concomitant reductions in oxygen consumption; functional reserve for oxygen delivery is thus generally reduced in this circulatory bed as well (Libonati *et al.*, 1973). These flow reductions are worsened by abdominal surgery, hyperventilation and both hyper- and hypocarbia (Strunin, 1980).

The changes in liver blood flow produced by inhalational anaesthetic agents are complex. For example, in a recent study in dogs it was shown that portal blood flow was reduced by both halothane and isoflurane, whereas hepatic arterial flow was maintained at 1 MAC halothane, reduced at 2 MAC halothane and increased during isoflurane anaesthesia (Gelman, Fowler and Smith, 1984). As there was no consistent correlation of these changes with systemic haemodynamic variables such as cardiac output and mean arterial pressure, it suggests that a number of local factors may be important. However, in this study with both agents there was still a progressive dose-dependent reduction in total hepatic blood flow; this was substantially greater with halothane (30 per cent at 1 MAC and 50 per cent at 2 MAC) than with isoflurane (10 per cent at 1 MAC and 30 per cent at 2 MAC). Indocyanine green half-life also increased progressively with increasing doses of both agents, but did not correlate with flow changes, suggesting altered distribution or that hepatic extraction ratios must have changed independently. That different patterns of blood flow distribution occur with different anaesthetic agents, and that these may change with pertubations such as hypovolaemia, was also emphasized in a study on the effects of ketamine, halothane, enflurane and isoflurane on regional haemodynamics in rats (Seyde and Longnecker, 1984).

The effects of the intravenous anaesthetic agents have not been as well documented. Interpretation of the studies which have been done is rendered difficult both because other drugs were frequently used simultaneously and because effects were not studied under conditions of steady-state blood concentration of the drug in question (Roberts, 1980). The barbiturates all cause dose-related myocardial depression, the neurolept techniques, benzodiazepines and opioid analgesics usually have little effect on the circulation if administered slowly to well-hydrated patients, and ketamine usually produces a moderate increase in cardiac output. Effects on hepatic and renal blood flow are poorly documented.

The implications of flow changes produced by either inhalational or intravenous agents on drug distribution *per se* are difficult to interpret because there are nearly always concomitant changes in drug clearance. In a study by White *et al*. (1976) it was shown that distribution of ketamine into muscle and skin of the rat was significantly slower after intravenous injection under halothane anaesthesia than in controls. However, concentrations in plasma and brain were significantly higher under halothane anaesthesia as plasma half-life was doubled. Ideally, the sites and rates of drug clearance should be determined at the same times as tissue concentration measurements, so that effects on distribution and on clearance may be evaluated separately.

Changes in drug binding and uptake processes

Changes may occur in the perioperative period in the concentrations of albumin and α_1-acid glycoproteins, and changes in the percentage of total drug bound to these plasma proteins have been reported for propranolol, phenytoin and quinidine (Bax and Woods, 1985).

It has also been shown that the free fraction of propranolol doubled during cardiopulmonary bypass, but was restored to preoperative values with heparin reversal (Wood, Shand and Wood, 1979). Cardiopulmonary bypass is associated with reduced clearance of a variety of drugs (Holley, Ponganis and Stanski, 1982). Because of its complexity it is difficult to apportion the effects to altered distribution, binding and clearance but it seems that most of these changes are probably associated more with factors such as haemodilution, hypothermia and response to surgery and stress than with anaesthesia *per se*, and are probably of little clinical significance, as no associated pharmacodynamic effects have been reported. Some of the factors have been studied separately. For example, normovolaemic haemodilution with dextran 40 has been shown to shift the dose–response curve of pancuronium and tubocurarine to the left, possibly because of an increase in the free concentrations of these drugs (Schuh, 1981).

It is possible that the steady-state volume of distribution of certain drugs could be altered by anaesthesia through changes in the kinetics of drug binding to tissue sites, but no clinically significant instances appear to have been reported to date. This would not be expected to occur with drugs which distribute only into body water, as it has been shown that the volume of total body water does not usually change significantly over the perioperative period (Elfstrom, 1979). Thus, it would seem that there is no evidence to date that loading doses of drugs used in the perioperative period should be modified.

Studies on the rate and pattern of drug distribution in relation to anaesthesia are generally difficult to interpret, as the necessary parameters have not usually been measured. It was recently reported that halothane reduced propranolol distribution and that this would contribute to the increased blood concentrations found during anaesthesia (Gordon, Wood and Wood, 1985). This conclusion was reached on the basis of a 62 per cent increase in femoral arterial propranolol concentrations, which was associated with a 36 per cent increase in the femoral arteriovenous propranolol extraction ratio. However, conclusions regarding the net flux of propranolol cannot be drawn without knowing blood flow through the limb, and, preferably, propranolol clearance as well, as both arterial and venous propranolol concentrations were still rising progressively at the end of the studies. In fact, the rate constants and limiting factors governing entry of drugs into and exit of drugs from tissues may differ appreciably and may vary independently in their response to anaesthesia. Detailed input–output drug concentration profiles, combined with simultaneous blood flow and drug clearance measurements, are necessary before conclusions can be drawn regarding drug distribution (Mather and Runciman, 1985; Upton *et al.*, 1986). Such studies indicate that anaesthesia may indeed alter the distribution patterns of some drugs with large apparent volumes of distribution (Runciman, Mather and Upton, 1985, unpublished observations). Although these are of theoretical interest, further studies are necessary to determine whether such changes are likely to have any clinical significance.

Anaesthetic agents may also interfere with the uptake of substances subject to active transport processes. The uptake of 5-hydroxytryptamine by lung *in vitro* has been shown to be significantly reduced by halothane, isoflurane and enflurane, so there may be substantial increases in circulating concentrations, with possible implications for both pulmonary and systemic vascular resistance (Hede and Post, 1981; Cook and Brandom, 1982). The removal of circulating noradrenaline by the lungs has also been shown to be inhibited by halothane (Naito and Gillis, 1973). Interference with such processes may contribute to the loss of circulatory homoeostatic mechanisms under anaesthesia (Runciman et al., 1984c). More studies are needed in this area to examine the effects of anaesthetic agents on other vasoactive agents such as angiotensins and prostaglandins.

Drug clearance and metabolism

Anaesthetic agents may alter drug clearance or metabolism by altering the rate of delivery of the drug in question to the sites of clearance or metabolism, or by altering the quantity or specific activity of enzymes responsible for the active transport or metabolism of the drug. Reports documenting such alterations have been summarized in Tables 4.1–4.4 (the references here have been numbered to simplify their citation).

Changes in rate of drug delivery

The changes in the rate and distribution of blood flow which occur under anaesthesia have been summarized in the previous section. For high clearance drugs the rate of delivery of the drug to the organ(s) of elimination may be the rate-limiting factor (Nies, Shand and Wilkinson, 1976).

Pulmonary blood flow is equal to cardiac output and, for substances cleared by the lung, clearance may be reduced by the same amount as cardiac output under anaesthesia. In principle, some compensation for reduced flow may occur by a proportionate increase in extraction ratio. However, in studies reported to date the extraction ratio under anaesthesia has either remained unchanged or has also been substantially reduced (see 23, 39). Although a wide range of endogenous substances (including several biogenic amines, adenine nucleotides, steroids, prostaglandins and peptide hormones) and drugs (including opioids, local anaesthetic agents, β-blockers, phenothiazines and tricyclic antidepressants) have been reported to be 'taken up' by the lung (Roth and Wiersma, 1983), experimental design in these drug studies has generally been inadequate to discriminate properly between distribution into the lung and elimination or clearance by the lung. Convincing evidence for substantial lung clearance of non-volatile drugs in man is lacking, except possibly for chlormethiazole (Mather et al., 1981); evidence for endogenous substances is far better. However, it is likely that it will be found that a range of drugs are cleared by the lung, and that reduced cardiac output will contribute significantly to the decreased clearance of these drugs under anaesthesia.

There are a number of intermediate and high clearance drugs metabolized in the liver for which reductions in hepatic blood flow are reflected by decreased clearance and increased blood concentrations (George, 1983). These include several antiarrhythmic agents (e.g. lignocaine, tocainide, verapamil), local anaesthetic agents (e.g. mepivacaine, bupivacaine), lipid-soluble β-blockers (e.g. alprenolol, labetalol, metoprolol, oxprenolol and propranolol), opioid analgesics (e.g. morphine, pethidine, pentazocine, dextro-propoxyphene), antidepressants (e.g imipramine, nortriptyline) and

Table 4.2 Reports documenting reduction of drug clearance or metabolism by halothane

	Author(s), year	Anaesthetic agent(s)/test drug(s)	Species	Experimental method used	Conclusions*
11	Arakawa et al., 1979	Halothane/pentazocine	Dog	Pharmacokinetic study of pentazocine after intramuscular injection	Halothane produced no change in half-life. However, clearance as calculated by dose/ area under curve was 74% of control value with the same dose of pentazocine*
12	Aune et al., 1983	Halothane, enflurane/ sulphanilamide, antipyrine, paracetamol	Rat	In vitro study of the metabolism of test drugs in the presence and absence of halothane or enflurane	Halothane and enflurane induced a strong concentration-related inhibition of antipyrine oxidation (40–70%) and of paracetamol conjugation (20–40%), and a significant dose-related reduction in cell viability and protein synthesis. There was a slight augmentation of sulphanilamide acetylation
13	Bell, Slattery and Calkins, 1985	Halothane/diazepam	Rat	Pharmacokinetic study of diazepam and its metabolites in blood and bile	Halothane produced a 42% reduction in the intrinsic clearance of diazepam. It was concluded that halothane inhibits intrinsic clearance by inhibiting oxidation, conjugation and biliary excretion
14	Bentley, Glass and Gandolfi, 1983	Halothane – nitrous oxide, fentanyl – nitrous oxide/lignocaine	Man	Pharmacokinetic study comparing lignocaine disposition with two different anaesthetic regimens	Lignocaine clearance was significantly reduced (by 34%) in the group with halothane–nitrous oxide anaesthesia as compared to the group with 'balanced' anaesthesia.
3	Bombeck et al., 1969	Halothane/ N,N-dimethylaniline	Calf	Metabolism study on biopsies taken from isolated perfused calves' livers	Halothane produced proliferative lesions of the smooth endoplasmic reticulum, and uncoupled oxidative N-demethylation in hepatic microsomal fractions
15	Borel et al., 1982	Halothane/fentanyl	Dog	Pharmacokinetic study of fentanyl kinetics in a control group and during 1.25% end-tidal halothane anaesthesia	Halothane reduced fentanyl clearance by 48% as compared to the value in the control group

	Author(s), year	Anaesthetic agent(s)/test drug(s)	Species	Experimental method used	Conclusions*
16	Brown, 1971	Halothane/amylobarbitone, hexobarbitone, pentobarbitone, aminopyrine, aniline	Rat	Metabolism study of rat microsomal enzyme activity in the presence and absence of halothane	Halothane depressed the metabolism of all the type I substrates by a dose-dependent, reversible, non-competitive inhibition of enzymes. In contrast, halothane enhanced the metabolism of aniline, a type II substrate
17	Burney and DiFazio, 1976	Halothane, nitrous oxide/lignocaine	Dog	Lignocaine pharmacokinetics studied in the presence of halothane or of nitrous oxide	Lignocaine blood concentrations were significantly higher and clearance was lower with halothane than with nitrous oxide anaesthesia
18	Cousins et al., 1982	Halothane, enflurane, pethidine/antipyrine	Man	Antipyrine kinetics were determined 24 hours before and 48 hours after halothane, enflurane and pethidine supplementation of nitrous oxide–oxygen anaesthesia	There was a significant (35%) reduction in antipyrine clearance 48 hours after halothane–nitrous oxide–oxygen anaesthesia, a non-significant reduction after enflurane and no change after pethidine supplementation
19	Dale et al., 1983	Halothane, enflurane on liver, kidney and lung microsomal enzyme activity	Rat	Rats were exposed to halothane or enflurane in concentrations from 50–1000 p.p.m. 6 hours a day for 3–11 days, and the effects on microsomal enzymes were determined at intervals	500 p.p.m. (0.05 MAC) halothane induced the activity of NADPH–cytochrome c reductase in the liver, decreased the concentration of cytochrome P450 in the kidney, and decreased all the enzyme concentrations measured in lung microsomes. Exposure to halothane 50 p.p.m. (0.005 MAC) and enflurane produced only minor changes
20	Denson et al., 1982	Halothane/bupivacaine	Rat	Metabolism study of effects of halothane on isolated rat hepatocytes	Halothane produced a significant dose-dependent inhibition of bupivacaine metabolism. The products of N-dealkylation were not reduced, suggesting that the principal effects were inhibition of metabolism by aromatic oxidation

*A statement followed by an asterisk indicates further comment in interpretation of the data by the authors of this chapter.

Table 4.2 *continued*

	Author(s), year	Anaesthetic agent(s)/test drug(s)	Species	Experimental method used	Conclusions*
21	Feely *et al.*, 1980	Halothane – nitrous oxide, fentanyl – nitrous oxide/propranolol	Man	Study of propranolol kinetics before, during and after operation in both euthyroid and hyperthroid patients	A marked reduction in propranolol clearance was shown in the postoperative period. However, this may have been due to factors other than anaesthesia; there was no difference in this respect between the halothane–nitrous oxide and the fentanyl–nitrous oxide groups
22	Fish and Rice, 1983	Halothane/enflurane	Rat	Pharmacokinetic study on effects of halothane on enflurane metabolism	Prior exposure to halothane reduced the rate of enflurane metabolism, possibly because of an interaction between halothane and cytochrome P450
23	Hede and Post, 1981	Halothane/5-hydroxytryptamine (5HT)	Rat	Study of effects of halothane on 5HT uptake in an isolated perfused ventilated rat lung preparation	Halothane was shown to reversibly inhibit the pulmonary uptake of 5HT, probably by reversible membrane stabilization of the capillary endothelial cellular membrane
24	Holstein-Rathlou, Christensen and Leyssac, 1982	Halothane, inactin, nitrous oxide/inulin, renin, prostaglandins	Rat (both Sprague-Dawley and Wistar)	Study of effects of each anaesthetic technique (compared to controls) on inulin clearance, overall renal and tubular function, plasma renin concentration and urinary prostaglandin excretion rates	With both anaesthetic techniques inulin clearance and proximal tubular reabsorption were significantly reduced, and urinary PGE_2 and $PGF_{2\alpha}$ excretion rates and plasma renin concentrations were elevated. There were differences with respect to anaesthetic technique and to strain of rat for effects on renal plasma flow, urine flow and solute excretion
25	Karlin and Kutt, 1970	Halothane/phenytoin	Man	Case report of phenytoin toxicity and hepatic dysfunction after halothane anaesthesia in a child	Phenytoin toxicity and hepatic dysfunction attributed to halothane anaesthesia

	Author(s), year	Anaesthetic agent(s)/test drug(s)	Species	Experimental method used	Conclusions*
26	Knights, Gourlay and Cousins, 1983	Halothane/cytochrome P450 concentration and aminopyrine	Rat	Animals (some induced with phenobarbitone) exposed to halothane in air, 14% or 10% oxygen, and sacrificed at 1, 2, 4, 6, 12, 24 or 48 hours after exposure, and cytochrome P450 and enzyme activities then determined	Exposure to 1% halothane in air produced no significant changes. In the enzyme-induced animals there were reduced cytochrome P450 concentrations, paralleled by reductions in aminopyrine demethylase activity for 6 hours after halothane–air exposure, 24 hours after halothane–14% oxygen exposure and 48 hours after halothane–10% oxygen exposure. There were no changes in aniline hydroxylase or NADPH–cytochrome c reductase activities
26b	Knights et al., 1983	demethylase, aniline hydroxylase and NADPH–cytochrome c reductase activities			
27	Lehmann et al., 1982	Halothane, enflurane/fentanyl	Rat, man	The effects of halothane and enflurane on the biotransformation of fentanyl were studied in vitro in rat liver and kidney homogenates, as well as after exposure of the rats to halothane or enflurane in vivo. Fentanyl kinetics were also studied in man under halothane or enflurane anaesthesia and compared with those under neurolept anaesthesia	Halothane and enflurane were strong inhibitors of fentanyl metabolism in vivo and in vitro in the rat, and fentanyl plasma concentrations were markedly elevated with enflurane and halothane anaesthesia in man. Fentanyl plasma concentrations under halothane anaesthesia were more than twice those under neurolept anaesthesia in man
28	Massarrat and Massarrat, 1979	Halothane, neurolept, epidural/bromosulphthalein (BSP)	Man	BSP kinetics were compared before and during vaginal hysterectomy under three different anaesthetic techniques	BSP elimination was significantly prolonged under halothane and neurolept anaesthesia, but was unchanged under epidural anaesthesia
29	Mather et al., 1986a	Halothane, spinal anaesthesia/pethidine	Sheep	Pharmacokinetic studies of effects of halothane or spinal anaesthesia with measurements of regional blood flows with drug extraction ratios	Under halothane anaesthesia hepatic clearance was reduced to 60% of control values, and renal clearance was abolished; both hepatic extraction ratio and blood flow were reduced. No changes under spinal anaesthesia

cont'd

*A statement followed by an asterisk indicates further comment in interpretation of the data by the authors of this chapter.

Table 4.2 continued

	Author(s), year	Anaesthetic agent(s)/test drug(s)	Species	Experimental method used	Conclusions*
30	Mather et al., 1986b	Halothane/lignocaine	Sheep	Pharmacokinetic studies of effects of halothane anaesthesia with measurements of regional blood flows with drug extraction ratios	Under halothane anaesthesia lignocaine hepatic clearance was essentially unaltered, despite a reduction in hepatic blood flow
31	Miller et al., 1979	Halothane, enflurane, ketamine, phenobarbitone/ pancuronium	Cat	Combined pharmacokinetic and pharmacodynamic study of pancuronium with different anaesthetic techniques	Onset time and duration of neuromuscular blockade were longer during enflurane and halothane anaesthesia, and clearance was reduced to about 70% of the values under ketamine or phenobarbitone anaesthesia. Plasma concentrations of pancuronium required for neuromuscular blockade were less with enflurane than with the other three agents
32	Nishida, 1979	Halothane/pentazocine	Dog	Study of pentazocine kinetics after IM injection of three different doses in both awake dogs and dogs anaesthetized with halothane. MAC also determined at each pentazocine dose	Pentazocine pharmacokinetics (after intramuscular injection) were not changed by halothane anaesthesia. There was a dose-dependent reduction of MAC for halothane by 20% at the low pentazocine dose to 40% at the high pentazocine dose
33	Pearson, Bogan and Sanford, 1973	Halothane/pentobarbitone	Sheep	Study of pentobarbitone kinetics with and without halothane anaesthesia	Halothane increased pentobarbitone half-life in sheep by a mean of 71%
34	Pessayre et al., 1978	Halothane (combined with various other agents)/ antipyrine	Man	Antipyrine kinetics determined before and 3 days after surgery	With operations less than 2 hours long, antipyrine clearance increased by an average of 48%. With operations 2–4 hours long, antipyrine clearance decreased by an average of 36%. With operations greater than 4 hours, antipyrine clearance decreased by an average of 47%

	Author(s), year	Anaesthetic agent(s)/test drug(s)	Species	Experimental method used	Conclusions*
35	Rahn, Dayton and Frederickson, 1969	Halothane/thiopentone	Man	Pharmacokinetic study of the effects of halothane on thiopentone kinetics	No effect of halothane shown on thiopentone kinetics. However, it has been shown subsequently that sampling was not continued for long enough to delineate changes in the elimination half-life of thiopentone*
36	Reilly et al., 1985	Halothane/propranolol	Dog	Pharmacokinetic study of the effects of halothane on propranolol kinetics	Intrinsic clearance of propranolol reduced by 62% under halothane anaesthesia and remained reduced by 48% 24 hours later. Bioavailability doubled both during anaesthesia and 24 hours later
37	Runciman et al., 1984c	Halothane, spinal anaesthesia/iodohippurate	Sheep	Pharmacokinetic studies of effects of halothane or spinal anaesthesia with measurements of regional blood flows and regional drug extraction ratios	Under halothane anaesthesia renal blood flow was reduced to 50% of control values and iodohippurate renal extraction ratio was reduced to 88% of control values; iodohippurate renal clearance was reduced to 45% of control values
38	Runciman et al., 1985	Halothane, spinal anaesthesia/cefoxitin	Sheep	Pharmacokinetic studies of effects of halothane or spinal anaesthesia with measurements of regional blood flows and regional drug extraction ratios	Under halothane anaesthesia both renal blood flow and cefoxitin renal extraction ratio were reduced to 50% of control values. Clearance thus was reduced by 75%. There were no changes under spinal anaesthesia
39	Runciman et al., 1986a	Halothane, spinal anaesthesia/chlormethiazole	Sheep	Pharmacokinetic studies of effects of halothane or spinal anaesthesia with measurements of regional blood flows and regional drug extraction ratios	Under halothane anaesthesia, hepatic extraction ratio and clearance were reduced to, respectively, 82% and 56% of control values, whilst pulmonary and renal clearances were abolished. There were no changes under spinal anaesthesia
39a	Runciman et al., 1986c	Halothane/tocainide	Sheep	Pharmacokinetic studies of effects of halothane on regional blood flows and regional drug extraction ratios	Under halothane anaesthesia, hepatic blood flow and tocainide extraction ratio were each reduced by about 25%; hence hepatic clearance was reduced to 50% of control values

cont'd

*A statement followed by an asterisk indicates further comment in interpretation of the data by the authors of this chapter.

Table 4.2 continued

	Author(s), year	Anaesthetic agent(s)/test drug(s)	Species	Experimental method used	Conclusions*
40	Selby et al., 1985b	Halothane/cefoxitin, pethidine	Sheep	Pharmacokinetic studies of effects of halothane with measurements of regional blood flows and regional extraction ratios both during and for 8 hours after anaesthesia	Under halothane anaesthesia hepatic clearance for pethidine was reduced to 55% of control values due to reduced hepatic blood flow, and recovered within 1 hour of the cessation of anaesthesia. Under halothane anaesthesia renal cefoxitin clearance was reduced to 46%, and slowly recovered to 68% from that value by 8 hours after cessation of anaesthesia. Both renal blood flow and cefoxitin renal extraction ratio were reduced during and after anaesthesia
41	Steffey et al., 1977	Halothane/pethidine	Dog	Pharmacokinetic study of pethidine kinetics after IM injections	The MAC of halothane was reduced by increasing doses of pethidine. Pethidine blood concentrations were increased under halothane anaesthesia, and pethidine clearances were reduced*
42	White et al., 1976	Halothane/ketamine	Rat	Combined pharmacokinetic and pharmacodynamic study in vivo; also a study on the effects of halothane on the hepatic microsomal metabolism of ketamine and its principal N-demethylated metabolites in vitro	Halothane prolonged the plasma and brain half-life of ketamine, increased the duration of ketamine-induced ataxia, increased plasma and brain ketamine concentrations and reduced the overall rate of in vivo metabolism in a concentration-dependent manner. In vitro hepatic microsomal metabolism of ketamine and its principal N-demethylated metabolite was inhibited non-competitively by halothane in a dose-dependent manner
43	Wood and Wood, 1984	Halothane, isoflurane, enflurane/aminopyrine	Rat	Pharmacokinetic study of the effects of different anaesthesic agents on aminopyrine kinetics in vivo	Halothane inhibited the rate of aminopyrine elimination in a dose-dependent fashion for at least 24 hours. Isoflurane had a smaller effect which was not as long lasting, whereas enflurane had no effect

*A statement followed by an asterisk indicates further comment in interpretation of the data by the authors of this chapter.

other drugs acting on the CNS (e.g. chlormethiazole, methohexitone). Representatives of each of these groups of drugs have been shown to have reduced clearance under anaesthesia, and reduced delivery of drug to the liver is a likely contributory mechanism in each case (see Tables 4.1–4.3). Unequivocal evidence that reduced drug delivery is an important factor in the reduced clearance has been documented in studies in which liver blood flow has been measured at the same time as drug clearance (29, 30, 39, 40).

There are also a wide range of high or intermediate clearance drugs eliminated by the kidney which are eliminated not only by glomerular filtration but also by tubular secretion (Duchin and Schrier, 1983). Some of these, such as the antibiotics, cefoxitin and gentamicin, are commonly used in the perioperative period. The clearance of both of these has been shown to be reduced by anaesthesia (6). Unequivocal evidence that reduced kidney blood flow contributes to reduced drug clearance under anaesthesia has been shown for iodohippurate, cefoxitin, inulin and lithium (24, 37, 38, 40, 55, 58).

Many drugs are metabolized to a more polar derivative in the liver, and are then excreted by the kidney. Some of these more polar metabolites are themselves pharmacologically active and/or may produce side effects (Drayer, 1983). Thus, for example, with inadequate renal function, increased antiarrhythmic effects may be seen with procainamide treatment due to accumulation of N-acetylprocainamide, and twitching and irritability may be seen due to accumulation of norpethidine with pethidine treatment. Increased side effects may also occur with clofibrate, allopurinol and sulphonamide treatment due to the accumulation of toxic metabolites. Although most of these problems are seen only in patients with compromised renal function, some, such as norpethidine accumulation, have been described in normal patients in the perioperative period (Austin, Stapleton and Mather, 1981). Large increases in norpethidine blood concentration have also been shown experimentally under halothane anaesthesia (Mather et al., 1986a). The profound depression of renal blood flow and loss of autoregulation which occur with general anaesthesia have recently been shown experimentally to persist for several hours into the postoperative period (Selby et al., 1985a, b), and may contribute to the incidence of these problems.

Changes in the rate of active transport or metabolism

Changes in the rate of active transport or metabolism may have contributed to altered clearance in most of the cases referred to in Tables 4.1–4.4 because, when drug extraction ratios across organs, intrinsic clearance, rate of metabolism or enzyme activity were specifically determined, significant alterations were shown in the great majority of cases. These will be considered in greater detail below, where the effects of each anaesthetic agent will be considered in turn.

Reductions of drug clearance or metabolism by diethyl ether (ether)

Ether in anaesthetic concentrations has been shown to inhibit the clearance or excretion of a number of drugs metabolized predominantly by oxidative pathways, such as hexobarbitone (10), pentobarbitone (2), antipyrine (1, 7), aminopyrine (5) and phenytoin (9) (Table 4.1). On the other hand, ether in subanaesthetic concentrations was shown to have no consistent effect on aminopyrine metabolism (8).

Conjugation of paracetamol has been shown to be inhibited *in vivo* both after a brief exposure to ether and during continuous ether anaesthesia (7), and to be inhibited by ether *in vitro* (1). Biliary secretion has also been shown to be inhibited by ether (4). Inhibition of metabolism *per se* was shown for antipyrine, paracetamol and pentobarbitone (1, 2).

Ether and pentobarbitone both reduced the renal clearance of gentamicin and tobramycin (6); these effects persisted for 2 hours after anaesthesia. Pentobarbitone was also shown to reduce the biliary excretion of iopanate (4) and both the metabolism and the excretion of sulphanilamide (6). Urethane, on the other hand, was either without effect or had markedly less effect than ether or pentobarbitone (4, 9).

Reductions of drug clearance or metabolism by halothane

There are some 30 reports of halothane reducing drug clearance and/or inhibiting metabolism (Table 4.2). These include studies in the rat, dog, cat, sheep, calf and in man.

Evidence of reduced clearance or metabolism of high clearance drugs predominantly metabolized by oxidative pathways has been reported for lignocaine (14, 17, 30), fentanyl (15, 27), bupivacaine (20), propranolol (21, 36), pethidine (29, 40, 41), chlormethiazole (39) and ketamine (42). Evidence for reduced clearance of low or intermediate clearance drugs has been reported for antipyrine (12, 18, 34) diazepam (13) (Kanto and Philajamaki, 1973), hexobarbitone (16), phenytoin (25), pancuronium (31), pentobarbitone (16, 33), enflurane (22), aminopyrine (16, 43), amylobarbitone (16), tocainide (39a), and N, N-dimethylaniline (3).

There is direct evidence for the inhibition of conjugation of paracetamol (12) and *p*-nitrophenol (Brown, 1972), and inferential evidence for the inhibition of conjugation of the products of oxidation of diazepam (13). There is indirect evidence for the inhibition of biliary secretion by halothane in studies demonstrating reduced elimination of bromosulphthalein (28) and of diazepam and its metabolites (13).

Evidence for inhibition of hepatic metabolism *per se* or of significant reductions in intrinsic clearance has been obtained for high clearance drugs, such as bupivacaine (20), fentanyl (27), pethidine (29, 40), propranolol (36) and ketamine (42), as well as for intermediate and low clearance drugs such as N, N-dimethylaniline (3), paracetamol (12), antipyrine (12), hexobarbitone (16), amylobarbitone (16), pentobarbitone (16), diazepam (13), enflurane (22), tocainide (39a) and aminopyrine (43). The hepatic extraction ratio of lignocaine was reported to be reduced in one study (Boyce, Cervenko and Wright, 1978) but in another remained essentially unchanged (30). Halothane was also shown to have a direct inhibitory effect in studies examining concentrations and/or activities of enzymes such as cytochrome P450 and NADPH–cytochrome *c* reductase (19, 26).

Halothane has been reported to reduce the renal clearance of drugs such as inulin (24), pethidine (29), iodohippurate (37), cefoxitin (38, 40) and chloromethiazole (39). Inhibition of active transport or metabolism was shown in each of these studies, and direct inhibition of renal microsomal enzymes by halothane has also been reported (19).

Halothane has been shown to reduce the pulmonary clearance of 5-hydroxytryptamine (23), chlormethiazole (39) and catecholamines (Naito and Gillis, 1973). A reduction in intrinsic clearance has been reported for chlormethiazole (39) and direct inhibition of lung microsomal enzymes was shown by Dale *et al*. (1983) (19).

That these inhibitory effects of halothane persist well into the postanaesthetic period has been reported both for some drugs cleared by the liver, such as propranolol (36), pethidine (40) and aminopyrine (43), and for cefoxitin, a drug cleared by the kidney (40).

On the other hand, it has been reported that there was little or no change under halothane anaesthesia in the half-life of thiopentone after intravenous injection or that of pentazocine after intramuscular injection (35, 11, 32). However, blood sampling was not continued for long enough to separate adequately the distribution and elimination half-lives in the former case, and in the latter there was some evidence of a reduction in pentazocine clearance.

Reductions of drug clearance or metabolism by enflurane, isoflurane, barbiturates, opioids, diazepam and nitrous oxide

Enflurane has been shown *in vitro* to inhibit the oxidation of antipyrine and the conjugation of paracetamol (12). However, a non-significant reduction in antipyrine clearance was reported in one study in man (18), and no consistent changes were shown in two other studies (43, 53). Enflurane had no effect on thiopentone kinetics (48) or fentanyl clearance in three of four groups of patients studied both intraoperatively and for 24 hours postoperatively (46). Clearance was, however, significantly reduced in the fourth group of patients (undergoing cardiac surgery) in this study. Enflurane was shown to produce only minor changes in the concentration of cytochrome P450 and in the activity of NADPH–cytochrome *c* reductase (19) and no changes in aniline hydroxylase activity (45), but did significantly inhibit aminopyrine demethylase activity (45). Enflurane was also shown to significantly reduce kidney blood flow and cefoxitin extraction ratio (55); however, these returned to control values by 8 hours after anaesthesia (55).

Isoflurane appears not to have been studied much in this context. However, it has been reported to inhibit the oxidative metabolism of halothane (47), to inhibit antipyrine clearance (but to a smaller extent than halothane) (43) and to have very similar effects as enflurane on renal blood flow and cefoxitin extraction ratio both during and after anaesthesia (55).

Barbiturates have also been reported to reduce the clearance of a number of drugs. Quinalbarbitone has been shown to reduce ketamine clearance both in the rat and man (51), pentobarbitone has been shown to reduce gentamicin and tobramycin clearance by the kidney, and sulphanilamide clearance and biliary secretion by the liver (4, 6), and amylobarbitone has been shown to reduce inulin clearance (58).

Morphine has been shown to increase the brain half-life of thiopentone in the rat (44), and to reduce bromosulphthalein clearance by the liver (49). Pethidine supplementation of nitrous oxide–oxygen–relaxant anaesthesia in man, on the other hand, was shown not to affect antipyrine clearance measured

Table 4.3 Reports documenting reductions of drug clearance or metabolism by enflurane, isoflurane, nitrous oxide, opioids, diazepam, neurolepts and barbiturates

	Author(s), year	Anaesthetic agent(s)/test drug(s)	Species	Experimental method used	Conclusions*
12	Aune et al., 1983	Enflurane, halothane/ sulphanilamide, antipyrine, paracetamol	Rat	Study of the metabolism of test drugs in the presence and absence of enflurane or halothane	Enflurane and halothane induced a strong concentration-related inhibition of antipyrine oxidation (40–70%) and of paracetamol conjugation (20–40%). They also produced a significant dose-related reduction in cell viability and protein synthesis. There was a slight augmentation of sulphanilamide acetylation
44	Cherksey and Altszuler, 1974	Morphine/thiopentone	Rat	Combined pharmacokinetic and pharmacodynamic study	Morphine lowered the brain threshold for thiopentone-induced sleep, but also prolonged the brain thiopentone half-life
4	Cooke and Cooke, 1983	Pentobarbitone, ether, urethane/iopanoate	Rat	Pharmacokinetics and metabolism of each iopanoate enantiomer studied with each anaesthetic agent in vivo	Pentobarbitone and ether significantly depressed the biliary secretion of each enantiomer compared with urethane
18	Cousins et al., 1982	Enflurane, pethidine, halothane/antipyrine	Man	Antipyrine kinetics were determined 24 hours before and 48 hours after halothane, enflurane or pethidine supplementation of nitrous oxide–oxygen anaesthesia.	There was a significant (35%) reduction in antipyrine clearance 48 hours after halothane supplementation, a non-significant reduction after enflurane and no change with pethidine supplementation
19	Dale et al., 1983	Enflurane, halothane/ on liver, kidney and lung microsomal enzyme activity	Rat	Rats exposed to halothane or enflurane in concentrations from 50 to 1000 p.p.m. 6 hours per day for 3–11 days, and effects of microsomal enzymes determined at intervals	Exposure to enflurane produced only minor changes, whereas exposure to halothane 500 p.p.m. produced significant effects (see Table 4.2)
45	DaRocha-Reis and Hipolito-Reis, 1982	Enflurane/on aniline hydroxylase activity, aminopyrine demethylase activity	Rat	Rats exposed to enflurane, 1%, 2% or 3% for 1 hour per day for 3, 7, 10, 14, 21 or 24 days, then sacrificed and liver microsomal protein weighed and tested	Enflurane exposure produced no increase in fractional liver or microsomal protein weights, and no changes in aniline hydroxylase activity. Aminopyrine demethylase was decreased after a number of exposures to an extent which varied with the dose

	Author(s), year	Anaesthetic agent(s)/test drug(s)	Species	Experimental method used	Conclusions*
46	Duthie and Nimmo, 1985	Enflurane/fentanyl	Man	Pharmacokinetic and pharmacodynamic study both intraoperatively in four groups of surgical patients (orthopaedic, upper abdominal, prolonged surgery and cardiac surgery) and postoperatively for 24 hours	Fentanyl by constant IV infusion at 100 μg per hour provided effective analgesia after surgery without significant respiratory depression. Clearance of fentanyl was reduced only in the cardiac surgery group, which had not reached steady-state blood concentrations by 24 hours after surgery
47	Fiserova-Bergerova, 1984	Isoflurane, nitrous oxide/halothane	Rat	Rats exposed to subanaesthetic concentrations of anaesthetic agents, after which concentrations of halothane and its metabolites were determined in the tissue of rats	Isoflurane produced a significant concentration-dependent inhibition of the oxidative metabolism of halothane, but enhanced the reductive metabolism of halothane. Exposure to nitrous oxide had no effect on halothane metabolism
48	Ghoneim and van Hamme, 1978	Enflurane–nitrous oxide/thiopentone	Man	Pharmacokinetic study of thiopentone kinetics in man both in volunteers and under anaesthesia	Neither enflurane–nitrous oxide anaesthesia nor the stress of surgery affected the distribution or clearance of thiopentone from plasma
6	Higashi *et al.*, 1982	Pentobarbitone/ gentamicin, tobramycin sulphanilamide	Rat	Pharmacokinetic study in rats on effects of pentobarbitone or ether on test drug disposition. See Table 4.1 for studies on ether	Pentobarbitone significantly reduced the clearance of both gentamicin and tobramycin, and greatly reduced both metabolism and excretion of sulphanilamide. However, there was a slight increase in the acetylated fractions of sulphanilamide excreted into the urine in 24 hours
49	Hurwitz and Fischer, 1984	Morphine/ bromosulphthalein (BSP)	Rat	Effects of morphine, hypoxia, hypercapnia and acidosis on BSP disposition were studied *in vivo*	Morphine halved the plasma clearance of BSP and tripled hepatic BSP concentration. Respiratory depression with hypoxia could have contributed to some of these effects, but did not account for them

cont'd

*A statement followed by an asterisk indicates further comment in interpretation of the data by the authors of this chapter.

Table 4.3 continued

	Author(s), year	Anaesthetic agent(s)/test drug(s)	Species	Experimental method used	Conclusions*
50	Idvall et al., 1983	Diazepam/ketamine—nitrous oxide	Man	A complex study on pharmacodynamic and pharmacokinetic interactions between diazepam and ketamine. For evidence of enzyme induction see Table 4.4	In the diazepam premedicated group of patients, haemodynamic stimulation by ketamine was significantly reduced, a lower rate of ketamine infusion was required during the first 30 minutes of anaesthesia, the biological half-life of ketamine was significantly increased and there were low levels of hydroxylated metabolites
51	Lo and Cumming, 1975	Diazepam, hydroxyzine, quinalbarbitone/ketamine	Man, rat	Combined pharmacokinetic and pharmacodynamic study of ketamine and these three premedicants in man. The effects of these three agents on ketamine metabolism were also studied in isolated perfused rat livers	Premedication with each of three agents studied significantly increased ketamine-induced sleep time in man. Mean plasma half-lives of ketamine were longer in patients premedicated with diazepam or quinalbarbitone. Ketamine half-life in the perfusate of isolated perfused rat livers was prolonged 30–50% by the addition of diazepam, quinalbarbitone or hydroxyzine
52	Nunn, 1984	Nitrous oxide/vitamin B_{12}	Rat, man	Toxicological, epidemiological and kinetic studies in man and rats	Nitrous oxide oxidizes and inactivates vitamin B_{12} in the form of methylcobalamin, the bound co-factor of methionine synthase, resulting in reduced methionine turnover and lowered serum methionine levels. This probably explains the toxic effects which may be produced on the fetus, the bone marrow and the nervous system by nitrous oxide
53	Oikkonen, Rosenberg and Neuvonen, 1984	Enflurane—nitrous oxide —fentanyl, droperidol—nitrous oxide, spinal/antipyrine	Man	Antipyrine kinetics compared with three anaesthetic techniques. All patients also had pethidine, diazepam and atropine premedication	There were marked individual differences in antipyrine half-life between patients, but there were no systematic significant differences between the groups subjected to different anaesthetic techniques

	Author(s), year	Anaesthetic agent(s)/test drug(s)	Species	Experimental method used	Conclusions*
54	Reiche and Frey, 1981	Chloramphenicol/ thiopentone, methohexitone, etomidate, propranidid and ketamine	Mouse	Pharmacodynamic study on the effects of chloramphenicol pretreatment on sleeping time after various induction doses of the anaesthetic agents	Sleeping time was prolonged with some doses of thiopentone, methohexitone and etomidate, but not with propranidid or ketamine. Termination of effect was probably by redistribution rather than metabolism and, although chloramphenicol has been shown to prolong barbiturate action by inhibition of liver mixed function oxidases, this effect was probably of no importance in this study*
55	Runciman et al., 1986b	Enflurane, isoflurane/ cefoxitin	Sheep	Pharmacokinetic studies of effects of enflurane or isoflurane on regional blood flows and regional extraction ratios both during and for 8 hours after anaesthesia	Both clearance and extraction ratio were reduced significantly under anaesthesia, but progressively recovered after anaesthesia and had approached control values by 8 hours after cessation of anaesthesia
56	Schuttler et al., 1983	Enflurane–nitrous oxide, fentanyl–nitrous oxide/ etomidate	Man	Pharmacokinetic study on the effects of four different anaesthetic techniques on etomidate kinetics	Etomidate kinetics in volunteers in the enflurane–nitrous oxide group were similar. However, volumes of distribution were reduced twofold and plasma clearance of etomidate was reduced threefold with fentanyl–nitrous oxide anaesthesia
57	Sear et al., 1984	Nitrous oxide/ etomidate	Man	Combined pharmacokinetic and pharmacodynamic study in patients undergoing anaesthesia by a constant rate etomidate infusion	In patients breathing nitrous oxide 67%, as compared to those breathing oxygen-enriched air, recovery was delayed fourfold, plasma etomidate concentrations were elevated by 37% and plasma clearance was reduced by 31%

*A statement followed by an asterisk indicates further comment in interpretation of the data by the authors of this chapter.

cont'd

Table 4.3 *continued*

	Author(s), year	Anaesthetic agent(s)/test drug(s)	Species	Experimental method used	Conclusions*
58	Thomsen and Olesen, 1981	Amylobarbitone, inactin/sodium, lithium and inulin kinetics	Rat	Comparison of urine flow and sodium, lithium and inulin clearances in two strains of awake unoperated rats, awake catheterized rats and rats anaesthetized with amylobarbitone or inactin	Both anaesthesia and surgery affected kidney function to different degrees in different rat strains. Inactin reduced urine flows and clearances in both rat strains, and amylobarbitone did so in Wistar rats. Awake catheterized and amylobarbitone-anaesthetized Sprague-Dawley rats showed few changes
42a	Wood and Wood, 1982a	Isoflurane, halothane, enflurane/aminopyrine	Rat	Pharmacokinetic study of the effects of different anaesthetic agents on aminopyrine kinetics *in vivo*	Halothane inhibited the rate of aminopyrine elimination in a dose-dependent fashion for at least 24 hours. Isoflurane had a smaller effect which was not as long lasting, whereas enflurane had no effect

*A statement followed by an asterisk indicates further comment in interpretation of the data by the authors of this chapter.

48 hours postoperatively in man (18).

Diazepam has been shown to prolong the half-life and effects of ketamine (50), and nitrous oxide to prolong those of etomidate (57). Chronic or repeated exposure to nitrous oxide has been shown to inactivate vitamin B_{12} and produce toxic effects on the fetus, bone marrow and the nervous system (52).

That there were direct effects on metabolism or intrinsic clearance was shown for the effects of enflurane on antipyrine (12), paracetamol (18), aminopyrine demethylase activity (45) and cefoxitin (55), for the effects of isoflurane on cefoxitin (55), for the effects of secobarbitone and ketamine on diazepam (51) and for the effects of pentobarbitone on sulphanilamide (6).

Studies examining possible enzyme induction by anaesthetic agents

Fourteen reports on studies examining possible enzyme induction are summarized in Table 4.4. Both the *in vitro* and the *in vivo* studies indicate that the effects are complex, and that they depend on the timing and extent of exposure, on the agent used, and on how and when the studies were carried out.

Of the eight *in vitro* studies reported, both enzyme induction and enzyme inhibition were shown to occur in five (12, 16, 19, 46, 65), enzyme inhibition only was shown in one (45) and enzyme induction only was shown in two (62, 64). Different anaesthetic agents had different effects on the same enzymes and different effects were produced by the same agent in different studies. For example, cytochrome P450 concentrations were reduced by halothane in one study (19), were unaffected by halothane in a second study (64), and were reduced by halothane but increased by ether in a third study (65). In the same studies, NADPH–cytochrome c reductase activity was increased only with the highest concentration of halothane in the first (19), was increased in a dose-dependent manner in the second (64) but was not affected in the third (65).

The studies in man are also difficult to interpret, with effects apparently depending on the anaesthetic agents used, on the duration of anaesthesia (or surgery), on the drugs or pathways studied and on the timing of the study. In most studies the issue was complicated by many uncontrolled variables and small samples.

In one study, antipyrine clearance was shown in a group of five patients to be increased by 50 per cent 1 week after surgery of 1 hour's duration under halothane anaesthesia, but had returned to preanaesthetic values by 4 weeks after surgery (63). In a second study under halothane anaesthesia, antipyrine clearance was increased by a similar amount 3 days after surgery, but only if surgery was of less than 2 hours' duration; if surgery was of greater than 4 hours in duration antipyrine clearance was significantly depressed (34). In a third study (60) antipyrine clearance was measured 4 and 8 days after surgery; there were statistically significant but clinically small reductions in antipyrine clearance after halothane and neurolept anaesthesia (20 per cent and 16 per cent, respectively). In a fourth study (61) of similar design to the third, no consistent changes in antipyrine clearance were found after enflurane anaesthesia.

Berman *et al.* (1976) studied steroid anaesthesia in six healthy male volunteers and concluded that there was evidence of enzyme induction in five out of six of the subjects (59), and Idvall *et al.* (1983) showed high levels of

Table 4.4 Studies examining possible enzyme induction by anaesthetic agents

	Author(s), year	Anaesthetic agent(s)/test drug(s)	Species	Experimental method used	Conclusions*
12	Aune *et al.*, 1983	Halothane, enflurane/ sulphanilamide, antipyrine, paracetamol	Rat	*In vitro* study of the metabolism of test drugs in the presence and absence of halothane or enflurane	Halothane and enflurane induced a strong concentration-related inhibition of antipyrine oxidation (40–70%) and of paracetamol conjugation (20–40%), and a significant dose-related reduction in cell viability and protein synthesis. There was a slight augmentation of sulphanilamide acetylation
59	Berman *et al.*, 1976	Enflurane/steroid metabolism	Man	Ratios of 6-β-hydroxycortisol (6-OHF) to 17-hydroxycorticosteroids (17-OHCS) in 24-hour urine specimens were compared before and after enflurane anaesthesia	The ratio of 6-OHF to 17-OHCS increased markedly in five and decreased slightly in one volunteer following anaesthesia, suggesting enzyme induction
16	Brown, 1971	Halothane/amylobarbitone, hexobarbitone, pentobarbitone, aminopyrine, aniline	Rat	Metabolism study of rat microsomal enzyme activity in the presence and absence of halothane	Halothane depressed the metabolism of all the type I substrates by a dose-dependent, reversible, non-competitive inhibition of enzymes. In contrast, halothane enhanced the metabolism of aniline, a type II substrate
19	Dale *et al.*, 1983	Halothane, enflurane/on liver, kidney and lung microsomal enzyme activity	Rat	Rats were exposed to halothane or enflurane in concentrations from 50 to 1000 p.p.m. 6 hours per day for 3–11 days, and the effects on microsomal enzymes were determined at intervals	500 p.p.m. (0.05 MAC) halothane induced the activity of NADPH–cytochrome *c* reductase in the liver, decreased the concentration of cytochrome P450 in the kidney and decreased all the enzyme concentrations measured in lung microsomes. Exposure to halothane 50 p.p.m. (0.005 MAC) and enflurane produced only minor changes
45	DaRocha-Reis and Hipolito-Reis, 1982	Enflurane/on aniline hydroxylase activity, aminopyrine demethylase activity	Rat	Rats exposed to enflurane 1%, 2% or 3% for 1 hour per day for 3, 7, 10, 14, 21 or 24 days, were then sacrificed and their liver microsomes were weighed and tested	Enflurane exposure produced no increase in liver or microsomal weights, and no changes in aniline hydroxylase activity. Aminopyrine demethylase was decreased after a number of exposures to an extent which varied with the dose

	Author(s), year	Anaesthetic agent(s)/test drug(s)	Species	Experimental method used	Conclusions*
47	Fiserova-Bergerova, 1984	Isoflurane, nitrous oxide/halothane	Rat	Rats were exposed to subanaesthetic concentrations of anaesthetic agents, after which concentrations of halothane and its metabolites were determined in the tissues of rats	Isoflurane produced a significant concentration-dependent inhibition of the oxidative metabolism of halothane, but enhanced the reductive metabolism of halothane. Exposure to nitrous oxide had no effect on halothane metabolism
60	Duvaldstein et al., 1981	Halothane, neurolept/antipyrine	Man	Antipyrine clearance was determined before and 4 or 8 days after surgery under halothane or neurolept anaesthesia	Statistically significant but clinically small increases in antipyrine clearance of 20% and 16% were shown in the halothane and neurolept groups, respectively. The mechanism was not clear
61	Duvaldstein, Mauge and Desmonts, 1981	Enflurane/antipyrine	Man	Antipyrine clearance was determined before and 4 or 8 days after surgery under enflurane anaesthesia	Enflurane anaesthesia had no significant effects on antipyrine half-life or clearance
50	Idvall et al., 1983	Diazepam/ketamine—nitrous oxide	Man	A complex study on pharmacodynamic and pharmacokinetic interactions between diazepam and ketamine on four groups of patients. One group of 4 patients had been on oral diazepam or barbiturates for 1–14 years (see table 4.3 for other groups)	The group of 4 patients were premedicated with atropine alone, and this group, as compared to controls, had high concentrations of hydroxylated metabolites, with levels higher than those of norketamine. The group of patients pretreated with diazepam had low levels of hydroxylated metabolites
62	Linde and Berman, 1971	Nitrous oxide, cyclopropane, diethyl ether, isopropyl ether, fluroxene, enflurane, isoflurane, chloroform, halothane and ethyl vinyl ether/hexobarbitone	Rat	Hexobarbitone sleeping time was determined after exposure to each anaesthetic agent for 7 hours each day for 1, 2, 3, 4 or 5 days. Rats were also exposed to ether (1.6% for 7 hours on 1 day) or halothane (0.4% for 7 hours on 2 consecutive days), and hydroxylation and demethylation activity of the liver were determined	Exposure to subanaesthetic concentrations of the ethers, halothane and chloroform enhanced the ability of rats to metabolize hexobarbitone, as evidenced by a reduction in sleeping time (cyclopropane and nitrous oxide did not). Pretreatment with ether or halothane led to increased rate of hexobarbitone and aniline hydroxylation by rat liver homogenates. Pretreatment with ether, but not halothane, enhanced the demethylase activity of rat liver homogenates

cont'd

*A statement followed by an asterisk indicates further comment in interpretation of the data by the authors of this chapter.

Table 4.4 continued

	Author(s), year	Anaesthetic agent(s)/test drug(s)	Species	Experimental method used	Conclusions*
63	Nimmo, Thompson and Prescott, 1981	Halothane (combined with various other agents)/antipyrine	Man	Antipyrine kinetics compared before and after halothane anaesthesia	Antipyrine clearance increased by about 50% after halothane anaesthesia
34	Pessayre et al., 1978	Halothane (combined with various other agents)/antipyrine	Man	Antipyrine kinetics determined before and 3 days after surgery	With operations less than 2 hours long, antipyrine clearance increased an average of 48%. With operations 2–4 hours long, antipyrine clearance decreased an average of 36%. With operations greater than 4 hours, antipyrine clearance decreased an average of 47%
64	Rietbrock, Lazarus and Otterbein, 1972	Halothane/hexobarbitone, cytochrome P450, NADPH–cytochrome c reductase	Rat	Effects of pretreatment of rats with 2% halothane in oxygen for 1 or 2 hours once daily for 5 days were determined on hexobarbitone sleeping time and on enzymes.	Exposure for 1 hour decreased hexobarbitone sleeping time by half and increased NADPH–cytochrome c reductase activity by one-third, whereas the amount of cytochrome P450 was not altered. Doubling the daily halothane exposure doubled the increase in NADPH–cytochrome c reductase activity
65	Ross and Cardell, 1978	Ether, halothane/smooth endoplasmic reticulum, cytochrome P450, cytochrome b_5, NADPH–cytochrome c reductase	Rat	Hepatic drug-metabolizing enzymes and ultrastructure were studied in rats after 2 hours of anaesthesia with 1 MAC halothane or ether	Smooth endoplasmic reticulum was increased by both agents in centrilobular hepatocytes. Halothane decreased cytochrome P450 and cytochrome b_5. Ether increased cytochrome P450 and cytochrome b_5. Neither agent changed NADPH–cytochrome c reductase

*A statement followed by an asterisk indicates further comment in interaction of the data by the authors of this chapter.

hydroxylated metabolites of diazepam in four patients who had been on long-term diazepam or barbiturate therapy (50). In these two studies it is possible that inhibition of the clearance of metabolites could have played a role.

Some conclusions

There are many reports documenting that anaesthesia or anaesthetic agents may alter drug availability and drug metabolism or clearance. Many drugs used for premedication (e.g. anticholinergics, phenothiazines, opioids and neurolepts) may cause changes in gastric emptying and thus in drug availability, and some (e.g. diazepam, morphine) may subsequently alter the kinetics of other drugs given later. The inhalational and intraveneous anaesthetic agents which have been studied to date may delay the absorption of drugs given intramuscularly, may delay redistribution of drugs to tissues, may cause significant reductions in the rate of delivery of drugs to the organs of drug clearance or metabolism, and may inhibit drug metabolism, active transport into renal tubules and biliary excretion. Some of these changes may persist for several hours after the termination of anaesthesia. Of the currently used inhalational agents, halothane appears to produce more profound disturbances than enflurane or isoflurane (Runciman *et al.*, 1986b), but more work is required in this area.

There is also some evidence that enzyme induction may occur in the days following anaesthesia and surgery. This is a much less consistent effect, and the changes are not as profound or as widespread as the inhibitory effects under anaesthesia. Both enzyme induction and enzyme inhibition appear to vary according to the anaesthetic agent used, the drug or metabolic pathway that is affected and the species studied.

It has been pointed out that many classic enzyme inhibitors and enzyme-inducing agents may have a biphasic effect on drug-metabolizing enzymes both *in vivo* and *in vitro*, usually causing immediate relatively short-lived inhibition and then going on to produce induction some 36–48 hours later (Kato, Chiesara and Vassanelli, 1964). It has also been pointed out that lipid-soluble drugs tend to be more potent enzyme inhibitors and inducers than water-soluble drugs. Thus it is not surprising that anaesthetic agents should have these properties.

It is difficult to propose a unifying hypothesis, on the information available to date, for a mechanism by which these effects may be mediated. It does seem that acute reductions in drug clearance are commonplace, that both reduced blood flow and metabolism play a role, and that different anaesthetic agents may have different qualitative and quantitative effects. Some influence on the macromolecular matrix in the immediate vicinity of the enzyme, or possible changes in the quaternary structure of the enzyme itself, would seem to be possible mechanisms for these effects. This view is consistent with observations that the effects are mediated through dose-dependent non-competitive mechanisms (Linde and Berman, 1971; White *et al.*, 1976).

Overall, the clinical relevance of all these observations is not yet clear. If the usual loading and maintenance doses are initiated under anaesthesia it is likely that, for many drugs, blood concentrations will be produced which are several-fold higher than those which would be produced in the same subject under normal circumstances. There is also some evidence that the relative importance of different metabolic pathways may alter under anaesthesia, and that the combination of a relative increase in production with a decrease in clearance of an active or toxic metabolite (e.g. norpethidine) may have clinically significant effects. It has been suggested that, because reports of such problems are very rare in the literature, because drugs are not identified as causing deaths in the perioperative period and because drug manufacturers usually make no mention of possible alterations in disposition under anaesthesia, there may be no significant clinical problem (Bax and Woods, 1985).

There are in fact reasons why such problems may not have been identified. First, the doses of many drugs used by anaesthetists are based on sound clinical experience which takes into account many variables such as age, pre-existing diseases, likely duration of surgery and the effects of other drugs used simultaneously. The doses of drugs which have identifiable effects are usually titrated by the anaesthetist against these effects. Secondly, if long-standing therapy of a drug with a large volume of distribution is continued through anaesthesia and surgery, large changes in clearance will produce only small changes in the blood concentration of the drug, due to the buffering effects of the large volume of distribution. Thirdly, if the blood concentration of many drugs is somewhat higher than usual for a few days, there may be no significant consequences and the situation may remain undetected.

Nevertheless, a knowledge of the likely effects of anaesthesia on drug disposition is of importance where therapy is initiated in the perioperative period with drugs with steep blood concentration–response curves and low therapeutic indices. For example, if anaesthesia has been supplemented by a pethidine infusion and naloxone has been used postoperatively, it would be valuable to know that the pethidine blood concentration may be much higher than usual, that naloxone clearance may be much lower and that renarcotization may occur considerably later than expected.

In summary, predictions about drug behaviour based on data obtained from volunteers or non-surgical patients should not be extrapolated to patients in the perioperative period. Where there is cause for concern about impending drug toxicity or poor liver and/or kidney function, regional anaesthesia should be considered whenever possible, as it has been shown to have no significant effects on the clearance or metabolism of drugs eliminated by the lungs, liver or kidneys (Mather, Runciman and Ilsley, 1980, 1982; Runciman *et al.*, 1982, 1984a–d, 1985, 1986a–c; Mather *et al.*, 1986a, b). Whilst it is likely that certain drug combinations will be identified for which special caution should be exercised, the practice of titrating dose against effects, whenever possible, will continue to remain the ideal approach.

References

Adjepon-Yamoah, K.K., Scott, D.B. and Prescott, L.F. (1973) Impaired absorption and metabolism of oral lignocaine in patients undergoing laparoscopy. *British Journal of Anaesthesia* **45**, 143–147

Arakawa, Y., Bandoh, M., Osagawara, H. *et al.* (1979) Pharmacokinetics of pentazocine in dogs under halothane anaesthesia. *Chemical and Pharmaceutical Bulletin* **27**, 2217–2220

Aune, H., Olsen, H. and Morland, J. (1981) Diethyl ether influence on the metabolism of antipyrine, paracetamol and sulphanilamide in isolated rat hepatocytes. *British Journal of Anaesthesia* **53**, 621–626

Aune, H., Bessesen, A., Olsen, H. and Morland, J. (1983) Acute effects of halothane and enflurane on drug metabolism and protein synthesis in isolated rat hepatocytes. *Acta Pharmacologica et Toxicologica* **53**, 363–368

Austin, K.L., Stapleton, J.V. and Mather, L.E. (1981) Rate of formation of norpethidine from pethidine. *British Journal of Anaesthesia* **53**, 255–258

Baekeland, F. and Greene, N.M. (1958) Effects of diethyl ether on tissue distribution and metabolism of pentobarbital in rats. *Anesthesiology* **19**, 724–732

Bastron, R.D. (1980) Renal haemodynamics and the effects of anaesthesia. In: *The Circulation in Anaesthesia. Applied Physiology and Pharmacology* (Ed. Prys-Roberts, C.), pp. 228–239. Blackwell Scientific: Oxford

Bax, N.D.S. and Woods, H.F. (1985) Effects of anaesthesia and surgery on drug kinetics and action. In: *Care of the Postoperative Surgical Patient* (Eds. Smith, J.A.R. and Watkins, J.), pp. 58–72. Butterworths: London

Bell, L.E., Slattery, J.T. and Calkins, D.F. (1985) Effects of halothane–oxygen anaesthesia on the pharmacokinetics of diazepam and its metabolites in rats. *Journal of Pharmacology and Experimental Therapeutics* **233**, 94-99

Benet, L.Z., Massoud, N. and Gambertoglio, J.G. (1984) *Pharmacokinetic Basis for Drug Treatment*. Raven Press: New York

Benowitz, N.L. and Meister, W. (1983) Pharmacokinetics in patients with cardiac failure. In: *Handbook of Clinical Pharmacokinetics* (Eds. Gibaldi, M. and Prescott, L.), section III, pp. 182–200. Adis Health Science Press: New York

Bentley, J.B., Glass, S. and Gandolfi, A.J. (1983) The influence of halothane on lidocaine pharmacokinetics in man. *Anesthesiology* **59**, A246

Berman, M.L., Green, D.C., Calverley, R.K., Smith, N.T. and Eger, E.I. II (1976) Enzyme induction by enflurane in man. *Anesthesiology* **44**, 496–500

Blaschke, T.F. (1983) Protein binding and kinetics of drugs in liver diseases. In: *Handbook of Clinical Pharmacokinetics* (Eds. Gibaldi, M. and Prescott, L.), section III, pp. 126–139. Adis Health Science Press: New York

Bombeck, C.T., Aoki, T., Smuckler, E.A. and Nyhus, L.M. (1969) Effects of halothane, ether and chloroform on the perfused bovine liver. *American Journal of Surgery* **117**, 91–107

Borel, J.D., Bentley, B.J., Nenad, R.E. and Gillespie, T.J. (1982) The infleunce of halothane on fentanyl pharmacokinetics. *Anesthesiology* **57**, A239

Boyce, J.R., Cervenko, F.W. and Wright, F.J. (1978) Effects of halothane on the pharmacokinetics of lidocaine in digitalis toxic dogs. *Canadian Anaesthetists' Society Journal* **25**, 323

Brown, B.R. (1971) The diphasic action of halothane on the oxidative metabolism of drugs by the liver. *Anesthesiology* **35**, 241–246

Brown, B.R. (1972) Effects of inhalational anesthetics on hepatic glucuronide conjugation: a study of the rat *in vitro*. *Anesthesiology* **37**, 483–488

Burney, R.G. and DiFazio, C.A. (1976) Hepatic clearance of lidocaine during N_2O anesthesia in dogs. *Anesthesia and Analgesia* **55**, 322–325

Cherksey, B.D. and Altszuler, N. (1974). On the mechanism of potentiation by morphine of thiopental sleeping time. *Pharmacology* **12**, 362–371

Cook, D.R. and Brandom, B.W. (1982) Enflurane, halothane, and isoflurane inhibit removal of 5-hydroxytryptamine from the pulmonary circulation. *Anesthesia and Analgesia* **61**, 671–675

Cooke, W.J. and Cooke, L. (1983) Effects of anesthetics on the hepatic metabolism and biliary secretion of iopanoic acid enantiomers in rat. *Journal of Pharmacology and Experimental Therapeutics* **225**, 85–93

Cousins, M.J., Skowronski, G.A. and Plummer, J.L. (1983) Anaesthesia and the kidney. *Anaesthesia and Intensive Care* **11**, 292–320

Cousins, M.J., Gourlay, G.K., Knights, K.M., Hall, P.M., Lunam, C.A. and O'Brien, P. (1982) Randomized prospective controlled study of metabolism and hepatotoxicity of halothane in man. *Anesthesiology* **57**, A223

Cullen, B.F. and Miller, M.G. (1979) Drug interactions and anesthesia: a review. *Anesthesia and Analgesia* **58**, 413–423

Dale, O., Nielsen, K., Westgaard, G. and Nilsen, O.G. (1983) Drug metabolizing enzymes in the rat after inhalation of halothane and enflurane. *British Journal of Anaesthesia* **55**, 1217–1223

DaRocha-Reis, M.G.F. and Hipolito-Reis, C. (1982) Effects of the inhalation of enflurane on hepatic microsomal enzymatic activities in the rat. *British Journal of Anaesthesia* **54**, 97–101

Denson, D.D., Myers, J.A., Watters, C. and Raj, P.P. (1982) Selective inhibition of the aromatic hydroxylation of bupivacaine by halothane. *Anesthesiology* **57**, A242

Drayer, D.E. (1983) Pharmacologically active drug metabolites. In: *Handbook of Clinical Pharmacokinetics* (Eds. Gibaldi, M. and Prescott, L.), section I, pp. 114–132. Adis Health Sciences Press: New York

Duchin, K.L. and Schrier, R.W. (1983) Interrelationship between renal haemodynamics, drug kinetics, and drug action. In: *Handbook of Clinical Pharmacokinetics* (Eds. Gibaldi, M. and Prescott, L.), section I, pp. 183–197. Adis Health Science Press: New York

Duthie, D.J.R. and Nimmo, W.S. (1985) The pharmacokinetics of fentanyl by constant rate IV infusion for pain relief after surgery. *Anesthesiology* **63**, A282

Duvaldstein, P., Mauge, F. and Desmonts, J-M. (1981) Enflurane anesthesia and antipyrine metabolism. *Clinical Pharmacology and Therapeutics* **29**, 61–64

Duvaldstein, P., Mazze, R.I., Nivoche, Y. and Desmonts J-M. (1981) Enzyme induction following surgery with halothane and neurolept anesthesia. *Anesthesia and Analgesia* **60**, 319–323

Elfstrom, J. (1979) Drug pharmacokinetics in the postoperative period. *Clinical Pharmacokinetics* **4**, 16–22

Fabre, J. and Balant, L. (1983) Renal failure, drug pharmacokinetics and drug action. In: *Handbook of Clinical Pharmacokinetics* (Eds. Gibaldi, M. and Prescott, L.), section III, pp. 212–234. Adis Health Science Press: New York

Feeley, J., Forrest, A., Gunn, A., Hamilton, W., Stevenson, I. and Crooks, J. (1980) Influence of surgery on plasma propranolol levels and protein binding. *Clinical Pharmacology and Therapeutics* **28**, 759–764

Fiserova-Bergerova, V. (1984) Inhibitory effect of isoflurane upon oxidative metabolism of halothane. *Anesthesia and Analgesia* **63**, 399–404

Fish, J.K. and Rice, S.A. (1983) Halothane inhibits metabolism of enflurane in Fischer 344 rats. *Anesthesiology* **59**, 417–420

Gelman, S., Fowler, K.C. and Smith, L.R. (1984) Liver circulation and function during isoflurane and halothane anesthesia. *Anesthesiology* **61**, 726–730

George, C.F. (1983) Drug kinetics and hepatic blood flow. In: *Handbook of Clinical Pharmacokinetics* (Eds. Gibaldi, M. and Prescott, L.), section I, pp. 97–113. Adis Health Science Press: New York

Ghoneim, M.M. and van Hamme, M.J. (1978) Pharmacokinetics of thiopentone: effects of enflurane and nitrous oxide anaesthesia and surgery. *British Journal of Anaesthesia* **50**, 1237–1242

Gordon, L., Wood, A.J.J. and Wood, M. (1985) Acute effects of halothane on drug distribution in the dog. *Anesthesia and Analgesia* **64**, 219 (abstract)

Hanew, T., Schenker, S., Meredith, C.J. and Henderson, G.I. (1984) The pharmacokinetic interaction of diethyl ether with aminopyrine in the rat. *Proceedings of the Society for Experimental Biology and Medicine* **175**, 64–69

Hede, A.R. and Post, C. (1981) Halothane inhibits the pulmonary clearance of 5-hydroxytryptamine in isolated perfused rat lungs. *Acta Pharmacologica et Toxicologica* **49**, 239–240

Hickey, R.F. and Eger, E.I. II (1980) Circulatory effects of inhaled anaesthetics. In: *The Circulation in Anaesthesia. Applied Physiology and Pharmacology* (Ed. Prys-Roberts, C.), pp. 441–457 Blackwell Scientific: Oxford

Higashi, Y., Notoji, N., Yamajo, R. and Yata, N. (1982) Effect of anesthesia on drug disposition in the rat. *Journal of Pharmacobio-Dynamics* **5**, 112–119

Holley, F.O., Ponganis, K.V. and Stanski, D.R. (1982) Effects of cardiopulmonary bypass on the pharmacokinetics of drugs. *Clinical Pharmacokinetics* **7**, 234–251

Holstein-Rathlou, N.-H., Christensen, P. and Leyssac, P.P. (1982) Effects of halothane–nitrous oxide inhalation anesthesia and inactin on overall renal and tubular function in Sprague-Dawley and Wistar rats. *Acta Physiologica Scandinavica* **114**, 193–201

Hurwitz, A. and Fischer, H.R. (1984) Effects of morphine and respiratory depression on sulfobromophthalein disposition in rats. *Anesthesiology* **60**, 537–540

Idvall, J., Aronsen, K.F., Stenberg, P. and Paalzow, L. (1983) Pharmacodynamic and pharmacokinetic interactions between ketamine and diazepam. *European Journal of Clinical Pharmacology* **24**, 337–343

Johannessen, W., Gadeholt, G. and Aarbakke, J. (1981) Effects of diethyl ether anaesthesia on the pharmacokinetics of antipyrine and paracetamol in the rat. *Journal of Pharmacy and Pharmacology* **33**, 365–368

Kanto, J. and Philajamaki, K. (1973) Interactions of diazepam and halothane in rats. *Annales Chirurgiae et Gynaecologica* **62**, 247–250

Karlin, J.M. and Kutt, H. (1970) Acute diphenylhydantoin intoxication following halothane anesthesia. *Journal of Pediatrics* **76**, 941–944

Kato, R., Chiesara, E. and Vassanelli, P. (1964) Further studies on the inhibition and stimulation of microsomal drug-metabolizing enzymes of rat liver by various compounds. *Biochemical Pharmacology* **13**, 69–83

Kehlet, H. (1984) The stress response to anaesthesia and surgery: release mechanisms and modifying factors. In: *Vasoactive amines, Clinics in Anaesthesiology* **2**(2), 315–340

Knights, K.M., Gourlay, G.K. and Cousins, M.J. (1983) Changes in rat hepatic microsomal mixed function oxidase activity following exposure to halothane. *Clinical and Experimental Pharmacology in Physiology* **10**, 655

Knights, K.M., Gourlay, G.K., Hall, P. and Cousins, M.J. (1983) The predictive value of changes in antipyrine pharmacokinetics in halothane and paracetamol induced hepatic necrosis in rats. *Research Communications in Chemical Pathology and Pharmacology* **40**, 199–216

Lehmann, A., Weski, C., Hunger, L., Heinrich, C. and Daub, D. (1982) Akute arzneimittelinteraktionen – untersuchungen bei ratte und mensch. *Anaesthesist* **31**, 221–227

Libonati, M., Malasch, E., Price, H.L., Cooperman, L.H., Baum, S. and Harp, J.R. (1973) Splanchnic circulation in man during methoxyflurane anesthesia. *Anesthesiology* **38**, 466–472

Linde, H.W. and Berman, M.L. (1971) Nonspecific stimulation of drug-metabolizing enzymes by inhalation anesthetic agents. *Anesthesia and Analgesia* **50**, 656–667

Lo, J.N. and Cumming, J.T. (1975) Interaction between sedative premedicants and ketamine in man and in isolated perfused rat livers. *Anesthesiology* **43**, 307–312.

Lockwood, G.F. and Houston, J.B. (1982) Effects of cold stress and ether stress on aminopyrine demethylation kinetics *in vivo*. *Journal of Pharmacy and Pharmacology* **34**, 777–781

Marsh, R.H.K., Spencer, R. and Nimmo, W.S. (1984) Gastric emptying and drug absorption before surgery. *British Journal of Anaesthesia* **56**, 161–164

Massarrat, S. and Massarrat, S. (1979) Transient liver deterioration induced by general anesthesia. *Acta Hepato-Gastroenterologica* **26**, 106–111

Mather, L.E. and Runciman, W.B. (1985) The physiological basis of pharmacokinetics: concepts and tools. In: *Quantitation, Modelling and Control in Anaesthesia* (Ed. Stoeckel, H.O.). Georg Thieme: Stuttgart

Mather, L.E., Runciman, W.B. and Ilsley, A.H. (1980) Cefoxitin clearance studied by physiological and compartment modelling techniques. *Clinical and Experimental Pharmacology and Physiology* **8**, 629–630

Mather, L.E., Runciman, W.B. and Ilsley, A.H. (1982) Anesthesia-induced changes in regional blood flow. Implications for drug disposition. *Regional Anesthesia* suppl. 7, S23–S33

Mather, L.E., Runciman, W.B., Ilsley, A.H., Thompson, K. and Goldin, A. (1981) Direct measurement of chlormethiazole extraction by liver, lung and kidney in man. *British Journal of Clinical Pharmacology* **12**, 319–325

Mather, L.E., Runciman, W.B., Ilsley, A.H., Carapetis, R.J. and Upton, R.N. (1986a) A sheep preparation for studying interactions between blood flow and drug disposition. V. The effects of general and spinal anaesthesia on blood flow and pethidine disposition. *British Journal of Anaesthesia* **58**, 888–896.

Mather, L.E., Runciman, W.B., Carapetis, R.J., Ilsley, A.H. and Upton, R.N. (1986b) Hepatic and renal clearances of lidocaine in conscious and anesthetized sheep. *Anesthesia and Analgesia* (in press)

Mazze, R.I. (Ed.) (1983) *Inhalational anaesthesiology. Clinics in Anaesthesiology* **1** (2), 239–524

Miller, R.D., Agoston, S., van der Pol, F., Booij, L.H.D.J. and Crul, J.F. (1979) Effect of different anaesthetics on the pharmacokinetics and pharmacodynamics of pancuronium in the cat. *Acta Anaesthesiologica Scandinavica* **23**, 285–290

Naito, H. and Gillis, C.N. (1973) Effects of halothane and nitrous oxide on removal of norepinephrine from the pulmonary circulation. *Anesthesiology* **39**, 575–580

Nies, A.S., Shand, D.G. and Wilkinson, G.R. (1976) Altered hepatic blood flow and drug disposition. *Clinical Pharmacokinetics* **1**, 135–155

Nimmo, W.S. (1983) Drugs, diseases and altered gastric emptying. In: *Handbook of Clinical Pharmacokinetics* (Eds. Gibaldi, M. and Prescott, L.), section III, pp. 1–16. Adis Health Science Press: New York

Nimmo, W.S., Thompson, P.G. and Prescott, L.F. (1981) Microsomal enzyme induction after halothane anaesthesia. *British Journal of Clinical Pharmacology* **12**, 433–434

Nishida, N. (1979) Halothane–pentazocine interaction in dogs. *Hokkaido Igaku Zasshi* **54**, 71–80

Nunn, J.F. (1984) Interaction of nitrous oxide and vitamin B_{12}. *Trends in Pharmacological Sciences* **4**, 225–228

Oikkonen, M., Rosenberg, P.H. and Neuvonen, P.J. (1984) Hepatic metabolic ability during anaesthesia. *Anaesthesia* **39**, 660–665

Pearson, G.R., Bogan, J.A. and Sanford, J. (1973) An increase in the half-life of pentobarbitone with the administration of halothane in sheep. *British Journal of Anaesthesia* **45**, 586–589

Pessayre, D., Allemand, H., Benoist, C., Afifi, F., Francois, M. and Benhamou, J-P. (1978) Effect of surgery under general anaesthesia on antipyrine clearance. *British Journal of Clinical Pharmacology* **6**, 505–513

Prys-Roberts, C.P. (1980) *The Circulation in Anaesthesia. Applied Physiology and Pharmacology*. Blackwell Scientific: Oxford

Prys-Roberts, C.P. and Hug, C.C. Jr (1984) *Pharmacokinetics of Anaesthesia*. Blackwell Scientific: Oxford

Rahn, E., Dayton, P.G. and Frederickson, E.L. (1969) Lack of effect of halothane on the metabolism of thiopentone in man. *British Journal of Anaesthesia* **41**, 503–505

Reiche, R. and Frey, H.H. (1981) Interactions between chloramphenicol and intravenous anaesthetics. *Anaesthesist* **30**, 504–507

Reilly, C.S., Wood, A.J.J., Koshakji, R. and Wood, M. (1985) The effect of halothane on drug disposition: contributions of changes in intrinsic drug metabolizing capacity and hepatic blood flow. *Anesthesiology* **63**, 70–76

Rietbrock, I., Lazarus, G. and Otterbein, A. (1972) Effect of halothane on the hepatic drug metabolizing system. *Naunyn-Schmiedeberg's Archives of Pharmacology* **273**, 422–426

Roberts, J.G. (1980) Beta-adrenergic blockade and anaesthesia with reference to interactions with anaesthetic drugs and techniques. *Anaesthesia and Intensive Care* **8**, 318–335

Ross, W.T. and Cardell, R.R. (1978) Proliferation of smooth endoplasmic reticulum and induction of microsomal drug-metabolizing enzymes after ether or halothane. *Anesthesiology* **48**, 325–331

Roth, R.A. and Wiersma, D.A. (1983) Role of the lung in total body clearance of circulating drugs. In: *Handbook of Clinical Pharmacokinetics* (Eds. Gibaldi, M. and Prescott, L.), section I, pp. 169–182. Adis Health Science Press: New York

Runciman, W.B. Ilsley, A.H., Mather, L.E., Upton, R.N. and Carapetis, R.J. (1982) A comparison of the effects of general and spinal anaesthesia on chlormethiazole kinetics in the chronically catheterised sheep. *Clinical and Experimental Pharmacology and Physiology* **9**, 399

Runciman, W.B., Ilsley, A.H., Mather, L.E., Carapetis, R.J. and Rao, M.M. (1984a) A sheep preparation for studying the interaction between blood flow and drug disposition. I. Physiological profile. *British Journal of Anaesthesia* **56**, 1015–1028

Runciman, W.B., Mather, L.E., Ilsley, A.H., Carapetis, R.J. and McLean, C.F. (1984b) A sheep preparation for studying the interaction between blood flow and drug disposition. II. Experimental applications. *British Journal of Anaesthesia* **56**, 1117–1129

Runciman, W.B., Mather, L.E., Ilsley, A.H., Carapetis, R.J. and Upton, R.N. (1984c) A sheep preparation for studying the interaction between blood flow and drug disposition. III. Effects of general and spinal anaesthesia on regional blood flow and oxygen tensions. *British Journal of Anaesthesia* **56**, 1247–1258

Runciman, W.B., Mather, L.E., Ilsley, A.H., Upton, R.N., McLean, C. and Carapetis, R. (1984d) The effects of general and spinal anaesthesia on drug clearance by lung, liver, kidney, gut and extravisceral sites. *Clinical and Experimental Pharmacology and Physiology* suppl. **8**, 68

Runciman, W.B., Mather, L.E., Ilsley, A.H., Carapetis, R.J. and Upton, R.N. (1985) A sheep preparation for studying interactions between blood flow and drug disposition. IV The effects of general and spinal anaesthesia on blood flow and cefoxitin disposition. *British Journal of Anaesthesia* **57**, 1239–1246

Runciman, W.B., Mather, L.E., Ilsley, A.H., Carapetis, R.J. and Upton, R.N. (1986a) A sheep preparation for studying interactions between blood flow and drug disposition. VI The effects of general and spinal anaesthesia on blood flow and chlormethiazole disposition. *British Journal of Anaesthesia* (in press)

Runciman, W.B., Selby, D.G., Mather, L.E., Ilsley, A.H., Carapetis, R.J. and McLean, C.F. (1986b) Duration of depression of cefoxitin elimination after general anaesthesia in the sheep. *Clinical and Experimental Pharmacology and Physiology* (in press)

Runciman, W.B., Mather, L.E., Carapetis, R.J., Ilsley, A.H. and McLean, C.F. (1986c) The effects of general anaesthesia on tocainide clearance in the sheep. *Xenobiotica* (in press)

Schuh, F.T. (1981) Influence of haemodilution of the potency of neuromuscular blocking drugs. *British Journal of Anaesthesia* **53**, 263–264

Schuttler, Z., Wilms, M., Stoeckel, H., Schwilden, H. and Lauven, P. (1983) Pharmacokinetic interaction of etomidate and fentanyl. *Anaesthesiology* **59**, A247

Sear, J.W. (Ed.) (1984) *Intravenous anaesthesiology. Clinics in Anaesthesiology* **2** (1)

Sear, J.W., Walters, F.J.M., Wilkins, D.G. and Willats, S.M. (1984) Etomidate by infusion for neuroanaesthesia. *Anaesthesia* **39**, 12–18

Selby, D.G., Carapetis, R.J., Upton, R.N. *et al*. (1985a) Duration of depression of cefoxitin renal extraction after halothane anaesthesia in the sheep. *Clinical and Experimental Pharmacology and Physiology* suppl. 9, 25

Selby, D.G., Ilsley, A.H., Runciman, W.B. and Mather, L.E. (1985b) Magnitude and duration of depression of drug clearance from halothane anaesthesia in the sheep. *Canadian Anaesthetists' Society Journal* **32**, 598

Seyde, W.C. and Longnecker, D.E. (1984) Anesthetic influences on regional hemodynamics in normal and hemorrhaged rats. *Anesthesiology* **61**, 689–698

Stanski, D.R. and Watkins, W.D. (1982) *Drug Disposition in Anesthesia*. Grune & Stratton: New York

Steffey, E.P., Howland, R., Asling, J.H., Eisele, J.H. and Hirsch, C. (1977) Meperidine–halothane interaction in dogs. *Canadian Anaesthetists' Society Journal* **24**, 459–467

Strunin, L. (1980) The splanchnic, hepatic and portal circulations. In: *The Circulation in Anaesthesia. Applied Physiology and Pharmacology* (Ed. Prys-Roberts, C.), pp. 241–251. Blackwell Scientific: Oxford

Thomsen, K. and Olesen, D.V. (1981) Effect of anaesthesia and surgery on urine flow and electrolyte excretion in different rat strains. *Renal Physiology* **4**, 165–172

Umeda, T. and Inaba, T. (1978) Effects of anesthetics on diphenylhydantoin metabolism in the rat: possible inhibition by diethyl ether. *Canadian Journal of Physiology and Pharmacology* **56**, 241–244

Upton, R.N., Mather, L.E., Runciman, W.B. and Nancarrow, C. (1986) The use of arteriovenous drug concentration differences for the model independent description of drug fluxes between organs and blood and the calculation of organ drug concentrations. *Clinical and Experimental Pharmacology and Physiology* (in press)

Vermeulen, N.P., Danhof, M., Setiawan, I. and Breimer, D.D. (1983) Disposition of hexabarbital in the rat. Estimation of first-pass elimination and influence of ether anesthesia. *Journal of Pharmacology and Experimental Therapeutics* **226**, 201–205

White, P.F., Marietta, M.P., Pudwill, C.R., Way, W.L. and Trevor, A.J. (1976) Effects of halothane anesthesia on the biodisposition of ketamine in rats. *Journal of Pharmacology and Experimental Therapeutics* **196**, 545–555

Wood, M. and Wood, A.J.J. (1982a) Contrasting effects of inhalational anesthetics on *in vivo* drug metabolism. *Anesthesiology* **57**, A245

Wood, M. and Wood, A.J.J. (1982b) *Drugs and Anesthesia*. Williams & Wilkins: Baltimore, MD

Wood, M. and Wood, A.J.J. (1984) Contrasting effects of halothane, isoflurane and enflurane on *in vivo* drug metabolism in the rat. *Anesthesia and Analgesia* **63**, 709–714

Wood, M., Shand, D.G. and Wood, A.J.J. (1979) Propranolol binding in plasma during cardiopulmonary bypass. *Anesthesiology* **51**, 512–517

Part two
Specific Mechanisms of Action

5

Hypnotics

Walter S. Nimmo

Hypnotics are drugs which produce sleep. Since earliest recorded history, man has sought sleep (and release into hallucinatory states) by means of drugs and alcohol. The Aztecs of South America used sacred mushrooms; orientals used cannabis and opium, and one of the most popular of all naturally occurring drugs to induce sleep was hyoscine obtained from the root of the mandrake.

Until the mid nineteenth century, remarkably little attention had been given by pharmacologists or doctors to the subject of sleep, but the use of chloral hydrate at that time as the first synthetic hypnotic has been followed by the synthesis of many different types of hypnotic drugs, much research into their actions and a phenomenal increase in their usage.

Neurotransmitters and sleep

Sleep is a state of low general vigilance with reduced activity and reactivity. However, this low general activity is not spread equally throughout all the functions of the organism: for example, circulation and respiration react similarly while asleep or awake whereas mental and sensory motor functions perform at severely impaired rates during sleep. Thus sleep is a state characterized by a set of generally but unequally reduced and discrete vigilances.

Sleep is not a constant state. It fluctuates both qualitatively and quantitatively. The familiar rapid eye movement (REM) sleep is characterized by dreams in contrast to orthodox or non-rapid eye movement (NREM) sleep. Thus sleep can be defined as a state of regularly changing (generally but not uniformly), low vigilance profiles.

It is convenient to look on the state of sleep or vigilance as the manifestation of the interaction of two opposing forces. The 'sleep system' involves the nucleus of the solitary tract, the medial thalamus, the basal forebrain and parts of the limbic system. A special system including parts of the pontine tegmentum is involved in REM sleep. The opposing forces or 'waking system' are located mainly in the brainstem reticular formation, its ascending and descending projections and, to some extent, in the limbic system.

This concept recognizes sleep to be a decrease in activity of the waking system *and* an increase in activity in the sleep system. There is some evidence for a mutually inhibiting feedback between the two systems (Koella, 1981).

In a similar fashion to other opposing forces within the central nervous system (e.g. sympathetic and parasympathetic systems, cholinergic and dopaminergic pathways), it seems likely that each neuronal system is characterized by its own transmitter substance although it is quite clear that there is no specific 'sleep transmitter' or 'waking transmitter'. Nevertheless, a considerable number of neurotransmitters have been shown to be involved in the adjustment of the level of various discrete vigilances.

5-Hydroxytryptamine (5HT, serotonin)

Injection of 5HT into the fourth ventricle of cats induces sleep which appears in two distinct phases. Shortly after injection, sleep occurs for a period of 30 minutes and is followed by a short period of wakefulness. Sleep then ensues for at least 8 hours. REM sleep occurs during this period. 5HT crosses the blood–brain barrier slowly. However, intravenous injection of 5HT precursors enhances slow wave sleep in cats and rabbits. In humans, L-tryptophan (a 5HT precursor) in small doses enhances slow wave sleep and in high doses it increases the amount of REM sleep (Williams, 1971).

In contrast, inhibition of 5HT synthesis by the tryptophan hydroxylase inhibitor p-chlorophenylalanine produces a dose-dependent drop in brain 5HT and a dose-dependent reduction of total sleep in cats. Slow wave sleep and REM sleep are affected equally. The effect on sleep is of very long duration and 3–4 weeks may elapse before sleep returns to control values. 5HT precursors antagonize this effect. Sleep returns to normal before the 5HT concentrations do, and if the inhibitor of 5HT synthesis is given 'chronically', sleep will still return to normal, suggesting a negative feedback mechanism.

The 5HT content of the brain may vary with the level of locomotor activity each day. In experiments in rodents, concentrations are highest at the end of a period of high activity.

Noradrenaline (NA)

Using a variety of methods of increasing brain NA pharmacologically it is known that NA has a central activating effect. For example, amphetamine releases catecholamines and produces arousal which can be demonstrated by behaviour and the EEG. This is inhibited by inhibitors of catecholamine synthesis.

Inhibition of catecholamine synthesis on its own induces a state of sedation. Clonidine, a central α_2-agonist, reduces NA release and has a sedating effect. It reduces REM sleep (Leppavuori and Putkonen, 1980).

Dopamine

Dopaminergic stimulation results in increased motor activity. The effect of dopamine injected into the brain of rats is inhibited by imipramine, which suggests that dopamine's activity may result from its incorporation into neurons to be converted to NA.

Acetylcholine (ACh)

Intravenous injection of ACh or a cholinomimetic such as nicotine or physostigmine is followed by electrocortical activation and arousal of the animal. Application of ACh to the ascending tegmentoforebrain produces arousal whilst the intraventricular injection of ACh induces behavioral and slow electrographic sleep. Brainstem neurons, whose activity is necessary for the induction of atonia and REM sleep, are probably cholinergic in nature. Cholinergic antagonists and agonists may both suppress cholinergic transmission – the former through receptor antagonism and the latter through an 'overload' effect. Atropine suppresses REM sleep in cats and rabbits. Hemicholinium, an inhibitor of ACh synthesis, reduces waking and suppresses REM sleep.

γ-Aminobutyric acid (GABA)

GABA is one of the major inhibitory substances within the brain. It has a role in the metabolism of brain cells and thus is distributed widely throughout nervous tissue. It is released from nervous tissue on electrical stimulation of the brain surface but removal of calcium ions prevents this release.

The effect of GABA is predominantly to produce postsynaptic hyperpolarization at synapses in the cerebral cortex, hippocampus and the cerebellum. This in turn results from an increased chloride conductance of the postsynaptic membrane.

Antagonists of GABA-ergic transmission such as picrotoxin or bicuculline produce generalized seizures. The role of GABA in the mode of action of hypnotics will be discussed later.

Polypeptides

Vasotocin, a nonapeptide found in the pineal gland, produces sleep when injected into the third ventricle of cats, and REM sleep is completely suppressed while slow wave sleep occurs. However, vasopressin and oxytocin do not seem to affect sleep. Some polypeptides are involved with waking; for example, D-ala-met-enkephalinamide (DALA) injected to the brain of rats increases locomotor activity – the effect is antagonized by naloxone. In mice and rats, thyrotropic-hormone-releasing factor (TRH, a tripeptide) reverses the depressant effects of pentobarbitone, and in man it has some antidepressant effects.

Knowledge of these various transmitters has allowed a better understanding of the influence of some drugs on sleep and, at times, an identification of the mode of action of hypnotics. However, precise mechanisms remain unclear for many substances.

Classification of hypnotics

Older hypnotics include choral hydrate, inorganic bromides and paraldehyde. Shortly after the beginning of this century, the barbiturates were introduced

Table 5.1   Classification and examples of hypnotics

Chemical class	Examples
	Chloral hydrate
	Bromide
	Paraldehyde
Barbiturates	Thiopentone
	Methohexitone
	Phenobarbitone
Acylureas	Carbromal
Carbamates	Ethinamate
Piperidinediones	Glutethimide
	Methylprylone
Acetylenic carbinols	Methylpentynol
Benzodiazepines	Diazepam
	Midazolam
Imidazole derivative	Etomidate
Phencyclidine derivative	Ketamine
Phenols	Propofol

and were popular for many years. Newer non-barbiturate hypnotics belong to a variety of chemical classes: acylureas, carbamates, piperidinedione, carbinols and benzodiazepines (Table 5.1). The benzodiazepines are the most popular.

Older hypnotics

Chloral hydrate is converted rapidly in the body to trichlorethanol, which is probably the active metabolite. It has been shown not to disturb the balance of REM and NREM sleep but little information is available. Chloral hydrate itself has some anticholinesterase activity but trichlorethanol does not have this property.

Bromide salts were used first to depress the central nervous system in the treatment of epilepsy and later were used as hypnotics. They are given orally as the sodium or potassium salts and act by replacing the chloride ion; peripheral tissues are less sensitive to this replacement than brain tissue. The exchange increases with repeated doses, and toxicity accompanies accumulation of the drug.

Paraldehyde is a cyclic ether which is toxic to nerves if placed near them. It has many problems and is seldom used.

Barbiturates

Barbituric acid is obtained from the condensation of malonic acid and urea (Fig. 5.1). All barbiturates used clinically are substituted water-soluble salts of barbituric acid and the chemical structures are given in Fig. 5.2. Barbituric acid itself is not a central nervous system depressant, and substitution of the hydrogens on the carbon atom at position 5 with alkyl or aryl groups is essential

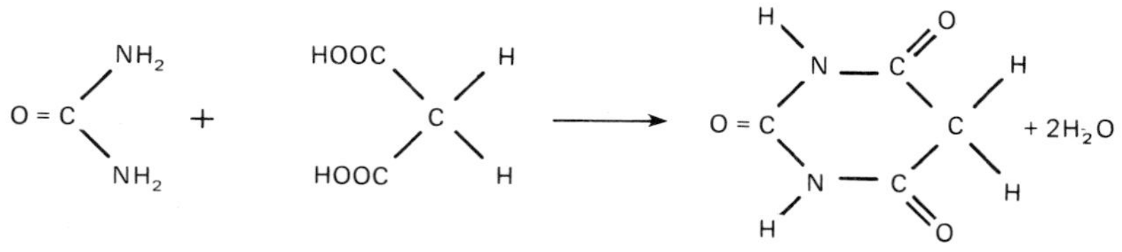

Fig. 5.1   Structure of barbituric acid.

for hypnotic or sedative activity. Both hydrogen atoms must be substituted and the two side chains are usually different.

A phenyl group on C5 or one of the nitrogens of the barbituric acid ring gives the drug anticonvulsant properties. Increasing the length of one or both of the alkyl side chains at C5 increases hypnotic potency until the side chains are increased to five or six carbons when hypnotic activity is reduced and convulsant properties may result.

Compounds with branched chains on C5 have a short duration of action. If the groups on C5 are derived from secondary alcohols and have unsaturated bonds, depressant potency is increased.

The substitution of a methyl or ethyl group on N1 often results in a more rapid onset of action and more rapid recovery but at the same time may result in excitatory effects such as tremor and muscle movements.

If the oxygen on C2 is replaced with sulphur, more rapid onset and shorter duration of action occur.

Barbiturates are general depressants. In large doses, they depress the activity of all cells in addition to neurons. However, nervous tissue is sensitive to barbiturate activity and, in normal doses, direct actions on other tissues are negligible.

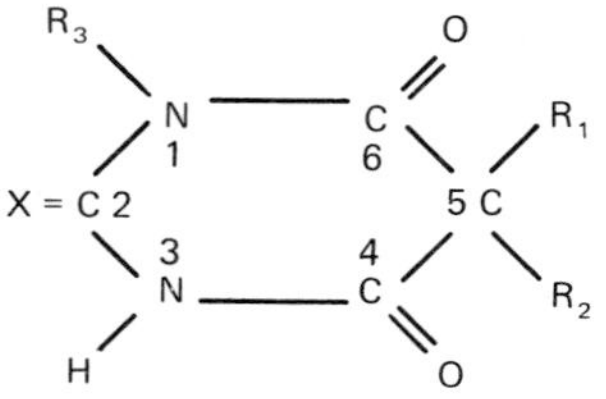

Drug	R_1	R_2	R_3	X
Phenobarbitone	ethyl	phenyl	H	O
Thiopentone	ethyl	1-methylbutyl	H	S
Methohexitone	allyl	1-methyl-2 pentynyl	CH_3	O

Fig. 5.2   Structures of barbiturates used clinically.

Barbiturates induce sleep probably by depressing the reticular activating system of the brainstem but other regions are affected also. Small doses depress monosynaptic pathways in the spinal cord. Although they depress conduction in axons, in the smallest effective doses their action is confined to synapses. At synapses, they first depress postsynaptic sensitivity to chemical transmitters and in larger doses they act presynaptically to impair the release of chemical transmitters.

In the central nervous system, barbiturates depress the responses of single neurons to ACh, 5HT, NA and glutamate. They also inhibit the release of ACh from the surface of the cortex and increase ACh concentrations within the brain. Some barbiturates increase GABA concentrations.

Multisynaptic pathways are depressed more readily than are pathways with few synapses (e.g. dorsal columns and medial lemnisci). The repetitive after-discharges of the reticular activating system in response to a single stimulus is depressed by barbiturates in very small doses. In larger doses they enhance presynaptic inhibition in the spinal cord and brain.

In isolated axons, barbiturates exert a membrane-stabilizing action. They increase the threshold to electrical stimulation, delay the increase in permeability to sodium ions, decrease sodium and potassium conductance, reduce the action potential amplitude and slow the rate of conduction. There is little change in resting membrane potential.

It seems likely that barbiturates (which are weak acids) enter the membrane in their non-ionized form and, once in the membrane, a proportion of the molecules become ionized and active within the cell (this is similar to the mode of action of local anaesthetic drugs). Membrane-stabilizing properties occur at higher barbiturate concentrations than are found in clinical use but it is possible that lower concentrations stabilize the pre- and postsynaptic membranes at synapses.

Again in high concentrations, barbiturates depress dehydrogenase enzymes involved in glucose oxidation and reduce the formation of energy-rich phosphates. During deep barbiturate-induced anaesthesia, brain oxygen consumption is decreased but with light anaesthesia it is affected very little.

The initial effect of barbiturate administration is clouding of consciousness accompanied by fast activity in the EEG, due probably to the drug depressing preferentially the medullary sleep centres. As consciousness is lost, the EEG becomes synchronized into large amplitude waves of low frequency (2–8 Hz) which resemble those of natural sleep. Barbiturates disturb the balance of the phases of sleep. With regular administration the proportion of REM sleep each night is reduced but then returns to normal with continued administration. When the drug is withdrawn, there is a rebound increase in the proportion of REM sleep and this continues for many nights. The patient experiences nightmares and feels he is sleeping badly. This type of interference with the normal phases of sleep is an important factor in the development of tolerance and dependence.

In small doses, barbiturates may increase sensitivity to pain and produce restlessness.

Many differences between various barbiturates can be explained on differences in lipid solubility and pharmacokinetic properties.

Table 5.2   Benzodiazepines in clinical practice

Drug	Active metabolites
Diazepam	Desmethyldiazepam Oxazepam Temazepam
Chlorazepate	Desmethyldiazepam
Prazepam	Desmethyldiazepam
Clonazepam	
Clobazam	Desmethylclobazam
Bromazepam	
Chlordiazepoxide	Desmethylchlordiazepoxide Demoxepam Desoxydemoxepam
Lorazepam	
Oxazepam	
Nitrazepam	
Flurazepam	Desalkylflurazepam
Flunitrazepam	7-Amino derivative Desmethyl derivative
Temazepam	
Triazolam	7-Hydroxy derivative
Midazolam	

Benzodiazepines

The most popular hypnotics in current use are the benzodiazepine compounds. Examples of this series are given in Table 5.2

These drugs exert anxiolytic, sedative, amnesic, anticonvulsant and central muscle relaxant activity as well as hypnotic actions. All of them possess a similar spectrum of activity but differ in the degree to which they produce the various effects.

The mechanism of action of benzodiazepines has been investigated and is presented in greater detail in Chapter 10. This information suggests a primary involvement of several neurotransmitters such as 5HT, NA and ACh. Electrophysiological studies have indicated that GABA is involved and, more recently, it seems that the drugs exert their actions by interacting with specific benzodiazepine receptors on the nerve cell membranes in the central nervous system (Braestrup and Nielsen, 1980).

Brain tissue binds benzodiazepines specifically. The highest degree of binding is found in cortical areas but there is some binding also in the amygdala and frontal cortex. There is a good correlation between the drug's affinity for these binding sites and its potency. No other drug or putative neurotransmitter binds significantly to these receptors.

Benzodiazepines enhance the inhibitory effect of GABA on neurons in the spinal cord where GABA mediates presynaptic inhibition and on neurons in the cuneate nucleus where GABA mediates both pre- and postsynaptic inhibition. Interaction between GABA receptors and benzodiazepine receptors can be shown at molecular level. GABA and all GABA agonists change the formation of GABA receptors and cause the chloride channels to open (hyperpolarization). The affinity of benzodiazepine receptors is thus increased.

Partial GABA agonists are often rigid molecules and thus produce less conformational change in the GABA receptor, so the benzodiazpine receptors are not fully activated while the chloride channels may open. Picrotoxin antagonizes GABA by a direct action on the chloride channels and thus does not interfere directly with the GABA/benzodiazepine interaction.

GABA-modulin is a protein which may be responsible for another interaction between benzodiazepine receptors and GABA receptors. GABA-modulin is present in brain and is a competitive inhibitor of both GABA receptor and benzodiazpine receptors. Benzodiazepines may increase the affinity of GABA receptors by displacing GABA-modulin from the receptor complex.

The identification of benzodiazepine receptors has, of course, led to a search for endogenous ligands analogous to the enkephalins. These ligands might represent a neurotransmitter or a neuromodulator. This search has had some success and several endogenous substances active at benzodiazepine receptors have been identified. In addition, a specific benzodiazpine antagonist has been synthesized and is undergoing clinical trials before being available for general use.

As for the barbiturates, many of the differences between the benzodiazepines may be explained on their pharmacokinetic differences.

The mode of action of other hypnotics and intravenous anaesthetic agents is less well identified, partly as a result of their use by a single bolus dose rather than in chronic therapy. Great strides have been made in drug analysis and in pharmacokinetic knowledge but much work remains to be done in elucidating their mode of action.

References

Braestrup, C. and Nielsen, M. (1980) Benzodiazepine receptors. *Arzneimittel-Forschung* **30**, 852–857

Koella, W.P. (1981) Neurotransmitters and sleep. In: *Psychopharmacology of Sleep* (Ed. Wheatley, D.), pp. 19–52. Raven Press: New York

Leppavuori, A. and Putkonen, P.T.S. (1980) Alpha-adrenoceptive influences on the control of the sleep–waking cycle in the cat. *Brain Research* **193**, 95–115

Williams, H.L. (1971) The new biology of sleep. *Journal of Psychiatric Research* **8**, 445–478

6

General anaesthetics

Keith W. Miller

General anaesthesia is caused by a wide range of substances which are administered at high concentrations and gain access to all parts of the body. They exert actions on peripheral organs, such as the neuromuscular junction and the heart, as well as on their primary target(s) in the central nervous system (CNS). The CNS is extremely complex and our rudimentary understanding of its physiology has prevented elucidation of how general anaesthetics reversibly depress consciousness. Faced with this ignorance two primary strategies have been employed to reveal the underlying molecular mechanisms. The first strategy is a pharmacological one which seeks information from the relative potencies of general anaesthetics in intact animals. The second strategy is to study the action of anaesthetics on accessible and well-defined structures which provide model systems whereby mechanisms may be discovered. Such mechanisms may be unique to the system studied or may occur more generally. In the latter case the mechanism may be related to that which causes general anaesthesia at some unknown site.

The fact that the mechanisms responsible for maintaining consciousness have resisted the efforts of physiologists leaves pharmacologists in a rather familiar position. Their response to such a situation is to study the molecular nature of the molecules having a common action and to deduce the complementary structure which will interact with such molecules – the 'lock and key' analogy. Information about mechanisms may also be deduced, especially if antagonists are available. Such an approach has led to breakthroughs in our knowledge in other fields. For example, studies of opiate action suggested the existence of opiate receptors, a hypothesis which was confirmed when naloxone-binding sites were found in the CNS and shown to interact with the same drugs as the putative opiate receptors. What were these opiate receptors for? The answer to this question came with the discovery by Hughes, Kosterlitz and their co-workers (Hughes *et al.*, 1975) of the existence of endogenous peptides which mimicked the action of opiates.

The phenomenon of general anaesthesia can be brought about by a remarkable range of substances – from the inert gas xenon to the steroid Althesin (Fig. 6.1) – suggesting that no single, structurally specific receptor for general anaesthetics exists. Given this, there are two possible overall classes of mechanisms which might give rise to anaesthesia. The first mechanism assumes that a non-specific locus of action is involved, one with which general

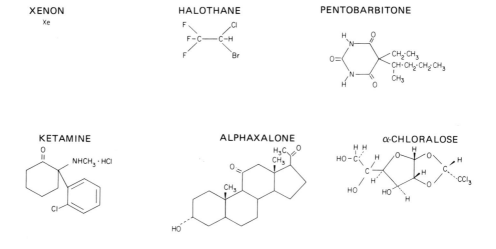

Fig. 6.1 The structures of some general anaesthetics. (Reproduced, with permission, from Janoff and Miller, 1982.)

anaesthetics of all molecular classes can interact. For example, the lipid bilayer of neuronal membranes would provide such a site. This is consistent with there being no known chemical antagonist of general anaesthesia and leads to the so-called unitary hypothesis, which states that a single molecular mechanism underlies general anaesthesia. The second mechanism assumes that there are a number of different ways of causing general anaesthesia. For example, one structural class of anaesthetic might act on a binding site on a protein in one region of the brain and another structural class on a differently shaped protein site elsewhere in the brain. Alternatively, one protein might possess a number of different binding sites, each capable of interacting with one structural class of general anaesthetic. This has been called the degenerate perturbation hypothesis of general anaesthetic action (Richards, 1980).

The first mechanism is the most attractive, but we shall see below that general anaesthetics can exert both types of action. This should not be too surprising when one considers the high concentrations at which general anaesthetics are administered and the number of side effects they exert. Indeed, it is not controversial that general anaesthetics act by several mechanisms; what is controversial is whether general anaesthesia *per se* is produced by a mechanism consistent with the unitary or with the degenerate perturbation hypothesis. Until these questions are resolved a reasonable position to take is that there is a single class of sites (perhaps in lipid bilayers) where all general anaesthetics act to cause general anaesthesia and perhaps some pharmacologically unspecific side effects, and that there is another class of sites (most probably on proteins) which interacts only with selected general anaesthetics and which mediates their non-anaesthetic actions. This is a hopeful situation because, if different mechanisms are involved in central and some peripheral actions, it may be possible when seeking new anaesthetics to design out undesirable side effects.

The pharmacology of general anaesthesia

All theories of general anaesthesia are based on relative potency data obtained in animals. Considerable effort has been expended to obtain reliable data free of such experimental artefacts as might arise from failure adequately to control such variables as temperature, partial pressure of carbon dioxide and so on (J.C. Miller and Miller, 1975; Quasha, Eger and Tinker, 1980). The potency of an anaesthetic is measured by determining whether an animal does or does not respond to a well-defined stimulus. Two end-points have been commonly used: the ability of an animal either to right itself when turned over (the righting reflex) or to respond with a gross purposeful, rather than reflex, movement to a *painful* stimulus, usually a tail clamp. The righting reflex has been used with small animals, mainly mice, which equilibrate rapidly with the anaesthetic and allow large numbers to be tested conveniently. Concentration–response curves can be obtained readily and potency is defined as ED_{50}, the concentration at which half the animals have lost their righting reflex. The slope of this curve provides a good check that the experiment was well controlled. On the other hand, the tail clamp has been employed with large mammals where the physiological state can be monitored easily. However, equilibration with inspired anaesthetic is slow and the alveolar anaesthetic concentration must be determined. Consequently, Eger and his colleagues have called this end-point 'MAC' for minimum alveolar concentration required to just prevent response. Their data are usually presented as an average of individual MACs, thus throwing away the useful check provided by the slope of the concentration–response curve.

Obviously potency will depend, up to a point, on the strength of the applied stimulus. For example, 0.66% halothane abolishes purposeful response to electrical stimulation at 10 volts, but 0.84% is required for 50 volts (Eger, Saidman and Brandstater, 1965). It follows that potency might appear to vary if the *perceived* stimulus changed. For example, MAC involves a painful stimulus so that variable *analgesic* potency in a group of anaesthetics might introduce an artefact into their relative anaesthetic potencies. Comparison of righting reflex with MAC suggests that considerations of this sort introduce an uncertainty which does not exceed a factor of 2 (Deady *et al.*, 1981; Kissin, Morgan and Smith, 1983), but if a wider range of anaesthetics, including barbiturates and steroids, is considered the uncertainty can approach a factor of 10 (Paton, 1974).

Table 6.1 summarizes some representative data for gaseous and volatile general anaesthetics. More extensive information can be found in the reviews referenced in the above paragraphs and in Firestone, Miller and Miller (1986). Such data are the touchstone against which theories of general anaesthesia are judged. It is obviously desirable to include anaesthetics from a wider variety of structural classes, but these are often intravenous agents which have complex pharmacokinetics (Fig. 6.1). To circumvent the pharmacokinetic problem, workers have traditionally turned to the tadpole. The drug

Table 6.1　The anaesthetic potency of some representative agents

	Chemical formula	Anaesthetic partial pressure (% of atm)	
		MAC in man	ED_{50} for loss of righting reflexes in mice
Halothane	$CF_3.CHClBr$	0.77	0.77
Isoflurane	$CF_3.CHCl.O.CHF_2$	1.15	0.57
Enflurane	$CHF_2.O.CHCl.CF_3$	1.68	2.0
Diethyl ether	$(C_2H_5)_2O$	1.92	3.0
Cyclopropane	C_3H_6	9.2	15
Xenon	Xe	71	95
Nitrous oxide	N_2O	105	140
Nitrogen	N_2	–	3800

concentration in the water bathing this small animal can be easily controlled. General anaesthetics gain access to the brain rapidly, inducing a stable level of anaesthesia and providing an accurate index of potency for every class of anaesthetic. Although the clinician may prefer to deal with mammals (indeed this is essential for detailed physiological studies), fortunately general anaesthetic potency varies little with the species employed (Quasha, Eger and Tinker, 1980).

The general anaesthetic potency data available for tadpoles have been tabulated recently (Firestone, Miller and Miller, 1986). Potency does not differ significantly from that in mammals (compare nitrogen in Tables 6.1 and 6.2). One feature which is immediately apparent is that although the concentration required to cause general anaesthesia varies over a wide range it rarely falls below 10 μmol/l. These are not very potent agents; for comparison most opiates are active at concentrations between 1 nmol/l and 1μ mol/l.

The normal alcohols increase in potency (i.e. concentration causing anaesthesia falls) as the number of carbon atoms increases, but this trend does not proceed unabated. Tridecanol is paradoxically less potent than dodecanol, and tetradecanol is totally devoid of activity. This is the so-called cut-off phenomenon noted by Ferguson (1939). It occurs in other homologous series (e.g. the alkanes and the fluorocarbons) and is not just a function of size. Note that putting a double bond between the ninth and tenth carbon of tetradecanol to form tetradecenol restores anaesthetic activity, postponing the cut-off by three carbons (Pringle, Brown and Miller, 1981).

Tridecanol is an example of what Paton (1974) termed a partial anaesthetic; even in a saturated solution only 70 per cent of the animals were anaesthetized (Pringle, Brown and Miller, 1981). Other examples are hexadecenol, perfluoropropane, some opiates and tetrahydrocannabinol.

Geometric isomers sometimes have equal potency (e.g. the *cis* and *trans* isomers of tetradecenol) and sometimes have unequal potency (e.g. β-chloralose and Betaxolone, analogues of agents shown in Fig. 6.1) and are without activity.

Optical isomers generally have equal potency; for example *d* and *l*-halothane

Table 6.2   Anaesthetic potency in tadpoles

Agent	ED_{50} for loss of righting reflexes	Agent	ED_{50} for loss of righting reflexes
Ethanol	190 mmol/l	Helium	Not anaesthetic
Butanol	12 mmol/l	Neon	Not anaesthetic
Hexanol	700 μmol/l	Argon	24 atm
Octanol	60 μmol/l	Hydrogen	198 atm
Decanol ·	13 μmol/l	Nitrogen	42 atm
Dodecanol	5 μmol/l		
Tridecanol	37 μmol/l		
Tetradecanol	Not anaesthetic		
cis-Tetradecenol	30 μmol/l		
trans-Tetradecenol	30 μmol/l		

(Kendig, Trudell and Cohen, 1973). Some intravenous agents may show modest stereoselectivity (Ryder, Way and Trevor, 1978) but it is difficult to exclude that this results from differential metabolism.

Although theories of general anaesthesia must primarily aim at accounting for the large variation in potency between different agents, superimposed on this are small variations, rarely exceeding a factor of 2, which can be induced in the potency of a given agent by various manipulations (Quasha, Eger and Tinker, 1980). One of the most influential of these in mechanistic studies has been the so-called pressure reversal of anaesthesia.

Pressure reversal of anaesthesia

First discovered in tadpoles by Johnson and Flagler (1950), it has since been demonstrated in many vertebrate species. Figure 6.2 shows dose–response curves for phenobarbitone, which is very long acting in mice and yields a stable level of anaesthesia. As the total pressure is raised with the non-anaesthetic gas helium, the dose–response curve is progressively displaced to the right (much higher pressures than this cause profound effects of their own). The effect is quite dramatic because the concentration–response curves are so steep. The group of mice anaesthetized with 140 mg/kg have all lost their righting reflexes at 2 atm, but have all regained them at 100 atm. However, the actual shift in ED_{50} over this range is less than a factor of 2 (Miller and Wilson, 1978).

Pressure reversal of anaesthesia has been demonstrated with all general anaesthetics studied. The degree of pressure reversal may vary among intravenous agents or this may be a pharmacokinetic artefact – unfortunately, in many studies dose–response curves have not been presented (for a review, see Dluzewski, Halsey and Simmonds, 1983).

Studies in mammals require a non-anaesthetic gas to be used to elevate the pressure. This leaves open the question whether pressure or helium is responsible for pressure reversal. Figure 6.3 shows the results of experiments

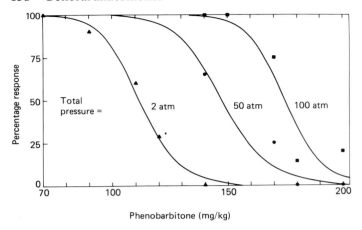

Fig. 6.2 The pressure reversal of anaesthesia in mice. Groups of 14 mice injected intraperitoneally with phenobarbitone were exposed to high pressures of the non-anaesthetic gas helium in the presence of 1 atm of oxygen. The percentage of animals with intact righting reflexes is given on the ordinate and the dose on the abscissa.

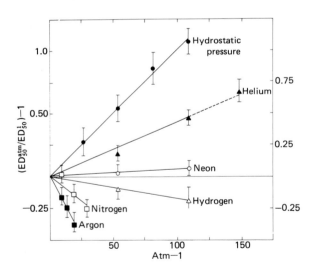

Fig. 6.3 The anaesthetic concentration (ED$_{50}$) of urethane is changed by raising the pressure on tadpoles swimming in a pressure bomb. This change is expressed by the ratio on the ordinate. For example, the ED$_{50}$ of urethane at 110 atm hydrostatic pressure is twice that at 1 atm. Thus hydrostatic and helium pressure reduce the potency of urethane (the pressure reversal effect), whilst neon does not change it and the anaesthetic gases hydrogen, nitrogen and argon increase urethane's potency. Atm − 1 = absolute pressure in atmospheres minus 1; thus ambient pressure is represented as zero. (Reproduced, with permission, from Dobson, Furmaniuk and Miller, 1985.)

with tadpoles which answer this question. $ED_{50}s$ for urethane (ethyl carbamate) were determined in a pressure bomb filled with urethane solutions at 1 atm and at a number of pressures up to 110 atm. The ED_{50} of urethane doubled over this range. When a space was left in the bomb and it was pressurized with a gas, which was allowed to dissolve in the remaining solution, the degree of pressure reversal decreased. The anaesthetic gases argon and nitrogen, not surprisingly, decreased the ED_{50} of urethane. However, although helium pressure increased the ED_{50} of urethane relative to the 1 atm value, it *decreased* the ED_{50} relative to the control value at the same *hydrostatic* pressure. Thus helium actually contributes an anaesthetic effect of its own – if only we could induce it to dissolve without having to raise the pressure, it would be an anaesthetic.

Is pressure reversal of any mechanistic significance? It could arise from an indirect physiological stimulation or from a direct antagonism of the anaesthetic's primary action. Many theories of general anaesthesia boldly assume that the latter is true and that those sites where pressure reversal of anaesthesia occurs are more probable sites for general anaesthetic action than sites where pressure reversal is not observed. Consistent with this, the effect of urethane on both the motor and the sensory responsiveness of the CNS was reversed by pressure (Angel *et al.*, 1980). Kendig and Grossman (1986) have reviewed other studies recently. They conclude that pressure reversal of anaesthetic-induced block of axonal conduction, which occurs at the level of sodium channel inactivation, shares some of the features of pressure reversal *in vivo*. However, at a number of other sites, notably the nicotinic acetylcholine receptor, pressure reversal was not observed. Those sites where pressure reversal of anaesthesia occurs are more probable sites for general anaesthetic action than sites where pressure reversal is not observed. A contrary view, based on recent studies in shrimp, is taken by Smith, Bowser-Riley and Daniels (1986).

Physical theories based on solvent models

Physical theories of general anaesthesia attempt to define the nature of the site with which general anaesthetics interact by examining correlations between physical properties and anaesthetic potency. The physical principles involved are outside the scope of this chapter, but have been reviewed in some detail elsewhere (Miller and Smith, 1973; Miller, 1974). The basic idea is to find a model where the configuration of the molecules surrounding the anaesthetic resembles closely that between the anaesthetic and its real, but unknown, site of action. When these conditions are fulfilled a good correlation will result. Unfortunately, many physical properties correlate with one another, and this fact has allowed many meaningless correlations to be proposed over the years. As a general rule, any correlation which includes only volatile anaesthetics must be regarded with suspicion (Miller, 1986). Luckily, it has been found that inclusion of a wider range of inhaled agents, particularly fully fluorinated gases such as carbon tetrafluoride and sulphur hexafluoride, destroys many spurious correlations (Miller and Smith, 1973; J.C. Miller and Miller, 1975; Koblin and

Eger, 1981). One of the correlations which survives such destructive testing is that with lipid solubility.

From the beginning the lipid solubility of general anaesthetics was invoked to explain their action (reviewed in Dluzewski, Halsey and Simmonds, 1983). Meyer and Overton at the turn of the century independently put forward the lipid hypothesis of general anaesthetic action. In a lecture in New York, Meyer (1906) stated 'The narcotizing substance enters into a loose physico-chemical combination with the vitally important lipoids of the cell, perhaps with the lethicin, and in so doing changes their normal relationship to the other cell constituents . . .'. The concept of the cell membrane had not yet emerged so Meyer used solubility in olive oil to support his hypothesis. The hypothesis can be written

$$C^{50} = S \cdot P^{50} \tag{6.1}$$

where C^{50} is the concentration in lipid (or olive oil) at anaesthesia, S is the anaesthetic's solubility in lipid when its partial pressure is 1 atm and P^{50} is the partial pressure of anaesthetic which anaesthetizes half a group of animals. Taking logarithms and rearranging leads to the test shown in Fig. 6.4, which illustrates that the correlation holds over five orders of magnitude of anaesthetic potency and includes the critical fully fluorinated gases. Systematic studies reveal that solubility in octanol, but not in alkanes, also provides a good correlation with potency (Miller, Wilson and Smith, 1978; Franks and Lieb,

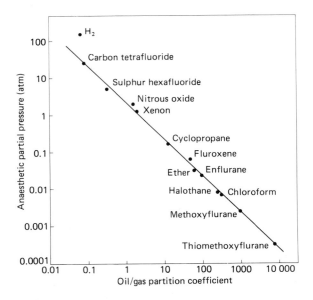

Fig. 6.4 Anaesthetic potency correlates with oil solubility. Anaesthetic partial pressure in mammals (MAC, see text) correlates over a 73 300-fold range of potency with the olive oil/gas partition coefficient at 37°C. The concentration in oil for each anaesthetic at its MAC averages 0.1 mol/l. Hydrogen deviates from the correlation because of the pressure reversal effect. (Redrawn with permission from Tanifuji, Eger and Terrell, 1977.)

1982). Thus we can conclude that the site of action of general anaesthesia is relatively, but not completely, non-polar in nature.

The lipid solubility hypothesis (Fig. 6.4) says that general anaesthesia occurs when the concentration of any lipid-soluble compound reaches a value of about 100 mmol/l in a hydrophobic phase such as olive oil. Mullins (1954) suggested that the volume of the anaesthetic molecule was also important because anaesthetics might act by filling a certain amount of free space in a membrane. This hypothesis would predict that pressure would enhance anaesthetic potency by forcing more anaesthetic molecules into the free space. This is obviously incorrect for general anaesthesia, but not necessarily for other actions of anaesthetics. For example, the interaction of xenon with myoglobin does involve filling empty cavities (Tilton, Kuntz and Petsko, 1984).

Can the lipid solubility hypothesis explain pressure reversal of anaesthesia? To do so, anaesthetic would have to be squeezed out of the model solvent as pressure increases. It turns out that any such squeezing out is of too small a magnitude to explain pressure reversal (Miller *et al.*, 1973). Another model, the critical volume hypothesis, circumvents this problem by noting that there are no holes in solvents, so when anaesthetics dissolve they actually cause solvents to expand. The critical volume hypothesis states that anaesthesia occurs when the volume of a hydrophobic region is caused to expand beyond a certain critical amount by absorption of molecules of an inert substance. Pressure reversal of anaesthesia occurs because pressure will counteract this expansion by simple mechanical compression. When olive oil is used as a model, general anaesthesia occurs in mice when the expansion exceeds 0.4 per cent. Pressure reversal of anaesthesia is accounted for quantitatively if the compressibility of the site is 2.4×10^{-5}/atm, a value which is close to that found for most simple solvents (Miller *et al.*, 1973).

Note that we have not needed in this section to worry about what the real nature of the anaesthetic site is beyond the fact that it behaves as a solvent rather like octanol. In the following sections we will be concerned with whether octanol is mimicking a lipid bilayer or a hydrophobic region of a protein.

Membranes as sites of general anaesthetic action

There is a strong consensus that general anaesthetics act by altering excitability of neuronal membranes. Inhibitory synapses may be enhanced, excitatory synapses may be depressed and axonal conduction may be inhibited (for reviews, see Richards, 1980; Koblin and Eger, 1981; Krnjevic, 1986). These studies do not add to our knowledge of the *molecular* mechanisms of general anaesthetic action and will not be reviewed here. They do, however, point to the plasma membrane of neurons, and particularly to excitable channels, as likely sites of action.

The last two decades have seen an explosion in knowledge about membranes (for reviews, see Bretscher, 1985; Storch and Kleinfeld, 1985). This aids considerably the task of understanding anaesthetic action. Membranes are composed of two building blocks, lipids and proteins. The basic structural feature is the lipid bilayer which can exist in the absence of proteins. Bilayers form spontaneously when phospholipids are vigorously dispersed in water.

This happens because of the phospholipid's amphipathic character: one end of the molecule is polar, often charged, and prefers to be in an aqueous environment; the other consists of two long hydrocarbon chains which will not mix with water. Over all, the molecule is roughly cylindrical in shape and thus many molecules can be close-packed side by side in rows. This results in a planar structure which is polar on one side and non-polar on the other. If two such structures are placed back to back with the tips of their hydrocarbon tails touching, the problem of dispersion in water is solved. There is now a sheet two molecules thick which has polar groups to interact with water on each side and the hydrocarbon chains tucked inside, out of contact with the water. The only remaining problem is exposure of hydrocarbon to water at the edges of the sheet. This is solved by wrapping the sheet round to form a spherical shell which has no edge, hence a lipid vesicle is a fundamentally stable structure (Fig. 6.5a). One other important feature of the lipid bilayer is that it is a fluid structure, the lipid molecules being in incessant motion.

The lipid bilayer forms a barrier round a cell which is impermeable to ions, but all the specialized tasks of the cell require proteins. Excitability depends on energy-consuming ion pumps which establish an electrochemical gradient across the cell membrane. These gradients can be transiently discharged by ion channels spanning the membrane, which open briefly to allow the ions to flow down their electrochemical gradients. The command to open these channels can come from a neurotransmitter (e.g. in postsynaptic membranes) or from a change in the voltage gradient across the membrane (e.g. in axons or presynaptic terminals). Electrophysiological studies suggest that these channels, particularly those activated by neurotransmitters, are sensitive to general anaesthetics.

Membrane proteins can be classified into two classes: extrinsic proteins which are loosely attached to the surface of the lipid bilayer, and intrinsic proteins which are embedded in the lipid bilayer. Intrinsic proteins are so intimately associated with the lipid bilayer that their activity can be retained during purification only if lipids are always present (for reviews, see Guidotti, 1978; Berman, 1981; Unwin and Henderson, 1984). Since ion channels must pass right through the lipid bilayer they are intrinsic proteins (Fig. 6.5b). Thanks to advances in molecular biology, the amino acid sequences of some of these channels have become available.

The nicotinic acetylcholine receptor has been sequenced (Noda et al., 1983). It consists of five subunits, two of which are identical, with a total molecular weight of 280 000. Theoretical analysis suggests that all these subunits have a similar arrangement in the lipid bilayer. In each case there are thought to be five α-helices which pass through the lipid bilayer. Three of them are non-polar, and two are polar or charged on one face and non-polar on the other. The latter group of two α-helices may be involved in lining the ion channel passing through the middle of the protein, with the non-polar group of α-helices making an outer annulus between the channel and the bilayer (Fairclough et al., 1983). The lipid composition is typical of plasma membranes, with some 17 per cent of the phospholipid carrying a net negative charge and 46 per cent of the total lipid being cholesterol (Popot et al., 1978). There are about 150 lipid molecules in contact with the protein, with cholesterol being a higher proportion of these than would be expected from

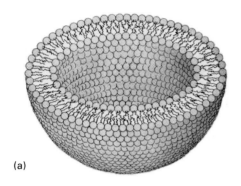

(a)

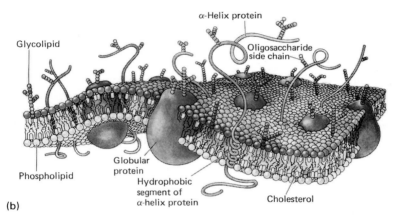

α-Helix protein

Glycolipid

Oligosaccharide
side chain

Phospholipid

Globular
protein

Hydrophobic
segment of
α-helix protein

Cholesterol

(b)

Fig. 6.5 Diagrammatic representation of the fundamentals of membrane structure. (a) A cross-section through a spherical lipid bilayer shell, the basic building block of all membranes. The polar headgroups of the phospholipids (represented by balls) face the aqueous phase on both sides of the bilayer, whilst the hydrocarbon chains form the interior of the bilayer. (b) A plasma membrane consists of such a lipid bilayer, composed of various phospholipids, in which cholesterol and proteins are embedded. The cytoplasmic side of this membrane faces down. Not shown are extrinsic proteins attached to this surface (see text). An example of an intrinsic protein embedded in the membrane is shown in Fig. 6.6. (Reproduced, with permission, from Bretscher, 1985.)

the composition of the lipid bilayer (for reviews, see Conti-Tronconi and Raftery, 1982; Popot and Changeux, 1984). Experiments in which the native lipids are totally replaced by synthetic ones show that the presence of cholesterol is essential for recovery of activity. Furthermore, increasing the cohesive pressure in the lipid bilayer encourages single receptor oligomers to cluster and form arrays in which the receptors act in concert (reviewed in Levitzki, 1985).

The axonal sodium channel differs from the acetylcholine receptor in being a single subunit of around 280 000 molecular weight, but shares the feature of having many hydrophobic α-helices which presumably pass through the lipid

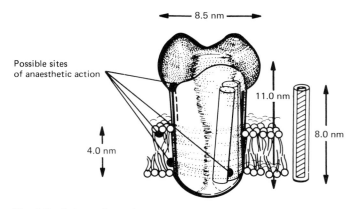

Fig. 6.6 A three-dimensional model for the funnel-shaped acetylcholine receptor molecule in the lipid bilayer. The protein is about 11 nm long perpendicular to the plane of the lipid bilayer which is 4 nm thick. Nearly half the protein projects well out into the extracellular space (top) and the binding sites for acetylcholine are thought to be at the top of the protein. Cylinders indicate α-helices which are probably packed perpendicular to the plane of the bilayer. Solid circles indicate possible sites of anaesthetic action in the lipid bilayer, lipid–protein interface intramembranous region of the protein or a hydrophobic cleft in the extramembranous region of the protein. (Redrawn, with permission, from Kistler *et al.*, 1982.)

bilayer (Noda *et al.*, 1984). Specific lipids are required to restore complete function in the reconstituted channel (Catterall *et al.*, 1984).

　　Thus excitable membranes, which are the target of general anaesthetic action, consist of lipid bilayers, 5 nm or so thick and extensive in two dimensions, composed of phospholipids and cholesterol and spanned by ion channels. These channels are large proteins having some two dozen hydrophobic and amphipathic α-helices passing through the lipid bilayer, but with a large proportion of their mass projecting well beyond the lipid bilayer. Putative hydrophobic sites of action for general anaesthetics (diameter about 0.5 nm) are found in the lipid bilayer, the lipid/protein interface, the hydrophobic membrane-spanning portion of the protein and the hydrophobic core of the extramembranous portion of the protein (Fig. 6.6).

Lipid solubility hypothesis of general anaesthesia

General anaesthetics should cause equal degrees of anaesthesia at equal concentrations in the lipid bilayer of neuronal membranes if the lipid solubility hypothesis is correct (Meyer, 1937). Figure 6.7 compares the ability of solubility in olive oil and in a lipid bilayer to correlate with general anaesthetic potency in mice. The fit of the fluorinated gases is noteworthy – they fail to fit on the line when solubility in a hydrocarbon is considered. Some 40 per cent of the mass of the phospholipid molecule is polar and the rest is hydrocarbon so it behaves as the moderately polar liquid which bulk solvent studies indicate to be the site of general anaesthesia. Workers have tested a wide range of anaesthetics, including gaseous and liquid inhalational anaesthetics, alcohols, ketones, carbamates and barbiturates. The potency of all these agents

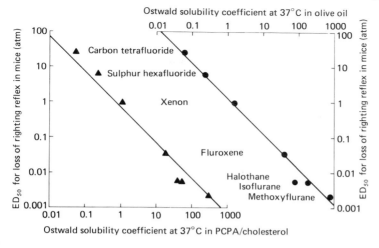

Fig. 6.7 A comparison of the classic correlation of general anaesthetic potency in mice with olive oil partitioning (right) and the same correlation with lipid bilayer partitioning. The lipid bilayer consists of egg lecithin and phosphatidic acid (25:1) containing 30 mol% cholesterol.

correlates very well with their solubility in lipid bilayers. The concentration of anaesthetic within the lipid bilayer which causes general anaesthesia depends on the lipid composition but is in the range 25–50 mmol/l. Solubility in lipid bilayers also explains why long chain alcohols fail to cause general anaesthesia; it turns out rather unexpectedly that they cannot achieve high enough concentrations in the bilayer (reveiwed in Janoff and Miller, 1982).

The success of the lipid solubility hypothesis of general anaesthetic action is quite impressive, although a number of tests remain to be made. Meyer's and Overton's intuition is amply vindicated now that olive oil can be replaced with a lipid bilayer!

A problem that the hypothesis does not address is why, if all lipid bilayers absorb anaesthetic, not all membrane processes are depressed. Another problem is that it cannot explain the pressure reversal of anaesthesia. These problems indicate the direction in which the hypothesis must be developed if it is to provide a more complete description of anaesthetic action.

Lipid perturbation hypotheses

The missing ingredient in the lipid solubility hypothesis is any notion of how the anaesthetic, once in the lipid bilayer, perturbs protein function. Many attempts have been made to address this problem. Their relative success has been reviewed recently (Roth, 1979; Franks and Lieb, 1982; Janoff and Miller, 1982; Dluzewski, Halsey and Simmonds, 1983; Goldstein, 1984). All these theories share the feature that anaesthetics are assumed to perturb the lipid bilayer's structure in some way and this perturbation is then transmitted to those membrane proteins whose function is altered. One can write a general statement of all lipid perturbation hypotheses as

$$E^{50} = C^{50} \cdot P_L \cdot T_P \qquad\qquad (6.2)$$

where E^{50} represents some functional change in an excitable membrane which leads to half of a group of animals being anaesthetized; C^{50} was defined above, P_L is a perturbation of the lipid bilayer produced by unit concentration of anaesthetic in the lipid bilayer and T_P describes the transmission of that lipid perturbation to the function of a membrane protein.

When the last two terms in equation (6.2) are ignored, it reduces to the lipid solubility hypothesis. The lipid perturbation hypotheses assume the last term is constant and ascribe various different meanings to P_L. Since C^{50} is usually constant it follows that if the hypothesis is correct, P_L will usually be constant, too; that is, the size of the perturbation will be directly proportional to the concentration of anaesthetic in the lipid bilayer (this is what is referred to as a colligative property). We might expect exceptions when:

1. C^{50} deviates from a constant when P_L would be expected to deviate in the opposite direction in order to keep E^{50} constant (e.g. this could account for the pressure reversal of anaesthesia);
2. the lipid composition differs from that at the site of general anaesthesia, for if P_L then takes on a small value it would explain why most proteins are unaffected by anaesthetics. The value of T_P should be independent of the anaesthetic but dependent on the protein in order to explain why some proteins are more sensitive than others to anaesthetics.

Finally, there is no reason to suppose, as most theories do, that anaesthesia results from a single lipid perturbation. A given protein might be sensitive to a number of different changes in its surrounding lipid bilayer (see, for example, Haydon et al., 1986).

Membrane expansion theories

The simplest lipid perturbation which accounts for pressure reversal and suggests a mechanism is membrane expansion. This is simply the critical volume hypothesis with the hydrophobic phase redefined as a lipid bilayer. Early experiments had shown that the area of erythrocytes increased when they were exposed to anaesthetics (Seeman, 1972; Roth, 1979), and this has been confirmed by more direct measurements (Bull, Brailsford and Bull, 1982). Volume measurements on lipid bilayers and erythrocytes (Kita and Miller, 1982) show that the expansion required to cause anaesthesia depends on the membrane and on the species and is in the range 0.2–0.6 per cent. Paradoxically, the measurements of erythrocyte area (above) reveal changes three to five times greater than this. The reason for this discrepancy is unknown. It might be due to the membrane getting thinner as its area increases, or to interactions with the cytoskeleton or to conformational changes in proteins (for a discussion, see Janoff and Miller, 1982).

How would proteins react to membrane expansion? Little is known about this, but studies in axons suggest some possibilities (Haydon *et al.*, 1986; and see under 'Lipid–protein interactions' below).

Membrane disordering theories

These theories evolved from early spectroscopic studies which showed that, when general anaesthetics dissolved in the close-packed parallel array of lipid molecules constituting the lipid bilayer, they forced the lipids to take up a more disordered arrangement (reviewed in Seeman, 1972). Although we remain profoundly ignorant about lipid–protein interactions, it can be argued that membrane order may modulate protein function (see, for example, Chapman, 1982, and Goldstein, 1984). Thus, it has been reported that a 6 per cent change in order parameter caused a tenfold change in $(NA^+ + K^+)$–stimulated ATPase activity (Sinensky *et al.*, 1979).

Spectroscopic studies of lipid order parameter are relatively easy to carry out using electron spin resonance (ESR) and spin-labelled lipids. Consequently a wider range of anaesthetics and membranes have been studied in pursuit of this theory than of any other (reviewed in Franks and Lieb, 1982; Janoff and Miller, 1982; Goldstein, 1984). The main conclusions are that:

1. Only lipid bilayers which contain phospholipids and cholesterol in a roughly equal molar ratio are consistently disordered by all general anaesthetics (including all the classes shown in Fig. 6.1) in proportion to their anaesthetic potency.
2. Lipid bilayers with no cholesterol are disordered by volatile anaesthetics but ordered by barbiturates, alphaxalone and ketamine (see Janoff and Miller, 1982).
3. Pressure and the non-anaesthetic gas helium order lipid bilayers and reverse the effects of anaesthetics (Chin, Trudell and Cohen, 1976).
4. The order parameter change corresponding to anaesthesia is about 0.6 per cent, but may be larger depending on the lipid composition of the bilayer (Harris and Groh, 1985).

There are some encouraging features to these studies; for example, the lipid composition required by the theory is comparable to that in excitable membranes, and the dependence on lipid composition provides some basis for expecting selective action of anaesthetics on membranes. Indeed, the cholesterol distribution in a given plasma membrane is not uniform, and some membrane proteins exclude cholesterol from their immediate surroundings, whilst others prefer to include it (Marsh and Watts, 1982; Levitzki, 1985). Nevertheless, it has yet to be securely demonstrated that anaesthetic-induced changes in lipid order provide a mechanism by which protein function can be modulated.

Lipid phase transition theories

The lipids of biomembranes are quite heterogeneous and evidence is accumulating that they are not distributed randomly either within a single leaflet of a bilayer or across the bilayer (Storch and Kleinfeld, 1985). Lateral phase separations occur in simple mixtures of lipids. A homogenous mixture of two lipids can be induced to separate into two phases of different composition by proteins, pH, or a change in temperature, ionic strength or calcium concentration (for reviews, see Boggs, 1970; Janoff and Miller, 1982). In some bacteria growth occurs optimally only in the same temperature range as lateral phase separation exists in the membrane lipids. Anaesthetics lower both the optimal growth temperature and the temperature over which lateral phase separation occurs (Janoff, Haug and McGroarty, 1979). Evidence that similar phenomena might occur in the mammalian nervous system is harder to come by, but the possibility has not been ruled out.

Trudell (1977) has proposed that the lipid surrounding an excitable protein exists in two phases: a solid, high density (called gel) phase, and a liquid, low density (called liquid crystalline) phase. Opening of a channel through the protein requires lateral expansion of the protein, compressing the surrounding lipids. This compressing force is accommodated by converting some of the expanded liquid crystalline lipid to compressed gel state lipid (Fig. 6.8).

The depression of a lipid phase transition temperature will be proportional to the concentration of anaesthetic in the lipid bilayer in the same way as freezing point depression depends on solute concentration in a bulk solvent. During anaesthesia the concentration of anaesthetic in lipid bilayers is a constant, independent of the anaesthetic, and therefore the depression in phase transition temperature will be also. Furthermore, because 'melting' involves a volume increase it will be opposed by pressure.

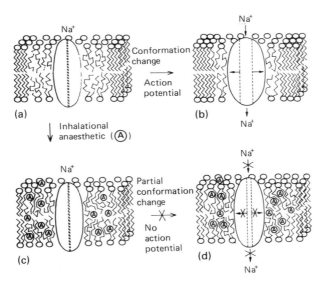

Fig. 6.8 The lateral phase separation theory of anaesthesia. (a) A phospholipid bilayer containing a sodium channel in the closed conformation. (b) The channel has undergone a hypothetical conformational change which is accomplished by packing some high-volume disordered lipid into low-volume arrays. (c) Anaesthetic molecules have melted regions of ordered lipid. (d) The protein is now unable to expand or change conformation and the excitation process does not occur. (Reproduced, with permission, from Trudell, 1977.)

Thus the theory is able to account for the main features of general anaesthesia. Most tests of the theory have looked at the temperature dependence of lateral phase separation. When one considers that many proteins select particular lipids to reside in close proximity to them (see above), it would make more sense to study lateral separations induced by proteins and other agents at constant temperature. The only such study examined the lateral phase separation induced in phosphatidic acid–phosphatidylcholine mixtures by polymyxin with encouraging results (Galla and Trudell, 1981).

Critique of lipid theories

Solubility in lipid bilayers accounts for the general anaesthetic potency of a vast range of anaesthetic molecules and provides a very satisfactory explanation for Meyer's and Overton's original observations. The theories have been very successful in suggesting lipid perturbations (P_L in equation 6.2) which account for the pressure reversal of anaesthesia and partially successful in suggesting mechanisms which might lead to selective perturbation of membranes. They have yet to get to grips seriously with the latter problem, however, and this makes it difficult to assess the significance of their major weakness, which is that the structural perturbations in the lipid bilayer are usually observed to be less than 1 per cent. Is this a big enough change to have functional consequences? Would it be bigger in bilayers of other lipid composition (Harris and Groh, 1985)?

One argument which is used against this change being sufficient is that comparable changes might be caused by changes in temperature of a degree Celsius or less. The rebuttal is that anaesthetics change only the lipid bilayer, so there would be, for example, a differential expansion between lipid and protein, whereas heat enters all components of the system equally, expanding both lipid and protein. This is a valid argument, but doubts must remain until either a mechanism coupling anaesthetic-induced lipid perturbations to changes in protein function is demonstrated or larger lipid perturbations are discovered.

Lipid–protein interactions

An anaesthetic at the lipid–protein interface experiences a dual environment. On the one hand it interacts with the lipid bilayer, and on the other with the protein. It might act on the protein either indirectly by perturbing the lipid or directly by perturbing the protein's structure.

The lipid–protein interface has proved difficult to study in detail. Rarely, it may be studied in orientated bilayers and then it can be shown that the lipid's acyl chains are not parallel to those in the bulk bilayer, but, rather, lie on the protein's surface in a disordered fashion. These lipids are in dynamic equilibrium with those in the lipid bilayer (for a review, see Marsh and Watts, 1982). Theoretical studies suggest that the surface which the protein exposes to the bilayer is rough (Guy, 1984). Thus lipids may wrap themselves round the protein so as to fill in the pits and present a smoother surface to the next layer of lipids. Anaesthetics could lodge in some of these pits, releasing segments of the acyl chains.

Little work has been undertaken in this area. In one study, ether perturbed the mobility of boundary lipid more than that of the bulk lipid bilayer or the protein (Bigelow and Thomas, 1984), suggesting the importance of lipid–protein interactions. Some mechanisms which might allow membrane proteins to respond selectively to such perturbations have been discussed recently (Miller, 1985).

Lipid—protein coupling in axonal membranes

The action of general anaesthetics on axonal conduction has been studied in great detail by Haydon and his colleagues (for full reviews, see Urban, 1985; Haydon *et al.*, 1986). They found, for example, that steady state inactivation curves (in Hodgkin–Huxley terminology, $h_\vee$ versus voltage) were shifted to the left by hydrocarbons but not at all by alcohols. This could be explained if the hydrocarbons, but not the alcohols, increased membrane thickness. An inactivation voltage sensor in the membrane would then experience a decreased voltage gradient only with hydrocarbons. This interpretation was consistent with capacitance measurements which suggested that, indeed, only hydrocarbons changed the axonal membrane's thickness. That hydrocarbons and alcohols might perturb a lipid bilayer differentially is quite consistent with recent studies reviewed by Simon, McIntosh and Hines (1986). Thus, in terms of equation (6.2), P_L is the bilayer thickness and T_P is the relationship of the voltage sensor to the voltage gradient across the bilayer.

Steady state activation was also affected by anaesthetics, but this could be explained only if a different lipid perturbation was invoked. The picture which emerges from these studies is one in which quite complex effects can be explained consistently within the framework of the lipid theories, provided that the complexity of anaesthetic–lipid interactions is taken into account.

Anaesthetic—protein interactions

General anaesthetics are known to interact with proteins. This is not surprising because about half the amino acids of proteins have hydrophobic side chains. In membrane proteins these amino acids may be in the lipid bilayer (see above), but in regions of the protein outside the membrane, or in cytoplasmic proteins, they will be internalized to avoid contact with water. Sometimes hydrophobic residues may be folded round an often rigid co-factor (e.g. nicotinamide or flavin nucleotides). Alternatively, proteins may aggregate to form oligomers with opposed hydrophobic faces (Williams, 1979).

Two types of anaesthetic–protein interactions can be distinguished. In the first there is great specificity and only a few anaesthetics take part. In the second there is less specificity and the site may appear to mimic that of general anaesthesia.

Specific interactions

The best example of the first type is provided by myoglobin. This protein may be crystallized and its structure studied by X-ray diffraction (Settle, 1973; Tilton, Kuntz and Petsko, 1984). Xenon at a partial pressure of 2.5 atm binds near the haem in an empty pocket surrounded by non-polar amino acid side chains. Difluorordichloromethane, which is slightly larger than xenon, can bind in the same pocket only by pushing some of these side chains aside. Further increase in the anaesthetic's size prevents binding. Some molecules such as ethane, which are the right size, fail to bind because their intermolecular forces are too weak; others such as krypton are simply too small. There are other sites for xenon at higher partial pressures, and the higher affinity of the haem site is probably attributable to haem's high polarizability.

It is interesting to note the similarity of these sites to those proposed by Mullins in 1954. Such sites probably exist on proteins of more physiological significance. For example, brain acetylcholinesterase is inhibited by volatile anaesthetics, but their ability to do so is unrelated to their anaesthetic potency (Braswell and Kitz, 1977). Other examples are reviewed in J.C. Miller and Miller (1975) and K.W. Miller (1985).

Non-specific interactions

Typical of the much less selective type of anaesthetic–protein interaction are the luciferases of bacteria and fireflies. In the bacterial enzyme anaesthetics cause two effects. First, they rapidly inhibit luminescence by competing with an alkyl aldehyde co-factor, which presumably occupies a hydrophobic cleft on the enzyme (its structure is unknown). Since this is a competitive inhibition, the anaesthetic concentration required will increase with the co-factor concentration. In whole cells inhibition occurs during the log phase of growth at concentrations comparable to those causing general anaesthesia, but higher concentrations are required in other phases. Second, during the early and late phases of growth low concentrations of anaesthetics may enhance luminescence on a slow time scale by a process requiring enzyme turnover. This effect may arise from facilitation of reduced flavin binding to the enzyme. Pressure reversal occurs but only in the early and late stages of the cell cycle (for a review, see Smith, Bowser-Riley and Daniels, 1986).

Recent work on the firefly enzyme shows that here inhibition is also competitive, but with a different co-factor, luciferin (the aldehyde does not seem to occur in this rather different luciferase). The anaesthetic potency of a wide range of volatile anaesthetics and alcohols correlates with their inhibitory action on the enzyme (Franks and Lieb, 1984). The cut-off in potency in the alkanols is correctly predicted within a few carbons, but the alkanes exhibit complex behaviour (Franks and Lieb, 1985). However, it remains to be seen whether the ability of the luciferase to mimic the site of general anaesthesia extends to all the agents in Fig. 6.1.

The luciferases provide as good a model of the site of general anaesthesia as any protein studied to date. Unfortunately, they have not been crystallized, so their structure is unknown, but co-factors often bind in hydrophobic clefts which may be hinged at their closed end. This might explain how the site on the luciferase accommodates a wider variety of anaesthetics than most proteins.

Some mechanisms at specific sites

Allosteric modulation by barbiturates

Barbiturates are now known to act as allosteric modulators at the GABA and acetylcholine (ACh) receptors and at voltage-sensitive sodium channels (Miller *et al.*, 1986; Olsen, 1982; Willow, Kuenzel and Catterall, 1984).

What is an allosteric effect? Imagine a protein which exists in two conformational states. It has a binding site for its primary ligand, an endogenous neurotransmitter, but this ligand binds only one conformation (the active conformation, conformation A) of the protein with high affinity. Since the two conformations are in equilibrium with each other, there will always be some protein in conformation A. When neurotransmitter is added it will bind to conformation A, increasing the proportion of protein in that active conformation (there are now two species having conformation A – one with ligand bound, the other without). Assume now there is a second site which binds an allosteric inhibitor with high affinity only when the protein is in the inactive conformation B. The inhibitor will act by increasing the proportion of protein in the inactive state, reducing the proportion in the active conformation. This concept was evolved in enzymology, but has been adapted to explain non-competitive inhibition in pharmacology (for a fuller description, see Burgen, 1981, and references cited therein) and on the ACh receptor (Changeux, Devillers-Thiery and Chemouilli, 1984).

Because allosterism is well understood, it is possible to infer with some confidence from the behaviour of a protein in the presence of inhibitors that an allosteric site exists. This is the case with the GABA receptor and the voltage-sensitive sodium channel (see above paragraph). One would not expect to be able to detect the binding of an anaesthetic to a membrane protein because such binding would be lost amid a high background of anaesthetic dissolved in the membrane's lipid. However, ACh receptors occur at unusually high density in certain electric fish, there being only a few hundred lipid molecules per receptor in cholinergic membranes isolated from the electroplaques of *Torpedo* (this is about 10 000-fold less lipid per receptor than is found in brain). This advantageous situation was exploited to directly demonstrate that [^{14}C]pentobarbitone bound in a saturable, stereoselective manner to an allosteric site on ACh receptors (Miller, Sauter and Braswell, 1982). Subsequent studies (Miller *et al.*, 1986) have shown that [^{14}C]amylobarbitone is a better ligand for detecting this site, and some typical data are given in Fig. 6.9.

The ACh receptor can exist in a number of different conformational states. At rest the ACh binding site has low affinity for ACh. When ACh binds to it a series of conformation changes are set in motion, including transient opening of the channel, and the receptor ends up in a state which has high affinity for ACh and which is functionally desensitized. After ACh dissociates, the

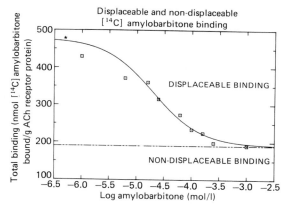

Fig. 6.9   [^{14}C]amylobarbitone (★) binds to a specific site on the ACh receptor from which it can be displaced by higher concentrations of barbiturates, in this case unlabelled amylobarbitone (▫). Not all the 'binding' can be displaced in this way; the residual binding represents that dissolved in the lipid bilayer. (Reproduced, with permission, from Miller *et al.*, 1986.)

receptor remains in this state for a time, slowly reverting to the resting state. If one measures ACh binding at equilibrium, when all the receptors are desensitized, high affinity binding is found. However, amylobarbitone binds more strongly to the resting state, so addition of it to the assay leads to conversion of some receptors from the desensitized to the resting state, effectively lowering ACh's affinity. Conversely, when ACh is added to the amylobarbitone-binding assay, converting some receptors to the desensitized state, less amylobarbitone binding is seen (Fig. 6.10).

This barbiturate site is of the 'hard' or specific variety. It does not bind alcohols, for example. Barbiturates bind to it stereoselectively and their affinities for the site do not correlate with their anaesthetic potencies (Dodson and Miller, 1985b). This lack of correlation with general anaesthesia is also characteristic of the barbiturate site on the GABA receptor (Ticku and Rastogi, 1986) and the sodium channel (Willow, Kuenzel and Catterall, 1984).

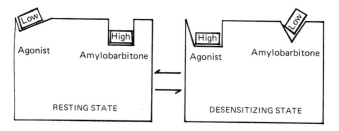

Fig. 6.10   This simple two-state model represents a possible mechanism for the effect of amylobarbitone on the ACh receptor. Amylobarbitone binds with high affinity to the resting state of the receptor, whereas ACh binds with higher affinity to the desensitized state. The relative concentrations of ACh and amylobarbitone would then determine the proportion of the receptor in each conformational state. (This is a simplified representation which accounts only for equilibrium effects of these two agents; see text. (Reproduced, with permission, from Miller *et al.*, 1986.)

Modulated receptor hypothesis

The barbiturate site on the ACh receptor is a physical entity and will be present on all of that protein's conformations. As the protein changes conformation the shape of the site will vary and, with it, the affinity for a given barbiturate. There is no reason why all barbiturates should bind most tightly to the same receptor conformation; indeed, this seems unlikely. In fact, in both the GABA and the ACh receptors cited above, different barbiturates bind preferentially to different conformations. Thus the situation can become quite complex, with each conformation having a different rank order for barbiturate binding.

A similar situation occurs for the local anaesthetic-binding site on sodium channels (Bean *et al.*, 1986) and ACh receptors (Cohen, Medynski and Strnad, 1985).

Conclusion

General anaesthesia

The physiological mechanism of general anaesthesia is enigmatic and may remain so pending a deeper understanding of the central nervous system. Meanwhile a well-characterized pharmacological definition of general anaesthesia is available. Unfortunately, the simplicity of a specific antagonist is missing (pressure is non-specific), so that to thoroughly characterize an effect as general anaesthetic-like requires a wider range of agents to be examined than in other fields. Thus to proceed critically we must proceed slowly and completely.

The lipid hypotheses have withstood a wider range of pharmacological tests than any protein model has been subjected to. Indeed most protein models fail early in such tests. A few protein models have fared better, notably the luciferases, but rigorous pharmacological tests have yet to be completed. However, the lipid hypotheses will remain unproven until a direct mechanistic link can be demonstrated experimentally between a lipid perturbation and a change in a protein's function.

Non-anaesthetic actions

It is proving easier to provide mechanisms for effects mediated by direct anaesthetic–protein interactions, particularly the more specific ones. The allosteric actions of barbiturates are the prime examples. Further progress is to be expected here because the underlying mechanisms are well established and the pharmacology is usually more restricted. This holds out some hope for avoiding side effects when designing new agents.

Future directions

The development of a more critical and analytical approach to anaesthetic mechanisms has replaced the old cavalier approach with a more detailed and systematic one. A classification of the many ways in which anaesthetics act is emerging from detailed studies of an increasingly mechanistic nature. This will clearly lead to new insights and perhaps new uses for anaesthetic agents. What remains unclear is how far such studies will provide the key to general anaesthesia itself.

References

Angel, A., Gratton, D.A., Halsey, M.J. and Wardley-Smith, B. (1980) Pressure reversal of the effect of urethane on the evoked somatosensory cortical response in the rat. *British Journal of Pharmacology* **70**, 241

Bean, B.P., Cohen, C.J., Tan, R.C. and Tsien, R.W. (1986) Lidocaine block of sodium channels in heart cells. In: *Molecular and Cellular Mechanisms of Anesthetics* (Eds. Roth, S.H. and Miller, K.W.), pp. 191–215. Plenum Medical: New York

Berman, M.C. (1981) Properties of cell membranes relevant to anaesthesiology. *South African Medical Journal* **59**, 403

Bigelow, D.J. and Thomas, D.D. (1984) Molecular dynamics and enzymatic activity in sarcoplasmic reticulum: a comparison of the effects of ether and temperature. *Biophysical Journal* **45**, 320a

Boggs, J.M. (1980) Intermolecular hydrogen bonding between lipids: influence on organization and function of lipids in membranes. *Canadian Journal of Biochemistry* **58**, 755

Braswell, L.M. and Kitz, R.J. (1977) The effects *in vitro* of volatile anesthetics on the activity of cholinesterases. *Journal of Neurochemistry* **29**, 665

Bretscher, M.S. (1985) The molecules of the cell membrane. *Scientific American* **253**, 100

Bull, M.H., Brailsford, J.D. and Bull, B.S. (1982) Erythrocyte membrane expansion due to the volatile anesthetics, the *l*-alkanols, and benzyl alcohol. *Anesthesiology* **57**, 399

Burgen, A.S.V. (1981) Conformational changes and drug action. *Federation Proceedings* **40**, 2723

Catterall, W.A., Messner, D.J., Hartshorne, R.P. *et al.* (1984) Molecular pharmacology of the sodium channel of mammalian brain. In: *IUEPHAR Proceedings*, vol. 1 (Eds. Paton, W., Mitchell, J. and Turner, P.), p. 219. Macmillan: London

Changeux, J.-P., Devillers-Thiery, A. and Chemouilli, P. (1984) Acetylcholine receptor: an allosteric protein. *Science* **225**, 1335

Chapman, D. (1982) Protein–lipid interactions in model and natural biomembranes. *Biological Membranes* **4**, 179

Chin, J.H., Trudell, J.R. and Cohen, E.N. (1976) The compression-ordering solubility-disordering effects of high pressure gases on phospholipid bilayers. *Life Sciences* **28**, 489

Cohen, J.B., Medynski, D.C. and Strnad, N.P. (1985) Interactions of local anesthetics with nicotinic acetylcholine receptors. In: *Effects of Anesthesia* (Eds. Covino, B.G., Fozzard, H.A., Rehder, K. and Strichartz, G.), pp. 13–28. American Physiological Society: Bethesda, MD

Conti-Tronconi, B.M. and Raftery, M.A. (1982) The nicotinic cholinergic receptor: correlation of molecular structure with functional properties. *Annual Review of Biochemistry* **51**, 491

Deady, J.E., Koblin, D.D., Eger, E.I. II, Heavner, J.E. and D'Aoust, B. (1981) Anesthetic potencies and the unitary theory of narcosis. *Anesthesia and Analgesia* **60**, 380

Dluzewski, A.R., Halsey, M.J. and Simmonds, A.C. (1983) Membrane interactions with general and local anaesthetics: a review of molecular hypotheses of anaesthesia. *Molecular Aspects of Medicine* **6**, 459

Dodson, B.A. and Miller, K.W. (1985a) Evidence for a dual mechanism in the anesthetic action of an opioid peptide. *Anesthesiology* **62**, 615

Dodson, B.A. and Miller, K.W. (1985b) Relative potencies for barbiturate binding to the acetylcholine receptor. *Anesthesiology* **63**, A383

Dodson, B.A., Furmaniuk, Z.W. Jr and Miller, K.W. (1985) The physiological effects of hydrostatic pressure are not equivalent to those of helium pressure. *Journal of Physiology* **362**, 233

Eger, E.I., Saidman, L.J. and Brandstater, B. (1965) Minimum alveolar anesthetic concentration: a standard of anesthetic potency. *Anesthesiology* **26**, 756

Fairclough, R.H., Finer-More, J., Love, R.A., Kristofferson, D., Desmeules, P.J. and Stroud, R.M. (1983) Subunit organization and structure of an acetylcholine receptor. *Cold Spring Harbor Symposia on Quantitative Biology* **58**, 9

Ferguson, J. (1939) The use of chemical potentials as indices of toxicity. *Proceedings of the Royal Society, B* **127**, 387

Firestone, L.L., Miller, J.C. and Miller, K.W. (1986) Tables of physical and pharmacological properties of anesthetics. In: *Molecular and Cellular Mechanisms of Anesthetics* (Eds. Roth, S.H. and Miller, K.W.), pp. 453–470. Plenum Medical: New York

Franks, N.P. and Lieb, W.R. (1982) Molecular mechanisms of general anaesthesia. *Nature* **300**, 487

Franks, N.P. and Lieb, W.R. (1984) Do general anaesthetics act by competitive binding to specific receptors? *Nature* **310**, 599

Franks, N.P. and Lieb, W.R. (1985) Mapping of general anaesthetic target sites provides a molecular basis for cutoff effects. *Nature* **316**, 349

Galla, H.J. and Trudell, J.R. (1981) Perturbation of peptide-induced lateral phase separations in phosphatidic acid bilayers by the inhalation anaesthetic methoxyflurane. *Molecular Pharmacology* **19**, 432

Goldstein, D.B. (1984) The effects of drugs on membrane fluidity. *Annual Review of Pharmacology and Toxicology* **24**, 43

Guidotti, G. (1978) Membrane proteins: structure and arrangement in the membrane. *Physiology of Membrane Disorders*, vol. 3, p. 49. Plenum Medical: New York

Guy, H.R. (1984) A structural model of the acetylcholine receptor channel based on partition energy and helix packing calculations. *Biophysical Journal* **45**, 249

Harris, R.A. and Groh, G.I. (1985) Membrane disordering effects of anesthetics are enhanced by gangliosides. *Anesthesiology* **62**, 115

Haydon, D.A., Elliott, J.R., Henry, B.M. and Urban, B.W. (1986) The action of nonionic anesthetic substances on voltage-gated ion conductances in squid giant axons. In: *Molecular and Cellular Mechanisms of Anesthetics* (Eds. Roth, S.H. and Miller, K.W.), pp. 265–275. Plenum Medical: New York

Hughes, J., Smith, T.W., Kosterlitz, H.W., Fothergill, L.A., Morgan, B.A. and Morris, H.R. (1975) Identification of two related pentapeptides from the brain with potent opiate agonist activity. *Nature* **258**, 577

Janoff, A.S. and Miller, K.W. (1982) A critical assessment of the lipid theories of general anaesthetic action. In: *Biological Membranes*, vol. 4 (Ed. Chapman, D.), pp. 417–476 Academic Press: London

Janoff, A.S., Haug, A. and McGroarty, E.J. (1979) Relationship of growth temperature and thermotropic lipid changes in cytoplasmic and outer membranes from *Escherichia coli* K12. *Biochimica et Biophysica Acta* **555**, 56

Johson, F.H. and Flagler, E.A. (1950) Hydrostatic pressure reversal of narcosis in tadpoles. *Science* **112**, 91

Kendig, J.J. and Grossman, Y. (1986) Homogeneous and branching axons: differing responses to anesthetics and pressure. In: *Molecular and Cellular Mechanisms of*

Anesthetics (Eds. Roth, S.H. and Miller, K.W.), pp. 331–338. Plenum Medical: New York

Kendig, J.J., Trudell, J.R. and Cohen, E.N. (1973) Halothane stereoisomers: lack of stereospecificity in two model systems. *Anesthesiology* **30**, 518

Kissin, I., Morgan, P.L. and Smith L.R. (1983) Anesthetic potencies of isoflurane, halothane, and diethyl ether for various end points of anesthesia. *Anesthesiology* **58**, 88

Kistler, J., Stroud, R.M., Klymkowsky, M.W., LaLancette, R.A. and Fairclough, R.H. (1982) Structure and function of an acetylcholine receptor. *Biophysical Journal* **37**, 371

Kita, Y. and Miller, K.W. (1982) The partial molar volumes of some *n*-alkanols in erythrocyte ghosts and lipid bilayers. *Biochemistry* **21**, 2840

Koblin, D.D. and Eger, E.I. II (1981) How do inhaled anesthetics work? In: *Anesthesia* (Ed. Miller, R.D.), pp. 283–308. Churchill Livingstone: New York

Krnjevic, K. (1986) Cellular and synaptic effects of general anesthetics. In: *Molecular and Cellular Mechanisms of Anesthetics* (Eds. Roth, S.H. and Miller, K.W.), pp. 3–16. Plenum Medical: New York

Levitzki, A. (1985) Reconstitution of membrane receptor systems. *Biochimica et Biophysica Acta* **822**, 127

Marsh, D. and Watts, A. (1982) Spin labeling and lipid–protein interactions in membranes. In: *Lipid–Protein Interactions*, vol. 2 (Eds. Jost, P.C. and Griffith, O.H.), pp. 53–126. John Wiley: New York

Meyer, H.H. (1906) The theory of narcosis. *Harvey Lectures* 11–17

Meyer, K.H. (1937) Contributions to the theory of narcosis. *Transactions of the Faraday Society* **33**, 1062

Miller, J.C. and Miller, K.W. (1975) Approaches to mechanisms of action of general anesthetics. *MTP International Review of Sciences: Physiological and Pharmacological Series*, Biochemistry Series I, 12, 33. Butterworths/University Park Press: Baltimore MD

Miller, K.W. (1974) Intermolecular forces. *British Journal of Anaesthesia* **46**, 190

Miller, K.W. (1985) The nature of the site of general anesthesia. *International Review of Neurobiology* **27**, 1

Miller, K.W. (1986) Are lipids or proteins the target of general anaesthetic action? *Trends in Neurosciences* **9**, 49

Miller, K.W. and Smith, E.B. (1973) Intermolecular forces and the pharmacology of simple molecules. In: *A Guide to Molecular Pharmacology–Toxicology*, part II. (Ed. Featherstone, R.M.), pp. 427–476. Marcel Dekker: New York

Miller, K.W. and Wilson, M.W. (1978) The pressure reversal of a variety of anesthetic agents in mice. *Anesthesiology* **48**, 104

Miller, K.W., Sauter, J.F. and Braswell, L.M. (1982) A stereoselective pentobarbital binding site in cholinergic membranes from *Torpedo californica*. *Biochemical and Biophysical Research Communications* **105**, 659

Miller, K.W., Wilson, M.W. and Smith, R.A. (1978) Pressure resolves two sites of action of inert gases. *Molecular Pharmacology* **14**, 950.

Miller, K.W., Paton, W.D.M., Smith, R.A. and Smith, E.B. (1973) The pressure reversal of anaesthesia and the critical volume hypothesis. *Molecular Pharmacology* **9**, 131

Miller, K.W., Braswell, L.M., Firestone, L.L., Dodson, B.A. and Forman, S.A. (1986) General anesthetics act both specifically and nonspecifically on acetylcholine receptors. In: *Molecular and Cellular Mechanisms of Anesthetics* (Eds. Roth, S.H. and Miller, K.W.), pp. 125–137. Plenum Medical: New York

Mullins, L.J. (1954) Some physical mechanisms in narcosis. *Chemical Reviews* **54**, 289

Noda, M., Takahashi, H., Tanabe, T. *et al.* (1983) Structural homology of *Torpedo californica* acetylcholine receptor subunits. *Nature* **302**, 528

Noda, M., Shimizu, S., Tanabe, T. *et al.* (1984) Primary structure of *Electrophorus electricus* sodium channel deduced from cDNA sequence. *Nature* **312**, 121

Olsen, R.W. (1982) Drug interactions at the GABA receptor–ionophore complex. *Annual Review of Pharmacology and Toxicology* **22**, 245

Paton, W.D.M. (1974) Unconventional anaesthetic molecules. In: *Molecular Mechanisms in General Anaesthesia* (Eds. Halsey, M.J., Millar, R.A. and Sutton, J.A.), pp. 48–64. Churchill Livingstone: Edinburgh

Popot, J.-L. and Changeux, J.-P. (1984) Nicotinic receptor of acetylcholine: structure of an oligomeric integral membrane protein. *Physiological Reviews* **64**, 1162

Popot, J.L., Demel, R.A., Sobel, A., Van Deenen, L.L.M. and Changeux, J.-P. (1978) Interaction of the acetylcholine (nicotinic) receptor protein from *Torpedo marmorata* electric organ with monolayers of phospholipids. *European Journal of Biochemistry* **85**, 27

Pringle, M.J., Brown, K.B. and Miller, K.W. (1981) Can the lipid theories of anaesthesia account for the cut-off in anaesthetic potency in homologous series of alcohols? *Molecular Pharmacology* **19**, 49

Quasha, A.L., Eger, E.I. II and Tinker, J.H. (1980) Determination and applications of MAC. *Anesthesiology* **53**, 315

Richards, C.D. (1980) In search of the mechanisms of anaesthesia. *Trends in Neurosciences* **3**, 9–13

Roth, S.H. (1979) Physical mechanisms of anesthesia. *Annual Review of Pharmacology and Toxicology* **19**, 159

Ryder, S., Way, W.L. and Trevor, A.J. (1978) Comparative pharmacology of the optical isomers of ketamine in mice. *European Journal of Pharmacology* **49**, 15

Seeman, P. (1972) Membrane actions of anesthetics and tranquillizers. *Pharmacological Reviews* **24**, 583

Settle, W. (1973) Function of the myoglobin molecule as influenced by anesthetic molecules. In: *A Guide to Molecular Pharmacology–Toxicology*, part II (Ed. Featherstone, R.M.), pp. 477–494. Marcel Dekker: New York

Simon, S.A., McIntosh, T.J. and Hines, M.L. (1986) The influence of anesthetics on the structure and thermal properties of saturated lecithins. In: *Molecular and Cellular Mechanisms of Anesthetics* (Eds. Roth, S.H. and Miller, K.W.), pp. 295–306. Plenum Medical: New York

Sinensky, M., Pinkerton, F., Sutherland, E. and Simon, F.R. (1979) Rate limitation of $(Na^+ + {}^+)$-stimulated adenosine-triphosphatase by membrane acyl chain ordering. *Proceedings of the National Academy of Sciences of the USA* **76**, 4893

Smith, E.B., Bowser-Riley, F. and Daniels, S. (1986) New observations on the mechanisms of pressure–anesthetic interactions. In: *Molecular and Cellular Mechanisms of Anesthetics* (Eds. Roth, S.H. and Miller, K.W.), pp. 339–352. Plenum Medical: New York

Storch, J. and Kleinfeld, A.M. (1985) The lipid structure of biological membranes. *Trends in Biochemical Sciences* **10**, 418–421

Tanifuji, Y., Eger, E.I. and Terrell, R.C. (1977) Some characteristics of an exceptionally potent inhaled anesthetic: thiomethoxyflurane. *Anesthesia and Analgesia* **56**, 387

Ticku, M.K. and Rastogi, S.K. (1986) Barbiturate-sensitive sites in the benzodiazepine–GABA receptor–ionophore complex. In: *Molecular and Cellular Mechanisms of Anesthetics* (Eds. Roth, S.H. and Miller, K.W.), pp. 179–188. Plenum Medical: New York

Tilton, R.F. Jr, Kuntz, I.D. Jr and Petsko, G.A. (1984) Cavities in proteins: structure of a metmyoglobin–xenon complex solved to 1.9 Å. *Biochemistry* **23**, 2849

Trudell, J.R. (1977) A unitary theory of anesthesia based on lateral phase separations in nerve membranes. *Anesthesiology* **46**, 5

Unwin, N. and Henderson, R. (1984) The structure of proteins in biological membranes. *Scientific American* **250**, 78

Urban, B.W. (1985) Modifications of excitable membranes by volatile and gaseous anesthetics. In: *Effects of Anesthesia* (Eds. Covino, B.G., Fozzard, H.A., Rehder, K. and Strichartz, G.), pp. 13–28. American Physiological Society: Bethesda, MD

Williams, R.J.P. (1979) The conformational properties of proteins in solution. *Biological Reviews* **54**, 389

Willow, M., Kuenzel, E.A. and Catterall, W.A. (1984) Inhibition of voltage-sensitive sodium channels in neuroblastoma cells and synaptosomes by the anticonvulsant drugs diphenylhydantoin and carbamazepine. *Molecular Pharmacology* **25**, 228

7
Neuromuscular blocking agents

S.A. Feldman

Although Claude Bernard demonstrated that curare produced paralysis of the muscles of a frog without a direct effect on either the motor nerves or the muscle, it was only following Kuhne's demonstration of the morphology of the neuromuscular end-plate that Vulpian (1866), a pupil and follower of Claude Bernard, postulated that curare produced its paralytic effect by an action localized to the end-plate of the neuromuscular junction. In 1906, Langley demonstrated that curare blocked the response of the neuromuscular junction to nicotine. As a result of these experiments he postulated that, within the end-plate, curare reacted with a specific nicotine receptor substance blocking normal neuromuscular transmission. It was not until the 1930s that a team of physiologists at the National Institute for Medical Research, London, composed of Dale, Feldberg, Brown and Bacq, demonstrated the importance of acetylcholine in neuromuscular transmission and the manner in which its effect was prevented by the prior administration of curare (Dale and Feldberg 1934; Dale, Feldberg and Vogt, 1936; Bacq and Brown, 1937). It was these experiments which led to the concept of curare acting by preventing access of physiological neurotransmitter to specific matching receptor sites. The 'key in the lock' theory was strengthened by the demonstration of similarities in the chemical structure of acetylcholine (ACh) and curare, as both compounds possess positively charged quaternary ammonium groups.

The original structural formula of d-tubocurarine proposed by King (1935) (Fig. 7.1a) suggested that the drug was a bisquaternary compound. In 1970, Everett and co-workers, working in Burroughs Wellcome Laboratories, using the then new technique of nuclear magnetic resonance spectroscopy demonstrated that d-tubocurarine was, in fact, a monoquaternary, monotertiary compound (Fig. 7.1b). However, at physiological pH the charge density on the tertiary group is very high, so its physicochemical properties approach that of the quaternary structure. The basic bisquaternary structure of potent neuromuscular blocking agents was supported by the work of Barlow and Ing (1948) and Paton and Zaimis (1949) on the bisquaternary polymethylene series; they showed that when the interonium distance was ten methylene groups, as in decamethonium (C=10), the compound had the greatest activity at the neuromuscular junction. Although active compounds exist with shorter interonium distances (e.g. fazadinium 0.7 nm, pancuronium 1.0 nm), it may well be that these compounds require two molecules acting

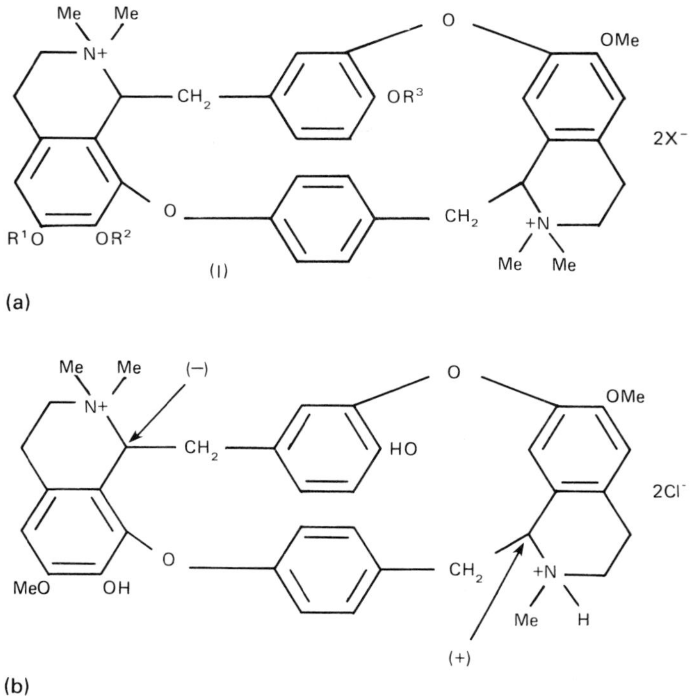

Fig. 7.1 (a) Original King (1935) formula for *d*-tubocurarine – bisquaternary compound. (b) Everett, Lowe and Wilkinson (1970) formula for *d*-tubocurarine – monoquaternary/monotertiary compound.

together to bridge a matrix of receptors placed 1.2–1.4 nm apart, or, alternatively, agents with longer interonium distances such as *d*-tubocurarine and C.10 bridge two reactive centres each 0.6–0.7 nm apart. A similar structural activity concept would explain the potent neuromuscular blocking activity of some compounds which are monoquaternary in structure.

Some monotertiary compounds such as the erythrina alkaloids have strong neuromuscular blocking properties. Because these compounds are lipophilic they penetrate the blood–brain barrier and have marked effects on the central nervous system, which makes them unsuitable for clinical use. It is interesting to note that quaternization of the tertiary compound dihydro-β-erythroidine results in a considerable reduction in potency (Irwin and Trams, 1962). Thus not all agents with active neuromuscular blocking properties are bisquaternary ammonium compounds nor does forming a bisquaternary compound from a monoquaternary or tertiary ion necessarily increase its potency. Some of the monotertiary monoquaternary compounds such as vecuronium, the monoquaternary derivative of pancuronium, are even more potent than the bisquaternary analogues. Not all agents acting at the neuromuscular junction causing transmission block are tertiary or quaternary amines. Indeed, some of the most active of neuromuscular blocking agents – the biotoxins such as the bungarotoxins and cobra venoms – are polypeptides rather than alkaloids. Some of the biotoxins are so potent that prolonged (12 to 24-hour) block may follow exposure to a 5 p.p.m. concentration of drug. Nevertheless it was the general similarity between the chemical structure of ACh and the quaternary ammonium structure of most potent neuromuscular blocking agents which gave support to the key in the lock concept of mechanism of action of the non-depolarizing neuromuscular blocking agents.

The neuromuscular junction

The studies of Birks, Huxley and Katz (1960), Birks and McIntosh (1961) and Robertson (1956) demonstrated the detailed morphology of the neuromuscular junction. The autoradiographic studies of Waser (1970, 1972, 1983) showed that the ACh receptors and the site of fixation of the muscle relaxants lay on the postsynaptic membrane of the neuromuscular junction on the crests of the gutters which traverse the end-plates. They are especially concentrated around the openings into secondary folds which dip down from the crests into the sarcoplasm of the muscle (Figs. 7.2 and 7.3). Using thioacetate stain to demonstrate cholinesterase, it can be shown that the areas which have a high affinity for radioactive neuromuscular blocking agents are also rich in cholinesterase (Davis and Koelle, 1967). At higher magnification it can be demonstrated that the highest density of receptors on the postsynaptic membrane is located directly opposite specific areas of the presynaptic membrane from which ACh is released. The ACh-releasing sites form a lattice over the presynaptic membrane, through the interstices of which ACh vesicles discharge their contents into the synaptic cleft directly opposite the receptor sites. It now seems probable that the siting of the receptors is at least partly determined by a trophic effect, possibly associated with the release of ACh.

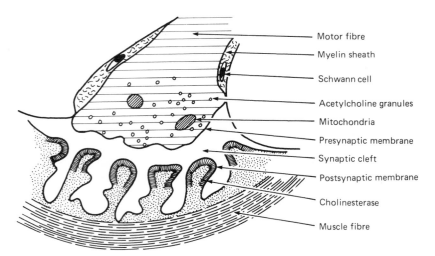

Fig. 7.2 Schematic view of neuromuscular junction showing receptor areas using cholinesterase stains.

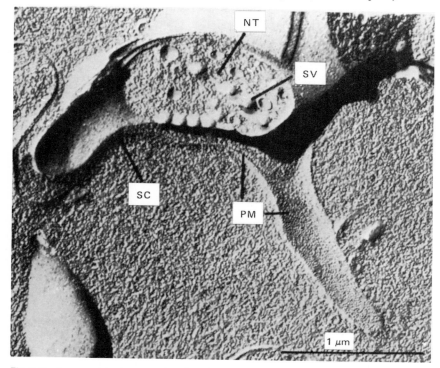

Fig. 7.3 Freeze-etched preparation showing nerve terminal (NT), synaptic vesicle (SV), synaptic cleft (SC) and receptor–cholinesterase rich area on postsynaptic membrane (PM). (After Waser, 1975, with permission.)

The cholinergic receptor (cholinoceptor)

Our knowledge of the structure and function of the postsynaptic cholinoceptor owes much to studies upon the nicotinic receptors in the electric sting organs (electroplaques) of the giant electric ray (*Torpedo marmorata*) and the electric eel (*Electrophorus electricus*). By attaching radioactive α-bungarotoxin or α-cobra venom to these organs, labelled extract of receptor substance can be separated in an ultracentrifuge and studied *in vitro*.

An alternative approach to the study of the nature of the receptor under more physiological conditions has been the use of autoradiography. Some workers (such as Miledi and Potter, 1971; Fambrough and Harzell, 1972; Fambrough, 1979) have labelled the receptors with radioactive α-bungarotoxin and other biotoxins and then studied autoradiographs of the receptors using the electron microscope. Waser and his co-workers (1975–1983) have studied autoradiographs of rat tissue labelled with radioactive curare-like compounds including curare, decamethonium and other relaxants. More recently, specific labelled receptor antibody has been used to identify and study mammalian receptors (Rash, Hudson and Ellisman, 1978). All these methods of research,

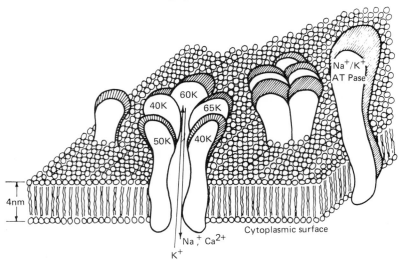

Fig. 7.4 The subunits which compose the receptor substance and which encircle the ionophore. (After Standaert, F.G., 1984. The donut and its hole. Proceedings of Harvard Medical School Symposium.)

together with improvements in imaging techniques such as the use of freeze-dried etching studies, have contributed greatly to our present concept of the structural arrangement of receptors and of the specific dynamics of these agents during drug-receptor responses.

From all these studies emerges a picture of the receptor as a large protein moiety composed of five subunits of a protein complex rich in glycoprotein and having a total size of about 10 nm. Of these five subunits, situated longitudinally through the ionophore, two have an identical structure, the two α-subunits. On one side of this pair lies a large δ unit whilst a β- and a γ unit lie on the other side causing asymmetry of the structure. The pentamer sits like a raised collar around the pore and extends inside the membrane around the ionophore at right angles to the surface (Fig. 7.4). Waser concluded from his work that the dynamics of the ACh receptor reaction are such as to indicate that cholinesterase itself must be intimately associated with the receptor substance. Although this has not been supported by studies of the receptor substance, both autoradiographic and dynamic studies confirm a close physical association of cholinesterase with the receptor. Recent work suggests that in order to open a sodium channel it is necessary for ACh molecules to react with specific recognition sites on the α-subunits. If opposite pairs of these sites are activated simultaneously, a rotational force is applied to the α-subunits. If this force produced is sufficient it will cause distortion of the receptor molecule, the ionophore will then be opened sufficiently to allow sodium influx to take place. It is possible that this process can be impaired if a small but critical number of these recognition sites are occupied by a non-depolarizing drug.

The conformational changes produced by the action of ACh may cause allosteric deformation, as suggested by Cohen and Changeux (1975) and

Changeux *et al.* (1976). This process is rate limited and would determine the maximum rate at which depolarization can take place.

With the complete elucidation of the amino acid sequence of the five subunits which make up the collar lining the ionophore ring (Changeux, Devilliers-Thiery and Chemonilli, 1984) has come the appreciation that the action of non-depolarizing blocking agents is particularly associated with the two α-subunits each with a molecular size of 40 000. Taylor, Brown and Johnson (1984) have suggested that the asymmetry of the arrangements of these two units, separated on one side by a subunit 65 000 molecular weight (δ) and on the other by two subunits of 50 000 and 60 000 (β and γ), contribute to some of the pharmacodynamic properties of the receptor. This has been taken further by Waud and Waud (1985), who have suggested that the reason why some non-depolarizing relaxants potentiate the effect of others, such as pancuronium and metacurarine (Lebowitz *et al.*, 1980) whilst others do not, is because of the different abilities of each drug to gain access to the receptor on the α-subunits and not, as previously suggested, due to different sites of action at the neuromuscular junction. As a result, occupation of the receptor sites on the two α-subunits is more likely with combinations of two matched drugs, resulting in a greater possibility of stabilizing each ionophore and achieving neuromuscular block. Evidence suggests that the likely bonding sites on the α-subunits of the receptor pentamer are in the region of the disulphide linkage in the amino acid chain.

Receptor activation

Within the complex cholinoreceptor it is not established with certainty whether the receptor sites for curare-like drugs are different from those for ACh or whether they are merely ACh receptors in an altered mode or special position. The activation of a cholinoreceptor by ACh causes opening of the ionophore and an increase in sodium, potassium and calcium conductance. It is estimated that this will cause the sodium channel to open for about 1 millisecond (in frog muscle at 20°C). In this time about 12 000 sodium ions can traverse the membrane. A single vesicle of ACh (quantum) would therefore need to open about 1700 channels to produce its depolarizing effect. When sufficient ACh is released to effect a sodium flux adequate to reach a triggering threshold a propagated action potential ensues. The longer the channel remains open the greater the number of ions which may pass. A fall in temperature delays channel closure, as do various agents such as 4-aminopyridine. However, muscle activity and neural stimulation shorten the duration of the channel opening, thereby reducing the sodium flux.

In normal neuromuscular transmission an excess of ACh is produced following motor nerve stimulation. There also exist many more receptors than necessary to produce the total increase in cation conductance required to effectively trigger an action potential. This is reflected in the large 'margin of safety' of neuromuscular transmission described by Paton and Waud (1967). Only when this margin is reduced by disease such as myasthenia gravis or by drugs such as tubocurarine which reduce receptor availability is this margin of safety decreased to an extent which affects neuromuscular transmission. As a result of this safety margin a degree of receptor occupancy less than 80 per cent cannot be detected by monitoring the twitch response of a limb muscle or 60 per cent if a tetanic response is studied. Whilst this concept is useful to explain some of the pharmacological effects of muscle relaxants, it probably represents an oversimplification of the actual physiological events within all the neuromuscular junctions following stimulation of a large motor nerve.

Drug receptor reaction

It is customary to consider two types of neuromuscular block: *curare-like block*, variously termed *non-depolarizing, antagonist or competitive block*, and *depolarizing* or *agonist block*. In addition, various other terms have been used to define special circumstances in which drug-induced failure of neuromuscular transmission occurs; these include *desensitization block, channel block* and *presynaptic block*. Each type of block must be considered in relation to its role in the interruption of neuromuscular transmission produced in clinical practice.

Non-depolarizing, antagonist or competitive block

This type of block results when the drug reduces the degree of depolarization of the postsynaptic membrane caused by ACh following motor nerve stimulation. When the reduction in the extent of depolarization is such that threshold depolarization is not reached, a neuromuscular block is present. As the effect is 'all or none' for each neuromuscular junction, what is seen in any particular muscle during this type of block represents a spectrum of these thresholds. For complete suppression of the response to occur even the most resistant junctions must be blocked; these are the ones with the greatest margin of safety. Because of this variation in sensitivity, increasing doses of non-depolarizing drugs cause progressively more depression of twitch response of muscles until finally complete suppression occurs.

Depolarizing or agonist block

Critical depolarization of the postsynaptic membrane from the resting value of 90 mV to 57 mV or less causes the membrane to become electrically inexcitable. Decamethonium has been shown to produce depolarization approaching this figure; however, suxamethonium causes a somewhat lesser degree of depolarization (Gissen and Nastuk, 1970). Sustained depolarization will lead to inactivation of sodium channels and hence will prevent impulses being generated in the muscle. It was the observation that the block induced can outlast the duration of the depolarization *in vitro* which led Thesleff (1955) to propose the existence of 'desensitization block'. Others have suggested that this effect is the result of a progressive loss of intracellular ion caused by a continuing depolarization in an *in vitro* preparation.

Presynaptic sites of action

The presence of presynaptic ACh recognition sites and their importance in regulating the mobilization of adequate stores of readily available ACh to meet increased neural activity have been proposed by Bowman and Webb (1976) and reviewed by Bowman, Marshall and Gibb (1984) and others. They are believed to be important in influencing the development of post-tetanic fade and the train-of-four response. For many years a presynaptic site of action of non-depolarizing neuromuscular blocking agents has been postulated (Standaert, 1964; Hubbard, Wilson and Miyamoto, 1969; Blaber, 1973; Gibb and Marshall, 1984). The principal evidence in favour of this site of action is the ability of some drugs in low doses to influence tetanic fade. This is quite easily demonstrated with tubocurarine whilst pancuronium is far less active in this respect. It is possible, therefore, that at least part of the neuromuscular blocking effect produced by some agents is due to an action at presynaptic sites. The importance of this mechanism in the establishment of neuromuscular block is uncertain and its contribution to the observed block with clinical doses of non-depolarizing relaxants varies from drug to drug.

Channel block

The possibility that under certain circumstances neuromuscular block may be achieved or influenced by blocking the ion channel has to be considered. The demonstration that drugs such as local anaesthetics, the alcohols and ethers potentiate the action of non-depolarizing blocking drugs by actions at sites within the ionophore, or on the cytoplasmic side of the membrane, lends support to this as a possible site of action for neuromuscular blocking drugs. The characteristic of this type of block is that the molecule must be small enough in its hydrated form to penetrate the open channel. The block will develop when the channel is open. It is a use-dependent block (Rang, 1981). This activity is demonstrated more easily in hyperpolarized membranes or following repetitive stimulation. The finding that gallamine is capable of producing increased block following neuromuscular activity suggests that molecules may actually penetrate into the channel during the phase of increased conductance producing channel block. Drugs such as pancuronium and vecuronium produce an effect only when the membrane is hyperpolarized or in concentrations far in excess of that needed to produce clinical block (Bowman, 1985). It would seem that, with the possible exception of gallamine and decamethonium, most neuromuscular blocking drugs exhibit this activity only in high doses or in unusual circumstances.

It has been suggested that phase II block following prolonged suxamethonium depolarization is the result of channel block developing to an extent that produces clinical neuromusclar block (Standaert, 1982). This would explain many of the phenomena associated with this type of block; however, if it were a true channel block then neostigmine would be expected to potentiate its activity as it is an 'in use' channel block. The reverse is found in clinical practice. In conditions where a pure phase II exists (e.g. after prolonged administration of a suxamethonium infusion or the use of suxamethonium in patients with myasthenia gravis) neostigmine, 4-aminopyridine and edrophonium actually reverse the block.

Desensitization block

This was the term introduced by Thesleff (1955) to explain the observation that the membrane depolarization produced by depolarizing drugs such as suxamethonium wore off some time before normal neuromuscular conduction had been re-established. It seems likely that this observation, which was made *in vitro*, may have been influenced by continuing ion flux producing a net depletion of intracellular cation. A situation of true desensitization (e.g. one where the block is neither enhanced nor antagonized by ACh) is not found in normal muscle in clinical practice.

The dynamics of non-depolarizing block

It has long been the custom to consider the type of reaction achieved by non-depolarizing neuromuscular blocking drugs as being competitive in nature. In accordance with this concept the action of increasing doses of antagonist can be reversed by increasing concentrations of agonist. By plotting the log dose–response curves at increasing concentrations of antagonist a family of parallel curves are produced (Fig. 7.5 and see also Chapter 1).

Studies carried out on isolated organ preparations in a water bath using carbachol as the agonist and various non-depolarizing drugs as antagonists support this concept. The rat or mouse phrenic nerve diaphragm preparation has been most commonly used in these experiments. These are poor preparations for the study of pharmacodynamic phenomena, as the access of drug to the receptor is by diffusion into the muscle tissue rather than from the blood perfusing the vessel-rich neuromuscular junction area. In the organ bath experiments the concentration of drug in the environment is constant whilst it is rapidly diminishing in the *in vivo* situation. Unfortunately, the validation of the classic concept rests almost entirely upon this particular laboratory preparation and is not readily reconciled with the following observations in patients during clinical usage of the non-depolarizing neuromuscular blocking agents.

1. In the presence of subparalytic plasma concentration of non-depolarizing muscle relaxants (this is particularly well documented following the administration of gallamine to anuric or oliguric patients), it may be impossible to reverse the action of the drug by neostigmine, irrespective of dose (Fairley, 1950; Montgomery and Bennett Jones, 1965). The fact that neostigmine does reverse the paralysis following the lowering of the blood level of drug (Feldman and Levi, 1963) suggests that the failure of reversal is not due to an abnormal receptor–gallamine reaction but is the result of a sustained plasma level of drug. This observation is supported by the evidence that it is not possible to reverse the action of tubocurarine, pancuronium or vecuronium (Katz and Katz, 1967; Baraka, 1977) in normal patients unless some degree of neuromuscular recovery is established, indicating a declining plasma level of drug. On the basis of the competition theory the effect of a modest plasma level of non-depolarizing drug should be readily overcome by the increased ACh following the administration of neostigmine, at least during the effective plasma half-life of the anticholinesterase.

2. Mixing 2 mg tubocurarine together with various doses of neostigmine from 0.5 mg to 2.5 mg and administering them diluted in saline into a vein in the forearm of volunteers immediately after inflating an arterial tourniquet to limit their spread to the isolated arm, does not modify the appearance of full neuromuscular block. The block starts to reverse only after intervals of 10–25 minutes, following the release of the cuff (Feldman

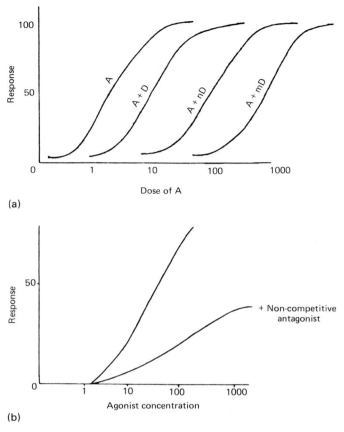

Fig. 7.5 Dynamics of (a) competitive block—agonist *vs* antagonist, and (b) non-competitive block—agonist *vs* non-competitive antagonist.

and Agoston, 1980). These isolated arm experiments are the closest replication in man of the conditions obtained *in vitro* during experiments with the phrenic nerve diaphragm preparation in a water bath.

It was the observation that, in patients with high but subparalytic plasma levels of non-depolarizing drugs, the response to neostigmine was not consistent with that of a competitive action which led Feldman and Tyrrell (1970) to re-examine the competitive hypothesis and to suggest the relationship more closely fitted a non-competitive action (Fig. 7.5). They administered very small doses of non-depolarizing (3 mg tubocurarine or 8 mg gallamine) muscle relaxants diluted in 40 ml of saline into the forearm immediately following application of an arterial tourniquet (the isolated arm technique), and demonstrated:

1. The recovery of the neuromuscular block produced did not parallel the rapid decline in plasma level of drug following the release of the tourniquet (Fig. 7.6).

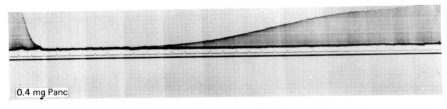

0.4 mg Panc

Fig. 7.6   Slow recovery (31 minutes) after release of arterial tourniquet following establishment of neuromuscular block by 0.4 mg pancuronium in 40 ml saline into isolated arm in conscious volunteer.

2. The rate of recovery depended upon the drug used and not upon its plasma concentration; that is, more rapid recovery occurred with gallamine than with pancuronium and that was more rapid than with tubocurarine (Table 7.1).

3. If a depolarizing drug such as decamethonium is used, the rate of recovery following release of the tourniquet is ten times quicker than that following gallamine although the usual duration of block following a bolus injection of an ED$_{95}$ dose of this drug in patients is similar to that of gallamine. This suggests a rapid washout of depolarizing drug from the receptor once the plasma level is reduced.

On the basis of this evidence they proposed that the action of these drugs is best explained in accordance with Paton's rate theory of drug action (1961). This theory proposed that agonist action is dependent upon rapid turnover of the agonist–receptor combination. Any slowly dissociating drug will tend to be antagonist in action as its presence at the receptor site impedes access of the biological transmitter to the receptor. The rapid recovery from decamethonium in the isolated arm experiments is caused by its relatively high dissociation rate. The slower the dissociation rate, the more likely is the drug to have antagonist properties.

To explain the reversal of non-depolarizing neuromuscular block by neostigmine, Feldman and Tyrrell (1970) suggested that ACh hastened the dissociation of drug from the receptor. They showed that repeated tetanic stimulation to one arm of patients, increased the rate of recovery from non-depolarizing neuromuscular block in that arm relative to the other side in the presence of identical plasma drug levels in the blood perfusing both arms.

Table 7.1   Comparison of the recovery index (25 – 75% recovery times) following 95% paralysis, using isolated arm and systemic injection

	Isolated arm (RI : N = 3 to 6)	Systemic (RI : N = 1 to 3)
d-Tubocurarine	12.8 ± 2.1	22.5 ± 3.2
Gallamine	9.8 ± 1.3	13.2 ± 2.8
Pancuronium	10.4 ± 1.4	19.4 ± 3.0
Alcuronium	9.6 ± 1.0	14.1 ± 3.6
Fazadinium	10.1 ± 1.2	14.8

The fundamental proposition that the affinity of the drug for the receptor is high in a non-depolarizing block is supported by the elegant work of Armstrong and Lester (1979). These workers showed that the association of curare with the receptor in frog muscle was 20 times quicker than the reversal produced by ionophoretic pulses of ACh. Armstrong and Lester explained these findings by the hypothesis that this effect was due to 'buffered diffusion'. This concept proposes a restricted microenvironment within the synaptic cleft, producing an attraction for positively charged ions by virtue of the high density of receptor substance in that area. They suggested that, once the drug was trapped inside this microenvironment, egress was very much slower than could be explained by simple diffusion. As a result, a high concentration of non-depolarizing drug remains close to the receptor. Within this microenvironment drug-receptor reaction might follow the dynamics of an equilibrium reaction. This attractive hypothesis is supported by the finding that the affinity of tubocurarine for the receptor is markedly decreased following saponification to destroy the synaptic membrane and the application of α-cobra venom which reduces the receptor population to approximately 10 per cent. However, it does not explain why the actions of non-depolarizing drugs are prolonged in myasthenia gravis where the receptor density is decreased by receptor antibody activity. It also fails to explain why agonist drugs such as C.10 are not affected by buffered diffusion in the same way as antagonist agents.

If antagonist drugs such as tubocurarine are bound to the receptor or are inhibited from freely leaving the synaptic cleft by buffered diffusion, then increasing the blood flow will be ineffective at 'washing out' the drug and reversing neuromuscular blockade. Agonist drugs such as C.10, however, should be readily removed from the receptor site by increasing the blood flow,

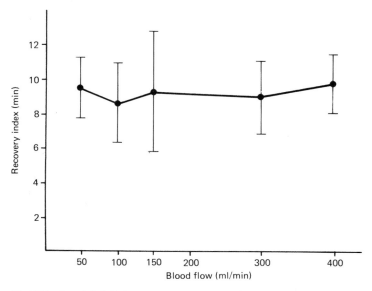

Fig. 7.7   An eightfold increase in blood flow does not influence the rate of recovery from gallamine neuromuscular block (Goat *et al.*, 1976).

provided a suitable concentration gradient exists between the perfusing blood and the receptor site. Churchill-Davidson and Richardson (1952), demonstrated that increasing the blood flow increased the recovery rate from decamethonium neuromuscular block; this is in keeping with the finding that the agonist drug is not firmly bound to the receptor. Goat *et al.* (1976) and Heneghan *et al.* (1978) demonstrated that there was no correlation between blood flow and recovery from non-depolarizing block (Fig. 7.7). In these studies the blood perfusing the leg contained significant, but decreasing, concentrations of antagonist drug which might have delayed recovery. However, White and Reitan (1984) confirmed that the recovery from tubocurarine block in dogs was uninfluenced by a four-fold increase in perfusion using blood from an extracorporeal oxygenator which contained no muscle relaxant in the perfusant, proving that, even when the concentration gradient between the blood and the receptor is maximal, recovery from non-depolarizing block is not affected by blood flow. This strongly supports the view that non-depolarizing neuromuscular blocking drugs are retained by physicochemical forces at the receptor site.

Pharmacokinetics

The importance of lowering the plasma level of drug so that reversal of neuromuscular block may take place has been established by many investigators (Baraka 1977; Katz and Katz, 1967; Feldman and Agoston, 1980). Agoston, Feldman and Miller (1979) showed that the rate of spontaneous recovery of pancuronium neuromuscular block is increased by a factor of 4 when the plasma–receptor gradient is increased by threefold (Fig. 7.8).

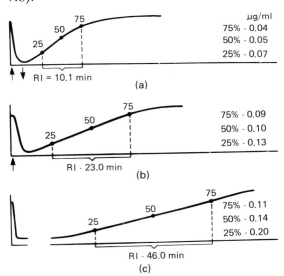

Fig. 7.8 Recovery from pancuronium block and blood levels: (a) 95 per cent block in isolated arm; (b) after bolus injection to 95 per cent block; (c) following 2 hours' continuous infusion to 90 per cent block. RI = recovery index. (Agoston, Feldman and Miller, 1979).

By various artifices, such as the isolated arm technique and unilateral tetanic stimulation, it is possible to produce the same degree of block with different plasma levels of drugs, even in the same person at the same time, due to the lag in recovery which follows reduction of the plasma concentration. However, in steady state conditions the plasma concentration producing 50 per cent block in most healthy patients is remarkably consistent. The large biological variations seen in the response to the same dose of neuromuscular blocking agent is largely due to different pharmacokinetic effects affecting both the rapid distribution phase and the slower clearance phase.

The reduction of the plasma concentration of all the highly charged neuromuscular blocking agents is effected to a varying extent by rapid redistribution and slower renal excretion. In addition, for particular agents, metabolism, biliary excretion and sequestration in the liver are important accessory pathways assisting the process of plasma clearance. The rapid distribution to the liver and kidney of all the neuromuscular blocking agents, as revealed by autoradiography, emphasizes the importance of these large distribution volumes. In the presence of normal renal blood flow a massive early appearance of drugs such as tubocurarine in the kidney is accompanied by excretion in the urine, even during the 5 minutes following injection into rats (Cohen, Hood and Golling, 1968). The effect of diminished renal and hepatic blood flow, decreased renal function, jaundice and liver disease may therefore cause significant changes in the pharmacokinetics of these drugs.

Special pharmacokinetic factors
In addition to redistribution, the reduction in plasma concentration of drug may involve three special pharmacokinetic processes: metabolism, sequestration and excretion.

Metabolic pathways
Plasma clearance of suxamethonium depends principally upon hydrolysis by plasma cholinesterase. Absence of this enzyme or its replacement by abnormal enzyme affects this process because the rate of hydrolysis varies with the log of the concentration up to that level at which enzyme saturation occurs.

The new benzyl isoquinoline esters of Saverase and Wastilla (1979) also use this method of hydrolysis, splitting the active bisquaternary compound into two inactive monoquaternary derivates. Some of these drugs are hydrolysed at rates giving a plasma half-life measured in seconds. It is interesting that the neuromuscular block they induce often considerably outlasts the anticipated plasma half-life of the drug.

Hofmann degeneration In this reaction, electron transport occurs in the presence of an alkaline milieu, splitting the quaternary amino bond into a less active or inactive tertiary compound (Fig. 7.9). The rate of reaction is also increased by a rise in temperature. As the process is physicochemical in nature the rate is related to the substrate concentration in a linear fashion. This process is principally responsible for the short plasma half-life of about 26 minutes for atracurium. In this reaction, raising the pH to that of the plasma causes spontaneous degradation of the parent drug. The reaction is modestly increased by further alkanization and by hyperthermia. The monotertiary product laudanosine penetrates the blood–brain barrier, and in high

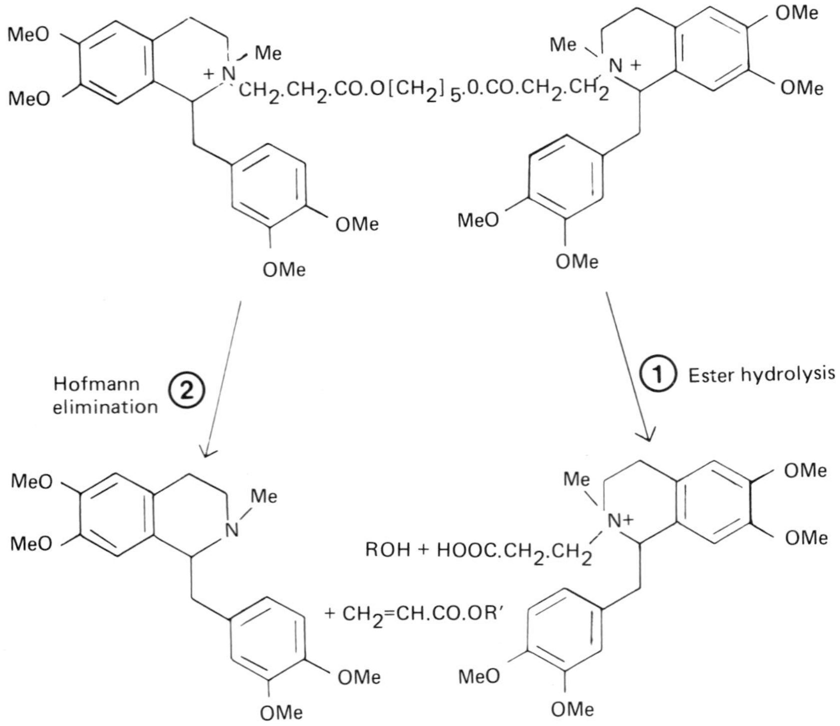

Fig. 7.9   Metabolic pathways for atracurium.

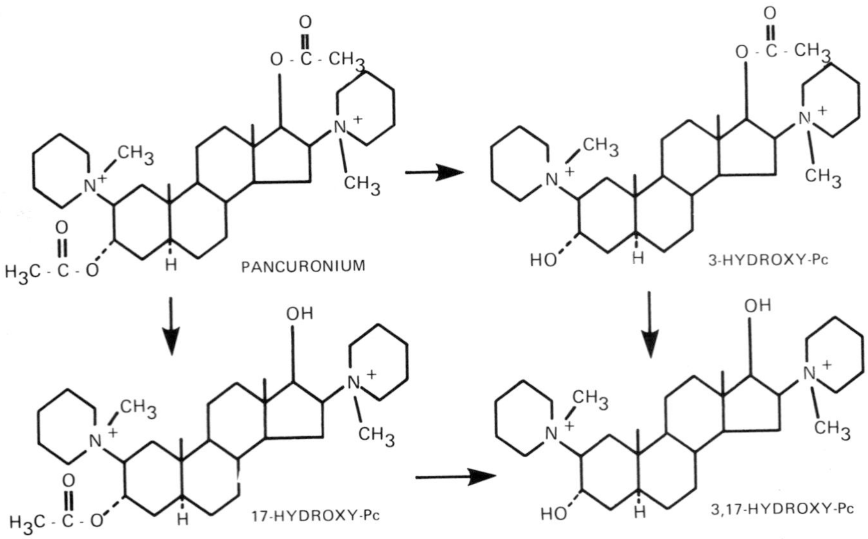

Fig. 7.10   Metabolic pathways for pancuronium.

concentration has a demonstrable analeptic effect, increasing the MAC requirements of volatile anaesthetic in animals (Hennis *et al.*, 1984).

Pancuronium and vecuronium   Metabolism in the liver at the 3- and 17-acetyl sites occurs to a limited extent (10–30 per cent), with pancuronium producing the 3-hydroxy, the 17-hydroxy and 3,17-hydroxy derivatives (Fig. 7.10). These less active metabolites are excreted principally in the urine but also to some extent in the bile.

Vecuronium is principally metabolized to the 3-hydroxy derivative, although all the metabolic processes described for pancuronium can occur. Metabolism probably contributes to the plasma clearance of about 20 per cent of an injected bolus dose of vecuronium.

Both metabolism and biliary excretion of the steroid muscle relaxants are significantly depressed by hepatic disease and by jaundice, causing a prolongation of the half-life of the drug. The effect of jaundice has been demonstrated *in vitro* to be associated with an increase in taurocholic acid, and it has been postulated that this competes with the drug for intracellular enzyme systems or carrier mechanisms (Vonk *et al.*, 1979).

Fazadinium   This azo dye based non-depolarizing muscle relaxant has a short plasma half-life in most animals as the bisquaternary structure is metabolized in the liver by azo reductase (Fig. 7.11). However, human liver has minimal capacity for reductive metabolism and as a result the drug has a much longer half-life and most of an injected dose is recoverable from the urine.

Sequestration
Although all the non-depolarizing muscle relaxants are rapidly distributed to the liver, spleen and kidneys, true sequestration in the liver producing almost a first-pass clearance occurs with some steroidal-based compounds. Rapid plasma clearance by organ uptake was demonstrated to occur in the liver with the pancuronium analogue ORG6368 (Agoston, 1984, personal communication). Large, rapid hepatic uptake of vecuronium has been demonstrated in animals and probably also occurs in man. The presence of only one fully quaternized onium group in this compound increases the potential for membrane penetration and therefore for organ sequestration. The difference between the α half-life of vecuronium and of pancuronium is largely attributable to sequestration causing the plasma concentration to fall.

Renal excretion
All the neuromuscular blocking drugs are concentrated in the kidneys. Up to 25 per cent of an initial bolus dose of tubocurarine is to be found in the kidneys of rats within 5 minutes (Cohen, Hood and Golling, 1968). It is not surprising, therefore, that all these water-soluble, almost fat-insoluble drugs, are excreted to a lesser or greater extent unchanged in the urine. Drugs such as gallamine and decamethonium are virtually only cleared by renal excretion. Alcuronium, pancuronium and metacurarine rely on renal clearance for removal of between 75 and 85 per cent of an injected dose. Up to 65 per cent of an injected dose of tubocurarine is normally recoverable in the urine; however, if the renal

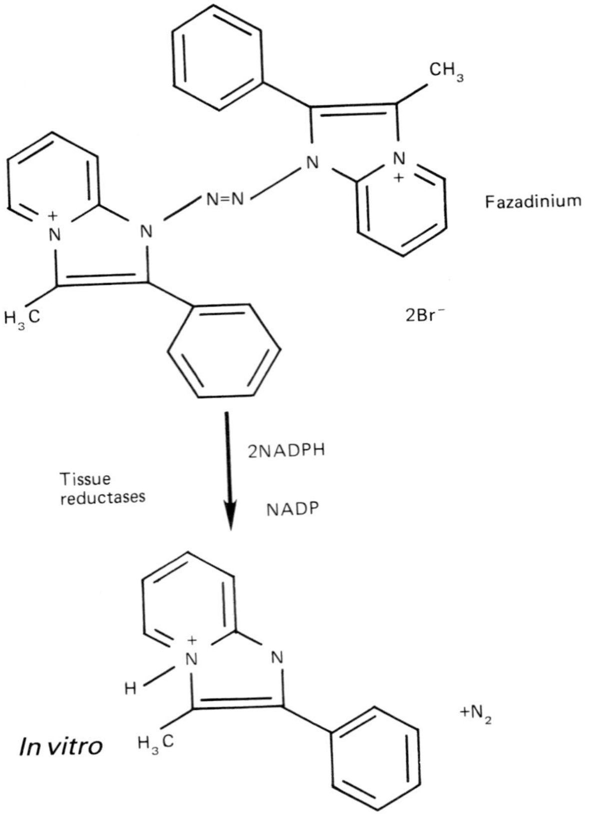

Fig. 7.11   Azo reductase metabolism of fazadinium.

pedicle of dogs is tied, up to 34 per cent of the drug may be recovered from the bile (Cohen, Brewer and Smith, 1967).

The plasma clearance of vecuronium appears to be associated with sequestration in the liver. Although some of the sequestrated drug undergoes metabolism and biliary excretion, the major portion of the injected dose appears in the urine. As a result there is a modest (about 10 per cent) increase in duration of action of the drug in patients with renal failure.

Atracurium, like suxamethonium, does not rely on renal function for plasma clearance of the drug and its action is not prolonged in renal failure.

Understanding the mechanism of action of the neuromuscular blocking drug thus requires a knowledge both of the nature of the receptor and of the manner in which these drugs interfere with normal receptor activation by ACh. Their action is terminated by their removal from the receptor and diffusion along a concentration gradient into the plasma from whence they are eliminated. Many physical, physiological, pharmacological and pathological factors can affect this process and modify their activity – the production of ACh, the sensitivity of the receptors and their number, the electrical threshold of the muscle and the rate of removal of the drug from the plasma. Understanding the nature of the process involved in the production of neuromuscular block allows a sensible interpretation of how these mechanisms may be altered by abnormal conditions and during anaesthetic practice.

References

Agoston, S., Feldman, S.A. and Miller, R.D. (1979) Plasma pancuronium and twitch response using the isolated arm, bolus injection and continuous infusion. *Anesthesiology* **51**, 119

Armstrong, D.L. and Lester, H.A. (1979) The kinetics of tubocurarine action and restricted diffusion within the synaptic cleft. *Journal of Physiology* **294**, 365

Bacq, Z.M. and Brown, G.L. (1937) Pharmacological experiments on mammalian voluntary muscle in relation to the theory of chemical transmission. *Journal of Physiology* **89**, 45

Baraka, A. (1977) Irreversible curarization. *Anaesthesia and Intensive Care* **5**, 244

Barlow, R.B. and Ing, H.R.C. (1948) Curare-like actions of polymethylene bis-quaternary ammonium salts. *British Journal of Pharmacology and Chemotherapy* **3**, 298

Birks, R. and McIntosh, F.C. (1961) Acetylcholine metabolism of a sympathetic ganglion. *Canadian Journal of Biochemistry and Physiology* **39**, 787

Birks, R., Huxley, H.E. and Katz, B. (1960) The fine structure of the neuromuscular junction of the frog. *Journal of Physiology* **150**, 134

Blaber, L.C. (1973) The prejunctional actions of some non-depolarising drugs. *British Journal of Pharmacology* **47**, 109

Bowman, W.C. (1985) The neuromuscular junction – recent developments. *European Journal of Anaesthesiology* **2**, 59

Bowman, W.C. and Webb, S.N. (1976) Tetanic fade during partial transmission failure produced by non-depolarising neuromuscular blocking drugs in the cat. *Clinical and Experimental Pharmacology and Physiology* **3**, 545

Bowman, W.C., Marshall, I.G. and Gibb, A.J. (1984) Is there feedback control of transmitter release at the neuromuscular junction? *Seminars in Anaesthesia* **3**, no. 4, 275

Changeux, J.P., Devillers-Thiery, A. and Chemonilli, P. (1984) Acetylcholine receptor. An allosteric membrane protein. *Science* **225**, 1335

Changeux, J.P., Benedetti, L., Bourgeois, J.P. *et al.* (1976) Some structural properties of the cholinergic receptor protein in its membrane environment relevant to its function as a pharmacological receptor. *Cold Spring Harbor Symposia on Quantitative Biology* **40**, 211

Churchill-Davidson, H.C. and Richardson, A.J. (1952) Decamethonium iodide (C_{10}) some observations using electromyography. *Proceedings of the Royal Society of Medicine* **45**, 179

Cohen, E.N., Brewer, W.M. and Smith, D. (1967) The metabolism and elimination of d-tubocurarine H^3. *Anesthesiology* **28**, 540

Cohen, E.N., Hood, N. and Golling, R. (1968) Use of wholebody autoradiography for determination of uptake and distribution of labelled muscle relaxants in the rat. *Anesthesiology* **29**, 987

Cohen, J.B. and Changeux, J.P. (1975) The cholinergic receptor protein in its membrane environment. *Annual Review of Pharmacology* **15**, 83

Dale, H.H. and Feldberg, W. (1934) Chemical transmission at motor nerve endings in voluntary muscle. *Journal of Physiology* **81**, 39

Dale, H.H., Feldberg, W. and Vogt, M. (1936) Release of acetylcholine at voluntary motor nerve endings. *Journal of Physiology* **86**, 353

Davis, R. and Koelle, G.B. (1967) Electron microscopic localization of acetylcholinesterase and non-specific cholinesterase at the neuromuscular junction by gold thiocholine and gold thioacetic acid methods. *Journal of Cell Biology* **34**, 157

Everett, A.J., Lowe, L.A. and Wilkinson, S. (1970) Revision of structure of (+)-tubocurarine chloride and chondrocurarine. *Journal of the Chemical Society* 1020

Fairley, H.B. (1950) Prolonged intercostal paralysis due to a relaxant. *British Medical Journal* **2**, 986

Fambrough, D.M. (1979) Control of acetylcholine receptors in skeletal muscle. *Physiological Review* **59**, 165

Fambrough, D.M. and Harzell, H.C. (1972) Acetylcholine receptors number and distribution at neuromuscular junction in rat diaphragm. *Science* **176**, 189

Feldman, S.A. and Agoston, S. (1980) Failure of neostigmine to prevent tubocurarine neuromuscular block in the isolated arm. *British Journal of Anaesthesia* **62**, 86

Feldman, S.A. and Levi, J.A. (1963) Prolonged paresis following gallamine. *British Journal of Anaesthesia* **35**, 804

Feldman, S.A. and Tyrrell, M.F. (1970) A new theory of the termination of action of the muscle relaxants. *Proceedings of the Royal Society of Medicine* **63**, 692

Gibb, A.J. and Marshall, I.G. (1984) Pre- and post-junctional effects of tubocurarine and other nicotinic antagonists during repetitive stimulation in the rat. *Journal of Physiology* **351**, 275

Gissen, A.J. and Nastuk, W.L. (1970) Succinylcholine and decamethonium comparison of depolarization and desensitization. *Anesthesiology* **33**, 611

Goat, V.A., Feldman, S.A., Yeung, M.L. *et al.* (1976) The effect of blood flow upon the activity of gallamine triethiodide. *British Journal of Anaesthesia* **48**, 69

Heneghan, C.P.A., Findley, I.L., Gilbe, C.E. and Feldman, S.A. (1978) Muscle blood flow and rate of recovery from pancuronium neuromuscular block in dogs. *British Journal of Anaesthesia* **50**, 1105

Hennis, P.J., Fahey, N.R., Miller, R.D., Canful, C. and Shi, W.Z. (1984) Pharmacology of laudanosine in dogs. ASA abstracts A305. *Anesthesiology* **61**, 3A

Hubbard, J.I., Wilson, D.F. and Miayamoto, M. (1969) Reduction of transmitter release by *d*-tubocurarine. *Nature* **223**, 531

Irwin, R.L. and Trams, E.G. (1962) Reduction of neuromuscular blocking activity of quaternary compounds by gangliosides. *Journal of Pharmacology and Experimental Therapeutics* **137**, 242

Katz, R.L. and Katz, G.J. (1967) Clinical considerations in use of muscle relaxants. In: *Muscle Relaxants* (Ed. Katz, R.L.), Advances in Anesthesiology. Elsevier: New York; Excerpta Medica: Amsterdam

King, H. (1935) Curare alkaloids. I. Tubocurarine. *Journal of the Chemical Society* 1381

Lebowitz, P.W., Ramsey, F.M., Savarese, J.J. and Ali, H.H. (1980) Potentiation of neuromuscular blockade in man produced by combinations of pancuronium and metacurarine or pancuronium and *d*-tubocurarine. *Anesthesia and Analgesia* **57**, 606

Miledi, R. and Potter, L.T. (1971) Acetylcholine receptors in muscle fibres. *Nature* **233**, 599

Montgomery, J.B. and Bennett Jones, W. (1965) Gallamine triethiodiode and renal disease. *Lancet* **2**, 1243

Paton, W.D.M. (1961) A theory of drug action based on the rate of drug-receptor combination. *Proceedings of the Royal Society, B* **154**, 21

Paton, W.D.M. and Waud, D.R. (1967) The margin of safety of muscle relaxant drugs. *Journal of Physiology* **191**, 59

Paton, W.D.M. and Zaimis, E.J. (1949) The pharmacological actions of polymethylene bis-methylammonium salts. *British Journal of Pharmacology and Chemotherapy* **4**, 381

Rang, H.P. (1981) Drugs and ionic channels: mechanisms and implications. *Postgraduate Medical Journal* **57**, suppl. 1, 89

Rash, J.E., Hudson, C.S. and Ellisman, M.H. (1978) Ultrastructure of acetylcholine receptors at mammalian neuromuscular junction. In: *Cell Membrane Receptors for Drugs and Hormones* (Eds. Straub, R.W. and Bolis, L.). Raven Press, New York

Robertson, J.D. (1956) Electron microscopies of the motor end plate and neuromuscular spindle. *Journal of Biophysical and Biochemical Cytology* **2**, 381

Savarese, J.J. and Wastilla, W.B. (1979) BW444V. Intermediate duration non-depolarizing neuromuscular blocking agent with significant lack of cardiovascular and autonomic effect. *Anesthesiology* **51**, 279

Standaert, F.G. (1964) The action of *d*-tubocurarine on the motor nerve terminal. *Journal of Pharmacology and Experimental Therapeutics* **143**, 181

Standaert, F.G. (1982) Sites of action of muscle relaxants. *ASA Refresher course abstracts* p.226

Taylor, P., Brown, R.D. and Johnson, D.A. (1983) The linkage between occupation and response of the nicotinic acetylcholine receptor. In: *Current Topics in Membranes and Transport*, vol. 18 (Eds. Martin, B.R. and Kleinzeller, A.). Academic Press: New York

Thesleff, S. (1955) The mode of neuromuscular block caused by acetylcholine, nicotine, decamethonium and succinylcholine. *Acta Physiologica Scandinavica* **34**, 218

Vonk, R.J., Westra, P., Houwertjes, M.C. and Agoston, S. (1979) Prolongation by bile salts of the duration of action of a steroidal neuromuscular blocking agent. *British Journal of Anaesthesia* **51**, 719

Vulpian, A. (1866) *Lecons sur la Physiologie Generale et comparee du systeme nerveux.* Faites à Museum d'Histoire Naturelle (Bailliere): Paris

Waser, P.G. (1970) Receptors on the postsynaptic membrane of the motor end plate. In: *Molecular Properties of Drug Receptors* (Eds. Porter, R. and O'Connor, M.), Ciba Foundation Symposium series. Churchill: London

Waser, P.G. (1972) Affinity labelling of cholinergic receptors with curarizing and depolarizing drugs. In: *Pharmacology Congress, San Francisco*. Karger: Basel

Waser, P.G. (1975) Molecular basis of curare action. In: *Muscle Relaxants* (Ed. Katz, R.L.), Monographs in Anesthesiology. Elsevier: New York; Excerpta Medica: Amsterdam

Waser, P.G. (1983) *Cholinergic Pharmakon-rezeptoren*. Ovell-Fussli Graphische: Berlin, Zurich

Waud, B.E. and Waud, D.R. (1985) Interaction amongst agents that block end-plate depolarization competitively. *Anesthesiology* **63**, 4

White, D.A. and Reitan, J.A. (1984) Effect of blood flow in the pharmacodynamics of non-depolarizing muscle relaxants using isolated limb model. Abstracts of ASA meeting. *Anesthesiology* **61**, A286

8

Adrenoceptor agonists

W.B. Runciman

In 1895, Oliver and Schafer described the profound cardiovascular effects of an extract of the adrenal medulla. They showed that a tiny amount of the extract caused a massive rise in blood pressure, not only by 'contraction of the arterioles' but also by 'increased rate and energy of the heart beat'. By the turn of the century, the active principle, adrenaline, had been isolated and identified (Abel and Crawford, 1897) and the similarities between its effects and those of stimulation of the sympathetic nerves had been noted (Lewandowsky, 1898).

In 1905, Elliot proposed that the release from sympathetic nerves of minute amounts of an adrenaline-like substance was a chemical step in the process of neurotransmission; Langley had already suggested in 1901 that effector cells might have excitatory and inhibitory 'receptive substances'. These workers would probably have found quite acceptable the modern definition of an adrenoceptor agonist as a compound with both affinity for and efficacy at specific cell membrane sites (termed 'adrenoceptors') (Lees, 1981).

In 1910, Barger and Dale studied a number of amines chemically related to adrenaline, determined the structural requirements for adrenaline-like activity and grouped the active compounds under the general heading of 'sympathomimetic amines'; those amines containing a catechol nucleus were termed 'catecholamines'. They also made the important observations that there were qualitative differences between some of the compounds, that some (but not all) of their effects could be blocked by certain alkaloids of ergot and that sympathetic nerve stimulation was mimicked more closely by noradrenaline than by adrenaline. Some of these observations were then overlooked for many years; indeed, Dale refrained from drawing the conclusion that noradrenaline was the natural transmitter for a number of years.

In 1921, Otto Loewi provided conclusive proof for the theory of chemotransmission with his classic experiments on the isolated frog heart. He showed that the perfusate of a heart which had undergone nerve stimulation would exert predictable effects on another, unstimulated, heart. This lent support to the general belief that adrenaline, the sympathetic chemotransmitter in the frog heart, was also that in man. In 1946, Von Euler showed that the peripheral sympathetic chemotransmitter in man was, in fact, noradrenaline, the biological precursor of adrenaline.

In 1948, Ahlquist proposed the existence of two different types of receptors – α-receptors, which were known to be blocked by compounds such as phenoxybenzamine, and β-receptors, for which no antagonists were known at that time. The sympathomimetic amines could then be classified according to their relative potencies as α- and/or β-agonists. In 1958 the first β-receptor blocker, dichloroisoprenaline, was described (Powell and Slater, 1958). In 1967, Lands et al. provided justification for the subdivision of β-adrenoceptors into β_1 and β_2 subtypes. Chemotransmitter theory has since undergone progressive refinement with the development of an increasingly selective range of agonists and antagonists, with advances in understanding of the mechanisms controlling the synthesis, storage, release, uptake and metabolism of catecholamines, in the mapping, identification and characterization of receptors, and with increased understanding of the steps between receptor activation and the production of biological effects.

Extensive noradrenergic, adrenergic and dopaminergic systems have been identified in the central nervous system. A host of pre- and postsynaptic regulatory mechanisms have been described. Alpha receptors have been divided into α_1 and α_2 subtypes. The discovery of the concomitant storage and release of one or more biologically active peptides in many peripheral sympathetic nerves has opened up a whole new field, and may provide explanations for a variety of previously unexplained phenomena, such as the failure of α-blockers to completely prevent, in some circulatory beds, vasoconstriction with sympathetic nerve stimulation. The demonstration that receptor number and affinity are subject to very substantial up- and down-regulation under a variety of pharmacological and pathophysiological influences has also explained a number of previously identified discrepancies. Finally, the recognition of the importance of protein phosphorylation as a final common pathway in biological regulation has raised the possibility of highly selective drug treatment, once the substrate proteins for the various protein kinases have been characterized, and once the molecular pathways have been identified by which specific physiological responses are elicited.

In the light of all this new information it is no longer adequate, for clinical practice, to simply classify sympathomimetic amines by their relative potencies as α- or β-agonists. The effects of these agents are superimposed on those of the endogenous catecholamines and they act through the same effector pathways, which are subject to many influences which alter their functions. The autonomic nervous system is an important regulator of the cardiovascular system, and an ever-increasing number of patients have abnormalities of both their cardiovascular and their autonomic nervous systems, and are on drug treatment affecting one or both of these systems. Anaesthesia and surgery may then further perturb these systems, and alter the effects of drugs acting upon them. Although the clinical significance of many of the factors known to influence the response to adrenoceptor agonists has not been established, some knowledge of these, and of the many interactions which may occur, is useful when using these potent compounds clinically.

As there have been well over 30 000 publications in this area in the last 20 years, selected papers and recent reviews are quoted only on topics not covered in standard texts (e.g. Bowman and Rand, 1980; Gilman, Goodman and Gilman, 1980).

Central nervous system

A detailed consideration of the central nervous system (CNS) catecholaminergic system is beyond the scope of this chapter but mention of some recent advances is appropriate. Extensive CNS adrenergic, noradrenergic and dopaminergic systems have been mapped and have been shown to play an important role in a variety of pathways and processes, including behaviour and memory (Vogt, 1984). Neurons originating in the compact locus ceruleus give rise to the dorsal noradrenergic bundle which innervates much of the cerebral cortex, and neurons situated more centrally in the medulla give rise to the ventral noradrenergic bundle, which supplies most of the limbic forebrain, a very important region in the control of emotion and behaviour. These neurons may each branch up to 100 000 times, suggesting that these systems provide background modulation for the activity of many other neurons, some with general and some with specialized local actions.

Recent work in the area of psychopharmacology promises both greater understanding and, ultimately, the possibility of rational effective treatment of common disorders such as depression and mania (Bunney and Garland, 1984). For example, biological markers have now been identified for discriminating between endogenous and non-endogenous depression, and for predicting the likely outcome of different forms of treatment (Wood and Rafaelsen, 1984). The identification of factors common to several successful methods of treatment of depression (including electroconvulsive therapy and treatment with tricyclic antidepressants, monoamine oxidase inhibitors and lithium), such as down-regulation of central β-adrenoceptors, suggests that elucidation of the mechanisms of these diseases may be possible in the future. New treatment strategies suggested by this information, such as the use of β-agonists to induce generalized down-regulation of β-receptors, have been shown to be clinically effective. To this end, lipophilic β-agonists have been developed which cross the blood–brain barrier better (e.g. clenbuterol). The overall situation is, however, likely to be complex, as there is evidence that this down-regulation of β-receptors is associated with interactions with central α_2-receptors as well as with cholinergic, serotoninergic and opioid systems (Wood and Rafaelsen, 1984).

It is now recognized that complex interactions between systems with different chemotransmitters are widespread, and it has been shown that many substances thought to have been peptide hormones are neurotransmitters, and vice versa. For example, somatostatin has been found in skin, gut and thyroid gland, and thyroid hormones have been shown to play a neuromodulator role in the brain (Dratman, Crutchfield and Gordon, 1984).

CNS catecholaminergic neurons are thus involved not only in the central integration of some homoeostatic mechanisms mediated by the autonomic nervous system but also in complex processes such as those controlling mood, behaviour and memory, and they interact with a wide range of systems incorporating cholinergic, serotoninergic, opioid and a variety of peptide-mediated neurons.

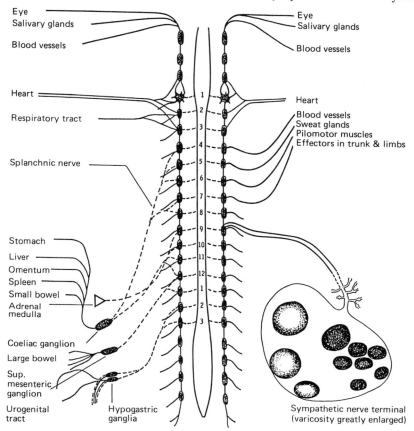

Fig. 8.1   Schematic representation of the peripheral (efferent) sympathetic nervous system. Nerves with preganglionic axons are shown as broken lines, and those with postganglionic axons as solid lines. The left side of the diagram shows both preganglionic and postganglionic sympathetic outflow, whereas the right side shows only postganglionic outflow to the eye and salivary glands and heart, and to the grey rami communicates to somatic nerves. A schematic representation of a postganglionic noradrenergic neuron, with one greatly enlarged varicosity, is also shown. This varicosity is depicted in greater detail in Fig. 8.2,

Peripheral sympathetic nervous system

A schematic representation of the peripheral (efferent) sympathetic nervous system is given in Fig. 8.1, and a diagram of a postganglionic sympathetic neuron in Fig. 8.2. The many physiological, pharmacological and pathophysiological influences on the peripheral sympathetic nervous system, and the factors which modify the effects of adrenoceptor agonists, may be considered systematically under the headings in Fig. 8.2.

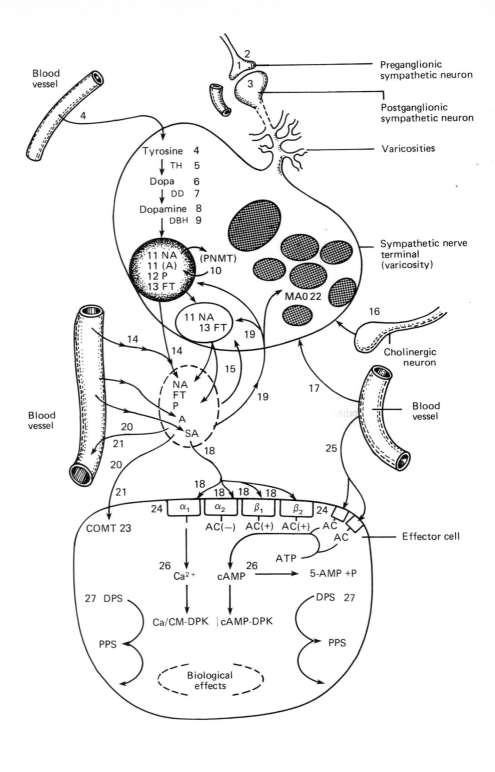

1. Preganglionic sympathetic neurons

Centres in the brainstem give rise to descending tracts which innervate the sympathetic preganglionic neurons in the intermediolateral column of the spinal cord; the intermediolateral column also receives input from cholinergic, serotoninergic, oxytocic and opioid neurons (Muldoon *et al.*, 1984). A single preganglionic sympathetic nerve fibre may impinge on a large number of postganglionic nerve cells in different ganglia, and each postganglionic nerve may innervate several thousand varicosities (see Fig. 8.1). An efferent sympathetic response may thus be somewhat 'diffuse', but extensive integration of efferent impulses occurs at the level of the spinal cord, medulla, hypothalamus and cortex, and different stimuli usually produce highly specific responses.

There is, therefore, continuous variation in the rate and pattern of discharge of these neurons. Some stimuli, such as postural blood pressure changes or light to moderate excercise, affect outflow to noradrenergic nerves rather than that to the adrenal medulla. In these instances activity correlates well with plasma noradrenaline levels (Lake, Chernow and Ziegler, 1984). On the other hand, stimuli such as psychological stress and hypoglycaemia mainly increase plasma adrenaline levels. There is evidence that complex central pathways are involved in the control of different patterns of discharge. For example, centrally acting opioids may cause a generalized increase in sympathetic outflow, whereas somatostatin or central cholinergic stimulation affect outflow to the adrenal medulla but not the noradrenergic nerves (Schultzberg, 1984).

There are several diseases in which preganglionic nerve traffic is reduced (Kopin, 1984; Lake, Chernow and Ziegler, 1984). These patients suffer from a variety of autonomic disturbances, including postural hypotension. However, as a result of reduced peripheral catecholamine release, receptors may up-regulate (see section 28 below) and the patients may also have hypertensive crises in response to endogenous adrenaline release and markedly exaggerated responses to exogenous sympathomimetic amines; thus α-agonists may cause severe hypertension and β_2-agonists dangerous

---

Fig. 8.2 Schematic representation of a postganglionic sympathetic neuron. The numbers 1–28 represent the levels at which physiological, pathophysiological and pharmacological factors may influence the effects of adrenoceptor agonists. The factors operating at each level are considered in the text. 1. Preganglionic neuron. 2. Ganglionic transmission. 3. Postganglionic neuron. 4. Tyrosine. 5. Tyrosine hydroxylase (TH). 6. Dihydroxyphenylalanine (Dopa). 7. Dopa decarboxylase (DD). 8. Dopamine. 9. Dopamine β-hydroxylase (DBH). 10. Phenethanolamine-*N*-methyltransferase (PNMT) (only in the adrenal medulla and CNS adrenergic neurons). 11. Storage of catecholamines: noradrenaline (NA); adrenaline (A). 12. Storage of peptides (P). 13. Storage of false transmitters (FT). 14. Release. 15. Prejunctional catecholamine and opioid influences. 16. Prejunctional cholinergic influences. 17. Other prejunctional influences. 18. Adrenoceptor agonists. 19. Neuronal uptake. 20. Redistribution and extraneuronal uptake. 21. Metabolism. 22. Monoamine oxidase (MAO). 23. Catechol-*O*-methyltransferase (COMT). 24. Adrenoceptors. 25. First messengers: adenyl cyclase (AC); inhibitor (−); facilitator (+). 26. Second messengers: cyclic adenosine monophosphate (cAMP); phosphodiesterase (PDE). 27. Third messengers and biological effects: calcium/calmodulin-dependent protein kinase (Ca/CM-DPK); cAMP-dependent protein kinase (cAMP-DPK); dephosphorylated protein substrates (DPS); phosphorylated protein substrates (PPS).

hypotension. Reduced peripheral catecholamine release may occur as a result of failure of the afferent limb of the baroreceptor reflex (as in familial dysautonomia), as a result of failure of central integration of the baroreceptor reflex (as in the Shy–Drager syndrome) or as a result of degeneration of the efferent limb (as in idiopathic orthostatic hypotension). It may also occur in some patients with Parkinson's disease, and in some spinal trauma patients before spinal autonomic reflexes have become stabilized. In other conditions, such as tetanus and the Guillain–Barré syndrome, very variable outflow may result in a labile blood pressure and dysrhythmias which are difficult to manage.

Some drugs, such as the α_2-agonist clonidine, produce selective alterations in sympathetic outflow patterns, whereas others, such as general anaesthetic agents, cause widespread disturbances, with some increasing outflow (e.g. diethyl ether and cyclopropane) and some decreasing it (e.g. halothane, isoflurane and enflurane) (Muldoon *et al.*, 1984). Both baro- and chemoreceptor reflexes are severely impaired with halothane anaesthesia (Nhill and Gelb, 1982; Seagard *et al.*, 1982).

2. Ganglionic transmission

Activation of postganglionic neurons is mediated primarily by acetylcholine, and may thus be blocked by ganglion-blocking drugs such as hexamethonium, mecamylamine and trimetaphan. The net effect of blockade is to produce postural hypotension and loss of other compensatory circulatory reflexes, to diminish sweating and reduce the flow of saliva and other gastrointenstinal secretions, to produce hypotonia of the bladder and bowel, and to produce dilated pupils and blurred vision. Ganglionic transmission may be modulated by both excitatory and inhibitory mechanisms. Prejunctional excitatory modulation is produced by muscarinic agonists and inhibitory modulation by α_2-agonists; both mediate these effects via second messengers, which may themselves be influenced by other first messengers (see section 25).

3. Postganglionic neurons

The synthesis of the enzymes and of the organelles necessary for the formation and release of noradrenaline (and probably enkephalins and other peptides) takes place in the cell body, followed by transport down the axon to nerve terminals, and may be subject to long-term neural and hormonal influences. For example, the activity of the enzyme tyrosine hydroxylase is increased by increased neural traffic, and that of the enzyme dopamine β-hydroxylase has been shown to be increased by testosterone and progesterone (Rutledge, 1984).

Axonal transport may be interfered with by the degenerative changes which occur in certain peripheral neuropathies, such as those which occur in diabetes, and propagation of the action potential may also be blocked in a number of ways. The nerve fibres may be divided surgically or chemically ablated, and temporary blockade may be achieved with local anaesthetic agents. Several other groups of drugs have some local anaesthetic effect, including the adrenergic neuron blockers, some opoids, and most antihistamines, but this effect is usually insignificant at the doses used clinically.

6-Hydroxydopamine causes selective destruction of sympathetic nerve terminals; this has been exploited experimentally. The drug has also been injected subconjunctivally in the treatment of glaucoma. However, the repeated injections which are necessary with recurrent regeneration of the nerve terminals result in inflammation and fibrosis. Widespread prolonged selective inhibition of axonal conduction is also caused by the puffer fish toxin, tetrodotoxin. With destruction, ablation or prolonged blockade of sympathetic nerves up-regulation of receptors occurs in the denervated area, leading to exaggerated responses to circulating sympathomimetic amines ('denervation hypersensitivity').

Synthesis of noradrenaline takes place in sympathetic nerve terminals, and of adrenaline in the adrenal medulla. The stages of catecholamine synthesis are shown in Fig. 8.3; each may be subject to a number of influences.

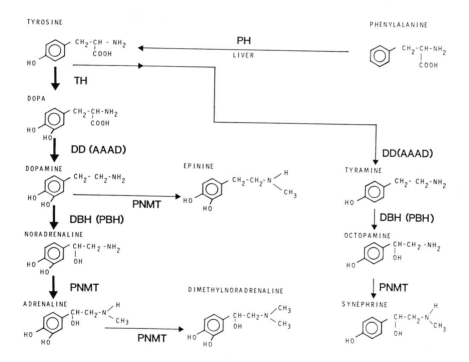

Fig. 8.3 Synthesis of catecholamines* and endogenous false transmitters. PH = phenylalanine hydroxylase. TH = tyrosine hydroxylase. DD = dopamine decarboxylase. AAAD = aromatic amino acid decarboxylase. DBH = dopamine-β-hydroxylase. PBH = phenylethylamine-β-hydroxylase. PNMT = phenylethanolamine-N-methyltransferase

*The term 'catechol' denotes a benzene ring with two hydroxyl groups on adjacent carbon atoms, compared with phenol which has only one hydroxyl group. The catechol derivatives occurring in nature have these hydroxyl groups on the 3 and 4 carbon atoms of the benzene ring; thus the sympathomimetic amines with this configuration in the benzene ring have become known as catecholamines.

4. Tyrosine and phenylalanine

The starting point for catecholamine synthesis is with either of the essential amino acids phenylalanine or tyrosine, which are derived from proteins in the diet. There is usually enough tyrosine in the diet, but, if not, it may be formed from phenylalanine in the liver. The disease phenylketonuria may be produced by congenital absence of the enzyme phenylalanine hydroxylase, and a similar condition by inhibition of this enzyme by compounds such as fluorophenylalanine.

Tyrosine is actively transported into cells, and other amino acids may compete for transport. Tyrosine availability may limit the rate of catecholamine synthesis with some rapidly firing systems (e.g. the adrenal medulla with severe hypotension), and may thus be a factor in some circumstances in patients with low tyrosine availability relative to other competing aromatic amino acids; some commercially available parenteral nutrition solutions contain relatively little tyrosine (Conlay and Maher, 1984).

5. Tyrosine hydroxylase (TH)

TH catalyses the addition of a 3-hydroxy group, thus converting the phenol tyrosine to its catechol analogue (see legend to Fig. 8.3). It is synthesized in the cell body and transported down the axon, is specific to catecholamine-producing tissues, and is the rate-limiting enzyme in catecholamine synthesis. As such, it is a logical target for pharmacological intervention. A number of tyrosine analogues will compete for the enzyme; one, α-methyl tyrosine, has been used clinically in the treatment of phaeochromocytoma to reduce catecholamine stores.

An acute increase in TH activity may be induced by increasing the concentration of the natural co-factor tetrahydrobiopterin (BH4). BH4 has been claimed to be effective clinically in some diseases thought to be due to CNS biogenic amine deficiencies such as Parkinson's disease and endogenous depression (Nagatsu and Nagatsu, 1984). The neuropeptides secretin and vasoactive intestinal peptide (VIP) have also been shown to increase TH activity.

TH plays an important role in the regulation of catecholamine synthesis. It is inhibited when noradrenaline concentrations rise because noradrenaline competes with essential co-factors (end-product regulation). There is also evidence for presynaptic regulation of TH via adreno- and cholinoreceptors and for trans-synaptic regulation by prostaglandins (see section 17).

6. Dihydroxyphenylalanine (dopa)

Dopa does not accumulate in adrenergic terminals because it is formed fairly slowly, as the product of the rate-limiting step in catecholamine synthesis, but is converted rapidly to dopamine. This conversion may be competitively inhibited by high levels of other substrates such as the drug methyldopa. In Parkinsons's disease, which is associated with inadequate amounts of dopamine in the substantia nigra of the CNS, this rate-limiting step is bypassed by the administration of large quantities of the L isomer of dopa, levodopa.

7. Dopa decarboxylase (DD)

DD is present in large quantities in the cytoplasm of many cells and converts dopa to dopamine. It also produces serotonin, tyramine and histamine from their corresponding precursor amino acids; thus the name 'aromatic amino acid decarboxylase' (AAAD) may be preferred. The drug methyldopa will compete for this enzyme, and is converted to α-methyldopa. Dopamine decarboxylase inhibitors such as benserazide are sometimes used in conjunction with levodopa in the treatment of Parkinson's disease. In low doses they selectively inhibit dopa decarboxylation in sympathetic nerves but not in the CNS, thus allowing the use of lower doses of levodopa (Da Prada *et al.*, 1984).

8. Dopamine

Dopamine is the end-point of catecholamine synthesis in dopaminergic neurons, but is further converted to noradrenaline in the adrenal medulla and in adrenergic and noradrenergic neurons. It is taken up and bound by storage vesicles in neurons and storage granules in chromaffin cells, and there is evidence that some dopamine is concomitantly released with noradrenaline and adrenaline. It has also been suggested that conjugated circulating dopamine may constitute a reserve pool of substrate for adrenaline or noradrenaline synthesis, which is available when necessary, and which bypasses the rate-limiting (TH) step in catecholamine synthesis (Lake, Chernow and Ziegler, 1984).

9. Dopamine-β-hydroxylase (DBH)

DBH catalyses the conversion of dopamine to noradrenaline; it is associated with the large noradrenaline storage vesicles (see section 11), and some is released with release of the contents of these vesicles. There is some evidence for an endogenous DBH inhibitor, which may act as a regulator in some neurons; DBH activity may be increased with prolonged neural traffic and by hormones such as progesterone and testosterone (Rutledge, 1984). DBH acts on a wide range of phenylethylamine substrates, thus allowing the formation of 'false transmitters' which then compete for storage in the vesicles with noradrenaline (see Fig. 8.3). Thus the name 'phenylethylamine-β-hydroxylase' (PBH) may be preferred. Tyramine is converted to octopamine and α-methyldopamine to α-methylnoradrenaline; only small amounts of octopamine are formed in mammals, but it is a major neurotransmitter in some invertebrates. α-Methylnoradrenaline acts as an α_2-agonist false transmitter in the treatment of hypertension with methyldopa.

10. Phenethanolamine-*N*-methyltransferase (PNMT)

PNMT is present in the adrenal medulla and CNS adrenergic neurons, and catalyses the conversion of noradrenaline to adrenaline by the transfer of a methyl group donated from adenosylmethionine. It acts on a range of hydroxylated phenylethylamines, and also forms synephrine from octopamine, epinine from dopamine, and dimethylnoradrenaline from adrenaline (see Fig. 8.3). The synthesis of PNMT is stimulated by the release of adrenocortical hormones into the adrenal portal system, and is decreased in Addison's disease. The envelopment of the adrenal medulla by the steroid-secreting cortical cells is a phylogenetically recent development, and this arrangement, with its portal vascular system, is found only in man and certain other mammals. PNMT has recently been found in some hypothalamic cells without tyrosine hydroxylase, implying the synthesis of other methylated amines (Sandler, 1984).

11. Storage of catecholamines

Adrenaline is stored in chromaffin granules in the adrenal medulla in association with adenosine triphosphate (ATP), with peptides such as enkephalins (Fried *et al.*, 1984) and with the proteins chromogranin A, chromomembrin B and cytochrome-b561. Adrenaline constitutes about 80 per cent of the catecholamine content of the chromaffin granules in man, with the balance made up of noradrenaline and small quantities of dopamine and other false transmitters. Met-, leu- and other as yet unidentified enkephalins have been shown to be concomitantly stored and released with adrenaline (Fried *et al.*, 1984). Also, in human phaeochromocytomas, large quantities of enkephalins have been found stored in the chromaffin granules of some adrenaline-secreting tumours (Schultzberg, 1984).

Noradrenaline is stored in both small (45–55 nm diameter) and large (75–90 nm diameter) dense-cored vesicles. There appear to be important differences between these vesicles (Fried *et al.*, 1984). Both the ratio of small to large vesicles and the overall number of vesicles vary between species, between tissues, within tissues and during development. The large vesicles are synthesized in the cell body, and are transported down the axon by a series of microtubules from their source in the Golgi apparatus to the terminal varicosities. The small vesicles appear to be synthesized by a specialized endoplasmic reticulum in the nerve terminals.

The large vesicles contain noradrenaline in association with ATP (in a molar ratio of about 30:1), dopamine (in a molar ratio of about 12:1), chromogranin A, chromomembrin B, cytochrome-b561, the enzyme DBH and, in certain fibres, one or more biologically active peptides. The small vesicles contain about one-tenth of the noradrenaline which the large vesicles contain (in association with ATP in about the same molar ratio) but virtually no dopamine, and have not been shown to contain any chromogranin A, DBH or neuropeptides. It is now thought that noradrenaline is synthesized only in large vesicles, with the overflow being taken up and stored in small vesicles, and that small vesicles preferentially discharge their contents at low rates of stimulation. This effect may be modulated locally by the overall number of vesicles, the ratio of small to large vesicles, the contents of the large vesicles and the rate of stimulation.

The binding of catecholamines in storage vesicles may be disrupted by drugs such as reserpine, guanethidine and bethanidine, and by some toxins. Treatment with reserpine leads to depletion of noradrenaline stores and loss of transmitter function; in low doses reserpine competes for storage, but in high doses it destroys the storage vesicles. Guanethidine and bethanidine affect nerve terminals in several ways, but deplete stores only when used in high doses, when they themselves are stored and act as false transmitters. The rate and extent of depletion in any particular tissue depend on noradrenaline turnover in that tissue. Thus, for example, a dose of reserpine which depletes the myocardial stores may have little effect on adrenal medullary stores. The rate of noradrenaline release with treatment with these drugs is not usually sufficient to cause any adrenoceptor agonist effects because the released noradrenaline is metabolized by monoamine oxidase in the cytoplasm of the nerve terminals. Decarborane (a rocket fuel and industrial catalyst), black widow spider venom and 6-hydroxydopamine also deplete catecholamine stores in nerve terminals as well as exerting other toxic effects.

12. Storage of peptides

A variety of neuropeptides have recently been shown to be stored in and released by sympathetic nerves associated with the heart and blood vessels of a range of mammals, including man (Furness et al., 1984). Met- and leu-enkephalins, neurotensin, substance P, somatostatin, vasoactive intestinal peptide (VIP) and neuropeptide Y (NPY) have all been found in sympathetic nerve terminals (Vogt, 1984). Some peptides have been shown to be stored in the large vesicles with noradrenaline and to be concomitantly released (e.g. enkephalins, neurotensin and NPY), whereas others may be stored in the non-granular vesicles found in sympathetic nerve terminals (Langer and Hicks, 1984). Some of these substances are also found in sensory nerves. There appear to be pathway-specific chemical 'codes' for functional subpopulations of neurons, as no peptides are found in some neurons, but one or more are found in others (Furness et al., 1984). For example, in noradrenergic nerves in which the fibres supplying mesenteric ganglia and blood vessels run together through the mesentery to the intestine, the neurons supplying the blood vessels contain NPY, whereas those supplying the ganglia do not (Furness et al., 1984).

A similar situation pertains in the submandibular gland in which fibres supplying vessels contain NPY, whereas those subserving secretion do not; α-adrenoceptor blockers totally block secretion but not vasoconstriction (Lundberg et al., 1984). The NPY-mediated vasoconstriction which persists after α-blockade is of much slower onset and longer duration than that mediated by noradrenaline; NPY is ten times more potent than noradrenaline as a vasoconstrictor.

In nerves which do contain peptides, the ratio of peptide to catecholamine may vary greatly between species (e.g. there is a 100-fold difference in the opioid/adrenaline ratio between the rat and man), and it may also vary within tissues and during development (Fried et al., 1984). Stores of peptides in these peripheral sympathetic nerve terminals have also been shown to be depleted by reserpine and β-hydroxydopamine (Furness et al., 1984).

13. Storage of false transmitters

A variety of endogenous and exogenous false transmitters may displace and be stored instead of noradrenaline or adrenaline. They are either stored after formation in the nerve terminals because of the lack of substrate specificity of the enzymes responsible for catecholamine synthesis (see Fig. 8.3) or are stored after neuronal uptake as phenylethylamine derivatives. Exogenous or released dopamine, tyramine and adrenaline are all taken up by sympathetic nerves to some extent, and may be stored, stoichiometrically displacing noradrenaline. Dopamine, dobutamine, tyramine and metaraminol, when administered in adequate doses, will all replace noradrenaline sufficiently rapidly to act, to some extent, as indirect sympathomimetic agents. Guanethidine and bethanidine, in high doses, will also compete for storage and act as false transmitters. Reserpine disrupts the storage of these false transmitters, and in high doses destroys the storage vesicles, but does not act as a false transmitter itself.

14. Release

Noradrenaline and adrenaline are normally rapidly released by nerve impulses, in contrast to the slowly acting depletion and displacement mechanisms outlined above. The excitation/release coupling mechanism has not been fully elucidated but is associated with an influx of Ca^{2+} ions which is necessary for the process to take place. This activates microtubular-associated contractile elements with movement of some vesicles to the axonal membrane, followed by the release of the catecholamine and peptide contents of the vesicles, and some ATP, chromogranins and DBH in ratios proportional to those found in the vesicles. However, the vesicle membrane lipids are not released, and this has generally been accepted as evidence for exocytosis. It has recently been suggested that the actual process of release may not be by exocytosis but by an ionic exchange mechanism (Uvnas, 1984). Because the amount of noradrenaline released represents the contents of only one or two vesicles of 1000 or more in a varicosity, it has been suggested that only a fraction of the contents of several vesicles may be released. It is proposed that, with the arrival of the nerve impulse, Ca^{2+} ions activate contractile elements to fuse the transmitter granule and axonal membranes, and that noradrenaline or adrenaline, which are ionically linked to protein carboxyl groups in the granular matrix, are then exchanged for Na^+ ions which flood in with the increase in Na^+ permeability which occurs with the action potential. With repolarization the Ca^{2+}, Na^+ and catecholamine ions are redistributed to their original sites by active transport mechanisms. The relative importance of the ion exchange and exocytotic mechanisms has not been established, but it is agreed that the synthesis, storage and reuptake machinery of vesicles is not destroyed with release of their contents. It has been suggested that, under normal physiological circumstances, the contents of the small vesicles are preferentially released and that those of the large vesicles are released only with rapid or prolonged firing. This would provide some economy, as the peptides and DBH released from large vesicles do not appear to be taken up again.

There are a large number of compounds which prevent the neural release of noradrenaline without abolishing end-organ responses. Bretylium and other calcium channel blockers prevent the influx of Ca^{2+} ions, which is the necessary first step in neurally mediated catecholamine release. There are several 'adrenergic neuron-blocking drugs', of which guanethidine and bethanidine are examples. They have a number of actions. Most exert some local anaesthetic effect, are weak DBH inhibitors, block neuronal uptake of catecholamines, displace the contents of vesicles and act themselves as false transmitters. However, they block neurally mediated release of catecholamines at doses at which they do not block sympathetic nerve conduction and at which they cause no significant reduction in catecholamine stores. The mechanism of their 'neuron-blocking' effect is poorly understood, but it is important at the doses used clinically; blockade of acetylcholine-mediated prejunctional facilitation of noradrenaline release via nicotinic receptors has been suggested as one possible mechanism (see section 16).

There are a group of compounds, the 'indirectly acting sympathomimetic amines', which cause release of noradrenaline, which then acts on receptors on effector cells. However, most exert at least some agonist effect on receptors themselves, and the mechanism of release is different from that with nervous stimulation. Tachyphylaxis occurs with repeated doses, indicating that a different, smaller, pool of noradrenaline is being released. This release is not as dependent on Ca^{2+} ions and is not associated with DBH release (Langer and Hicks, 1984).

15. Prejunctional catecholamine and opioid influences

There is now evidence that a number of mechanisms may regulate the release of noradrenaline (Langer and Hicks, 1984). There are prejunctional α_2-adrenoceptors which, when occupied by α_2-agonists, reduce noradrenaline release, thus constituting a 'negative feedback mechanism'. (There is some evidence that concomitantly released opioids may be involved in a similar feedback mechanism.)

Although there has been considerable debate (Kalsner, 1984; Westfall, 1984), α_2-receptor-mediated feedback is now thought to play a significant role in everyday regulation in man. It may be an important mechanism by which α_2-agonists exert some of their antihypertensive effect, and it probably also explains why neuronal uptake blockers and why α-blockers respectively increase and decrease the effects of exogenous noradrenaline more than those of endogenously released noradrenaline.

There are also prejunctional facilitatory β-adrenoceptors which, at very low concentrations of β_2-agonists, increase noradrenaline release. It has been suggested that circulating adrenaline may aggravate 'stress-induced' hypertension by this mechanism in some individuals, and that it may be a mechanism by which β-blockers exert some of their antihypertensive effect.

16. Prejunctional cholinergic influences

The involvement of cholinergic nerves in the regulation of noradrenaline release was first proposed by Burn and Rand in 1959. There is now evidence that acetylcholine released from parasympathetic nerve terminals plays a regulatory role via both muscarinic (inhibitory) and nicotinic (facilitatory) receptors, particularly in organs such as the heart, where cholinergic and adrenergic nerve terminals are in close proximity. The muscarinic receptors have been shown to be in very close association with the noradrenergic storage vesicles themselves (Rutledge, 1984).

17. Other prejunctional influences

There is also evidence that a variety of locally formed or blood-borne substances may regulate neurotransmission. Angiotensin, prostaglandin $F_{2\alpha}$ ($PGF_{2\alpha}$) and 5-hydroxytryptamine (5HT, serotonin) act as facilitators, whereas histamine, adenosine and several opioids (including enkephalins) act as inhibitors. In the latter case this may represent another negative feedback mechanism. Yet another feedback mechanism is represented by the release of PGE_2 formed by the effector end-organ with sympathetic nerve stimulation, which can feed back to inhibit further noradrenaline release ('trans-synaptic regulation').

18. Adrenoceptor agonists

Adrenoceptor agonists may be defined as substances which possess affinity for and exert effects at adrenoceptors, and they may be classified according to their relative potencies at each type of receptor (Table 8.1). They arrive at adrenoceptors either after release from adjacent sympathetic nerves or by diffusion from the blood stream. All endogenous adrenoceptor agonists act on more than one receptor type, but synthetic agonists which have a reasonable degree of specificity for individual receptor types are now known (see Table 8.1). For example, methoxamine, α-methylnoradrenaline, dobutamine and salbutamol each act fairly selectively on α_1-, α_2-, β_1- and β_2-receptors, respectively. However, even these 'selective' receptor agonists still exert a wide spectrum of biological effects, due to the wide range of tissue-specific third messengers (Table 8.2), and because they exert at least some effects at other receptors. For example, dobutamine, in the presence of extensive β - blockade, will not increase cardiac output, but will increase peripheral vascular resistance, indicating that it has at least some α_1 activity.

A wide variety of compounds have been produced by attaching different substituent groups to the carbon atoms or amine group of the phenylethylamine molecule. A detailed description of these is beyond the scope of this chapter; however, some general observations may be made with respect to the structure–activity relationships of these compounds, although there are exceptions to most of the 'rules' (see Table 8.1).

Substitution on the amine group generally reduces α activity, and increased bulk of this substituent generally enhances β activity. Thus isoprenaline is a more selective β-agonist than adrenaline, which in turn is a more selective β-agonist than noradrenaline; salbutamol, terbutaline and ephedrine all exert β-agonist effects. Phenylephrine, a selective α-agonist with a methyl substituent group, constitutes an exception to this rule.

Potency is generally increased by the presence of hydroxyl groups in the 3 and 4 positions on the aromatic nucleus, and by the presence of a hydroxyl group on the β-carbon atom. Thus phenylephrine is less potent than adrenaline, and dopamine and dobutamine are about 100 times less potent than adrenaline, noradrenaline and isoprenaline. The presence of hydroxyl

Table 8.1 Chemical structures and classification by adrenoceptor agonist activity of selected sympathomimetic amines

Selected sympathomimetic amines	Aromatic ring	β-Carbon −CH−	α-Carbon −CH−	Amine −NH−	Adrenoceptor agonist activity α_1	α_2	β_1	β_2
Phenylethylamine		H	H	H				
Dopamine	3−OH, 4−OH	H	H	H				
Noradrenaline	3−OH, 4−OH	OH	H	H				
Adrenaline	3−OH, 4−OH	OH	H	CH_3				
Isoprenaline	3−OH, 4−OH	OH	H	$CH(CH_3)_2$				
Terbutaline	3−OH, 5−OH	OH	H	$C(CH_3)_3$				
Salbutamol	3−CH_2OH, 4−OH	OH	H	$C(CH_3)_3$				
Dobutamine	3−OH, 4−OH	H	H	*				
α-Methylnoradrenaline	3−OH, 4−OH	OH	CH_3	H				
Methoxamine	2−OCH_3, 5−OCH_3	OH	CH_3	H				
Phenylephrine	3−OH	OH	H	CH_3				
Ephedrine		OH	CH_3	CH_3				
Amphetamine		H	CH_3	H				

The arrows denote the spectrum of agonist activity of each compound: solid arrows indicate direct agonist activity and broken arrows indicate that effects are exerted indirectly via release of noradrenaline. Another group of compounds, the imidazolines, act as α-agonists, and have a different general structure†. Naphazoline, oxymetazoline and the selective α_2-agonist clonidine are representative of this group.

* −CH−$(CH_2)_2$−◯−OH with CH_3

†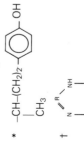

Table 8.2 Location of adrenoceptor subtypes and biological effects of occupancy by appropriate agonists

Location	Response	Adrenoceptor subtype
Heart	Increased force of contraction	β_1 (α_1)
	Increased automaticity and conduction velocity	β_2 (β_1)
	Increased glycogenolysis	β_1 (β_2)
Blood vessels	Constriction of most arteries and veins	α_1 (α_2)
	Dilation of most arteries and veins	β_2 (β_1)
Lung	Bronchodilatation	β_2 (β_1)
	Some bronchoconstriction demonstrable	α_1
Gut	Contraction of sphincters	α_1
	Relaxation of smooth muscle	β_1
Skeletal muscle	Tremor (increased rates of contraction of fast fibres)	β_2
	Increased glycogenolysis	β_2
Uterus	Contraction of pregnant uterus	α_1
	Relaxation of pregnant uterus	β_2
Eye	Contraction of radial muscles (mydriasis)	α_1
	Relaxation of ciliary muscle for far vision	β_2
Skin	Contraction of pilomotor muscles	α_1
	Increased secretion of sweat glands	α_1
Noradrenaline release	Prejunctional inhibition of release	α_2
	Prejunctional facilitation of release	β_2
Acetylcholine release	Inhibition at ganglia and enteric synapses	α_2
	Facilitation at skeletal neuromuscular junctions	α_2
Liver	Glycogenolysis	α_1
	Gluconeogenesis	α_1
Kidney	Renin secretion inhibited	α_2
	Renin secretion promoted	β_1
Pancreas	Insulin secretion inhibited	α_1
	Insulin secretion promoted	β_2
Adipose tissue	Lipolysis (white fat)	β_1
	Calorigenesis (brown fat)	β_1
Platelets	Aggregation promoted	α_2

The wide variety of responses by different tissues are mediated by tissue-specific third and subsequent messengers. This Table is incomplete, as most tissues probably have more than one receptor subtype, with the relative densities of the different subtypes varying both in different regions of the tissue and in relation to proximity to sympathetic nerve terminals (Lees, 1981; Minneman, Pittman and Molinoff, 1981; Louis *et al.*, 1982).

groups in the 3 and 5 positions generally confers β_2-selectivity on compounds with large amino substituent groups (e.g. terbutaline). Substitution on the α-carbon atom blocks oxidation by monoamine oxidase (MAO), and, in non-catecholamines such as methoxamine, ephedrine and amphetamine, greatly prolongs duration of action. However, the duration of action of α-methylnoradrenaline is not great because, as a catecholamine, it is still subject to metabolism by catechol-*o*-methyltransferase (COMT).

Adrenoceptor agonist effects may be produced by the endogenous release or by administration of directly acting agonists, by the release of false transmitters, or by the administration of sympathomimetic amines which displace noradrenaline from nerve terminals ('indirectly acting sympathomimetic amines'). Several compounds which exert their effects by direct action on receptors are shown in Table 8.1. False transmitters include tyramine, octopamine, synephrine, epinine and dimethylnoradrenaline; all are usually found only in small quantities and have weak direct and indirect effects (see Fig. 8.3). A typical indirectly acting sympathomimetic amine, amphetamine, is also shown in Table 8.1; note that it lacks both the hydroxyl groups on the ring and the β-hydroxyl group on the side chain. Being less polar and more lipophilic, these compounds usually have marked CNS effects. Compounds which lack hydroxyl groups on the aromatic ring but possess a β-hydroxyl group (such as ephedrine) and compounds which have hydroxyl groups on the ring but lack a β-hydroxyl group (such as dopamine and dobutamine) tend to have both direct and indirect effects. Although the indirectly acting sympathomimetic amines exert much of their effect by releasing noradrenaline, they do not mimic noradrenaline because they generally have agonist effects of their own and because they penetrate the CNS to varying extents. It is also important to note that, with compounds which act on more than one receptor type, different effects may be obtained at different doses. Thus with dopamine, noradrenaline and adrenaline, β effects predominate at low doses, but α effects predominate at high doses, and, with dopamine, renal and mesenteric vasodilator (dopaminergic) effects are evident only at very low doses.

19. Neuronal uptake

The main factor in the termination of the effects of noradrenaline as a chemotransmitter is its uptake back into sympathetic nerve terminals, where most of it is stored in vesicles for reuse. Neuronal uptake is an active process with a low threshold, and may take place against a gradient of up to 1 in 10 000; it is not substrate specific and is also important in terminating the effect of several other phenylethylamine derivatives. The rate and extent of uptake vary between tissues, and both these and the nature of the amine taken up influence the ultimate effects. Thus although dopamine is taken up and displaces noradrenaline, it is itself mostly converted to noradrenaline by DBH. Both tyramine and metaraminol are taken up and act as indirect sympathomimetics, but tyramine's effects are short lived as it is metabolized by MAO, whereas metaraminol, which is not metabolized by MAO, tends to be recycled and to accumulate in vesicles. Compounds with substituents on the amide nitrogen tend not to be taken up. Thus adrenaline is only taken up to some extent, and substances with bulky substituents on the amide nitrogen are not taken up at all (e.g. most selective β-adrenoceptor agonists).

Several drugs inhibit neuronal uptake and thus potentiate the action of directly acting sympathomimetic amines, but inhibit those of the indirectly acting sympathomimetic amines. However, each of these drugs possesses a number of other actions, and each may interfere with adrenergic transmission in a number of ways. Cocaine in low doses blocks uptake; however, in high doses it also blocks conduction, thus inhibiting endogenous neurotransmitter release whilst still enhancing the effects of exogenous catecholamines. The tricyclic antidepressants are potent uptake blockers but also have a broad spectrum of other actions. The phenothiazines block uptake but also act as adrenoceptor blockers and as adrenergic neuron blockers. Several of the adrenergic neuron blockers, such as guanethidine, also block neuronal uptake, as do a number of the indirectly acting sympathomimetic amines.

On the other hand, increased concentrations of extracellular fluid cations (such as Na^+ or Li^+) have been shown to increase central and peripheral neuronal uptake, which may explain the effectiveness of lithium salts in the treatment of mania and the decreased response of lithium-treated patients to exogenous catecholamines.

In summary, although uptake is important in terminating the effects of noradrenaline as a neurotransmitter, the biological effects of the neuronal uptake of the other amines or of uptake blockers also depend to a large extent on the other properties of the relevant amines or blockers.

20. Redistribution and extraneuronal uptake

Also important in terminating the effects of catecholamines and other sympathomimetic amines are local uptake into extraneuronal tissues, and diffusion into and distribution by the blood stream to other tissues and to sites of metabolism. Extraneuronal uptake has a higher threshold than neuronal uptake, and is saturable only with very high concentrations of amine. Also, the relative affinities of the various amines for extraneuronal uptake are different from those for neuronal uptake. Once taken up, amines may be metabolized by both MAO and COMT. Extraneuronal uptake may only be important in terminating the effect of locally released neurotransmitters when neuronal uptake is blocked or has been saturated by the presence of large concentrations of amines. However, it always plays a role in terminating the effects of exogenous amines, particularly those with large substituent groups on the amine nitrogen, which are not taken up neuronally.

Extraneuronal uptake is not affected by most of the drugs which affect neuronal uptake, but is markedly inhibited by the products of metabolism of adrenaline and noradrenaline by COMT (metanephrine and normetanephrine), and by some steroids. The α-blocker phenoxybenzamine is one drug which inhibits both neuronal and extraneuronal uptake.

21. Metabolism

Metabolism is relatively unimportant in terminating the effects of endogenous catecholamines under normal physiological circumstances, as evidenced by the much smaller effects of MAO and COMT inhibitors compared with those of neuronal uptake inhibitors. The functions of COMT and MAO are complementary to each other, but MAO is more important locally and may play a regulatory role in sympathetic nerve terminals, whereas COMT is generally more important in the metabolism of circulating amines. The major pathways are shown in Fig. 8.4. The 3-methoxy compounds formed by COMT and those with acid side chains formed by MAO are each, in turn, substrates

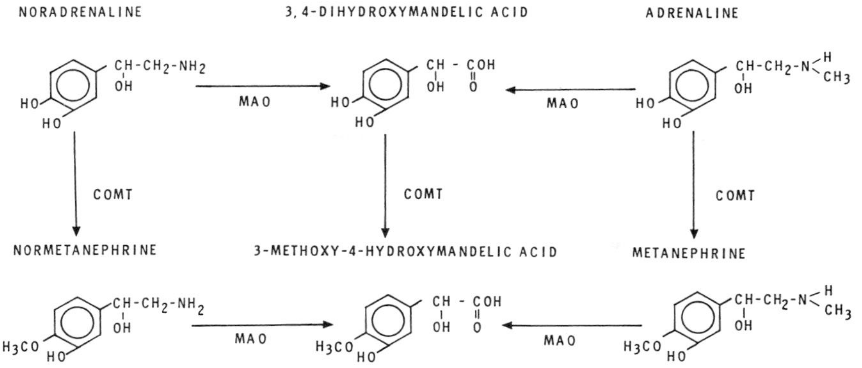

NORADRENALINE   3,4-DIHYDROXYMANDELIC ACID   ADRENALINE

CH-CH$_2$-NH$_2$ MAO   CH - COH   MAO   CH-CH$_2$-N$\langle$H CH$_3$

COMT   COMT   COMT

NORMETANEPHRINE   3-METHOXY-4-HYDROXYMANDELIC ACID   METANEPHRINE

CH-CH$_2$-NH$_2$ MAO   CH - COH   MAO   CH-CH$_2$-N$\langle$H CH$_3$

Fig. 8.4   Major pathways of catecholamine metabolism. MAO = monoamine oxidase. COMT = catechol-*O*-methyltransferase.

for MAO and COMT respectively. Thus, the common end-product, 3-methoxy-4-hydroxymandelic acid, constitutes the main metabolite found in urine (with some 3-methoxy-4-hydroxyphenylglycol), although both free and conjugated intermediary products from both of these pathways, products of other minor pathways and small amounts of the catecholamines themselves also appear in the urine. COMT and MAO are considered separately below, as there are clinically significant differences in their relative importance under different circumstances.

22. Monoamine oxidase (MAO)

MAO is present in almost all tissues, with particularly high concentrations in the intestinal mucosa and liver (important in the metabolism of active dietary amines), kidney and lung (important in the metabolism of circulating amines) and both central and peripheral neurons using monoamine transmitters (important in the local metabolism of catecholamines and serotonin). It catalyses the oxidative deamination of a wide range of amines to form the corresponding aldehyde derivatives, which in turn are oxidized or reduced to the corresponding acid or alcohol (the latter being important in the CNS). All these reactions take place in close association with mitochondria. It does not act on substances with a substituent group on the α-carbon atom, such as metaraminol or α-methylnoradrenaline, nor on substances with bulky substituent groups on the amine, such as the selective β-adrenoceptor agonists.

There are several groups of drugs which act as monoamine oxidase inhibitors (MAOIs), all of which possess other actions, including the inhibition of a wide range of other enzymes. Thus they markedly potentiate the action of many sedatives, hypnotics, opioids, anticholinergics, antihistamines, phenothiazines, tricyclic antidepressants and sympathomimetic amines, and may produce hepatotoxic effects.

The MAOIs produce an increase in the duration of effect of monoamines released both centrally and peripherally, which is thought to be responsible for their mood elevating and analgesic effects. Both hypotension and hypertension may complicate MAOI therapy. Hypotension may be produced by increased concentrations of less potent endogenous false transmitters such as octopamine and tyramine, which are normally produced in small quantities but are destroyed by MAO, by reduced noradrenaline stores due to end-product inhibition of tyrosine hydroxylase as a result of increased free noradrenaline concentrations in cytoplasm, and possibly also by effects on medullary and hypothalamic cardiovascular control centres. On the other hand, hypertensive crises may be produced by the ingestion of active amines or their precursors in foodstuffs such as beer, wine and preserved meat or fish, which are normally metabolized by MAO and liver microsomal enzymes. There may also be exaggerated responses to indirectly acting sympathomimetic amines which are not substrates for neuronal uptake and for which termination of effect depends on metabolism by MAO. In contrast, however, there are usually only modest increases in response to endogenous catecholamines because termination of effect is due mainly to neuronal uptake rather than to metabolism.

23. Catechol-*o*-methyltransferase (COMT)

COMT is widely distributed as a cytoplasmic enzyme, and catalyses the transfer of a methyl group from adenosylmethionine to the 3-hydroxy group of catecholamine compounds. Its presence in liver, kidney and lung, all organs with high blood flow, is important in metabolizing circulating catechol compounds, whereas its presence in some adrenergic nerves, the brain and some sympathetically innervated end-organs such as the heart and blood vessels may be important in modulating the effects of both endogenous and exogenous catecholamines (after uptake) at these sites. Several drugs which inhibit COMT are known and are used clinically, such as pyrogallol and rutin, but they are not used specifically as COMT inhibitors.

24. Adrenoceptors

The possibility of the existence of 'receptive substances' was first suggested by Langley in 1901, but the concept of different effects of sympathomimetic amines being mediated by different receptors only started to gain widespread acceptance with Ahlquist's proposal for the existence of α- and β-receptors in 1948, and with the subsequent progressive development of more selective adrenoceptor agonists and antagonists. It is now likely that radioligand labelling and monoclonal antibody techniques will lead to the complete characterization of the receptor macromolecules and their interactions with adrenoceptor agonists (Caron *et al.*, 1984). It has been suggested that, because adrenergic, dopaminergic and muscarinic cholinergic receptors have similarities with respect to biological function (all influencing adenyl cyclase and calcium flux), they may have a common ancestral gene, and a similar structure, with variable externally orientated regions for agonist binding, and constant internally orientated regions for interactions with adenyl cyclase and calcium channel control (Venter *et al.*, 1984). Thus although the adrenoceptor subtypes reside on different peptides, and although there is evidence for some polymorphism of receptor binding site structure between species, it is thought that the relevant regions of the molecules are similar (Seidman and Homcy, 1984).

Adenyl cyclase is a membrane-bound enzyme which catalyses the conversion of ATP to cyclic adenosine $3',5'$-monophosphate (cAMP); β_1- and β_2-receptor occupancy activates this enzyme, whereas α_2-receptor occupancy inhibits it. Thus, with β-receptor occupancy, intracellular cAMP levels are increased, whereas with α_2-receptor occupancy they are reduced. The α_1-receptor is poorly understood, but receptor occupancy produces an increase in membrane permeability to calcium, with a resultant increase in intracellular calcium, which activates contractile (and other) mechanisms (Caron et al., 1984). The biochemical nature of the interactions between receptor occupancy and adenyl cyclase or calcium channel control have not yet been elucidated (Seidman and Homcy, 1984). The kinetics of agonist and antagonist interactions with receptors and the role of guanine triphosphate are considered in Chapter 9.

The adrenoceptor agonists act as 'first messengers', acting via adenyl cyclase or calcium channel control mechanisms to produce changes in intracellular cAMP or calcium concentrations. Calcium and cAMP act as 'second messengers', acting via cAMP-dependent or calcium/calmodulin-dependent protein kinases to produce changes in specific protein substrates, which act as 'third messengers'; calcium also exerts effects via other mechanisms in various tissues. As there are a number of physiological and pharmacological influences which may act at each of these levels, they are considered separately.

25. First messengers

In addition to adrenoceptor agonists, there are a number of endogenous and exogenous substances which may, via different receptors or binding sites, activate or inhibit adenyl cyclase, and thus alter intracellular cAMP concentrations. Glucagon, prostaglandins, thyroid hormones, histamine, vasopressin, chlorpropamide and the new positive inotropic agent, amrinone, may all activate adenyl cyclase, whereas insulin, methacholine and the phenothiazines may inhibit it (Kones, 1973; Honerjager, Schafer-Korting and Reiter, 1981). Sympathomimetic amines, acting via adrenoceptors, therefore constitute only one of several groups of drugs which may act as first messengers to produce changes in cAMP concentrations. There are also a number of compounds other than adrenoceptor agonists which influence calcium channels, such as local anaesthetic agents, calcium channel blockers and some antiarrhythmic agents. Factors influencing calcium flux and the calcium-dependent effector mechanisms are dealt with in Chapter 16.

26. Second messengers

Calcium and cAMP play roles as second messengers in most cells. A further second messenger, of particular importance in the CNS, is cyclic guanosine $3',5'$-monophosphate (cGMP) which is produced from guanosine triphosphate (GTP) upon activation of the membrane-bound enzyme guanylate cyclase; GTP also plays a role in regulating adrenoceptor affinity for agonists (see Chapter 9). Most, if not all, of the second messenger actions of cAMP and cGMP are mediated via cAMP- and cGMP-dependent protein kinases. Many of the second messenger actions of calcium are also mediated via one of several calcium/calmodulin-dependent or calcium/phosphatidylserine-dependent protein kinases, although calcium also operates via other mechanisms.

Intracellular levels of the second messengers may be altered directly, as well as via a variety of first messenger systems. Inhibitors of phosphodiesterase, the enzyme responsible for cAMP breakdown, such as the methylxanthines (e.g. theophylline), the tricyclic antidepressants and diazoxide, all increase cAMP levels, whereas phosphodiesterase facilitators such as insulin and imidazole decrease them (Kones, 1973). Intracellular calcium concentrations, too, may be altered by drugs such as the cardiac glycosides. The situation is further complicated, with respect to calcium, by the fact that both voltage-dependent and slow calcium channels may be subject to some regulation by cAMP-dependent protein kinase mechanisms (Nestler and Greengard, 1984).

27. Third messengers

The second messengers, acting via protein kinases, phosphorylate a wide range of substrate proteins which act as third messengers. In some cases the third messenger is the immediate mediator of the biological effect, but more frequently it triggers a cascade of events which ultimately result in the biological effect. Some of these cascades have been well characterized (e.g. that mediating hepatic glycogenolysis) but most have yet to be defined.

Third and subsequent messengers produce the specific biological effects characteristic of different tissues. For example, at least 70 phosphoproteins which act as substrates for cAMP-, cGMP- or calcium-dependent protein kinases have been identified in nervous tissue alone. This is the mechanism by which adrenoceptor agonists, although acting via only four receptor subtypes, produce such a range of different effects in different tissues (see Table 8.2).

Thus, although β_1- and β_2-receptor occupancy both increase cAMP, each produces a variety of different effects (Lees, 1981). β_1-receptor occupancy increases myocardial contractility and glycogenolysis, but also relaxes smooth muscle in the gut and promotes renin secretion by the juxtaglomerular apparatus. β_2-receptor occupancy, in addition to generally producing smooth muscle relaxation, also increases automaticity of the heart, facilitates prejunctional noradrenaline release and promotes insulin release from the pancreas. α_2-receptor occupancy inhibits adenyl cyclase, and, in addition to inhibiting presynaptic noradrenaline release, produces vasoconstriction, influences renin secretion and renal tubular function, and enhances platelet aggregation (Louis et al., 1982). α_1-receptor occupancy, which does not appear to influence adenyl cyclase but leads to altered calcium flux, not only produces smooth muscle contraction in many tissues but also increases myocardial contractility, increases hepatic glycogenolysis and gluconeogenesis, and reduces insulin secretion by the pancreas (Scholz, 1984). It is in manipulation at the third or subsequent messenger level that the potential exists for highly specific therapeutic intervention.

28. Factors affecting receptor number and affinity

Both acute and chronic changes in receptor number and affinity may occur in response to different stimuli, with drug treatment, and in various disease states (Seidman and Homcy, 1984). Receptor numbers increase with low catecholamine background concentrations. This may occur generally in patients with diseases such as idiopathic orthostatic hypotension (see section 1), or regionally after sympathetic denervation. The reverse occurs in patients exposed to high catecholamine concentrations, such as those with a phaeochromocytoma. In these patients very large resting concentrations may have little biological effect.

Reduced β-receptor density and sensitivity have been demonstrated in the myocardium of patients with cardiac failure (Bristow et al., 1982); it is likely that this is an important part of the disease process. The situation may be further complicated by drug treatment. Generalized down-regulation of β-receptor numbers has also been shown both in cardiac failure patients and in asthmatic patients on adrenoceptor agonist treatment (Seidman and Homcy, 1984). Conversely, generalized up-regulation of β-receptor sensitivity has been shown to occur with β-blocker treatment (Wood and Rafaelsen, 1984). Both these effects may occur within a few hours or days, and may correlate with clinically observed attenuation of response to therapy (tachyphylaxis) (Hertel and Perkins, 1984; Seidman and Homcy, 1984).

Changes in adrenoceptors may also be produced by hormones. Increased β-receptor numbers have been found with glucocorticoid therapy (Davies and Lefkowitz, 1984) and increases in both receptor number and sensitivity have been shown to occur in hyperthyroidism in man (Anderson, Nilsson and Koo, 1983). Conversely, reductions in both receptor number and affinity have been shown in experimental models of hypothyroidism (Stiles and Lefkowitz, 1981).

Pharmacokinetics

Much effort has been expended in measuring blood catecholamine levels since the first attempts by Batelli in 1902, and many publications have appeared in recent years since the availability of sensitive, reproducible assay techniques. For this reason, readers are referred to review papers only (Runciman, 1980; Derbyshire and Smith, 1984; Lake, Chernow and Ziegler, 1984).

Endogenous amines

Catecholamines or false transmitters may be released from sympathetic nerve terminals either as a result of neural activity or, by a different mechanism, as the result of indirectly acting sympathomimetic amines. For factors influencing rates and patterns of release, see sections 1–17 above. Locally released amines reach a high concentration in the region of receptors on effector cells adjacent to sympathetic nerve terminals, and termination of effect is mainly by neuronal uptake, with some extraneuronal uptake, and with some diffusion into the blood stream (see sections 19–23). As the small amounts of noradrenaline which escape uptake are subject to metabolism by both COMT and MAO, resting blood noradrenaline levels are low, with venous concentrations (about

0.3 ng/ml) being higher than arterial. Arterial levels may be only 70 per cent of pulmonary artery concentrations, due to pulmonary metabolism, and hepatic vein levels only 30 per cent of arterial, due to metabolism in gut and liver. The plasma half-life of endogenously released noradrenaline has been calculated to be less than 1 minute.

Small amounts of adrenaline (and possibly tiny amounts of other catecholamines and false transmitters) are also normally released into the blood stream from the adrenal medulla. As adrenaline is also subject to some uptake and to metabolism by COMT and MAO, resting blood concentrations are also low (about 0.1 ng/ml), with pulmonary arterial levels being higher than arterial levels but arterial levels being higher than those in the venous effluent of most organs; plasma half-life is again less than 1 minute.

Because rates of uptake and metabolism are rapid and fairly constant, blood concentrations of adrenaline and noradrenaline provide some reflection of the level of sympathetic nervous system activity in normal individuals, particularly when large beds of tissue are being consistently activated for several minutes, such as during controlled sustained exercise (Lake, Chernow and Ziegler, 1984). Standing from the supine position doubles noradrenaline levels, and mild exercise increases them threefold. However, with severe or prolonged activity, and in most clinical situations, blood catecholamine levels are very variable. Drug treatment may influence resting catecholamine levels. They may be increased up to eightfold with drugs such as vasodilators, diuretics and uptake blockers, and may be decreased with drugs such as reserpine, guanethidine and the MAOIs. Levels may be increased two- to fivefold in the immediate postoperative period, and are usually still double control values 24 hours after an abdominal operation. Pain, hypovolaemia and myocardial infarction may increase plasma noradrenaline levels by up to ten- or even 20-fold, and septic or haemorrhagic shock may increase them 30- to 50-fold. There is no correlation between haemodynamic parameters (such as blood pressure and heart rate) and blood catecholamine concentrations, except possibly for brief periods after sudden severe perturbations. Thus, a correlation between changes in systolic blood pressure and catecholamine levels has been shown after endotracheal intubation, but, in the same patients in the postoperative period, haemodynamic parameters were normal whilst noradrenaline blood levels were double control values (Derbyshire and Smith, 1984).

Resting catecholamine levels may be increased tenfold or more in some patients with phaeochromocytomas, and may peak at greater than 100-fold normal resting values. In other patients, they may be within the normal range, at least intermittently. Effects on resting blood pressure are also very variable. Although resting blood pressure may be only moderately elevated in certain patients, 70 per cent of these suffer from orthostatic hypotension, presumably as a manifestation of substantial receptor down-regulation in response to chronically high average circulating blood catecholamine levels (Desmonts and Marty, 1984).

In summary, therefore, plasma levels of endogenous catecholamines do provide a crude index of general sympathetic nervous system activity, but correlate poorly with haemodynamic responses and provide no reflection of the concentration of noradrenaline near receptors in particular organs, especially at low levels of activity.

Exogenous amines

Sympathomimetic amines may be administered to patients or volunteers, usually by intravenous injection or infusion. These exogenous amines diffuse into the region of receptors from the blood stream, where their effects are superimposed on those of endogenously released amines.

With infusions of adrenaline or noradrenaline fairly predictable plasma concentrations may be achieved in most subjects. For each 0.01 $\mu g/kg$ per minute infused, plasma noradrenaline levels increase by about 1 ng/ml and plasma adrenaline levels by 0.5 ng/ml. Increases are linear with infusion rates of up to 40 μg per minute in adults (i.e. beyond the usual clinical dose range), and with infusion rates of greater than 1 μg per minute endogenous catecholamines usually make little contribution to plasma levels. In adults infusions of adrenaline or noradrenaline at rates of 1–10 μg per minute produce similar plasma concentrations to those produced endogenously with severe stress, shock or cardiac failure; both exogenous and endogenous catecholamines function as circulating hormones under these circumstances. It is significant that infusions in this dose range usually produce marked haemodynamic improvement in patients with septic or cardiogenic shock, but frequently produce little effect in volunteers with normal cardiovascular reserves and intact homoeostatic mechanisms.

With the infiltration of adrenaline with local anaesthetics, blood adrenaline concentrations may increase up to fourfold, which usually produces no changes in heart rate or blood pressure but which may increase liver blood flow significantly. The situation is much more complex with non-catecholamines and with indirectly acting sympathomimetic amines, because there is variable release of endogenous noradrenaline (with the potential for tachyphylaxis) and because different amines are subject to varying degrees of neuronal uptake, extraneuronal uptake and metabolism. For example, an amine which is subject to neuronal uptake but is not subject to metabolism by MAO, such as metaraminol, tends to be recycled and to act as a false transmitter for a relatively long period of time.

The most useful general conclusions which may be drawn are that the plasma half-lives of exogenous catecholamines are 1–2 minutes (whereas those of non-catecholamines are 1–4 hours), that with the usual rates of infusion they act as circulating hormones in concentrations similar to those produced endogenously with severe stress or shock, and that plasma levels correlate poorly with biological effects in both normal volunteers and in patients.

Pharmacodynamics

It might be hoped that the effects of a sympathomimetic amine could be predicted by correlating the information in Tables 8.1 and 8.2. However, this is not the case, for a number of reasons.

First, many of the primary effects of sympathomimetic amines are negated or minimized *in vivo* by homoeostatic mechanisms. Thus heart rate changes are usually negligible with adrenaline or noradrenaline infusions, due to reflex baroreceptor mediated responses. Likewise, in certain subjects a pressor response is not obtained even with the infusion of noradrenaline or adrenaline at rates beyond those usually used clinically (Runciman, 1980).

Secondly, many of the effects which are used to classify adrenoceptor agonists and which are prominent in pharmacological texts are not marked *in vivo* or are of little or no consequence clinically. With the systemic administration of sympathomimetic amines effects on sweating, pilomotor activity, salivary gland secretion, pupil size, and gut and bladder function generally fall into this category, although some of these signs may be useful as indices of endogenous sympathetic nervous system activity under anaesthesia.

Thirdly, the mechanisms by which biological responses are produced, even assuming constant predictable agonist concentrations at receptors, are complex, and the ultimate biological effects may be subject to many other influences. For example, in the heart both the overall numbers and the relative densities of α_1, β_1- and β_2-receptors vary progressively between the right and left sides, with greater numbers being found on the left side. There are also greater numbers of β_2-receptors in areas remote from sympathetic nerve terminals (Minneman, Pittman and Molinoff, 1981; Stiles and Lefkowitz, 1984). Thus the relative contributions of α- and β-receptors to, for example, an increase in myocardial contractility may vary regionally, and there may also be different patterns of response to circulating amines compared with those to amines released from nerve terminals. Vascular responses also may vary regionally within organs, and may respond differently to locally released and circulating amines due to regional variations in the relative densities of both α- and β-receptor subtypes (Alabaster and Davey, 1984; Cohen, Shepherd and Vanhoutte, 1984). Receptor number and sensitivity are also subject to both acute and chronic up- or down-regulation, and may be influenced by both the disease state and the drug treatment. Effects may also be greatly altered by other factors affecting first or second messengers, or by other drugs or processes affecting the end-organ. Calcium channel blockers, for example, oppose the effects of β-receptor agonists on the myocardium. Hormonal factors, concomitantly released peptides and local regulatory factors may all be important in normal individuals, and a host of locally produced or circulating biologically active substances are present and may exert profound effects in patients with shock (Runciman and Skowronski, 1984).

Effects and clinical use of sympathomimetic amines

'The specific circulatory responses to the administration of an autonomic drug are infinitely variable in any single experimental animal or human subject or patient' (Ahlquist, 1965).

In spite of the great variability in response to sympathomimetic amines, they have been used since the turn of the century in the treatment of cardiac failure, circulatory collapse and shock, bronchospasm and allergic conditions, and as haemostatics and vasoconstrictors (Schafer, 1908). Treatment has tended to remain empirical, in spite of the great increases in our understanding of their mechanisms of action. Progress in some areas has been greater than in others. For example, the synthesis of selective β_2-receptor agonists with durations of action suitable for outpatient use has proved to be a major advance in the treatment of asthma. However, the same advances have not been made in the treatment of circulatory failure. To some extent this has been due to a poor understanding of the complex, more variable pathophysiology involved, and to some extent because too much emphasis has been placed on expecting agents to act according to their pharmacological classification as agonists, rather than on objective examination of the actual effects produced in patients with particular diseases. As more information comes to light, it is evident that local influences are very important and that choice of agent and dose must be titrated against the desired biological end-point while also monitoring less desirable side effects.

The problem has been aggravated by the fact that the effects of adrenoceptor agonists in conditions such as septic shock vary greatly between individuals. The conduct of systematic studies which may be compared between centres has been hindered by the great variability in the types of patients treated in different centres, as well as by the lack of general agreement as to what biological end-points should be used to adjust infusion rates of adrenoceptor agonists. Thus, choice of agent is usually dictated by personal preference, and dose by a weighting of a combination of subjective parameters such as clinical assessment of tissue perfusion and objective parameters such as blood pressure, urine flow, cardiac output and oxygen consumption. As a better understanding of these disease processes is gained, a more rational approach will be allowed.

Adrenaline, noradrenaline and dopamine

In man, infusions of adrenaline, noradrenaline or dopamine all have similar effects on central haemodynamics, with β-agonist effects predominating at low doses and α-agonist effects becoming more evident at high doses. In adults, low doses are 1–5 μg per minute and high doses 15–25 μg per minute for adrenaline and noradrenaline; the corresponding doses are 100 times greater for dopamine.

Mean blood pressure and cardiac output tend to increase progressively with increasing doses, with a slight increase or no change in heart rate. It is traditional to state that dysrhythmias are a particular problem with adrenaline. There is no theoretical basis for this, and in clinical practice dysrhythmias are rare with all three agents, if given at reasonable rates by infusion.

Glomerular filtration rate and renal tubular function remain essentially unchanged; at higher doses renal blood flow may fall. At very low doses there may be an increase in renal blood flow with dopamine, mediated via dopaminergic receptors; however, α- and β-effects dominate with moderate and high dose rates, and the increase in urine flow seen in some patients seems to be due to interference with renal tubular function rather than to an increase in renal blood flow (Hilberman, 1982). There are usually increases in blood glucose, free fatty acids, cholesterol, low density lipoproteins and renin, and a reduction in insulin secretion.

In critically ill patients with septic shock, both adrenaline and dopamine are commonly used to maintain blood pressure and flow, and urine output. There is evidence that, in shock and severe heart failure, cardiac output and blood pressure are maintained only by increased sympathetic drive, and that exogenous catecholamines are simply replacing endogenous catecholamine drive which is failing at a number of levels (Runciman, 1980).

In patients with life-threatening bronchospasm or anaphylactic shock, adrenaline is the drug of choice due to its prominent β_2-agonist bronchodilatory effects and its inhibitory effect on the release of the mediators of anaphylaxis by mast cells. Furthermore, because of its short half-life, blood concentrations can be rapidly titrated up and down against effect.

Catecholamines are also one of the main lines of treatment for the life-threatening low cardiac output state which may follow cardiopulmonary bypass. Adrenaline and dopamine have been found to increase cardiac output with little increase in heart rate or afterload, and are thus suitable first-line drugs in this context. In cardiopulmonary resuscitation, α-effects appear to be important (Otto, Yakaitis and Blitt, 1981; Otto et al., 1981); adrenaline has become the drug of first choice, although theoretically noradrenaline or dopamine could be satisfactory alternatives.

In cardiogenic shock, both dopamine and dobutamine have been shown to improve blood pressure and cardiac output after myocardial infarction, but no increased long-term survival due to their use has been demonstrated (Bihari and Tinker, 1983). It is difficult to justify the use of adrenoceptor agonists in this context when β-adrenoceptor antagonists have been shown to reduce mortality after myocardial infarction (see Chapter 9).

Isoprenaline, dobutamine and prenalterol

Isoprenaline, as a selective β_1- and β_2-agonist with virtually no α-effects, produces an increase in cardiac output, an increase or decrease in mean blood pressure and, usually, an increase in heart rate. As a result of its tendency to cause a tachycardia both directly and reflexly, it is no longer considered a 'first-line' drug, and should be reserved for patients with excessive α-responses to adrenaline or dopamine (Kones, 1973; Lesch, 1976).

Dobutamine, as a selective β_1-agonist, was developed for use in cardiac failure and for patients emerging from cardiopulmonary bypass. However, it has a propensity for producing an increase in heart rate in some patients (Bohn et al., 1980; Chamberlain, Pepper and Yates, 1980). Prenalterol, a new relatively selective β_1-agonist, is reported to increase cardiac output without increasing heart rate, probably because it has some pressor effect. Although its clinical role has not yet been established, it may have a place in the treatment of cardiac failure as it is active orally as well as parenterally (Smith and Oldershaw, 1984).

Salbutamol, terbutaline and fenoterol

These and other similar selective β_2-agonists, have proved very useful in the treatment of asthma, and are also used to prevent uterine contractions in premature labour. Tremor, tachycardia and, occasionally, hypotension may be problems with large doses. They have been shown to cause less tachycardia for the same degree of bronchodilatation than isoprenaline or orciprenaline. They all have similar effects clinically, although fenoterol is twice as potent and has a slightly longer duration of action. None of the β_2-agonists is a catecholamine and thus their effects last for 4–8 hours. Controlled dose-response studies have shown conclusively that, if the drugs are inhaled, there is less increase in heart rate and less tremor for the same degree of bronchodilation than if given by the oral or intravenous route, although more than 75 per cent of inhaled drug has been shown to be swallowed eventually (Svedmyr and Simonsson, 1978).

Clonidine

The selective α_2-agonist clonidine is used in the treatment of hypertension. It exerts some of its antihypertensive effect by prejunctional α_2-mediated inhibition of noradrenaline release from sympathetic nerve terminals and by reducing renin secretion by the juxtaglomerular apparatus, but its effects on CNS α_2-receptors in medullary pathways involved in vasomotor control may be more important.

Phenylephrine and methoxamine

The selective α_1-agonists cause a sustained rise in blood pressure and a reflex bradycardia if used systemically. However, their main use is as nasal decongestants and mydriatics. Theoretically, they should be used to replace adrenaline in reducing local anaesthetic absorption. The imidazolines (see Table 8.1) have traditionally been used as nasal decongestants, but cause more 'rebound' effects, possibly due to some α_2-effect at low doses inhibiting local noradrenaline release.

Indirectly acting sympathomimetic amines

Agents with mixed direct and indirect actions are still in use, mainly because of the convenience of their long half-lives. Ephedrine has significant direct β_2-agonist effect as well and mimics adrenaline, whereas metaraminol mimics large doses of noradrenaline to a greater extent. Ephedrine is also widely used to reverse hypotension in obstetric patients after epidural blockade; this practice is based on the fact that it has been shown experimentally in the pregnant ewe not to decrease uterine blood flow (Ralston, Shnider and de Lorimer, 1974). Mephentermine also mimics noradrenaline, but has greater CNS effects. Amphetamine and methamphetamine act mainly indirectly and have powerful CNS effects as well as prolonged peripheral sympathomimetic effects.

References

Abel, J.J. and Crawford, A.C. (1897) On the blood-pressure-raising constituent of the suprarenal capsules. *Bulletin of the Johns Hopkins Hospital* **8**, 151–157

Ahlquist, R.P. (1948) A study of adrenotropic receptors. *American Journal of Physiology* **153**, 586–599

Ahlquist, R.P. (1965) Section 2, Circulation: In *Handbook of Physiology*, American

Society of Physiology, III. Williams & Wilkins: Baltimore, MD

Alabaster, V. and Davey, M. (1984) Precapillary vessels: effects of the sympathetic nervous system and of catecholamines. *Journal of Cardiovascular Pharmacology* suppl. 2. S365–S376

Anderson, R., Nilsson, J.F. and Koo, J. (1983) Beta-adrenoceptor-adenosine 3',5'-monophosphate system in human leukocytes before and after treatment for hyperthyroidism. *Journal of Clinical Endocrinology and Metabolism* **56**, 42–45

Barger, G. and Dale, H.H. (1910) Chemical structure and sympathomimetic action of amines. *Journal of Physiology* **41**, 19–59

Bihari, D.J. and Tinker, J. (1983) The management of shock. In: *Care of the Critically Ill Patient* (Eds. Tinker, J. and Rapin, T.), pp. 189–222. Springer Verlag: New York

Bohn, O.J., Poirier, C.S., Edmonds, J.F. and Barker, G.A. (1980) Hemodynamic effects of dobutamine after cardiopulmonary bypass in children. *Critical Care Medicine* **8**, 367–371

Bowman, W.C. and Rand, M.J. (1980) *Textbook of Pharmacology*, 2nd edn. Blackwell Scientific: Oxford

Bristow, M.R., Ginsburg, R., Minobe, W. *et al.* (1982) Decreased catecholamine sensitivity and beta-adrenergic-receptor density in failing human hearts. *New England Journal of Medicine* **307**, 205–211

Bunney, W.E. and Garland, B.L. (1984) A re-evaluation of the catecholamine hypothesis in affective disorders. In: *Catecholamines: Neuropharmacology and Central Nervous System – Therapeutic Aspects* (Eds. Usdin, E., Carlsson, A., Dahlstrom, A. and Engel, J.), pp. 3–9 Alan R. Liss: New York

Caron, M.G., Regan, J.W., Dickenson, K.E.J. *et al.* (1984) Molecular characterization of adrenergic receptor by affinity chromatography and photo affinity labeling. In: *Catecholamines: Basic and Peripheral Mechanisms* (Eds. Usdin, E., Carlsson, A., Dahlstrom, A. and Engel, J.), pp. 283–292. Alan R. Liss: New York

Chamberlain, J.H., Pepper, J.R. and Yates, A.K. (1980) Dobutamine, isoprenaline, and dopamine in patients after open heart surgery. *Intensive Care Medicine* **7**, 5–10

Cohen, R.A., Shepherd, J.T. and Vanhoutte, P.M. (1984) Effects of the adrenergic transmitter on the epicardial coronary arteries. *Federal Proceedings* **43**, 2862–2866

Conlay, L.A. and Maher, T.J. (1984) Neurotransmitter precursors and cardiovascular function. *Clinics in Anaesthesiology* **2** (2), 353–362

Da Prada, M., Keller, H.H., Pieri, L., Kettler, R. and Haefely, W.E. (1984) The pharmacology of Parkinson's disease: basic aspects and recent advances. *Experientia* **40**, 1165–1172

Davies, A.O. and Lefkowitz, R.J. (1984) Regulation of beta-adrenergic receptors by steroid hormones. *Annual Review of Physiology* **46**, 119–130

Derbyshire, D.R. and Smith, G. (1984) Sympathoadrenal responses to anaesthesia and surgery. *British Journal of Anaesthesia* **56**, 725–740

Desmonts, J.M. and Marty, J. (1984) Anaesthetic management of patients with phaeochromocytoma. *British Journal of Anaesthesia* **56**, 781–789

Dratman, M.B., Crutchfield, F.L. and Gordon, J.T. (1984) Thyroid hormones and adrenergic neurotransmitters. In: *Catecholamines: Neuropharmacology and Central Nervous System – Theoretical Aspects* (Eds. Usdin, E., Carlsson, A., Dahlstrom, A. and Engel, J.), pp. 425–440. Alan R. Liss: New York

Elliot, T.R. (1905) The action of adrenalin. *Journal of Physiology* **32**, 401–467

Fried, G.G., Lagercrantz, H., Klein, R. and Thureson-Klein, A. (1984) Large and small noradrenergic vesicles – origin, contents and functional significance. In: *Catecholamines: Basic and Peripheral Mechanisms* (Eds. Usdin, F., Carlsson, A., Dahlstrom, A. and Engel, J.), pp. 45–54. Alan R. Liss: New York

Furness, J.B., Costa, M., Papka, R.E., Della, N.G. and Murphy, R. (1984) Neuropeptides contained in peripheral cardiovascular nerves. *Clinical and Experimental Hypertension: Theory and Practice* **A6**, 91–106

Gilman, A.G., Goodman, L.S. and Gilman, A. (Eds.) (1980) *Goodman and Gilman's Pharmacological Basis of Therapeutics*, 6th edn. Macmillan: New York

Hertel, C. and Perkins, J.P. (1984) Receptor-specific mechanisms of desensitization of beta-adrenergic receptor function. *Molecular and Cellular Endocrinology* **37**, 245–256

Hilberman, U. (1982) Renal protection. In: *Critical Care – State of the Art* (Eds. Shoemaker, W.C. and Leigh Thompson, W.), pp. 111 (H): 1–28. Society of Critical Care Medicine: Fullarton, CA

Honerjager, P., Schafer-Korting, M. and Reiter, M. (1981) Involvement of cyclic AMP in the direct inotropic action of amrinone: biochemical and functional evidence. *Naunyn-Schmiedeberg's Archives of Pharmacology* **318**, 112–120

Kalsner, S. (1984) Limitations of presynaptic theory: no support for feedback control of autonomic effectors. *Federation Proceedings* **43**, 1358–1364

Kones, R.J. (1973) The catecholamines: reappraisal of their use for acute myocardial infarction and the low cardiac output syndromes. *Critical Care Medicine* **1**, 203–220

Kones, R.J. (1974) Cardiogenic shock. Therapeutic implications of altered myocardial energy balance. *Angiology* **25**, 317–333

Kopin, I.J. (1984) Catecholamines and the cardiovascular system: recent advances in biochemical evaluation of adrenergic activity. In: *Catecholamines: Basic and Peripheral Mechanisms* (Eds. Usdin, E., Carlsson, A., Dahlstrom, A. and Engel, J.), pp. 347–356. Alan R. Liss: New York

Lake, C.R., Chernow, B. and Ziegler, M.G. (1984) Clinical pharmacology of the sympathetic nervous system. *Clinics in Anaesthesiology* **2** (2), 269–288

Lands, A.M., Arnold, A., McAuliff, J.P., Luduena, F.P. and Brown, R.G. Jr (1967) Differentiation of receptor systems activated by sympathomimetic amines. *Nature* **214**, 597–598

Langer, S.Z. and Hicks, P.E. (1984) Physiology of the sympathetic nerve ending. *British Journal of Anaesthesia* **56**, 689–700

Langley, J.N. (1901) Observations on the physiological action of extracts of the suprarenal bodies. *Journal of Physiology* **27**, 237–256

Lees, G.M. (1981) A hitch-hiker's guide to the galaxy of adrenoceptors. *British Medical Journal* **283**, 173–177

Lesch, M. (1976) Inotropic agents and infarct size. Theoretical and practical considerations. *American Journal of Cardiology* **37**, 508–513

Lewandowsky, M. (1898). Uber eine wirkung des nebenniere tractes auf des Auge. *Zentralblatt für Physiologie* **12**, 599–600

Loewi, O. (1921) Uber Humorale übertragharkeit der Herznervenwirkung. *Pflügers Archiv für die gesamte Physiologie* **189**, 239–242

Louis, W.J., Summers, R.J., Dynon, M. and Jarrott, B. (1982) New developments in alpha-adrenoceptor drugs for the treatment of hypertension. *Journal of Cardiovascular Pharmacology* **4**, S168–S171

Lundberg, J.M., Terenius, L., Hokfelt, T. and Tatemoto, K. (1984) Catecholamines, neuropeptide Y (NPY), and the pancreatic polypeptide family: coexistence and interaction in the sympathetic responses. In: *Catecholamines: Neuropharmacology and Central Nervous System – Theoretical Aspects* (Eds. Usdin, E., Carlsson, A., Dahlstrom, A. and Engel, J.), pp. 179–190. Alan R. Liss: New York

Minneman, K.P., Pittman, R.N. and Molinoff, P.B. (1981) Beta-adrenergic receptor subtypes: properties, distribution, and regulation. *Annual Review of Neurosciences* **4**, 419–461

Muldoon, S.M., Moss, J., Freas, W. and Roizen, M.F. (1984) The effects of anaesthetics on the sympathoadrenal system. *Clinics in Anaesthesiology*, **2** (2), 289–306.

Nagatsu, T. and Nagatsu, I. (1984) Catecholamine-synthesizing enzymes: summary. In: *Catecholamines: Basic and Peripheral Mechanisms* (Eds. Usdin, E., Carlsson, A.,

Dahlstrom, A. and Engel, J.), pp. 219–221. Alan R. Liss: New York

Nestler, E.J. and Greengard, P. (1984) Protein phosphorylation in nervous tissue. In: *Catecholamines: Basic and Peripheral Mechanisms* (Eds. Usdin, E., Carlsson, A., Dahlstrom, A. and Engel, J.), pp. 9–22. Alan R. Liss: New York

Nhill, R.L. and Gelb, A.W. (1982) Peripheral chemoreceptors during anesthesia: are the watchdogs sleeping? *Anesthesiology* **57**, 151–152

Oliver, G. and Schafer, E.A. (1895) The physiological effects of extracts of the suprarenal capsules. *Journal of Physiology* **18**, 230–276

Otto, C.W., Yakaitis, R.W. and Blitt, C.D. (1981) Mechanism of action of epinephrine in resuscitation from asphyxial arrest. *Critical Care Medicine* **9**, 364–365

Otto, C.W., Yakaitis, R.W., Redding, J.S. and Blitt, C.D. (1981) Comparison of dopamine, dobutamine, and epinephrine in CPR. *Critical Care Medicine* **9**, 640–643

Powell, C.E. and Slater, I.H. (1958) Blocking of inhibitory adrenergic receptors by a dichloro analog of isoproterenol. *Journal of Pharmacology and Experimental Therapeutics* **122**, 480–488

Ralston, D.H., Shnider, S.M. and de Lorimer, A.A. (1974) Effects of equipotent ephedrine, metaraminol, mephentermine and methoxamine on uterine blood flow in the pregnant ewe. *Anesthesiology* **4**, 354–370

Runciman, W.B. (1980) Sympathomimetic amines. *Anaesthesia and Intensive Care* **8**, 289–309

Runciman, W.B. and Skowronski, G.A. (1984) Pathophysiology of haemorrhagic shock. *Anaesthesia and Intensive Care* **12**, 193–205

Rutledge, C.O. (1984) Uptake and storage: summary. In: *Catecholamines: Basic and Peripheral Mechanisms* (Eds. Usdin, E., Carlsson, A., Dahlstrom, A. and Engel, J.), pp. 149–150. Alan R. Liss: New York

Sandler, M. (1984) Shaking the kaleidoscope. In: *Catecholamines: Neuropharmacology and Central Nervous System – Therapeutic Aspects* (Eds. Usdin, E., Carlsson, A. Dahlstrom, A. and Engel, J.), pp. 231–234. Alan R. Liss: New York

Schafer, E.A. (1908) Present condition of our knowledge regarding the functions of the suprarenal capsules. *British Medical Journal* June 6, 1346–1351

Scholz, H. (1984) Inotropic drugs and their mechanisms of action. *Journal of the American College of Cardiology* **4**, 389–397

Schultzberg, M. (1984) Catecholamines and peptides: summary. In: *Catecholamines: Neuropharmacology and Central Nervous System – Theoretical Aspects* (Eds. Usdin, E., Carlsson, A. Dahlstrom, A. and Engel, J.), pp. 239–247. Alan R. Liss: New York

Seagard, J.L., Hopp, F.A., Donegan, J.H., Kalbfleisch, J.H. and Kampine, J.L. (1982) Halothane and the carotid sinus reflex: evidence for multiple sites of action. *Anesthesiology* **57**, 191–202

Seidman, C. and Homcy, C. (1984) Studies on the beta-adrenergic receptor: clinical and basic implications. *Clinics in Anaesthesiology* **2** (2), 341–352

Smith, L.D.R. and Oldershaw, P.J. (1984) Inotropic and vasopressor agents. *British Journal of Anaesthesia* **56**, 767–780

Stiles, G.L. and Lefkowitz, R.J. (1981) Thyroid hormone modulation of agonist–beta-adrenergic receptor interactions in the rat heart. *Life Sciences* **28**, 2529–2536

Stiles, G.L. and Lefkowitz, R.J. (1984) Cardiac adrenergic receptors. *Annual Review of Medicine* **35**, 149–164

Svedmyr, N. and Simonsson, B.G. (1978) Drugs in the treatment of asthma. *Pharmacology and Therapeutics B* **3**, 397–440

Uvnas, B. (1984) Chemical nature of vesicular NE storage and release – different theories. In: *Catecholamines: Basic and Peripheral Mechanisms* (Eds. Usdin, E., Carlsson, A., Dahlstrom, A. and Engel, J.), pp. 55–64. Alan R. Liss: New York

Venter, J.C., Fraser, C.M., Lilly, L., Seeman, P., Eddy, B. and Schaber, J. (1984) The structure of neurotransmitter receptors (adrenergic, dopaminergic and muscarinic cholinergic). In: *Catecholamines: Basic and Peripheral Mechanisms* (Eds. Usdin, E.,

Carlsson, A., Dahlstrom, A. and Engel, J.), pp. 293–302. Alan R. Liss: New York

Vogt, M. (1984) What about catecholamines now? In: *Catecholamines: Basic and Peripheral Mechanisms* (Eds. Usdin, E., Carlsson, A., Dahlstrom, A. and Engel, J.), pp. 5–7. Alan R. Liss: New York

Von Euler, U.S. (1954) Adrenaline and noradrenaline: distribution and action. *Pharmacological Reviews* **6**, 15–22

Westfall, T.C. (1984) Evidence that noradrenaline transmitter release is regulated by presynaptic receptors. *Federation Proceedings* **43**, 1352–1357

Wood, K. and Rafaelsen, O.J. (1984) Catecholamines in affective disorders: summary. In: *Catecholamines: Neuropharmacology and Central Nervous System – Therapeutic Aspects* (Eds. Usdin, E., Carlsson, A., Dahlstrom, A. and Engel, J.) pp. 29–30. Alan R. Liss: New York

9

Adrenoceptor antagonists

W.B. Runciman

Within a decade of the first description of the effects of 'extracts of the suprarenal capsules' (Oliver and Schafer, 1895), it had been discovered that some of the effects of adrenaline could be blocked by certain alkaloids of ergot, and the possibility of the existence of two types of receptor had been suggested by Dale. However, it was only in 1948, with Ahlquist's proposal for α- and β-receptors and the classification of the sympathomimetic amines on the basis of their relative potencies as α- and/or β-agonists, that the existence of β-blockers was postulated, and it was a further decade before the first β-blocker was described (Powell and Slater, 1958).

It is now recognized that there are a variety of compounds which have affinity for adrenoceptors but limited or no efficacy at these receptors. Compounds which occupy receptors, and therefore compete for occupancy with agonists, but produce only weak or attenuated effects, are termed partial antagonists, or are said to have some intrinsic sympathomimetic activity; those which occupy receptors and produce no typical adrenoceptor agonist effects are termed adrenoceptor antagonists or blockers. Relatively selective agonists and antagonists for α_1-, α_2, β_1- and β_2-adrenoceptors are now known (Table 9.1). The many factors which may influence the effects of the adrenoceptor

Table 9.1 Examples of relatively selective adrenoceptor agonists and antagonists

Relatively selective agonists and antagonists	Adrenoceptors			
	α_1	α_2	β_1	β_2
Agonists				
Methoxamine	←——→			
Clonidine		←——→		
Dobutamine			←——→	
Salbutamol				←——→
Antagonists				
Butoxamine				←——→
Metoprolol			←——→	
Yohimbine		←——→		
Prazosin	←——→			

agonists have been considered in the previous chapter. Some of these factors also modify the effects of the adrenoceptor antagonists, most of which also exert a number of other unrelated effects which influence the biological effects ultimately produced.

As adrenoceptor antagonists interfere with fundamental mechanisms involved in the regulation of the cardiovascular and respiratory systems, and as many patients presenting for anaesthesia and surgery are now being treated by these agents, a knowledge of their effects and their possible interactions with other drugs and with anaesthetic agents is essential for the practising anaesthetist. As in the previous chapter, selected papers and recent reviews are quoted only on topics not adequately dealt with in standard texts (e.g. Bowman and Rand, 1980; Gilman, Goodman and Gilman, 1980).

Mechanisms of action

Most of the adrenoceptor antagonists bind competitively to what are visualized as specific externally orientated drug-binding sites on the relevant receptor peptides. Each partial agonist has a specific affinity for each adrenoceptor subtype and a limited capacity to activate adenyl cyclase or to influence calcium channel control, and each antagonist likewise has a specific affinity for the binding site but has no capacity to activate any receptor mechanisms. Although each agonist or antagonist has a characteristic affinity for a particular receptor subtype, binding, except in the case of the haloalkylamines, is by weak ionic linkages and is competitive and reversible according to the relative affinities and concentrations of the competing compounds at each receptor subtype. Affinity for receptors, efficacy at receptors and the relative potency of each drug in terms of additional effects are generally unrelated to each other and are intrinsic properties of the drug in question. Each of these factors will be considered in turn for both α- and β-receptor antagonists.

α-Adrenoceptor antagonists

There are several groups of compounds which act as α-adrenoceptor blockers (Table 9.2). As most of these exert a wide spectrum of other effects, and as some are not used primarily for their α-adrenoceptor-blocking effects, the mechanisms of action of each group will be discussed separately.

Alkaloids of ergot

These are of historical interest only, as their capacity to exert some antiadrenaline effect was documented by Dale in 1906. There are six active naturally occurring alkaloids and several semisynthetic derivatives, which act to varying extents as partial agonists and antagonists on α-adrenergic, tryptaminergic and dopaminergic receptors. Ergotamine is a typical competitive partial agonist. It has 300 times the affinity of noradrenaline for α-adrenoceptors but produces less than one-third of the maximum response; the initial response to ergotamine is an increase in blood pressure due to this agonist effect. These compounds are used in the treatment of migraine and as oxytocics; none is clinically useful as an α-blocker.

Table 9.2 α-Adrenoceptor antagonists

Drug group	Drug
Ergot alkaloids	Ergotamine, dihydroergotamine
Haloalkylamines	Phenoxybenzamine, dibenamine
Imidazolines	Phentolamine, tolazoline
Tricyclics	Imipramine, desipramine, azapetine
Phenothiazines	Chlorpromazine, trifluoperazine
Butyrophenones	Haloperidol, droperidol
Benzodioxanes	Piperoxan, prosympal, dibozane
Prazosin	Prazosin
Phenoxyalkylamines	Thymoxamine, phenoxyethyldiethylamine
Yohimbine alkaloids	Yohimbine, indoramin

Haloalkylamines

Phenoxybenzamine is a clinically useful member of this group of drugs, which are chemically related to the nitrogen mustards. Initial antagonism is competitive, as the presence of adequate concentrations of an agonist prevents blockade; however, as a strong covalent bond is formed with the receptor (compared with the weak ionic bond formed by the α-agonists), blockade, once established, is only slowly reversible ('non-equilibrium blockade'). Such blockade is also produced on histamine, serotonin and acetylcholine muscarinic receptors. In addition, several other effects are produced on adrenergic mechanisms. Both neuronal and extraneuronal uptake of amines are blocked, thus potentiating the effects of adrenoceptor agonists at β-receptors but preventing noradrenaline release by indirectly acting sympathomimetic amines. β-Effects are further potentiated by the fact that more endogenous noradrenaline is released than usual, as the prejunctional α_2-receptors, which normally inhibit noradrenaline release, are also blocked.

Imidazolines

The imidazolines tolazoline and phentolamine closely resemble the imidazoline α-adrenoceptor agonists in chemical structure and are competitive antagonists at α-receptors. They have no effect on β-receptors. Although these compounds are pure antagonists in the pharmacological sense, low concentrations produce enhancement of the effects of endogenous sympathetic nerve activity because the α_2-receptors are more sensitive to competitive blockade than the α_1-receptors. Thus, at low doses, prejunctional inhibition of noradrenaline release is blocked and the increased local concentration of noradrenaline effectively competes with the imidazoline antagonists at α_1-receptors. At higher doses more complete α-receptor blockade is achieved, but there is still enhancement of the effects of β-agonists due to the increased local concentrations of endogenous noradrenaline produced by α_2-receptor blockade. The imidazolines have no effect on uptake mechanisms.

Tolazoline also exerts other effects, as it resembles histamine in structure.

It stimulates gastric acid secretion and causes peripheral vasodilation via H_1- and H_2-receptors, respectively. It also stimulates the gastrointestinal tract, causing diarrhoea, and increases sweating and the production of salivary and pancreatic secretions by a cholinergic mechanism. These side effects are less marked with phentolamine, which is also ten times more potent as an α-receptor antagonist than tolazoline.

Tricyclics, phenothiazines, butyrophenones and benzodioxanes

These groups of drugs all act as competitive α-receptor antagonists (see Table 9.2). The phenothiazines and tricyclics, in addition to having a variety of other effects, block neuronal uptake of amines. Azapetine is a tricyclic with a different arrangement of its dibenzazepine nucleus, and is a fairly selective α-blocker. Piperoxan, like the imidazolines, selectively blocks α_2-receptors at low doses, whereas prosympal appears to have high affinity for both α_1- and α_2-receptors and does not produce enhancement of endogenous sympathetic activity at low doses.

Prazosin

Prazosin is a relatively selective α_1-adrenoceptor antagonist. It produces less tachycardia for a given fall in blood pressure, possibly because it has no effect on the α_2-receptor-mediated prejunctional inhibition of noradrenaline release from cardiac sympathetic nerves (Graham, 1984).

Phenoxyalkylamines

Thymoxamine and phenoxyethyldiethylamine, in addition to being competitive α-antagonists, act as antihistamines and have local anaesthetic properties. Thymoxamine is a relatively selective α_1-antagonist.

Yohimbine alkaloids

Yohimbine and some related alkaloids and their semisynthetic derivatives are competitive α-antagonists which resemble the alkaloids of ergot in chemical structure. Yohimbine itself is a relatively selective α_2-receptor antagonist (Goldberg and Robertson, 1983). It also blocks serotonin receptors, has local anaesthetic properties, produces a number of CNS effects such as irritability, nausea and vomiting, and produces release of antidiuretic hormone.

Indoramin is an α_1- and α_2-receptor antagonist which also has antihistamine and local anaesthetic properties. It exerts some direct effects on the heart as well, as it produces a fall in blood pressure without a compensatory reflex tachycardia.

β-Adrenoceptor antagonists

The β-adrenoceptor antagonists are all isoprenaline analogues, and as such have greater chemical structural similarities to the β-agonists than most of the α-antagonists have to the α-agonists. As there is also considerable overlap with respect to their other properties (Table 9.3 and Fig. 9.1), they will be considered together. The factors influencing the interactions of β-antagonists with receptors and the relative importance of partial agonist, membrane-stabilizing and antiarrhythmic effects will each be considered in turn.

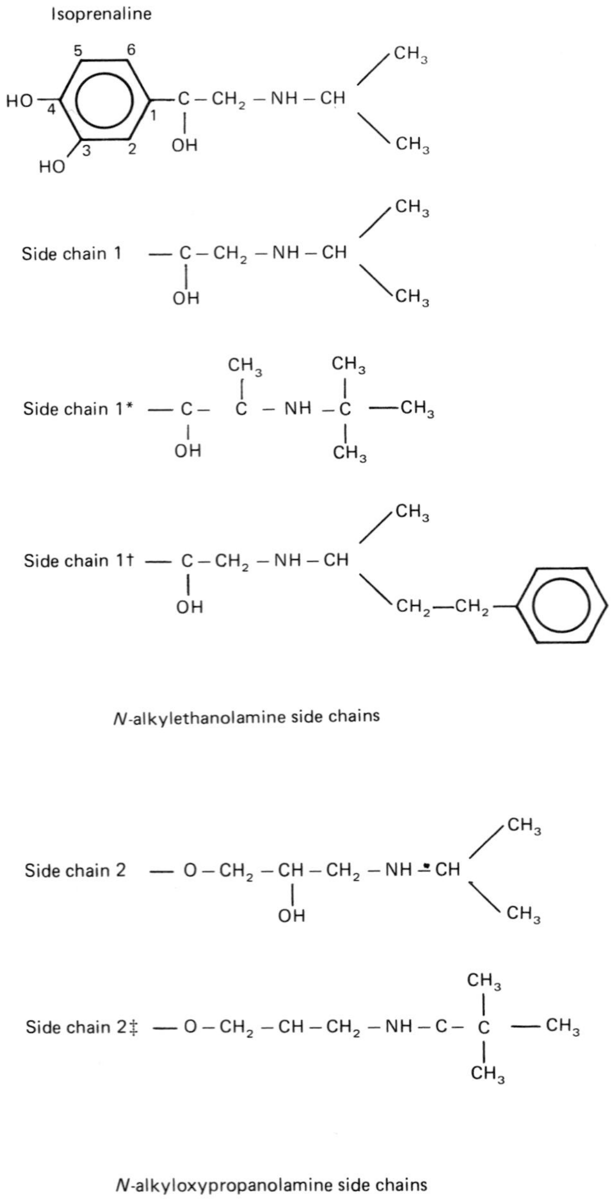

Isoprenaline

Side chain 1

Side chain 1*

Side chain 1†

N-alkylethanolamine side chains

Side chain 2

Side chain 2‡

N-alkyloxypropanolamine side chains

Fig. 9.1 Chemical structure of isoprenaline and side chains of β-adrenoceptor antagonists listed in Table 9.3.

Table 9.3 Chemical structure and properties of isoprenaline and selected β-adrenoceptor antagonists

Compound	Chemical structure R-side chain −1 or −2	Adrenoceptor antagonist activity	Partial agonist potency (as % of isoprenaline)	Membrane stabilization effect
Isoprenaline	R −1	−	100%	−
Acebutolol	R−2	β_1, β_2	−	+
Butoxamine	R−1*	β_2	−	+
Alprenolol	R−2	β_1, β_2	25%	+
Atenolol	R−2	β_1	−	−
Labetalol	R−1‡	$\alpha_1, \beta_1, \beta_2$	−	+
Metoprolol	R−2	β_1	−	+
Nadolol	R−2‡	β_1, β_2	−	−
Oxprenolol	R−2	β_1, β_2	30%	+ +
Pindolol	R−2	β_1, β_2	50%	+
Propranolol	R−2	β_1, β_2	−	+ + +
Sotalol	R−1	β_1, β_2	−	−
Timolol	R−2†	β_1, β_2	−	−

The β-blockers are all analogues of isoprenaline (Fig. 9.1), which has an aromatic ring with hydroxyl groups on the 3 and 4 carbon atoms, and an N-alkylethanolamine side chain (side chain 1). All the β-blockers have an aromatic ring with bulkier substituents than isoprenaline (R−1), and either an N-alkylethanolamine side chain (side chain 1) or an N-alkyloxypropranolamine side chain (side chain 2). *, †, ‡ denote additional structures (see Fig. 9.1).

Interactions with receptors

All the β-adrenoceptor antagonists bind competitively and reversibly with adrenoceptors by the same ionic bonds as the agonists. However, there are local factors which may influence agonist, but not antagonist, affinity for adrenoceptors. Studies with two cultured cell lines, one lacking the drug-binding site (the 'receptor unit') and the other lacking the capacity to activate adenyl cyclase (the 'enzyme unit'), have shown that these sites are two separate macromolecular units and that the synthesis of each is controlled by different genes (Carlsson and Hedberg, 1980). Binding of agonists to the receptor unit is thought to induce allosteric changes in the receptor protein and to activate the enzyme unit. The affinity of agonists for the receptor unit is increased both by this binding process and by guanine triphosphate (GTP). Hydrolysis of the membrane-bound enzyme GTP is thought to play an important role in terminating the agonist-induced hormonal signal. The kinetics of antagonist binding, however, are quite different; they are unaffected by GTP and do not cause the appropriate allosteric changes in the receptor unit to activate the enzyme unit (Carlsson and Hedberg, 1980). It is important to note, therefore, that *in vivo* the relative affinities of agonists and antagonists for a particular receptor subtype in a particular organ may be altered by local mechanisms. Such changes in receptor affinity as well as in receptor number have now been documented in a number of diseases and with a variety of drugs. These have been reviewed in the previous chapter.

As is the case with the β-agonists, there is an isopropyl or bulkier substituent on the amine, and substituents on the aromatic ring which appear to influence relative affinities for the different receptor subtypes. Hydroxyl substitution on a side chain carbon atom results in optical isomerism and seems essential for activity, with the laevoratory forms of both agonists and antagonists being much more active than the dextrorotatory forms. This is useful in determining mechanisms of action, as isomeric specificity influences binding on adrenoceptors but does not influence other properties such as those which produce membrane stabilization.

Some β-adrenoceptor antagonists may display some degree of selectivity for β_1 or β_2 subtypes (see Table 9.3). Metoprolol and atenolol have a degree of selectivity for β_1-receptors. However, this selectivity is only relative and in large enough doses these drugs will block β_2-receptors as well, and may, for example, precipitate severe bronchospasm in some individuals (Moulds, 1984). Butoxamine is a relatively selective β_2-antagonist. It has no useful clinical application but is an important experimental tool.

It is important to note that these subtype classifications are based on pharmacological determinations of relative agonist and antagonist affinities and specifities, and not on the biological effects resulting from receptor occupancy *in vivo* (Carlsson and Hedberg, 1980). The situation *in vivo* is very complex, as there are mixed populations of β_1- and β_2-receptors in most organs, as the relative and absolute subtype densities may vary in different regions of an organ, as their distances from sympathetic nerve terminals vary, and as different agonists have different affinities for receptor subtypes (Minneman, Pittman and Molinoff, 1981; Stiles and Lefkowitz, 1984).

Figure 9.2 demonstrates some of these complex interactions. In an *in vitro* study, propranolol, a non-selective β-blocker, shifted the dose–response curves for noradrenaline and adrenaline to the right to the same degree. However, metoprolol, a selective β_1-blocker, produced a preferential shift of the noradrenaline curves, whereas butoxamine, a selective β_2-blocker, produced a preferential shift of the adrenaline curves. Thus, in this study, heart rate responses were being predominantly mediated via β_2-receptors with exogenous adrenaline and via β_1-receptors with exogenous noradrenaline. Furthermore, *in vivo*, because relative receptor subtype densities vary with distance from sympathetic nerve terminals, the effect of β-receptor blockers will depend not only on the nature and concentration of the competing agonist but also on whether it has been released from a nerve terminal or has been blood borne.

These observations have some clinical implications. For example, metoprolol and propranolol are equipotent in inhibiting exercise tachycardia with normal endogenous release of noradrenaline from sympathetic nerve terminals in the heart. However, metoprolol is five times less potent in inhibiting heart rate responses to exogenous adrenaline (Carlsson and Hedberg, 1980). In the former case the heart rate responses were probably mainly β_1 mediated by receptors close to nerve terminals, whereas in the latter case they were probably β_2 mediated by receptors which may have been more remote from nerve terminals, and for which the particular agonist chosen,

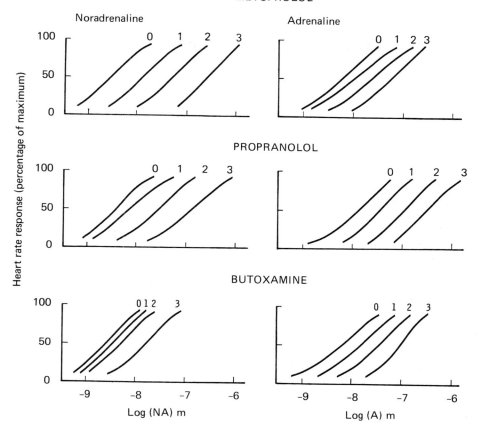

Fig. 9.2 Concentration–heart rate response curves to noradrenaline (NA) and adrenaline (A) in the isolated cat heart before (0) and after (1, 2, 3,) three increasing concentrations of metoprolol (0.01, 0.05 and 0.25 mg/ml), propranolol (0.001, 0.005 and 0.025 mg/ml) and butoxamine (0.1, 0.5 and 2.5 mg/ml). Note that responses to noradrenaline were not greatly affected by butoxamine, and that those to adrenaline were not greatly affected by metoprolol, implying that heart rate responses were being mediated by β_1-receptors in the former case, and β_2-receptors in the latter. (After Carlsson and Hedberg, 1980; reproduced with permission.)

adrenaline, had a greater affinity than noradrenaline. Thus, it is possible that the selective β_1-blockers may fail to confer protection in particularly stressful situations in which there may be high concentrations of circulating adrenaline.

Partial agonist effects

The non-selective β-antagonists pindolol, oxprenolol and alprenolol may all elicit up to 20–50 per cent of the effect of isoprenaline whilst competitively blocking receptors. There has been much debate as to whether this is an advantage or a disadvantage. It seems that, quantitatively, the effect exerted *in vivo* is usually similar to that exerted by normal sympathetic nervous system activity at rest (McCulloch, 1984). Thus, a fall in heart rate and cardiac output may be avoided at rest whilst responses to exercise or stress will still be affected. This does not appear to influence the efficacy of these agents as antihypertensives (Aellig, 1983) and may be an advantage in patients with borderline heart failure or chronic obstructive airways disease (Taylor, 1983; Foëx, 1984).

Membrane-stabilizing effects

The membrane-stabilizing or local anaesthetic potency of propranolol is about equal to that of lignocaine. Whilst that of most of the other β-blockers is considerably less than this, most of them will produce at least some membrane stabilization in the heart, as manifested by reduced rate of rise of action potentials. However, this quinidine-like effect is insignificant in the concentration range required clinically to produce adequate β-blockade. It has been shown that any reduced contractility or rate of conduction which may occur with β-blocker therapy is due not to this effect but to withdrawal of sympathetic tone (Foëx, 1984).

Antiarrhythmic effects

β-blockers may exert significant antiarrhythmic effects. However, as indicated above, reduction in rate of rise of the initial depolarization wave of the cardiac action potential does not occur in the usual dose range, and does not seem to be responsible for this effect. Blockade of the effects of catecholamines on the rate of spontaneous resting membrane potential decay contributes to this effect, and a further mechanism may be the increase in duration of the action potential which has been observed to occur with the 'chronic' administration of some β-blockers (Foëx, 1984).

Pharmacokinetics

α-Adrenoceptor antagonists

Only the kinetics of drugs commonly used clinically will be discussed.

Phentolamine

Phentolamine orally is only about one-fifth as active as when given parenterally, and anaesthetists should use this latter route. It has a half-life of only 10–15 minutes, and hence small incremental intravenous bolus doses (starting with 1 mg) should be given until the desired effect is achieved, followed by an infusion the rate of which can be titrated against effect. Several hundred milligrams may be necessary over a few hours. Great caution should be exercised with the initial doses as tachycardia, dysrhythmias and angina may be caused.

Phenoxybenzamine

Phenoxybenzamine is a relatively unstable compound and has erratic oral bioavailability, with only about one-fifth of an oral dose being absorbed in an active form. It has a slow onset of action (over about an hour), as it undergoes cyclization itself before alkylating the receptor by rearrangement. About 50 per cent of a dose is excreted in 12 hours, but it is very lipid soluble and some drug remains in fat and, possibly, attached to receptors for weeks. A satisfactory method of administration is to infuse 1 mg/kg body weight as a very dilute solution over at least an hour once a day, for several days. The patient should be monitored, and infusions of intravenous fluid may be necessary.

Prazosin

Prazosin is an effective oral antihypertensive agent. It is rapidly metabolized in the liver, and has a half-life of about 3 hours. Its bioavailability is only about 60 per cent, due to first-pass metabolism after oral administration, and its kinetics are not significantly altered in patients with renal failure. Half-life is prolonged in patients with cardiac failure, and treatment should be initiated slowly (e.g. with a 1 mg dose), as syncope may be produced by acute venodilation without reflex tachycardia.

β-Adrenoceptor antagonists

Under normal circumstances, after a single dose there is a relationship between the blood concentration of a β-blocker and parameters such as heart rate or systolic blood pressure (Regardh, 1980). However, this relationship is not maintained with long-term therapy in conditions such as angina or hypertension, and in fact there is also wide variability both in the pharmacokinetic characteristics of different β-blockers and in the manner in which different subjects handle some β-blockers (Regardh, 1980; Lennard *et al.*, 1982). Some of the reasons for this wide variability are evident if the pharmacokinetic characteristics of the β-blockers are considered in more detail. Duration of effect after the last oral dose, the effects of compromised liver and kidney function, and techniques for maintaining β-blockade parenterally are all of particular importance to the anaesthetist.

Absorption and bioavailability

There are large differences between the various β-blockers both in terms of percentage absorption from the gastrointestinal tract and in terms of the extent to which they are subject to 'first-pass' metabolism by the liver (Table 9.4). After ingestion, time to peak blood concentration varies from 1 to 4 hours; the hydrophilic agents atenolol, nadolol and sotalol are absorbed slightly more slowly than the lipophilic agents but the differences are not clinically significant. Controlled release preparations may halve the peak and double the trough blood concentrations between doses, and thus offer significant advantages in terms of less variability in effect and decreased dosing interval (Regardh, 1980).

With the hydrophilic drugs, all the absorbed drug is available although incomplete absorption limits the overall bioavailability of atenolol and nadolol. However, with all the other β-blockers there is substantial first-pass hepatic metabolism. The extent to which it occurs appears to be related to the lipophilicity of the drug. Very lipophilic drugs, such as alprenolol, oxprenolol

Table 9.4 Approximate values for some pharmacokinetic parameters of selected β-adrenoceptor antagonists after oral administration

Drug	Percentage of oral dose absorbed	Bioavailability as a percentage of oral dose	Major route of clearance (hepatic/renal)	Volume of distribution (l/kg body weight)	Elimination half-life (hours)	Total body clearance (l/min)	Percentage protein binding
Acebutolol	70*	50	Hepatic	2.3	3–4†	0.6	20
Alprenolol	90*	10	Hepatic	3.3	2–3†	1.2	80
Atenolol	50	50	Renal	0.7	5–7	0.1	0
Labetalol	70	30	Hepatic	11	3–4	2.4	50
Metoprolol	90	50	Hepatic§	5.0	3–4§	1.1	10
Nadolol	20	20	Both	2.0	10–12	0.2	30
Oxprenolol	90	30	Hepatic	1.2	1–3	0.4	80
Pindolol	90	60	Both	1.2	3–4	0.4	50
Propranolol	90	30	Hepatic	3.6	3–4†	1.0	90
Sotalol	90	100	Renal	1.4	10–15‡	0.2	0
Timolol	90	50	Hepatic§	2.0	3–4§	0.5	10

(Data from Regardh, 1980.)

* Dose-dependent bioavailability.

† Clinically important active metabolites formed.

‡ Dose dependent (increases with dose).

§ Probable genetically determined variability between subjects.

and propranolol have only 30–50 per cent bioavailability in spite of greater than 90 per cent being absorbed from the gastrointestinal tract. There may also be considerable intersubject variability in first-pass metabolism (see below).

Distribution and protein binding
Distribution half-lives of β-adrenoceptor antagonists are generally less than 10 minutes, indicating rapid distribution from blood to tissues. Steady-state volumes of distribution are large, so only 1–2 per cent of the drug is located in the blood. The incidence of CNS side effects, such as light-headedness and vivid dreams, has been claimed to be greater with lipid-soluble drugs, which more readily penetrate the blood–brain barrier, than with hydrophilic drugs. However, this has not been documented in controlled studies (Regardh, 1980).

Atenolol, metoprolol, sotalol and timolol are carried in the blood almost entirely as free drug. Acebutolol, labetalol, nadolol and pindolol are 20–50 per cent bound to plasma proteins, and oxprenolol and propranolol are 80–90 per cent bound. As only the unbound drug is effective, displacement from binding sites may, in theory, alter effects with the highly protein-bound drugs. For example, the free fraction of propranolol has been shown to double (from 6.5 to 13.5 per cent) during cardiopulmonary bypass, and to be restored essentially to preoperative values with heparin reversal by protamine (Wood, Shand and Wood, 1979).

Elimination
Polar hydrophilic drugs such as pindolol and nadolol are eliminated predominantly by the kidneys. Atenolol and sotalol are eliminated exclusively by the kidneys with clearances approximating glomerular filtration rate. Half-lives of all these drugs are increased in the presence of renal failure.

Because the more lipophilic compounds with larger volumes of distribution are subject to increased hepatic metabolism, these two effects tend to cancel each other, resulting in a fairly narrow range of average half-lives (2–4 hours) for these drugs. There may be genetically determined differences in the capacity of some individuals to metabolize β-blockers (e.g. metoprolol and timolol). In these individuals the elimination half-life may be prolonged up to threefold (Lennard et al., 1982; Lennard, 1985). Also with liver disease, clearance and plasma binding of lipophilic drugs may be greatly reduced. The half-life of propranolol has been reported to increase from 3 to 23 hours in severe cirrhosis. Kinetics do not appear to be affected as greatly for labetalol and metoprolol in severe cirrhosis, but bioavailability is increased (Regardh, 1980).

Propranolol, atenolol and metoprolol all have active metabolites which may contribute to the effects produced. With oral administration relatively more metabolites are present than with parenteral administration, due to the first-pass effect, and different relationships have been shown between plasma concentrations of parent drug and effect when comparing these two routes of administration for these compounds (Ablad et al., 1974). Other drugs form active metabolites, but these are not usually of any clinical significance because they either have very short half-lives or are very low in potency. As metabolites are usually more polar than parent drugs and are usually eliminated by the kidney, they may become of greater significance in renal failure. Increased retention of active metabolites in renal failure has been shown to increase β-blocking effect with acebutolol but not with metoprolol or propranolol (Regardh, 1980).

Doses of β-blockers should always be adjusted to suit the needs of individual patients, as there are many sources of variability. All the lipophilic drugs should be used with caution in hepatic failure, when atenolol and sotalol may be safest; all the drugs subject to substantial renal clearance (and acebutolol, with its active, renally cleared polar metabolites) should be used with caution in renal failure. Doses of all β-blockers should be reduced in the elderly, who have been shown to have higher blood concentrations than young or middle-aged individuals on the same doses (Regardh, 1980); also, the possibility of genetic differences between individuals in their capacities for oxidative metabolism should be borne in mind (Lennard, 1985).

Duration of β-blockade after the last oral dose

With normal doses the half-lives of the clinically important β-blockers range from 3 to 12 hours (see Table 9.4). Thus, for brief procedures, if the patient continues to take β-blockers up to the time of surgery and is able to continue to take them postoperatively, β-blockade effect continues to be reasonable. However, even with doses of propranolol of up to 240 mg per day, blockade, as assessed by isoprenaline dose–response curves, has been shown to have regressed completely by 24 hours (Prys-Roberts, 1984). Thus, in postoperative patients to whom drugs cannot be given orally or by nasogastric tube, β-blockers may have to be given intravenously.

Parenteral administration of β-blockers

β-Blockers should be given intravenously by infusion or in very small incremental doses because effects are produced in minutes and may be quite dramatic. The doses used by anaesthetists for the suppression of transient dysrhythmias or tachycardia, such as 1 mg increments of propranolol, are usually much smaller than those necessary to produce the blood concentrations which have been measured in patients on oral β-blocker treatment.

For the maintenance of β-blockade intravenous infusions should be used. It has been pointed out (Prys-Roberts, 1984) that about one-third of the calculated intravenous dose is all that is necessary, as the 'wasted' areas under the peaks of the blood concentration–time curves, which are characteristic of oral dosing regimens, are not produced with continuous intravenous infusions. Thus, a patient on 240 mg propranolol daily does not require the 72 mg per day calculated from the 30 per cent bioavailability of propranolol but only about 1 mg per hour. The same has been found for labetalol in patients presenting for aortic surgery. Calculation from oral dosing and bioavailability data yields a predicted infusion rate of 20 mg per hour, whereas in practice this rate has been found to be excessive, and about 5–10 mg per hour has been shown to produce the desired degree of blockade (Prys-Roberts, 1984).

If establishment of β-blockade is urgently indicated in a patient on no previous therapy, repeated small intravenous loading doses followed by infusions at the rates indicated above will rapidly and safely achieve the desired state.

Pharmacodynamics

The effects of adrenoceptor antagonists in low doses may be very variable (Astrom, 1980). Some of the factors influencing effects at adrenoceptors which were considered in the previous chapter contribute to this variability. There may be overall or regional variations in sympathetic nervous system activity which may be subject to a host of pathophysiological and pharmacological influences, and there may be different responses to endogenous and exogenous agonists. The use of antagonists will produce variable effects in different regions, depending on the balance between sympathetic and parasympathetic tone in that organ prior to introduction of the antagonist. Drugs such as phenoxybenzamine and phentolamine may selectively block α_2-receptors in low doses and enhance endogenous sympathetic activity, whilst receptor number and affinity may be altered in various disease states, with drug treatment and with endocrine status. With higher doses, more complete competitive blockade is established, and the effects are more predictable. However, other first messengers, biologically active peptides released from sympathetic nerves and other factors affecting the second and subsequent messengers may still be the source of considerable variability in response to adrenoceptor antagonists. Finally, as discussed above, each partial agonist or antagonist also exerts a number of other unrelated effects.

Effects and clinical use

α—Adrenoceptor antagonists

α-Adrenoceptor antagonists are not employed as widely as β-blockers, but there are some specific indications for their use in the operative and perioperative periods.

In general, the α-blockers reduce blood pressure, cause marked postural hypotension and produce a baroreceptor-mediated reflex tachycardia which is aggravated by increased endogenous noradrenaline release by phenoxybenzamine and other drugs which also block α_2-receptors. The high incidence of postural hypotension, a particularly disabling condition, and nasal stuffiness, a particularly irritating effect, have generally limited the clinical use of the non-selective α-blockers to the short-term management of particular problems in hospitalized patients. Great care should be exercised with these patients because cardiovascular homeostatic reflexes have been severely impaired, and catastrophic hypotension may follow the use of drugs which cause vasodilation, such as anaesthetic agents, opioid analgesics or local anaesthetics used for producing regional blockade.

Non-selective α-antagonists

Phentolamine is a weak competitive α-blocker with a rapid onset of action and a short duration (15–30 minutes) of effect. Because of its short half-life it is useful in controlling sudden increases in blood pressure which are expected to be of relatively short duration. In this context it may lower blood pressure, lower both right and left ventricular filling pressures, improve stroke volume output and subendocardial perfusion, and abolish α-receptor-mediated coronary artery spasm. It is used to control hypertension intra- and postoperatively, during operative manipulations of a phaeochromocytoma and to control perfusion pressure during cardiac surgery. It may also be used to reverse electrocardiographic evidence of myocardial ischaemia in these contexts. Baroreceptor-mediated reflex tachycardia frequently occurs, which may be controlled by small doses of a selective β_1-antagonist.

Phenoxybenzamine is a non-selective α-blocker with a slow onset and a long duration of action. It causes marked postural hypotension and is unsuitable for routine use in outpatients. However, it is a very valuable drug in the preoperative and operative management of patients with phaeochromocytomas. It has also been used in the long-term management of patients with inoperable phaeochromocytomas and for the short-term preservation of kidneys for transplantation.

Selective α₁-antagonists

The selective α_1-antagonist prazosin is useful in treating hypertensive patients with poor renal function because renal blood flow and cardiac output are unchanged and renin secretion is inhibited. It may also have a role in the treatment of congestive cardiac failure, as it has greater affinity for α-receptors in capacitance vessels than those in resistance vessels, and thus has haemodynamic effects which resemble those of glyceryl trinitrate rather than those of hydralazine. The relative lack of reflex tachycardia is also important in patients with severe arteriosclerotic disease. Thymoxamine, another relatively selective α_1-antagonist, has been used in the treatment of circulatory failure after cardiac surgery as well as to improve peripheral circulation in patients with peripheral vascular disease.

Selective α₂-antagonists

The α_2-antagonists tend to increase circulating catecholamine concentrations, to cause an increase in heart rate, blood pressure and motor activity and to cause nausea, vomiting, sweating and tremor. They have no clinical uses but have been useful experimentally.

β-Adrenoceptor antagonists

β-Adrenoceptor antagonists are now very widely used in the treatment of ischaemic heart disease and hypertension; they are also used during and after anaesthesia for the suppression of the severe short-lived episodes of tachycardia, dysrhythmias and hypertension which may occur in patients with cardiovascular disease. Because they modify circulatory homeostatic responses and because the patients in question usually already have significant cardiovascular disease, their effects on the cardiorespiratory system, both in the awake patient and under anaesthesia, are of particular interest to the anaesthetist.

The β-blockers all tend to reduce heart rate and cardiac output. The extent to which this occurs depends on the initial degree of endogenous sympathetic activity, with greater reductions occurring in patients with high levels of activity at the time of treatment. There are some differences in the cardiovascular effects of the non-selective and β_1-selective antagonists (see below).

All β-blockers tend to worsen obstructive airways disease, and may cause catastrophic bronchospasm in particular individuals; this is more likely to occur with non-selective β-blockers than with selective β_1-antagonists. There is very wide interindividual variability in this respect, which attests again to the many factors which may influence a biological effect in any particular end-organ.

The effects of β-blockers on intermediary metabolism are complex. They vary from species to species and tissue to tissue, and are also influenced by endogenous or exogenous adrenoceptor agonist activity and other factors influencing first and second messengers. β-Blockers do not normally affect blood glucose or insulin concentrations although they may occasionally produce marked increases in blood glucose levels in diabetics; also, sympathetic-nervous-system-mediated glycogenolysis and lipolysis are inhibited in response to stimuli such as hypoglycaemia (Kleinbaum and Shamoon, 1984). Although it is well recognized that β-blockers prolong recovery from hypoglycaemia in diabetics and patients with liver disease, they may also precipitate hyperglycaemia in these patients and in some normal fasting individuals, particularly soon after instigation of β-blocker therapy. These problems are exacerbated by the fact that tachycardia and sweating, which are part of the β-receptor-mediated sympathetic response to hypoglycaemia, are also blocked, and by the fact that there may be exaggerated responses (such as severe hypertension) to α-receptor-mediated responses. Careful instruction is necessary if β-blockers have to be given to patients who are susceptible to hypoglycaemia or who have to fast for an investigation soon after starting β-blocker therapy.

As would be anticipated from inspection of Table 8.2 in the previous Chapter, β-blockers also have other effects; however, most of these are usually of no clinical significance. They block catecholamine-mediated uterine relaxation (particularly in the non-pregnant state), and experimentally block the 'antianaphylactic effect' of catecholamines (Assem and Schild, 1971). β-Receptor-mediated skeletal muscle tremor is also blocked by these agents, but tremor originating in the CNS (e.g. parkinsonian tremor) is unaffected. Nausea, vomiting and mild diarrhoea occur occasionally and probably represent blockade of β-mediated relaxation of the gut. A variety of CNS symptoms have been attributed to CNS penetration by β-blockers, but in carefully controlled double blind trials these appear to occur with equal frequency with placebo treatment (Weiner, 1980).

Non-selective β-antagonists

Several non-selective β-blockers have been developed and marketed, the relevant features of several of which have been summarized in Tables 9.3 and 9.4. As they are widely used in the treatment of cardiovascular diseases, a more detailed consideration of their effects on the cardiovascular system is appropriate.

As stated above, cardiac output and heart rate are reduced. With the non-selective β-blockers cardiac output may be reduced by reductions in both heart rate and stroke volume output, and there may be a slight increase in peripheral vascular resistance due both to blockade of β_2-receptors mediating vasodilation and to compensatory sympathetic reflexes. Blood flow to all tissues except the brain is reduced (Nies, Evans and Shand, 1973). As outlined above, with the partial agonists (e.g. pindolol, oxprenolol and alprenolol) these reductions are minimized at rest but may be just as marked with exercise or stress as with the pure antagonists.

In patients with severe heart disease, and particularly in those dependent on increased sympathetic drive, the β-blockers may precipiate acute heart failure. This may be due to direct effects on the heart (manifested by increased end-diastolic volumes and pressures) as well as to salt and water retention which probably result from altered intrarenal haemodynamics.

However, beneficial effects normally predominate. There is a reduction in myocardial oxygen consumption, with preferential perfusion of subendocardial areas and reduced inotropic and chronotropic effects of both endogenous and exogenous catecholamines (Weiner, 1980). The effects of other drugs acting on first or on second messengers (e.g. calcium, the methylxanthines and digitalis) are unaltered.

β-Blockers are also used in the management of acute perioperative tachycardias and dysrhythmias, of thyroid crises, of phaeochromocytomas and of hypertrophic obstructive cardiomyopathies. They are also particularly useful as adjuncts to vasodilator therapy to minimize the reflex tachycardia and increase in cardiac output which occur with these agents.

Propranolol, the original β-blocker, is still widely used in oral doses of up to 480 mg per day. Its intravenous use has already been discussed. Some other non-selective β-blockers may have specific applications. For example, the renally excreted antagonists nadolol and sotalol may be useful in patients with compromised hepatic function; the partial agonist pindolol is used by some in patients with borderline left ventricular failure; and timolol (topically) has been shown to be useful in the treatment of glaucoma, although the mechanism by which it produces a reduction in intraocular pressure is still unclear.

Selective β_1-antagonists

Metoprolol and atenolol are relatively selective β_1-antagonists, neither of which has any agonist activity or significant membrane-stabilizing effect. Metoprolol is a lipophilic compound which is well absorbed, but has only 50 per cent bioavailability due to the first-pass effect. It has a large volume of distribution, a high clearance and low plasma protein binding. Atenolol, on the other hand, is a hydrophilic compound which is fairly poorly absorbed and thus has a bioavailability approximately equal to that of metoprolol although it is not subject to any first-pass effect. Its volume of distribution and clearance are each about ten times smaller than those of metoprolol, and it has a half-life of 5–7 hours compared to that of 3–4 hours for metoprolol (see Table 9.4).

In contrast to the non-selective β-antagonists, stroke volume is generally maintained with these agents, and there is usually little or no change in systemic vascular resistance although heart rate, cardiac output and blood pressure are usually reduced. Great caution should still be exercised in treating patients with severe cardiac disease, as acute heart failure may be precipitated. However, the tendency not to increase peripheral vascular resistance may be advantageous in this context.

The β_1-antagonists also usually cause less bronchospasm than the non-selective antagonists, but may still be catastrophic in certain individuals. They may also produce some degree of glucose intolerance, may prolong and very occasionally precipitate hypoglycaemia, and may produce CNS toxicity symptoms. Selective β_1-antagonists may also be tolerated better than non-selective antagonists in patients with peripheral vascular disease and Raynaud's disease, as they do not block β_2-mediated peripheral vasodilation.

Selective β_2-antagonists
Drugs such as butoxamine and the α-methyl analogue of dichloroisoprenaline are relatively selective β_2-antagonists. They are being used as experimental tools but have no accepted clinical role. Possible clinical applications which have been suggested are to minimize the β_2-mediated release of insulin, glucagon or parathyroid hormone, and to reduce tremor in skeletal muscles (Lees, 1981).

Labetalol
Labetalol is an α_1-, β_1- and β_2-antagonist. It has no intrinsic agonist activity but it does inhibit neuronal uptake of sympathomimetic amines to some extent. It is about one-tenth as potent as phentolamine as an α-blocker, and about one-third as potent as propranolol as a β-blocker. In man, it is more potent as a β-blocker than as an α-blocker (MacCarthy and Bloomfield, 1983). It is an effective antihypertensive agent for long-term oral use as well as for the establishment and maintenance of β-blockade parenterally in the perioperative period or in the intensive care unit.

References

Ablad, B., Carlsson, B., Carlsson, E., Dahlof, C., Ek., L. and Hultberg, E. (1974) Cardiac effects of beta-adrenergic antagonists. *Advances in Cardiology* **12**, 290–302

Ablad, B., Carlsson, E., Ek, L., Gillis, J. and Lundgren, B. (1980) General pharmacology of beta-adrenoceptor antagonists. In: *Beta-blockade and Anaesthesia* (Eds. Popper, P.J., van Dijk, B. and van Elzakker, A.H.M.), pp. 46–58. Lindgren: Molndal, Sweden

Aellig, W.H. (1983) Clinical pharmacology of beta-adrenoceptor blocking drugs possessing partial agonist activity with special reference to pindolol. *Journal of Cardiovascular Pharmacology* **5**, S21–S25

Ahlquist, R.P. (1948) A study of adrenotropic receptors. *American Journal of Physiology* **153**, 586–599

Assem, E.S.K. and Schild, H.O. (1971) Antagonism by beta-adrenoceptor blocking agents of the antianaphylactic effect of isoprenaline. *British Journal of Pharmacology* **42**, 620–630

Astrom, H. (1980) Haemodynamic properties of beta blockers. In: *Beta-blockade and Anaesthesia* (Eds. Popper, P.J., van Dijk, B. and van Elzakker, A.H.M.), pp. 59–64. Lindgren: Molndal, Sweden

Bowman, W.C. and Rand, M.J. (1980) *Textbook of Pharmacology*, 2nd edn. Blackwell Scientific: Oxford

Carlsson, E. and Hedberg, A. (1980) The beta-adrenoceptor concept. In: *Beta-blockade and Anaesthesia* (Eds. Popper, P.J., van Dijk, B. and van Elzakker, A.H.M.), pp. 17–28. Lindgren: Molndal, Sweden

Foëx, P. (1984) Alpha- and beta-adrenoceptor antagonists. *British Journal of Anaesthesia* 56, 751–765

Goldberg, M.R. and Robertson, D. (1983) Yohimbine: a pharmacological probe for study of the alpha 2-adrenoceptor. *Pharmacological Reviews* 35, 143–180

Gilman, A.G. Goodman, L.S. and Gilman, A. (Eds.) (1980) *Goodman and Gilman's Pharmacological Basis of Therapeutics*, 6th edn. Macmillan: New York

Graham, R.M. (1984) Selective alpha 1-adrenergic antagonists: therapeutically relevant antihypertensive agents. *American Journal of Cardiology* 53, 16A-20A

Kleinbaum, J. and Shamoon, H. (1984) Effect of propranolol on delayed glucose recovery after insulin-induced hypoglycaemia in normal and diabetic subjects. *Diabetes Care* 7, 155–162

Lees, G.M. (1981) A hitch-hiker's guide to the galaxy of adrenoceptors. *British Medical Journal* 283, 173–177

Lennard, M.S. (1985) Oxidation phenotype and the metabolism and action of beta-blockers. *Klinische Wochenschrift* 63, 285–292

Lennard, M.S., Silas, J.H., Freestone, S., Ramsay, L.E., Tucker, G.T. and Woods, H.F. (1982) Oxidation phenotype – a major determinant of metoprolol metabolism and response. *New England Journal of Medicine* 307, 1558–1560

MacCarthy, E.P. and Bloomfield, S.S. (1983) Labetalol: a review of its pharmacology, pharmacokinetics, clinical uses and adverse effects. *Pharmacotherapy* 3, 193–219.

McCulloch, M.W. (1984) Beta-blockers – mechanisms of action. *Australian Prescriber* 7, 25–28

Minneman, K.P., Pittman, R.N. and Molinoff, P.B. (1981) Beta-adrenergic receptor subtypes: properties, distribution, and regulation. *Annual Review of Neurosciences* 4, 419–461

Moulds, R.W.F. (1984) Beta-blockers – clinical pharmacology. *Australian Prescriber* 7, 28–31

Nies, A.S., Evans, G.H. and Shand, D.G. (1973) Regional haemodynamic effects of beta-adrenergic blockade with propranolol in the unanesthetized primate. *American Heart Journal* 85, 97–102

Oliver, G. and Schafer, E.A. (1895) The physiological effects of extracts of the suprarenal capsules. *Journal of Physiology* 18, 230–276

Powell, C.E. and Slater, I.H. (1958) Blocking of inhibitory adrenergic receptors by a dichloro analog of isoproterenol. *Journal of Pharmacology and Experimental Therapeutics* 122, 480–488

Prys-Roberts, C. (1984) Kinetics and dynamics of beta-adrenoceptor antagonists. In: *Pharmacokinetics of Anaesthesia* (Eds. Prys-Roberts, C. and Hug, C.C. Jr), pp. 293–309. Blackwell Scientific: Oxford

Regardh, C.-G. (1980) Pharmacokinetics of beta-adrenoceptor antagonists. In: *Beta-blockade and Anaesthesia* (Eds. Popper, P.J., van Dijk, B. and van Elzakker, A.H.M.), pp. 29–45. Lindgren: Molndal, Sweden

Stiles, G.L. and Lefkowitz, R.J. (1984) Cardiac adrenergic receptors. *Annual Review of Medicine* 35, 149–164

Taylor, S.H. (1983) Intrinsic sympathomimetic activity: clinical fact or fiction? *American Journal of Cardiology* 52, 16D–26D

Weiner, N. (1980) Drugs that inhibit adrenergic nerves and block adrenergic receptors. In: *Goodman and Gilman's Pharmacological Basis of Therapeutics* 6th edn. (Eds. Gilman, A.G. Goodman, L.S. and Gilman, A.), pp. 176–210. Macmillan: New York

Wood, M. Shand, D.G. and Wood, A.J.J. (1979) Propranolol binding in plasma during cardiopulmonary bypass. *Anesthesiology* **51**, 512–517

10

Drugs interfering with synaptic transmission in the central nervous system

T.W. Stone

A background to psychotropic drugs

The history of psychopharmacology is a story of accidental discoveries and incidental observations. Reserpine, for example, the use of which in western medicine was initially in the treatment of hypertension, was found to produce severe depression, resulting in a significant number of suicides. Iproniazid, used in the treatment of tuberculosis, was found on the other hand to produce an elevation of mood. From these fortuitous beginnings about 30 years ago a new realm of medicine has developed, accompanied by an immense industrial investment in 'psychotropic drugs' – drugs capable of modifying in some way man's reaction to and interaction with the environment and society. The development of this interest and investment has been possible only since the realization that many of these psychotropic agents interfere with the processes of synaptic transmission, and the function of this chapter is to illustrate some of the ways in which such interactions can occur. As an essential prelude to the discussion of drug mechanisms, the first part of this chapter presents a brief summary of current views on synapses and synaptic transmission.

Synaptic transmission in the central nervous system

In principle the phenomenon of synaptic transmission in the CNS is not greatly different from that in the periphery. At most central synapses there is a

Fig. 10.1 A schematic drawing of an idealized synapse, illustrating some of the potential sites of drug action. Drugs may interfere with the synthesis of the neurotransmitter (▲) or its precursor (△) (1), or the movement of precursor or formed transmitter into the synaptic vesicles (2). Compounds such as reserpine may also prevent the storage and retention of transmitter within the vesicles. Some substances such as colchicine which affect microtubule and microfilament function can inhibit the movement of vesicles to the presynaptic membrane (3), whereas some drugs may inhibit or promote (e.g. amphetamines) the release of transmitter (4). Many useful drugs act on the postjunctional receptors (5), either mimicking a neurotransmitter or blocking its effect, or altering the receptor sensitivity. This increase or decrease of postsynaptic responsiveness may also be exerted at sites beyond the membrane receptors, such as adenylate or guanylate cyclases, ionic channels, macromolecule metabolism, etc. (6). Most neurotransmitters are metabolized after being taken up into postjunctional cells (7) or associated tissue

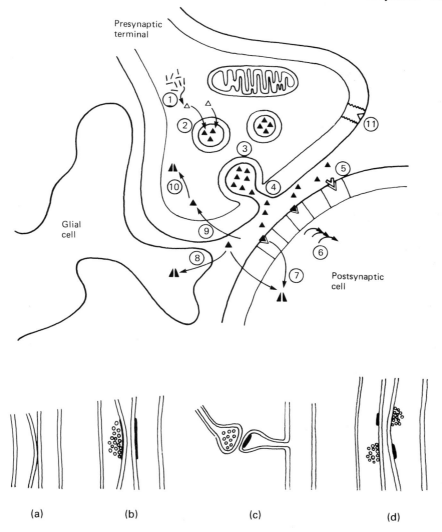

(a)   (b)   (c)   (d)

such as glial cells (8). Similarly, there are frequently uptake mechanisms for transmitters into the releasing terminal (9), sometimes linked to degradative metabolism (10). Many drugs are known to interfere with these various processes of membrane transport and metabolism of transmitters. Finally, there are presynaptic receptors for a number of transmitters which may stimulate or suppress further transmitter release. The best known of these are the presynaptic α_2-receptors which inhibit transmitter release (11). (a–d) A few of the morphological variants of synapses in the CNS. (a) A presumed electrically operated synapse, with no vesicles or other specialization but a fused region of the outer layers of the respective plasma membranes. (b) These synapses are often found between axons or dendrites en passant. (c) A conventional synapse made onto a dendritic spine – a specialized projection from the dendrite trunk. These are very common in neocortex and striatum. (d) Reciprocal synapses – usually dendrodendritic. They may function as local feedback regulatory circuits.

synaptic gap, vesicles presumed to contain the appropriate neurotransmitter exist in the presynaptic terminals, and upon the invasion of those terminals by an action potential the vesicles are believed to fuse with the plasma membrane of the terminal in such a way as to release the transmitter across the cleft onto the postsynaptic surface (Fig. 10.1).

There is, however, much more variation in the morphology of synapses in the CNS than in the periphery. Certainly there are synapses at which the synaptic cleft can be measured in ångstroms, as it can at the peripheral neuromuscular junction, and many of those axons responsible for releasing monoamines such as noradrenaline, 5-hydroxytryptamine (5HT) and dopamine do so from varicosities into a yawning micron-sized gap much as happens in the corresponding elements of the peripheral sympathetic nervous system. In addition, however, there are electrically operated synapses which do not involve a chemical transmitter, synapses formed *en passant* between axons or between dendrites, synapses onto specialized receiving areas in which there is an apparently two-way transmission between adjacent areas of neuronal membrane and so on (Fig. 10.1).

The functional significance of all this structural variety is a mystery, but it is unfortunately accompanied by an equally great variety of chemical neurotransmitters. About 50 compounds currently have enough experimental support to be considered seriously as possible transmitters, ranging from the simple amino acids such as glutamate and γ-aminobutyric acid (GABA), probably the most widely used excitatory and inhibitory transmitters respectively in the CNS, to amines such as noradrenaline, 5HT and dopamine and peptides such as vasopressin, cholecystokinin, enkephalins, endorphins, substance P and many others.

As if this diversity of chemical messengers were not enough of a complexity in itself, it appears that many of these substances may have two or more actions on postsynaptic cells. In the simplest case a transmitter may produce a change of membrane conductance which results in a hyperpolarization (inhibition) or depolarization (excitation) of the target cell. In some cases, however, transmitters may exert very little effect of their own, although they produce marked changes in the responses of cells to other transmitters; this kind of behaviour has led to the introduction of the term 'neuromodulator', but it has to be admitted that the distinction between transmitter and modulator is not always clear-cut, and many compounds show a repertoire of actions which include elements of both classes.

Indeed the concept of 'co-transmission' proposes that at some synapses a number of compounds may be released. Thyrotrophin, for example, appears to co-exist with 5HT in some central neuron terminals and to be released by suitable stimuli. Acetylcholine probably has a similar relationship with vasoactive intestinal polypeptide (VIP), GABA with motilin, dopamine with cholecystokinin, ATP with noradrenaline and so on. When released there is in some cases an interaction between the two compounds, such as a potentiation or antagonism, and the whole system then clearly functions as a safety mechanism to prevent excessive under- or overactivity of that particular synapse. In other cases the two substances have very distinct functions, one acting directly on the postsynaptic cell, for example, while the other changes local blood flow or glial metabolism to match or compensate for the change of neuronal activity. There is some evidence that the relative amounts of such co-transmitters released by a neuron may depend on the frequency and pattern of the axonal activity.

It has also become clear recently that synaptic transmitters and modulators have effects which not only affect neuronal behaviour on a time scale of milliseconds and seconds but also may produce changes over periods of hours or days. Thus transmitters in the hippocampus (probably glutamate or a similar substance) can produce changes of neuronal excitability which may persist for several days after a 1-second tetanic stimulation; this may be related to the role of the hippocampus in memory. Some of the peptide co-transmitters mentioned above can also produce long-term changes in the number or affinity of the synaptic receptors for amine or amino acid transmitters. In addition, the phenomenon of denervation supersensitivity, long recognized for example as an increase in the sensitivity to acetylcholine at the neuromuscular junction following nerve section, also occurs in the CNS. The increase in the number of transmitter receptors is then referred to as 'up-regulation'. The converse change, a decrease or 'down-regulation' of receptors, is also seen in response to an increase in the stimulation of those receptors.

It is this enormous diversity of chemical interactions which provides the awesome problems of trying to understand not only how CNS operates normally and what underlies the various disorders observed clinically but also of trying to modify its function to alleviate those disorders. Each neuron in the CNS, it must be realised, is under the influence of several hundred synapses, possibly releasing several dozen different chemicals. With statistics like these it is perhaps remarkable that we know so much and can often predict a great deal about the effects of drugs on the brain.

Methods

The remainder of this chapter summarizes a vast body of knowledge of the mechanisms of action of some of the most widely used drugs acting on the CNS. No attempt has been made to discuss in detail any of the methods used in this work, but passing reference will be made to behavioural studies, to electrophysiological methods (particularly those in which the effects of neurotransmitters or drugs are examined on single cell activity) and to binding studies in which the association between a radiolabelled transmitter or drug and a preparation of tissue membranes is studied *in vitro*. This last method is becoming used increasingly widely and routinely to study the 'pharmacology' of the CNS, but it must be emphasized that the relationship between these binding sites and the true receptors for transmitters and drugs is unknown, and only recently have investigators been compelled to come to terms with the artificiality of the method. While the technique has the advantage of reproducibility, simplicity and economy, and avoids the use of anaesthetized animals, these uncertainties must raise serious doubts about the validity of binding studies and their significance. There are several instances in the following discussion where binding studies give results opposite to those of electrophysiological and behavioural methods, and readers should always be wary of attempts to overemphasize the value of such experiments merely because of their technical advantages.

Benzodiazepines

As a group, the benzodiazepines are not easy to classify pharmacologically because different members of the series are most effective as anticonvulsants, muscle relaxants, anxiolytics, sedatives or 'minor' tranquillizers (a term now rarely used to indicate the use of these and similar drugs in non-psychotic states, mainly neuroses) (Usdin *et al.*, 1983; Burrows, Norman and Davies, 1984). Diazepam is probably among the best known anticonvulsant and anxiolytic benzodiazepines whereas nitrazepam is one of the commonest sedative benzodiazepines.

The GABA hypothesis

Among the earliest observations on the pharmacology of the benzodiazepines under experimental conditions was the finding that certain inhibitory processes in the CNS, including presynaptic inhibition in the spinal cord and brainstem, were enhanced by diazepam. These inhibitory phenomena were thought to be mediated by γ-aminobutyric acid (GABA), a simple amino acid which now appears to be the most widely used inhibitory neurotransmitter in the mammalian CNS. There is a vast literature documenting this facilitatory action of benzodiazpines on responses both to exogenously applied GABA and on the inhibitory postsynaptic potentials and conductance changes produced in neurons by stimulating afferent pathways believed to release GABA from their axon terminals (Usdin *et al.*, 1983).

The facilitation by benzodiazepines of GABA-ergic neurotransmission is not the result of any change of the biosynthetic or removal processes for GABA, for example by inhibiting GABA transaminase or the uptake mechanisms for GABA into neurons and glia. The interaction seems to occur rather at the postjunctional complex where the GABA receptor is coupled to ionic channels in the membrane. Thus activation of GABA receptors causes an increase in the membrane conductance for chloride ions. This effectively inhibits the ability of the neuron to respond to other synapses on its surface either by causing hyperpolarization (if the chloride equilibrium potential is higher than the resting membrane potential so that chloride ions pass into the cytoplasm) or simply as a result of the increase of membrane conductance, effectively producing a short circuit across the membrane. As revealed by studies of the effects of GABA and benzodiazepines on isolated neurons in tissue culture, where presynaptic mechanisms involving synthesis, metabolism, release or uptake are eliminated, it is the ability of the GABA receptor to open these chloride channels which is facilitated by benzodiazepines (Paul, Marangos and Skolnick, 1981; Olsen, 1982; Williams, 1984).

This interaction has been studied not only from the truly functional aspect of changes in neuronal inhibition but also by examining the factors which affect benzodiazepine binding to brain membranes. Radiolabelled benzodiazepines will bind with a very high affinity to fragments of brain membranes *in vitro* (Braestrup and Squires, 1977), and, whilst very few chemically and pharmacologically unrelated compounds will affect that binding, there is a remarkable correlation between the affinity or capacity of the benzodiazepine binding site for a series of benzodiazepines and the clinical efficacy of those same compounds, especially when considered as anticonvulsants or muscle relaxants. Using autoradiographic analyses of the distribution of radiolabelled benzodiazepines, the binding site has been localized to the region of the synapse, although it remains uncertain whether the site is restricted to the presynaptic, postsynaptic or associated glial cell membranes at the synapse.

GABA and several GABA-mimetic compounds active at the $GABA_A$ site (the normal inhibitory receptor for GABA) increase the binding affinity of these benzodiazepines, although compounds active at the $GABA_B$ site are ineffective. It is likely, though, that the interaction between benzodiazepines and GABA is not restricted to the GABA receptor module, since binding is also changed by the presence of chloride ions, and there are complex interactions between GABA, benzodiazepines and substances which are thought to interact directly with the chloride channel mechanism (the ionophore) such as pentobarbitone or picrotoxin (Olsen, 1982; Williams, 1984). Benzodiazepines, however, do not displace picrotoxin and therefore are unlikely to act directly at the chloride ionophore. Picrotoxin, on the other hand, probably does act at the level of the channel itself since it is a non-competitive inhibitor of the chloride activation produced by GABA and does not displace GABA binding.

The most popular overall view of the membrane complex responsible for these events includes the GABA receptor, activation of which results in an allosteric change of conformation such that an adjacent or closely coupled chloride ionophore is pulled into an open conformation (Fig. 10.2). The benzodiazepine receptor is then presumed to exist in a situation which allows it, when activated, to facilitate that GABA receptor–ionophore interaction, as well as permitting the GABA receptor complex to facilitate the attachment of benzodiazepines to their binding site (Olsen, 1982; Williams, 1984). Consistent with this picture is the finding that only those GABA agonists with flexible molecular structures able to take part in a conformational change of the receptor molecule, such as GABA itself and muscimol, can potentiate benzodiazepine binding. Rigid molecules such as isoguvacine, piperidine-4-sulphonic acid and the systemically active compound 4,5,6,7-tetrahydroisoxazolo-[5,4,c]-pyridin-3-ol (THIP) are unable to produce this potentiation. Indeed the rigid analogues of GABA may actually prevent the actions of GABA on benzodiazepine binding.

It is intuitively easy to understand how the various pharmacological actions of benzodiazepines, which are generally of a depressant nature, can be due to a potentiation of an endogenous inhibitory process, but it is worth emphasizing that benzodiazepines can be effective only where there is continuing inhibitory (specifically GABA-mediated) tone. Since most of the GABA is probably released by interneurons which form part of recurrent inhibitory feedback circuits (e.g. in the cerebral cortex, striatum, cerebellum, spinal cord, hippocampus), the effects of benzodiazepines will tend to be self-limiting. As a GABA-releasing synapse is potentiated, for example, the activity of the postsynaptic target neuron will be correspondingly diminished, and thus the activity of the GABA-releasing interneurons activated by it will also decrease. An equilibrium will therefore be established which will stop short of the total inhibition of a circuit. This is an important mechanistic difference from those

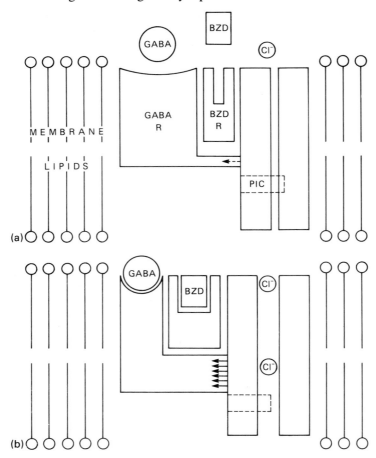

Fig. 10.2 A diagrammatic representation of the GABA–benzodiazepine receptor–chloride ionophore complex. In the resting state (a) the Cl⁻ channel is closed and benzodiazepine (BZD) binding to its receptor is relatively low. When GABA acts on its receptor site (b) an allosteric conformational change occurs which is simultaneously responsible for pulling open the chloride channel and for facilitating the binding of BZD. Conversely, at those complexes where a BZD molecule becomes bound to its receptor, the interaction of GABA with its receptor will be facilitated. Note the separate picrotoxin (PIC)-binding site associated with the chloride channel itself.

compounds which activate the GABA receptors directly because the latter compounds will be much more likely to produce depression of the nervous system with consequent unwanted, potentially hazardous, side effects. This has proved to be a major limitation on the development of direct-acting GABA agonists, such as THIP, as clinically useful anticonvulsants.

Excitatory amino acids

Whilst the 'GABA hypothesis' remains probably the best documented and most widely supported hypothesis of the mechanism of action of benzodiazepines, there have been many studies performed in which the results are not entirely consistent with this concept. For instance, in some areas of the CNS benzodiazepines do not enhance the effects of GABA at doses which reduce the excitatory effects of simple dicarboxylic amino acids such as glutamate or aspartate (Assumpcao et al., 1979). This phenomenon has been reported too often to be artifactual, and of course the functional result, a reduction of neuronal activity, would be similar to that resulting from the facilitation of GABA inhibition. As the evidence is quite strong for the involvement of glutamate, for example, in convulsant disorders such as epilepsy, it is conceivable that different mechanisms underlie the various pharmacological actions of benzodiazepines mentioned above. This would certainly be a more acceptable explanation of the differences of benzodiazepine pharmacology profiles than merely differences in their pharmacokinetic behaviour.

Adenosine and endogenous ligands

From the premise that a very high affinity binding site ('receptor') for the exogenous compound morphine might imply the existence of an endogenous compound acting at that site, a search was begun which culminated in the discovery of the enkephalin peptides. It was therefore a not unreasonable intellectual leap to the proposition that endogenous ligands may also exist for the equally high affinity benzodiazepine-binding sites. Among the first compounds to be isolated from brain which displaced benzodiazepine binding were the purine derivatives inosine and hypoxanthine (Tallman et al., 1980). It is still not clear whether these compounds are of any physiological relevance to the workings of the brain or whether they play any part in the actions of benzodiazepines. Both substances have rather poor ability to displace benzodiazepine binding, with the concentrations producing 50 per cent displacement being about 1 mmol/l, but it is very likely that both compounds can reach concentrations of this order, particularly during times of excessive CNS activity such as during convulsions.

Whilst the significance of these interactions between benzodiazepines, inosine and hypoxanthine remains unclear, it was soon found that other purine-related compounds would also interact with benzodiazepines. In particular, dipyridamole, an inhibitor of neuronal uptake of purines, showed a marked ability to displace benzodiazepines from their binding sites. This observation in turn led to the discovery that a number of benzodiazepines would themselves inhibit the uptake of purines, especially adenosine. Adenosine has become the object of many research programmes over the last 15 years, since the realization that this purine nucleoside is widely released from tissues during periods of activity and that it can then act to restrain both the activity of the tissue itself directly and the stimulating effect of nervous activity by depressing transmitter release; adenosine has thus come to be regarded as one of the most ubiquitous homoeostatic regulatory compounds in the body (T.W. Stone, 1981). The effect of benzodiazepines in inhibiting the uptake and thus the removal of adenosine from the tissues, therefore, would be to potentiate this overall depressant action on tissue activity. In the case of the CNS this is clearly an attractive explanation for the generally depressant properties of this class of drugs.

Pharmacological investigation has now refined the concept of adenosine involvement so that it is believed to play some role in the muscle relaxant and sedative effects of benzodiazepines but not the anxiolytic or anticonvulsant effects. It must be emphasized, however, that the importance of this role is still not clear, since some benzodiazepine derivatives which are antagonists of the behavioural effects of benzodiazepines do not antagonize the suppression of adenosine uptake (Morgan, Lloyd and Stone, 1983). Furthermore, the concentrations of benzodiazepines which are effective in depressing uptake are very high relative to the plasma concentrations occurring clinically: therapeutic levels would be able to produce only about 20 per cent inhibition of uptake in most test systems.

Xanthines

The possible involvement of purines in the actions of benzodiazepines is nevertheless of some practical importance in view of the fact that commonly used methylxanthines, such as caffeine and theophylline in tea, coffee, chocolate etc., are antagonists of the effects of adenosine, and can antagonize some of the effects also of benzodiazepines. Equally, the anticonvulsant actions of benzodiazepines can be demonstrated against seizures produced by the intake or administration of very high doses of xanthines. If benzodiazepines are being used for sedative or myorelaxant properties in particular, therefore, it may be advisable always to take into account variations in xanthine intake by patients.

Benzodiazepines do not interfere with most of the other enzyme systems associated with purine metabolism, such as adenosine kinase which regulates the synthesis of ATP, but they are quite effective inhibitors of phosphodiesterase. They can therefore increase the levels of cAMP within cells but, as elsewhere in the body, it is not known whether this result is of any relevance to their pharmacological actions.

GABA-modulin

An early hypothesis of the mechanism of benzodiazepine action arose from observations that procedures such as freezing and thawing of brain membranes, which disrupt protein complexes, would increase GABA binding. This led Costa's group to extract a protein component from membranes which, they theorized, normally occupied or covered part of the GABA receptor complex. This protein, which became known as GABA-modulin, was then thought to be displaced by benzodiazepines, thus producing the observed enhancement of GABA binding (Costa and Guidotti, 1979). The GABA-modulin hypothesis still boasts a small but distinguished band of supporters.

β-Carbolines

Most recently much excitement was generated when, in the search for endogenous ligands of the benzodiazepine receptor, a β-carboline derivative (β-carboline-3-carboxylic acid ethyl ester, or β-CCE) was isolated from human urine. This compound had an affinity for central benzodiazepine receptors comparable with the most potent benzodiazepines in clinical use (Braestrup, Nielsen and Olsen 1980). This particular compound, however, proved to be an artifact of the extraction process, and although a great deal of interest continues in the extraction and identification of related compounds which may act as endogenous ligands of the benzodiazepine receptor, no substantial further developments have been forthcoming.

Experimental compounds

The study of benzodiazepine mechanisms has been greatly facilitated by the discovery of benzodiazepine analogues with unusual profiles of pharmacological activity. There are, for example, benzodiazepine antagonists (invariably referred to by the manufacturer's code names such as Ro 15-1788 or CGS 8216). These compounds prevent all the behavioural effects of the benzodiazepines but do not, for instance, block the inhibition by the tranquillizers of adenosine uptake (one of the reasons why this particular mechanism is of doubtful importance clinically). There are also subdivisions such as 'inverse agonists' or 'contra-agonists', including compounds such as β-CCE which is not a benzodiazepine antagonist although it has opposite behavioural effects and can displace benzodiazepines from binding sites. Another of these substances is Ro 5-3663, which again is not an antagonist but it potently *induces* convulsions. This convulsant benzodiazepine is not anxiogenic, emphasizing that there is not necessarily any simple relationship between the anxiolytic and anticonvulsant properties of the benzodiazepines.

Some general considerations

It remains a matter of pure speculation whether the benzodiazepines in common use are agonists or antagonists at their central binding sites. It is possible, for example, that there is an endogenous compound whose physiological function is essentially anxiogenic, perhaps maintaining a degree of wary caution and alertness at times of danger. Benzodiazepines would presumably then act as antagonists at the receptors for that substance. It is equally feasible that the benzodiazepines are agonists at central receptors for a compound whose function is anxiolytic, reducing the stress reaction of the organism to danger.

It is interesting to note that, whatever the significance of the benzodiazepine 'receptor', it is presumably of some importance throughout the animal kingdom; benzodiazepine-binding sites have been found in many lower vertebrates and invertebrates, including schistosomes.

The process of ageing is associated with an increase in the amount of benzodiazepine binding, at least in animal studies, whereas there is a corresponding decrease in the amount of GABA binding and of the ability of GABA to potentiate benzodiazepine binding. Elderly subjects show an increased susceptibility to the anxiolytic actions of benzodiazepines, and it is possible therefore that this is related to a similar increase of benzodiazepine-binding sites.

Barbiturates

Various members of the barbiturate family of drugs are used for purposes similar to the benzodiazepines, ranging from sedation and anticonvulsant properties through, of course, to full anaesthesia. It was therefore natural to enquire whether the mechanism of action of these compounds had anything in common with the benzodiazepines. It is now known that pentobarbitone, for example, will enhance the chloride conductance increase produced by GABA and will also potentiate the enhancement of benzodiazepine binding produced by GABA (Olsen, 1982; Williams, 1984).

Antidepressants

As noted earlier in this chapter, some of the first observations of CNS pharmacology were the result of unwanted and unexpected effects of drugs in clinical use for peripheral disorders. Reserpine, for example, reduces the ability of neuron terminals to store amine neurotransmitters, thus producing an initial release and subsequent depletion of the transmitters. When used in the treatment of hypertension, reserpine was responsible for inducing severe depression in about 15 per cent of patients. Conversely, the antitubercular drug iproniazid was found to produce an elevation of mood in patients, and it was soon realized that this drug could produce the opposite effects to reserpine on aminergic neurons (i.e. it could increase the availability of amines in the synaptic gap as a result of inhibiting their destruction by monoamine oxidase). Observations such as these soon led to the formal statement of a hypothesis of the aetiology of depression – the 'catecholamine hypothesis' (Schildkraut, 1965). According to this view depression is the result of a lack of aminergic transmission, and recovery from the depressed state is associated with increased aminergic function.

From these beginnings two general classes of drugs with antidepressant activity were developed. These were the monoamine oxidase inhibitors such as iproniazid and tranylcypromine, and the amine uptake inhibitors such as imipramine and amitriptyline, the latter compounds becoming known as the tricyclic antidepressants because of their molecular structure.

The use of monoamine oxidase inhibitors (MAOIs) has declined a great deal because of the incidence of side effects and the frequency of interactions with foodstuffs such as wines and cheeses. However, with the realization that there are two distinct forms of the oxidase enzyme, interest has been aroused in the possibility of selective inhibition of only one form. Monoamine oxidase A attacks preferentially noradrenaline and 5HT and is inhibited by nialamide and clorgyline. Monoamine oxidase B has a greater selectivity for phenylethylamine and tryptamine and is inhibited by deprenyl. Dopamine and tyramine are metabolized by both A and B enzymes to some extent. Clearly, however, the preferential suppression of monoamine oxidase A should allow some potentiation of both noradrenergic and 5-hydroxytryptaminergic neuron pathways, whilst dietary increases of tyramine or phenylethylamine can still be dealt with by oxidase B. Clinical trials with potential selective inhibitors of monoamine oxidase A reveal clear antidepressant potential.

Both the monoamine oxidase inhibitors and the uptake inhibitors bring with them a number of very undesirable side effects, largely due to their potentiation of amine effects in the peripheral nervous system, although some of the tricyclics are also extremely potent histamine and acetylcholine antagonists. The last 20 years have therefore seen a massive effort to develop new antidepressant drugs with greater efficacy and selectivity of action, but although a number of such drugs have been discovered, the variety of their effects on the CNS is such that the classic catecholamine hypothesis has become untenable.

There have always been two disturbing difficulties with the original catecholamine hypothesis. First, many compounds with a clear ability to increase the functional concentration of amines in the synaptic cleft (e.g. cocaine, which inhibits neuronal uptake) do not have any significant antidepressant activity. This may, of course, simply be due to the gross non-specificity of such drugs, leading to pronounced changes in arousal and perception, and marked stimulation and euphoria.

The second, and greater, difficulty is that the inhibitory effect of antidepressant drugs on amine uptake occurs immediately *in vitro*, and is clearly evident within minutes or hours even after a single administration *in vivo*. The clinical, behavioural antidepressant effect itself, however, is not apparent for 1–4 weeks after beginning 'chronic' treatment. This latent period cannot be wholly explained on the basis of the pharmacokinetics of antidepressants, for example as slow penetration and accumulation in the CNS. A latent period of 6–10 days even exists for electroshock therapy of depression where kinetic considerations are clearly inappropriate.

These doubts about the validity of the catecholamine hypothesis have been amplified during the last 20 years as attempts have been made to produce antidepressant drugs with greater efficacy and selectivity, and without the very marked anticholinergic, antihistaminic and adrenergic side effects of the original drugs. One product of this research, for example, was the discovery of a large number of drugs such as iprindole, trazodone, zimelidine, mianserin and buproprion which have some antidepressant activity but do not inhibit amine uptake or monoamine oxidase. The classic catecholamine hypothesis therefore was in need of reappraisal.

Chronic effects of antidepressants

Catecholamines

β-Receptors

In view of the time lag between the acute biochemical and clinical effects of antidepressant drugs, attention was turned to the detection of changes of aminergic function occurring at the time antidepressant activity was demonstrable (i.e. several weeks after commencing chronic administration). It was known that noradrenaline in particular would activate adenylate cyclase in neuronal membranes, leading to an increase of intracellular cAMP concentrations, and although this effect, like uptake inhibition or monoamine oxidase inhibition, could be elicited acutely *in vivo* or *in vitro* in animals, it was found that the effect was less marked in animals treated for several days or weeks with antidepressants. In other words, there was a 'down-regulation' of noradrenaline-stimulated cyclase activity (Sulser, Vetulani and Mobley, 1978). In many species, including man, this stimulatory effect of noradrenaline on adenylate cyclase is mediated by β-receptors, and in many cases it has now been shown that the subsensitivity of the cyclase system is accompanied by a decrease of β-adrenoceptor ligand binding.

This down-regulation of β-mediated adenylate cyclase is probably the inverse equivalent to the phenomenon of denervation supersensitivity, in which a neuronal lesion or blockade of synaptic transmission is followed by an increase in the number of postjunctional receptors in an attempt to compensate for the underactivity of the tissue. The down-regulation of central β-receptors can then be understood as a compensatory reduction of neuronal sensitivity in response to the maintained elevation of extraneuronal catecholamine concentrations produced by the antidepressant drugs. This concept is supported by the finding that β-subsensitivity does not follow antidepressant treatment if the aminergic neurons are first destroyed or inactivated by lesions or reserpine: most antidepressants, therefore, are unlikely to produce the sensitivity changes by acting directly on the postsynaptic receptors.

This interplay between presynaptic neuronal activity and the compensatory up-regulation and down-regulation of postsynaptic receptors is not confined to the aminergic systems. It is widely recognized as a homoeostatic phenomenon in almost every kind of neuronal pathway so far studied.

In support of a major aetiological (and therapeutic) role in depression for changes in the β-receptor systems of the brain is the fact that most clinically useful antidepressants, including the newer compounds such as iprindole, trazodone, buproprion, etc. mentioned above, have a similar action. (Since iprindole does not increase amine availability at the synapse this implies that, for a few compounds, direct actions on the postjunctional receptor mechanism may be involved in the down-regulation.) Furthermore, electroconvulsive shock treatment, widely recognized as one of the most effective means of alleviating depression, also results in a down-regulation of β-receptors and its cyclase, and also prevents the up-regulation which follows amine depletion by reserpine or central lesions.

Unfortunately for the further understanding of depression and its treatment, the functional significance of this receptor regulation is not at all clear. The commonest view of the CNS is of a complex of neurons organized in such a way that the firing rate of any one cell is determined largely by the summation of postsynaptic potentials generated on its surface by incoming synapses. Whilst there is certainly abundant evidence for an involvement of adenylate cyclase in the regulation of cell firing, and the decrease of β-agonist sensitivity is indeed often accompanied by a diminished effect of β-agonists on cell firing, it is also quite certain that this nucleotide is important in long-term regulation of nucleic acid and protein synthesis, cell growth, development and differentiation. This point is made because several studies have shown that in spite of the reduced β-receptor number (mainly β_1) and β-stimulated cyclase, there is frequently a net *increase* in the size of observable responses to β-stimulation, including changes of cell firing and behavioural responses. The problem is not confined to the CNS: chronic administration of antidepressants produces a decrease of β-receptor number in peripheral tissues such as adipose, cardiac and endocrine tissues, but changes of postreceptor mechanisms occur which more than compensate for this, leaving some tissues with an enhanced sensitivity to aminergic stimulation (E.A. Stone, 1983).

It is interesting that β-receptor down-regulation has prompted several attempts to develop a theoretical framework for understanding the depressive state. Animals subjected to stressful situations, for instance, develop a subsensitivity of their CNS β-receptor systems, but chronic treatment with antidepressant drugs or electroconvulsive shocks, themselves producing a similar down-regulation, induce a resistance in these animals both to further changes of β-sensitivity and to the deleterious effects of stress on behaviour. It has therefore been proposed that β-receptor down-regulation represents an attempt on the part of the CNS to reduce the amount of aminergic stimulation (frequently associated with arousal and learning) in order to cope with stressful situations. Depression then arises as a result of an inability to generate that down-regulation: the patient is forced to remain in a stress-sensitive state. Antidepressant therapy then assists the patient by promoting the down-regulation he needs.

One of the most recent consequences of all the work on β-receptors has been the realization that β-agonists, such as salbutamol, also possess antidepressant properties, presumably because they are able to induce the receptor down-regulation more directly than conventional drugs. Certainly it is said that the latency to the emergence of clinical improvement is only 5 or 6 days, significantly shorter than with uptake inhibitors, monoamine oxidase inhibitors, etc.

α-Receptors

In the continuing search for better correlates of antidepressant activity, the discovery of β-receptor changes was naturally soon followed by an examination of α-receptors. There is a good correlation between the ability of tricyclic antidepressants to displace α-adrenoceptor ligands from central receptors and their relative ability to suppress psychomotor agitation and to produce sedation (and hypotension) (U'Prichard et al., 1978). An inverse correlation obtained for the ability of these compounds to produce psychomotor activation, a useful property of antidepressants in cases of retarded depression.

Most attention, however, has been focused specifically on the α_2-receptor (Fig. 10.3). This predominantly presynaptic receptor, which inhibits the release of noradrenaline, can be activated relatively selectively by clonidine and blocked by yohimbine. Around 1980 it was found that chronic treatment with some antidepressants, particularly desipramine, would produce a down-regulation of central α_2-sites whether studied by biochemical methods (by preventing noradrenaline release, clonidine administration produces a reduced concentration of amine metabolites in the CSF and urine), behavioural methods (clonidine produces sedation) or electrophysiological means (clonidine inhibits the firing of neurons in the locus ceruleus by activating 'autoreceptors' on the cell bodies) (Sugrue, 1981, 1983). Such a down-regulation of the inhibitory α_2-receptors would result in a net increase of resting noradrenaline release. Clearly this would produce an extraneuronal accumulation of amine and thus a secondary down-regulation of postjunctional

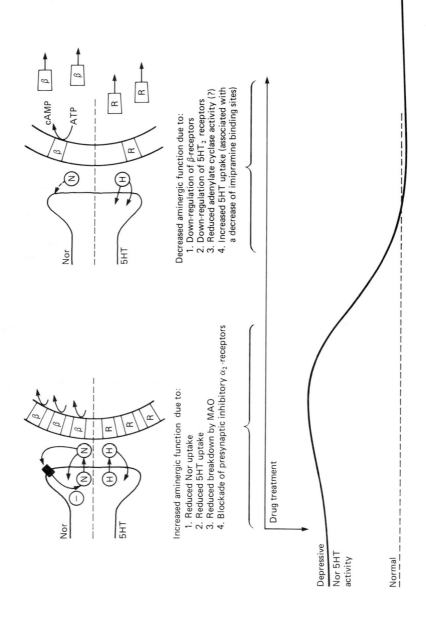

Fig. 10.3 A simplified summary of some of the changes of noradrenaline (Nor) and 5HT function associated with depression and its treatment. Note that the possible involvement of dopamine, histamine, adenosine, etc. mentioned in the text are not included here.

Increased aminergic function due to:
1. Reduced Nor uptake
2. Reduced 5HT uptake
3. Reduced breakdown by MAO
4. Blockade of presynaptic inhibitory α₂-receptors

Decreased aminergic function due to:
1. Down-regulation of β-receptors
2. Down-regulation of 5HT₂ receptors
3. Reduced adenylate cyclase activity (?)
4. Increased 5HT uptake (associated with a decrease of imipramine binding sites)

Drug treatment

Depressive

Nor 5HT activity

Normal

β-receptors, contributing to the β-subsensitivity discussed above.

Strongly supporting this proposed mechanism is the finding that the administration of a combination of an α_2-antagonist with a classic uptake inhibitor produces a down-regulation of the β-receptor far more rapidly than the uptake inhibitor alone. Indeed, significant down-regulation can occur after a single administration of this drug combination. The mixture also shortens appreciably the lag time to the onset of clinical improvement. It seems very likely that some of the antidepressant drugs whose mechanism of action is presently still uncertain will be found to act as α_2-antagonists. Such appears to be the case, for example, for mianserin.

5-Hydroxytryptamine (5HT, serotonin)

Among even the first groups of tricyclic antidepressants, interesting differences of clinical effects were observed which were found to correlate with a difference of biochemical activity. The tertiary amine tricyclics were particularly effective in treating depression with associated psychomotor agitation, and were found to be much more effective inhibitors of the neuronal uptake of 5HT than of noradrenaline. Tricyclics with a secondary amine group, on the other hand, were of greater value in producing a degree of psychomotor activation in retarded depressives, and were most effective at inhibiting cellular uptake of noradrenaline.

In addition, it has been found that tryptophan, the metabolic precursor of 5HT, has some antidepressant properties whereas depletion of central 5HT levels by the tryptophan hydroxylase inhibitor p-chlorophenylalanine tends to reduce the efficacy of antidepressant drugs.

These relationships have given rise to a series of 5HT theories of depression (Sugrue, 1981, 1983) and have also led to specific attempts to synthesize compounds with a higher selectivity for the 5HT uptake system than the classic compounds (Carlsson, 1984). The products of this research have included drugs such as zimelidine and fluoxetine which are indeed potent and highly effective antidepressants.

Following the same argument as for the catecholamine theories (e.g. that uptake inhibition by itself cannot account for the delayed clinical improvement) it has been found that chronic antidepressant treatment induces a down-regulation of 5HT binding sites. In particular, there is a decrease in the number of $5HT_2$ receptors in the neocortex (Peroutka and Snyder, 1980). As with the catecholamine system, this decrease of receptor number is accompanied by an *increase* in the electrophysiological and behavioural effects of 5HT activation and this lack of correlation is of some concern. Nevertheless, drugs such as mianserin and iprindole, whose mechanisms of action are at present unclear, do produce antagonism and down-regulation respectively of the 5HT receptor, and it seems probable that this action may contribute to their activity (Sugrue, 1983).

Although much less studied than the catecholamine systems, the role of 5HT in depression and its treatment has recently received a major boost with the discovery that highly specific binding sites exist for radiolabelled tricyclics in association with 5HT containing neuron terminals. Thus these binding sites, usually studied using tritiated imipramine, disappear if 5HT neurons are destroyed, and binding is dependent on sodium concentration in the incubation medium, just as is 5HT uptake. It is therefore likely that imipramine binding sites are associated with the 5HT uptake transporter. The potencies of a range of antidepressants in displacing the binding correlates well with their ability to depress 5HT uptake (Grabowsky, McCabe and Wamsley, 1983).

These imipramine 'receptors' also occur on platelets, and it has been shown that the number of these sites is reduced in untreated depressive patients (Briley *et al.*, 1980). Their number does not, however, increase as a result of treatment, suggesting that the phenomenon may be state independent; that is, a reflection not of the existence of depression but of the susceptibility of the patient to depression, a condition which presumably persists even during a drug-induced respite from the disease symptoms.

It has been argued that, by analogy with other systems discussed in this chapter, the existence of high affinity sites for imipramine may indicate an endogenous ligand. That ligand might function physiologically to promote or maintain 5HT uptake into neurons. If it became hyperactive it would lead to reduced 5HT function with up-regulation of receptors, and depression. Tricyclics might then act to displace the endogenous agent and produce the observed inhibition of uptake. Alternatively, the endogenous agent might itself be an inhibitor of reuptake but present in reduced amounts during depression. Imipramine and its analogues could then be envisaged as substitutes mimicking this physiological function.

Other mechanisms

Although histamine is not usually classed as a major CNS transmitter it does have widespread effects on the CNS, including the ability to activate adenylate cyclase. The finding that a number of antidepressants, including the rather anomalous ones such as iprindole, were able to block histamine stimulation of cyclase, and that some members of the group were more potent antagonists of H_1 and H_2 receptors than compounds used clinically for that purpose, led to some speculation that these effects were of primary importance in the control of depression (Kanof and Greengard, 1978). However, many of these phenomena have been demonstrated only in the test tube, and seem not to occur on intact cell systems. The role of histamine therefore remains an intriguing curiosity, but as yet of no practical value.

Similarly, since adenosine can interact with catecholamine receptors to modulate their sensitivity, it is conceivable that substances which produce a change of adenosine activity could indirectly influence amine responses. Thus it was of interest to find that several antidepressants, again including iprindole, could potentiate both the activation of adenylate cyclase and the electrophysiological effects of adenosine in the CNS, and the same result is seen following electroshock treatments. Again the hypothesis has some merits, but it has been shown that there is no change in the number of adenosine receptors as a result of antidepressant therapy, and the possible involvement of adenosine is now receiving less attention.

Finally, it should be noted that interest has arisen recently in possible contributions of several other transmitters or modulators to the control of depression. These include dopamine, for which there is some evidence of a down-regulation of presynaptic receptors and of an inhibition of uptake by antidepressants (Bunney and Garland, 1982), and peptides such as substance P, for which neuronal sensitivity is changed after antidepressant treatment. One of the most recently introduced antidepressant drugs, buproprion, is said to have no discernible effect on monoamine oxidases, noradrenaline or 5HT uptake, β-receptor or 5HT receptor density or adenylate cyclase. One of its few actions is to depress dopamine uptake.

The present state of knowledge of the mechanisms of action of antidepressant drugs may appear confused, but its very complexity serves to underline an important lesson which is being recognized increasingly by academic and clinical personnel alike. It is that, in trying to understand a complex system such as the brain and its disorders, it is of little value viewing single pathways or transmitter systems in isolation. The myriads of neurons, synapses and transmitters which make up the brain act in concert, controlling, modifying and compensating for activity to such a degree that errors or changes in any one system will induce a hundred others. Thus it is vital to realize that there probably is no single mechanism of antidepressant drug action, just as there is almost certainly no single mechanism of depression.

Stimulants

The use of CNS stimulants has declined somewhat over the past decade, largely because of the liability of abuse of the most effective family of such compounds, the amphetamines. The amphetamines were once widely used to promote alertness and an elevation of mood, actions which resulted from the ability of these substances to induce a release of amine transmitters from neuron terminals. This effect was rather non-selective, and involved noradrenaline, 5HT and dopamine. This resulted in a wide spectrum of behavioural results which undoubtedly contributed to their unpopularity.

Where stimulants are required today the drugs of choice are usually the amphetamine-like drugs pemoline or methylphenidate, both of which have amine-releasing actions similar to amphetamine but with less potential for abuse.

The commoner class of CNS stimulants is the methylxanthine group, including caffeine, theophylline and theobromine. These compounds were once thought to activate the CNS by inhibiting phosphodiesterase, thus producing an increase of cAMP levels in the brain, but it is now clear that they act by blocking the actions of adenosine.

Adenosine is released from almost all tissues (including neurons) during metabolic activity, and its effects are generally depressant. In the CNS, for example, it suppresses neuronal firing and inhibits transmitter release, as well as modulating responses to other neurotransmitters and producing local changes of metabolism and blood flow (Stone, 1981). Thus, by antagonizing these effects the methylxanthines are able to produce some CNS stimulation, and it should be recalled that if given in very high doses even these common dietary xanthines can produce convulsions.

Neuroleptics

As in the case of many other centrally acting drugs, the mechanism of action of the neuroleptics, or 'major tranquillizers' as they are occasionally known, is still not clear. These drugs are used in the treatment of major psychotic illnesses such as schizophrenia. Those drugs currently in use are primarily of value in combating the 'positive' symptoms of schizophrenia – delusions, hallucinations and disordered cognition, for example, which characterize so-called type I patients (Crow, 1980). The negative symptoms of type II patients are less amenable to pharmacological manipulation. The major groups of drugs presently available include the phenothiazines (fluphenazine), butyrophenones (haloperidol) and thioxanthines (*cis*-flupenthixol).

The dopamine hypothesis

For almost two decades the most convincing theory of the mechanism of action of the neuroleptics has been that they prevent excessive activity in aminergic pathways in the CNS. More specifically it has seemed that most neuroleptics were effective by virtue of their ability to block dopaminergic neurons in limbic regions of the brain (Jenner and Marsden, 1983). The main evidence in support of this hypothesis is presently of three kinds. First, compounds such as amphetamine, which increase the activity in central aminergic systems by promoting the release of the transmitters from nerve terminals, can mimic certain of the symptoms of schizophrenia. Indeed, the 'amphetamine psychosis' which results from chronic treatment of patients resembles schizophrenia so closely that it has frequently been considered a suitable model for the disease. Although amphetamine evokes the release of all the amine transmitters, animal experimentation has revealed that most of the effects of amphetamine relevant to human affective disorders are probably mainly due to the release of dopamine.

Secondly, most of the neuroleptics which were first available for clinical use are able to block the behavioural and electrophysiological effects in animals of compounds known to selectively activate dopamine receptors. These effects include, for example, the depression by dopamine agonists of cell firing in the substantia nigra. This response is mediated by dopamine 'autoreceptors' situated on the cell bodies of the nigral neurons. Dopamine agonists also inhibit the release of prolactin, for example, in both man and animals, and this action is similarly prevented by many neuroleptics.

Thirdly, and most recently, it has been discovered that postmortem brain from schizophrenic patients contains a higher density of dopamine receptors (studied by the radioactive ligand binding methods) than do control brains matched for age, sex, etc.

The difficulties with the dopamine hypothesis have come from several sources. First, it is clear that other neuron systems and transmitters are of great importance in modulating the effects of neuroleptics. Antagonists of 5HT, for instance, such as cyproheptadine, will diminish the dopamine antagonist actions of the neuroleptics. Secondly, it has been suggested that the apparent up-regulation of dopamine receptors in schizophrenic brains is not a true reflection of the disease process, but results from the neuroleptic treatment of the patients. In untreated patients it appears that there is a *reduction* of dopamine receptor numbers rather than an increase (Reynolds *et al.*, 1980). This would of course be consistent with the up-regulation of transmitter receptors seen in most neuronal systems following chronic administration of a suitable antagonist, lesion or depleting agent.

Certainly it is true that the chronic administration of neuroleptics will produce an up-regulation of dopamine receptors in all animal species studied. It even appears likely that such a change in the number of dopamine receptors may be the primary neurochemical event which leads to the involvement of the dopaminergic neurons in schizophrenia; those drugs which are able to block the effects of dopamine do so within minutes or hours of their acute administration, whereas the onset of clinical improvement does not occur for several weeks.

The increase of dopamine receptor number has also been proposed as the major factor underlying the prominent motor disorders which can arise after chronic treatment with neuroleptics. Over a period of weeks or months there may be involuntary movements of the body resembling Parkinson's disease, and these are attributable to the reduced activity of striatally released dopamine. However, usually after several years of neuroleptic medication, orofacial dyskinesia can occur. These have been attributed to the increased sensitivity to released dopamine resulting from the increase of receptor number, and they are very difficult to treat or reverse since they may be acutely exacerbated by reducing the neuroleptic dose.

These dyskinesias have nevertheless provided important clues to the behaviour of dopaminergic receptors. Even during the development of these movements the antipsychotic activity of the neuroleptics is not lost, presumably because a balance is established between the degree of blockade produced by the drugs and the increase of dopamine receptor number in the relevant areas of brain. The emergence of dyskinetic movements then may imply the involvement of a subpopulation of dopamine receptors which do not share the same sensitivity to neuroleptic blockade as the receptors responsible for the psychotic state (although they must be sufficiently sensitive for up-regulation to be stimulated). This opens the door to the concept of drugs which may act much more selectively on one or other subpopulation of dopamine receptors.

The hypoprolactinaemia which also accompanies antipsychotic therapy is presumably due to the up-regulation of dopamine receptors in the tuberoinfundibular system of dopaminergic neurons.

Dopamine receptors

Within the last decade several attempts have been made to categorize dopamine receptors into several subpopulations so as to explain the observations just described, as well as to account for the variety of clinical profiles obtained with different neuroleptics. It has been firmly established for several years that there are at least two varieties of dopamine receptor, referred to as D_1 and D_2 (Table 10.1). The former is positively linked to adenylate cyclase (increasing cAMP levels); the latter does not seem to be coupled to cyclase at all (Kebabian and Calne, 1979). However, many of the neuroleptics block the behavioural and neurochemical effects of activating the

Table 10.1 Properties of D_1 and D_2 dopamine receptors

	D_1	D_2
Effect on adenylate cyclase	Stimulation; increases cAMP	No effect
Location (see Fig. 10.4)	Striatonigral and intrinsic striatal neurons	Nigrostriatal neurons; corticostriate endings
Function	Unknown	Responsible for most electrophysiological and behavioural effects of dopamine agonists
Effect of dopamine	Agonist at micromolar levels	Agonist at nanomolar levels
Effect of apomorphine	Partial agonist (micromolar)	Full agonist (nanomolar)
Ergot alkaloids	Antagonists	Agonists
Selective antagonists	SCH 23390	Benzamides (sulpiride)
Effect of neuroleptics	Phenothiazines, butyrophenones and thioxanthines are non-selective antagonists at both sites	

D_2 site, while having little effect on the D_1 sites. Indeed, it has only recently become possible to begin probing the functional significance of the D_1 site with the development of selective D_1 antagonists (experimental compounds such as SCH 23390). It does appear, though, that both the D_1 and the D_2 receptor can have a presynaptic or a postsynaptic location (Fig. 10.4), so any difference of function is presumably more dependent on the situation of a particular neuron than on a more general functional distinction between the two receptors.

Nevertheless, even this simple division goes some way towards explaining different neuroleptic profiles and the incidence of side effects. The butyrophenones, diphenylbutylpiperidines (pimozide) and benzamides (sulpiride) are relatively specific D_2 antagonists whereas the phenothiazines and thioxanthines are rather non-selective blockers of D_1 and D_2. As illustrated in Fig. 10.4, the D_1 population exists on intrinsic neurons in the striatum, and it is presumably this group of receptors which is involved in the involuntary movements associated with chronic phenothiazine and thioxanthine treatment (Jenner and Marsden, 1983).

In addition, the clinical and animal behavioural effects of a range of neuroleptic drugs correlate well with their ability to displace binding of D_2 ligands, supporting the view that this class of receptor is primarily involved in the psychotic state. The dopamine agonist bromocriptine, derived from ergot, can produce a profound psychotic state closely resembling schizophrenia; bromocriptine is a selective agonist at D_2 receptors. Finally, the changes in dopamine receptor density mentioned above appear to be restricted to the D_2 population of sites.

The concept of D_1 and D_2 sites has thus become quite generally accepted and a summary of the main pharmacological properties of the two populations is given in Table 10.1. It is appropriate, however, to conclude this part of the discussion by noting that the two groups of receptors appear to be intimately linked. Agonists at D_2 receptors, for instance, will diminish a D_1 response initiated at about the same time. Similarly, a D_2 blocker will enhance a D_1

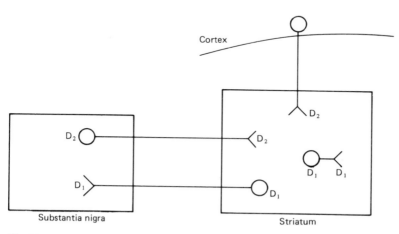

Fig. 10.4 A diagram of the locations of D_1 and D_2 dopamine receptors, as characterized in Table 10.1, in the corticonigrostriatal system.

effect. One suggested explanation for these phenomena is that D_1 and D_2 may be different forms of the same receptor molecule, possibly a normal and a desensitized form respectively.

Recently, more elaborate subclassifications of dopamine receptors have been attempted in which up to four species of receptor are said to be distinguishable (see Jenner and Marsden, 1983). However, much of the evidence for these divisions comes from binding studies which, as noted earlier, bear an unknown relationship to function. Only time will tell whether these newer classifications are of real value.

Dopaminergic pathways

Another factor determining the therapeutic and toxic effects of neuroleptics is that there are major differences in the regions of brain responsible for mediating the different effects of drugs. At present, dopaminergic neurons are recognized as forming at least four distinct pathways in the CNS. These include the mesostriatal, from substantia nigra to striatum, the mesocortical, from ventral tegmentum to cingulate and prefrontal cortex, the mesolimbic, from both substantia nigra and ventral tegmentum to the nucleus accumbens, tuberculum olfactorium and amygdala, and finally the tuberoinfundibular system from the arcuate and periventricular nuclei of the hypothalamus to the median eminence.

It is clearly an attractive idea that the mesolimbic and mesocortical pathways may be primarily involved in the antipsychotic aspects of neuroleptic action, and the striatal pathways in the movement difficulties.

New drugs

The earlier groups of neuroleptics thus block dopamine receptors and displace spiperone binding in most of the areas receiving a dopaminergic innervation. The newer compounds, however, such as sulpiride, clozapine and thioridazine block dopamine and displace spiperone only in limbic regions, not striatal. The D_2 antagonist sulpiride, for example, has no blocking activity against the classic locomotor effects of dopamine receptor stimulation such as stereotyped movements or circling behaviour following nigrostriatal lesions, both effects attributed to stimulation of striatal structures. It is the D_1 agonists, on the other hand, which can induce dyskinetic movements.

From these various considerations of dopamine function it becomes clear that the newer neuroleptic agents, such as sulpiride, represent a major advance over earlier drugs because many of them stimulate selectively D_2 receptors in limbic areas of the brain, with little effect on D_1 receptors in striatal areas. Most of these compounds also have little effect on receptors for 5HT, ACh, histamine, GABA and so on. But there are also enigmas.

Clozapine, for example, is one of the most selective antipsychotic drugs available. It has less tendency to lead to movement disorders than any other neuroleptic, although other toxic effects have limited its usefulness in the clinic to date. It can interact with dopamine receptors only at very high concentrations. On the other hand, clozapine is a potent antimuscarinic compound, and can readily displace muscarinic, $5HT_1$-, $5HT_2$- and histamine-related ligands from brain membranes. It therefore has a rather wide spectrum of pharmacological actions (reminiscent of some early neuroleptics) although lacking dopamine blockade, yet it is an effective antipsychotic agent. It is considered by many to be the starting point for a new generation of neuroleptics which will possess antipsychotic activity without the 'extrapyramidal' side effects of classic drugs.

Noradrenaline
Finally, it has been suggested that the role of amines other than dopamine may have been neglected for too long. Many of the useful neuroleptics, including compounds such as clozapine and thioridazine, are able to block the central effects of noradrenaline, for example, and it has now been shown that the postmortem brains of schizophrenic patients contain higher than normal levels of this amine. It is also the case that damage to the noradrenergic neurons in the brain prevents the development of supersensitivity of dopamine receptors, so there clearly must exist a close relationship between these amine systems, which could mean that a primary change in the noradrenaline system would affect brain function secondarily via its influence on dopamine neurons.

Against an involvement of noradrenaline in psychotic states is the fact that conventional α-adrenergic blockers do not seem to show significant antipsychotic activity. However, there is increasing evidence that β-blockers such as propranolol may indeed have some antipsychotic properties, and the selective α_2-agonist clonidine also shows similar activity. More selective interference with noradrenaline systems may therefore prove useful in the psychiatric clinic.

GABA
Although there is relatively little evidence for a major involvement of GABA in the antipsychotic properties of neuroleptic drugs, it has been suggested that destruction by chronically administered neuroleptics of GABA-releasing interneurons in the striatum might be involved in the development of involuntary movements. This suggestion originally arose from the observation that the increase in the number of dopamine- or neuroleptic-binding sites in striatum occurs within weeks of beginning neuroleptic therapy, whereas the dyskinetic movements appear only after many months or years of continued treatment. Furthermore, dopamine receptor up-regulation seems to be a universal consequence of neuroleptic medication whereas tardive dyskinesias occur only in a proportion of patients. According to the GABA hypothesis it is the toxic effects of neuroleptics on a population of (inhibitory) GABA neurons which leads to an imbalance in the excitatory and inhibitory systems of the striatum, the net result of which is an increased motor output (Fibiger and Lloyd, 1984).

Endogenous susbtances
The psychotic states have not been forgotten in the rush to find endogenous compounds responsible for mental health. Several groups of workers believe that an endogenous amphetamine-like or phenylethylamine-like substance may exist in the brain, concentrations of which could be elevated in psychotic states. This hypothesis should at present be considered very preliminary.

Anticonvulsants

Probably less is known about the mechanisms of action of the anticonvulsants than any other group of centrally acting drugs. Diazepam and pentobarbitone are possible exceptions to this, and they have been discussed in a previous section of this chapter.

Phenytoin

Diphenylhydantoin, one of the most widely prescribed antiepileptic medications, is still a mystery. The most common view of its mechanism of action is that it somehow stabilizes neurons so that paroxysmal activity is less likely to start, and, even if it does start, it is unlikely to spread far enough to become a generalized seizure. Phenytoin is known to interfere with many enzyme processes in the CNS, and some of these may contribute to the drug's anticonvulsant activity. For example, the stimulation of sodium/potassium ATPase (the 'sodium pump'), which has been reported many times, would result in a hyperpolarization of cells and a diminished tendency to fire action potentials.

One of the recent developments in the study of phenytoin has been the unveiling of a high affinity binding site in the CNS, which is being proclaimed as a potential indicator of the existence of an endogenous ligand. Phenytoin may therefore act by displacing an endogenous convulsant from that site, or by mimicking an endogenous anticonvulsant.

GABA

It is perhaps not unexpected that convulsions can readily be induced in animals by the administration of compounds such as strychnine, which blocks the inhibitory transmitter glycine, and bicuculline or picrotoxin, which block GABA. Similarly, inhibitors of GABA synthesis (by the enzyme glutamate decarboxylase) will produce convulsions. There is therefore much interest in developing compounds which will elevate GABA concentrations in the brain by inhibiting its destruction by GABA-transaminase. None of the currently available drugs works in this way, but two drugs are available which act on the GABA systems in other ways (Meldrum, 1984).

Sodium valproate is known to enhance the effects of GABA on CNS neurons. It does not interact with the membrane complex described in the section on benzodiazepines, and it does not seem to have marked effects on GABA metabolism. It is likely that the effect is mediated directly at the receptor, increasing the potency of GABA.

THIP (4,5,6,7-tetrahydroisoxazolo-[5,4,c]-pyridin-3-ol) is currently undergoing clinical trials as a systemically active compound capable of acting directly on GABA receptors. Whilst it is certainly anticonvulsant, its wide spectrum of side effects raises doubts as to its eventual therapeutic value.

Excitatory amino acids

An alternative approach to anticonvulsant therapy is to block the effects of the excitatory transmitters such as glutamate. This possibility is a subject of much research, and it has been suggested that this action may contribute to the effects of phenytoin and benzodiazepines.

Purines

As noted above, adenosine is generally depressant in its overall effects on the CNS, and xanthines which act as adenosine antagonists can cause convulsions. Compounds such as phenytoin and valproate have no interaction at all with such purines but the possibility that benzodiazepines may act by enhancing the effects of purines was discussed earlier. It has now also been found that carbamazepine, useful in a large proportion of epileptic patients to control or help to control their fits, can displace adenosine binding in the CNS. Since no other action of carbamazepine has so far been detected which could begin to explain its anticonvulsant activity, this phenomenon is being given a great deal of excited attention.

References

Assumpcao, J.A., Bernardi, N., Brown, J. and Stone, T.W. (1979) Selective antagonism by benzodiazepines of neuronal responses to excitatory amino acids in the cerebral cortex. *British Journal of Pharmacology* **67**, 563–568

Braestrup, C. and Squires, R.F. (1977) Specific benzodiazepine receptors in rat brain characterized by high affinity 3H-diazepam binding. *Proceedings of the National Academy of Sciences of the USA* **74**, 3805–3809

Braestrup, C., Nielsen, M. and Olsen, C.E. (1980) Urinary and brain β-carboline-3-carboxylates as potent inhibitors of brain benzodiazepine receptors. *Proceedings of the National Academy of Sciences of the USA* **77**, 2288–2292

Briley, M.S., Langer, S.Z., Raisman, R., Sechter, D. and Zarifian, E. (1980) Tritiated imipramine binding sites are decreased in platelets of untreated depressive patients. *Science* **209**, 303–305

Bunney, W.E. and Garland, B.L. (1982) A second generation catecholamine hypothesis. *Pharmacopsychiatria* **15**, 111–15

Burrows, G.D., Norman, T.R. and Davies, B. (Eds.) (1984) *Antianxiety Agents.* Elsevier: Amsterdam

Carlsson, A. (1984) Current theories on the mode of action of antidepressant drugs. *Advances in Biochemical Psychopharmacology* **39**, 213–221

Costa, E. and Guidotti, A. (1979) Molecular mechanisms in the receptor action of benzodiazepines. *Annual Review of Pharmacology* **19**, 531–545

Crow, T.J. (1980) Molecular pathology of schizophrenia: more than one process. *British Medical Journal* **280**, 66

Fibiger, H.C. and Lloyd, K.G. (1984) Neurobiological substrates of tardive dyskinesia: the GABA hypothesis. *Trends in Neurosciences* **7**, 462–464

Grabowsky, K.L., McCabe, R.T. and Wamsley, J.K. (1983) Localisation of [3H]-imipramine binding sites in rat brain by light microscopic autoradiography. *Life Sciences* **32**, 2355–2362

Jenner, P. and Marsden, C.D. (1983) Neuroleptics. In: *Psychopharmacology*, part I (Eds. Grahame-Smith, D.G. and Cowen, P.J.), pp. 180–247. Excerpta Medica: Amsterdam

Kanof, P.D. and Greengard, P. (1978) Brain histamine receptors as targets for antidepressant drugs. *Nature* **272**, 329–333

Kebabian, J.W. and Calne, D.B. (1979) Multiple receptors for dopamine. *Nature* **277**, 93–96

Meldrum, B.S. (1984) Amino acid neurotransmitters and new approaches to anticonvulsant drug action. *Epilepsia* **25**, suppl. 2, S140–S149

Morgan, P.F., Lloyd, H.G.E. and Stone, T.W. (1983) Benzodiazepine inhibition of adenosine uptake is not prevented by benzodiazepine antagonists. *European Journal of Pharmacology* **87**, 121–126

Olsen, R.W. (1982) Drug interactions at the GABA receptor–ionophore complex. *Annual Review of Pharmacology* **22**, 245–277

Paul, S.M., Marangos, P.J. and Skolnick, P. (1981) The benzodiazepine–GABA–chloride ionophore receptor complex: common site of minor tranquillizer action. *Biological Psychiatry* **16**, 213–229

Peroutka, S.J. and Snyder, S.H. (1980) Long-term antidepressant treatment decreases spiroperidol-labeled serotonin receptor binding. *Science* **210**, 88–90

Reynolds, G.P., Reynolds, L.M., Riederer, P., Jellinger, K. and Gabriel, E. (1980) Dopamine receptors and schizophrenia: drug effect or illness? *Lancet* **2**, 1251

Schildkraut, J.J. (1965) The catecholamine hypothesis of affective disorders: a review of supporting evidence. *American Journal of Psychiatry* **122**, 509–522

Stone, E.A. (1983) Problems with current catecholamine hypotheses of antidepressant agents. *Behavioral and Brain Sciences* **6**, 535–578

Stone, T.W. (1981) Physiological roles for adenosine and ATP in the nervous system. *Neuroscience* **6**, 523–555

Sugrue, M.F. (1981) Current concepts on the mechanisms of action of antidepressant drugs. *Pharmacology and Therapeutics* **13**, 219–247

Sugrue, M.F. (1983) Chronic antidepressant therapy and associated changes in central monoaminergic receptor functioning. *Pharmacology and Therapeutics* **21**, 1–33

Sulser, F., Vetulani, J. and Mobley, P.L. (1978) Mode of action of antidepressant drugs. *Biochemical Pharmacology* **27**, 257–261

Tallman, J.F., Paul, S.M., Skolnick, P. and Gallager, D.W. (1980) Receptors for the age of anxiety: pharmacology of the benzodiazepines. *Science* **207**, 274–281

U'Prichard, D.C., Greenberg, D.A., Sheehan, P.P. and Snyder, S.H. (1978) Tricyclic antidepressants: therapeutic properties and affinity for α-noradrenergic receptor binding sites in the brain. *Science* **199**, 197–198

Usdin, E., Skolnick, P., Tallman, J.F., Greenblatt, D. and Paul, S.M. (Eds.) (1983) *Pharmacology of Benzodiazepines*. Macmillan: London

Williams, M. (1984) Molecular aspects of the action of benzodiazepine and non-benzodiazepine anxiolytics: a hypothetical allosteric model of the benzodiazepine receptor complex. *Progress in Neuropsychopharmacology* **8**, 209–247

11

Local anaesthetics

Benjamin G. Covino

The basic pharmacological action of local anaesthetic drugs is to inhibit the excitation–conduction process of peripheral nerve fibres and nerve endings. The purpose of this chapter is to review our current knowledge regarding: (1) the basic mechanism of action of local-anaesthetic-induced conduction blockade; (2) the site of action in the nerve membrane; (3) the active form of local anaesthetic agents; (4) differential conduction blockade; and (5) the structure-active relationship of the clinically useful local anaesthetics. A brief review of the basic electrophysiological properties of the nerve membrane should prove useful in understanding the mechanism by which local anaesthetic agents produce conduction blockade.

Electrophysiology of peripheral nerve

At rest, a negative electrical potential of approximately −60 to −90 mν exists across the nerve cell membrane which represents the resting membrane potential. If a stimulus of sufficient intensity is applied to the nerve, the interior

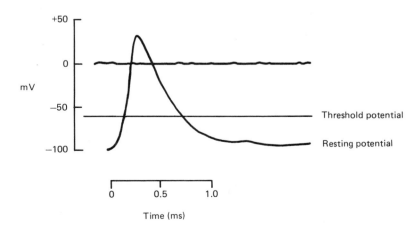

Fig. 11.1 Action potential of peripheral nerve.

of the cell becomes progressively less negative with respect to the exterior, resulting in a state of depolarization (Fig. 11.1). The cell membrane possesses a critical threshold potential or firing level which must be achieved before complete depolarization can occur. Normally, the threshold potential level is approximately 20 mv less then the resting potential. A cell with a resting potential level of -70 mv will have a threshold potential or firing level of approximately -50 mv. If the stimulus applied to the nerve is not sufficient to decrease the potential difference across the cell membrane from the resting to the threshold potential level, a localized incomplete state of depolarization occurs which is not adequate to produce a propagated action potential. Once the threshold potential level is achieved, an extremely rapid phase of depolarization commences, which is spontaneous in nature and not dependent on the strength of the applied stimulus. The nerve membrane essentially follows the 'all or none' rule; that is, an applied stimulus of sufficient strength is required to achieve the threshold potential level which, in turn, will result in complete depolarization (Fig. 11.1). Any additional increase in stimulus intensity has no effect on the degree of depolarization or the amplitude of the action potential because the triggering effect is 'all or none'. The development of the action potential results in a reversal of the electrical potential, such that at the end of the depolarization phase the interior of the cell actually moves to a positive electrical potential of $+40$ mv as compared to the exterior of the cell. Under normal conditions the total height of the action potential is approximately 110 mv; that is, the potential difference across the membrane has changed from a resting potential level of -70 mv to a peak level of $+40$ mv at the end of depolarization.

At the conclusion of the depolarization phase, repolarization of the cell membrane begins. During this time the electrical potential within the cell again becomes progressively more negative until the original resting potential of -60 to -90 mv is re-established. The period of repolarization is important electrophysiologically, since during this phase the membrane is in a state of refractoriness. During the early portion of the repolarization phase, the refractoriness is absolute in nature such that the cell will not respond to a stimulus regardless of strength. During the latter phase of repolarization the cell is in a state of relative refractoriness. During this time the cell will respond only to a stimulus whose intensity is greater than that normally required to produce depolarization. The refractory period is important, since it limits the number of impulses which can be conducted along a nerve fibre per unit time. The entire process of depolarization and repolarization occurs within 1 millisecond. The depolarization phase occupies approximately 30 per cent of the entire action potential, whereas repolarization accounts for the remaining 70 per cent. Frequently a brief period of hyperpolarization may be observed following the end of the repolarization phase. During this time the potential difference across the cell membrane is actually more negative than during the resting potential.

Propagation of the action potential from the area of initial excitation along the entire length of a nerve fibre does not require sequential stimulation of individual segments of the nerve. Once initial excitation occurs in a localized area of the nerve, a spontaneous and self-perpetuating system propagates the impulse along the entire length of the nerve fibre. This process is dependent on the change of electrical potential across the cell membrane at the area of excitation and on the ability of the nerve to function as an electrical cable. In unmyelinated C fibres, current will flow from the depolarized active region into the adjacent polarized segment (Fig. 11.2). This current flow will thereby reduce the charge and voltage in the inactive region which is sufficient to decrease the intracellular potential to the threshold level required for depolarization. Therefore, the local circuit flow of current between immediately adjacent areas of polarized and depolarized membrane results in spontaneous propagation of the impulse along the fibre at a constant velocity of approximately 1 m per second. In myelinated nerve fibres, the impulse proceeds from one node of Ranvier to the adjacent node. The conduction velocity is proportional to the size of the fibre and intranodal distances. Thus, in large myelinated A fibres impulse propagation occurs at the rate of 70–120 m per second whilst small, lightly myelinated B fibres conduct impulses at the rate of 3–15 m per second.

Ionic factors responsible for action potential

The electrophysiological properties of the nerve membrane are dependent on (1) the concentration of electrolytes in nerve cytoplasm and extracellular fluid, and (2) the permeability of the cell membrane to various ions, particularly sodium and potassium. The ionic composition of the cytoplasm and the extracellular fluid differs markedly. The intracellular concentration of potassium is approximately 110–170 mmol/l, whereas the intracellular concentration of sodium and chloride ions is approximately 5–10 mmol/l. In extracellular fluid the situation is reversed. The concentration of sodium is approximately 140 mmol/l and the concentration of chloride is 110 mmol/l. On the other hand, the extracellular concentration of potassium is only 3–5 mmol/l. The ionic asymmetry on either side of the cell membrane is due in part to the selective permeability characteristics of the membrane. At rest, potassium ions may diffuse easily across the cell membrane, indicating that the membrane is fully permeable to this particular ion. However, only limited diffusion of sodium ions across the membrane occurs at rest, indicating that the membrane

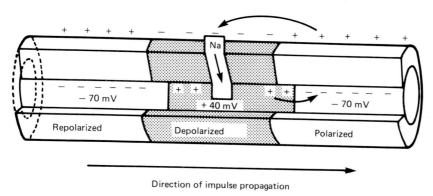

Direction of impulse propagation

Fig. 11.2   Mode of impulse propagation in an unmyelinated nerve fibre.

is relatively impermeable to sodium, which accounts for the high extracellular concentration and low intracellular concentration of sodium. Although the membrane is permeable to potassium ions, a high intracellular concentration of this ion in maintained by the attractive forces of the negative charges mainly on proteins which exist within the cell. These large negatively charged proteins are unable to diffuse across the cell membrane. The attraction of the negative charges on the proteins tends to counterbalance the tendency of the postively charged potassium ions to diffuse out of the cell by passive movement along a concentration gradient and through a freely permeable membrane. The electrical potential which should exist across the membrane separating two concentrations of the same ion was predicted by the Nernst equation.

$$E = -\frac{RT}{nF} ln \frac{[A]_i}{[A]_o}$$

Where E =membrane potential between inside and outside of cell
       R =gas constant in joules (8.315)
       T =absolute temperature
       n =valence of the ion
       F =Faraday's constant (96 500 coulombs)
       ln =natural logarithm

At room temperature (18°C) and assuming a K_i/K_o ratio across the nerve membrane of 30, the Nernst equation would predict the following:

$$E = -58 \log \frac{[30K]_i}{[K]_o}$$
$$E = -85.7 \, mv$$

This predicted resting membrane potential of $-85.7 \, mv$ agrees closely with the measured resting potential values of -60 to $-90 \, mv$ obtained from nerve preparations with intracellular electrodes. At rest, it would appear that the nerve fibre behaves as a potassium electrode, which should react to changes in intra- or extracellular potassium concentration. Indeed, it has been clearly shown that changes in the intracellular or extracellular concentration of

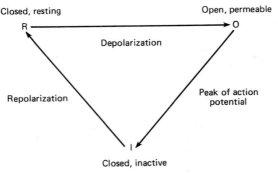

Fig. 11.3 Various states of sodium channel. R represents closed state at rest. O represents open state during depolarization. I represents inactive, closed state at the end of depolarization.

potassium will markedly alter the resting membrane potential. For example, as the extracellular concentration of potassium is increased, the resting membrane potential will tend to decrease. Studies have indicated that a decrease of 58 mv in resting potential occurs for a tenfold change in external potassium concentration. On the other hand, changes in sodium concentration appear to have little, if any, effect on the resting membrane potential.

Excitation of a nerve results in marked changes in the permeability of the cell membrane and ionic fluxes across the membrane. The movement of ions across the nerve membrane occurs through ion-specific pores or channels. Sodium channels have been studied most extensively. Efforts have been made to determine the size and density of these channels. In addition, physiological studies have indicated that sodium channels exist in various states (Hille, 1984). When the nerve membrane is quiescent the sodium channels are considered to be in a state of rest (R), and impermeable to the passage of sodium ions (Fig. 11.3). Following stimulation, the channels pass from a closed to an open state (O), thus permitting the passage of sodium ions across the membrane. When threshold potential is exceeded, most of the sodium channels are in an open state, allowing a maximum increase in the permeability of the cell membrane to sodium ions, and an explosively rapid influx of sodium ions into the axoplasm follows. This marked increase of sodium conductance is responsible for the rapid depolarization of the cell. As the potential difference changes from the threshold level of approximately -50 mv to $+40$ mv at the peak of the action potential, the open sodium channels become inactivated (I) leading to a decrease in sodium permeability. It is this sodium inactivation that ultimately terminates the depolarization phase. At the end of depolarization or at the peak of the action potential, the nerve membrane is essentially transformed from a potassium electrode to a sodium electrode, and the positive membrane potential of $+40$ mv can be calculated again from the Nernst equation by substituting the ratio of sodium ions between the inside and the outside of the nerve membrane (Na_i/Na_o) for the potassium ion ratio (K_i/K_o).

At the conclusion of the depolarization phase, the membrane starts to repolarize. The initial phase of repolarization and the absolute refractory period are related mainly to inactivation of sodium channels (I) resulting in a decrease in sodium flux. However, the remaining portion of the repolarization phase is a function of an increase in potassium conductance and efflux of this ion from the interior to the exterior of the cell. Potassium conductance is still somewhat greater than normal when repolarization is complete, which accounts for the phase of membrane hyperpolarization. When the membrane potential returns to its normal resting level, potassium and sodium channels have also returned to their normal resting states.

Although the fluxes of sodium and potassium are high during the depolarization and repolarization phases, the actual concentration changes across the cell membrane are very small because the time during which these flows occur is very short. Therefore, following return of the membrane to the resting potential level, only a slight excess of sodium ions is present within the cell and a slight excess of potassium ions exists outside the nerve cell. At the conclusion of the excitation period, a metabolically active period begins, although electrically the nerve cell is quiescent. Restoration of the normal ionic

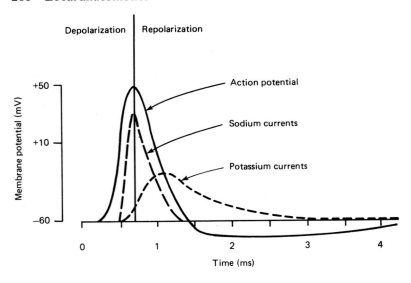

Fig. 11.4 Relationship between depolarization and repolarization phases of nerve action potential and sodium and potassium currents.

gradient across the nerve membrane requires the expenditure of energy for the active transport of sodium from the inside to the outside of the nerve cell against a concentration gradient. This active transport of sodium ions is made possible by the so-called 'sodium pump'. The energy required to drive the sodium pump is derived from the oxidative metabolism of adenosine triphosphate (ATP). This metabolic pump, which actively extrudes intracellular sodium ions, also is believed responsible, in part, for the transport of potassium ions from the extracellular space to the interior of the nerve cell.

The return of potassium to the interior of the nerve cell occurs against a concentration gradient, but down an electrogenic gradient. Thus, re-establishment of the potassium gradient across the cell membrane may be partly an active process and partly a passive phenomenon. Potassium will continue to return to the interior of the cell until the electrostatic attraction of the negative charges on the intracellular proteins balances the chemical concentration gradient. Figure 11.4 summarizes the relationship between electrical activity in the nerve and the alterations in ionic fluxes across the membrane.

Mechanism of local-anaesthetic-induced conduction blockade

Application of a sufficient concentration of local anaesthetic agent to peripheral nerve either *in vitro* or *in vivo* will inhibit impulse conduction. However, electrophysiological studies have shown that neither the resting membrane potential nor the threshold potential of isolated nerves is altered following exposure to various concentrations of local anaesthetic agents such as procaine or lignocaine.

The primary effect of local anaesthetic agents involves the depolarization phase of the action potential. A decrease in the rate and degree of depolarization is observed as the concentration of local anaesthetic agent applied to an isolated nerve is increased. Although a subliminal concentration of local anaesthetic agent will not prevent the development of a propagated action potential, rate of depolarization and repolarization is decreased, refractory period is prolonged and conduction velocity is decreased. As a result, the number of impulses transmitted per unit time in an isolated nerve exposed to a subliminal concentration of local anaesthetic agent will be decreased. When the minimum concentration (C_m) of a local anaesthetic agent required to cause complete conduction blockade is achieved, the rate and degree of depolarization are sufficiently depressed that the threshold potential level is not achieved. Studies by Aceves and Machne (1963) showed a 59 per cent decrease in the maximum rate of rise of the action potential of the isolated lumbar spinal ganglion of the frog after exposure to procaine. Similarly, Shanes et al. (1959) reported a 42 per cent decrease in the maximum rate of depolarization of the squid axon following the application of cocaine or procaine. In both studies, a concomitant decrease in the rate of depolarization of 37–55 per cent was also observed. The prolonged repolarization phase may reflect a direct local anaesthetic action or may be indicative of a direct relationship between the rate of repolarization and the rate of depolarization. In general, the primary action of local anaesthetic is a decrease in the rate and degree of depolarization.

Since the action potential of the nerve membrane is a function of changes in sodium and potassium permeability and conductance, a number of studies have been carried out to evaluate the effect of local anaesthetic on ionic permeability. Initially, Condouris (1961) observed a direct correlation between the concentration of sodium in the bathing solution and the concentration of cocaine required to reduce the height of the spike potential of the isolated frog sciatic–peroneal nerve trunk. For example, at a normal sodium concentration of 116 mmol, approximately 3.2 mmol of cocaine was required to produce a 50 per cent decrease in the height of the spike potential. When the sodium concentration was lowered to 12 mmol, only 0.15 mmol of cocaine was necessary to cause a similar reduction of 50 per cent in the amplitude of the spike potential.

The most direct evidence concerning the effect of local anaesthetic agents on sodium and potassium conductance has been obtained by means of voltage clamp techniques. Taylor (1959) and Shanes et al. (1959) demonstrated that procaine and cocaine are capable of decreasing the inward flow of sodium currents and the outward flow of potassium currents during voltage clamping of the membrane. However, both studies demonstrated a greater inhibitory effect on sodium conductance (g_{Na}) than on potassium conductance (g_K). For example, 0.05–0.1 per cent cocaine produced a 31–64 per cent decrease in g_{Na} compared to a 22–57 per cent decrease in g_K. Procaine (0.1 per cent) resulted in a 58 per cent decrease in g_{Na}, while at the same time reducing g_K by 21 per cent. Furthermore, studies on the isolated frog sciatic nerve by Hille (1966), in which the membrane potential was held at the normal resting potential of

-75 mv, demonstrated complete loss of sodium currents in the presence of 10^{-3} mol/l lignocaine with no discernible effect on outward potassium current. A concentration of 3.5×10^{-3} mol/l lignocaine was required to produce a 25 per cent decrease in g_K. In a subsequent study, Strichartz (1975) also demonstrated almost complete inhibition of g_{Na} with minimal change in g_K following application of lignocaine to a single myelinated frog sciatic nerve preparation. Definitive proof that local-anaesthetic-induced conduction blockade is due to an inhibition of sodium conductance was forthcoming from investigations with the biotoxins, tetrodotoxin and saxitoxin. These two substances are the most potent nerve conduction blockers found to date. Tetrodotoxin will prevent excitation of the isolated squid axon at a concentration of 10^{-7} mol/l. *In vivo* studies have shown that tetrodotoxin at a dose of 4 μg can produce spinal anaesthesia in sheep for 17–23 hours. In terms of ionic membrane permeability, these two biotoxins have been demonstrated in various biological preparations to specifically inhibit sodium conductance without an effect on potassisum conductance. For example, Hille (1966, 1968) reported that 3×10^{-7} mol/l tetrodotoxin completely inhibited g_{Na} in the isolated frog sciatic nerve without any discernible effect on g_K. Similarly, saxitoxin caused a dose-related decrease in g_{Na} with complete blockade occurring at approximately 10^{-7} mol/l whilst no change in g_K was observed at any concentration of saxitoxin.

In summary, the basic mechanism by which local anaesthetics cause conduction block in peripheral nerves involves inhibition of the increase in membrane permeability to sodium ions which results in a failure of membrane depolarization.

Site of action of local anaesthetic agents

In recent years attempts have been made to determine the specific site in the nerve membrane at which local anaesthetics exert their inhibitory action. Three specific sites have been suggested as possible locations for the action of local anaesthetics: (1) the surface of the nerve membrane; (2) within the nerve membrane; and (3) specific receptors within the sodium channel.

A brief review of the anatomy of peripheral nerves may be appropriate to a clearer interpretation of these various theories concerning the possible site of action of local anaesthetics.

Peripheral nerves are mixed nerves containing both myelinated and unmyelinated fibres which conduct afferent and efferent impulses subserving either sensory or motor functions. The structure of a peripheral nerve is shown in Fig. 11.5. The entire nerve is surrounded by an epineurium, or sheath, composed of connective tissue and tightly joined cells. Within this sheath, groups of nerve fibres are organized in fascicles surrounded by a second sheath, the perineurium. Finally, each individual axon is intimately surrounded by non-neuronal glial cells which form the endoneurium.

These various neuronal coverings serve as barriers which can influence the diffusion of local anaesthetics. The A and B nerve fibres are encased in a myelin sheath which extends, discontinuously, from the roots of the spinal cord to the region of entry at the target organ. Each segment or internode of myelin is formed by one Schwann cell which wraps round the axon, forming an insulating cylinder of as many as several hundred bilayer membranes (Fig. 11.5b and c). The myelin sheath of peripheral fibres accounts for more than half of the thickness of the fibre diameter. The myelin sheath is interrupted at intervals by narrow zones of constrictions (the nodes of Ranvier) which contain the structural elements essential for neuronal excitability (Fig. 11.6). These nodes are covered by a Schwann cell which projects to the surface of the axolemma and makes several intimate contacts with the neuron surface. The sodium channels of myelinated fibres are located at the nodes of Ranvier such that excitation proceeds from one node to the next in a saltatory fashion. The potassium channels are present almost exclusively in the internodal region, where they exert little influence on impulse propagation (Chiu and Ritchie, 1980). Between the extranodal Schwann cell and the axolemma lies nodal-gap substance, dense in negatively charged material, which may act as a reservoir to bind metal cations and basic drugs near the nodal membrane. Thus, at no point along the fibre is the axon membrane freely exposed to the surrounding medium.

All fibres of diameter greater than 1 μm are myelinated. Small C fibres are unmyelinated but are enclosed within a Schwann cell which forms an intimate cover around several fibres (see Fig. 11.5c). Cross-sectional electron micrographs of non-myelinated nerves show that individual axons are located

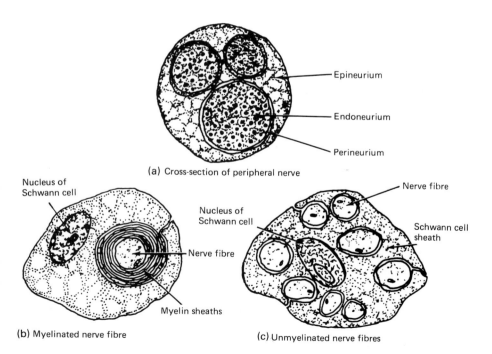

(a) Cross-section of peripheral nerve

Epineurium

Endoneurium

Perineurium

Nucleus of Schwann cell

Nucleus of Schwann cell

Nerve fibre

Nerve fibre

Schwann cell sheath

Myelin sheaths

(b) Myelinated nerve fibre

(c) Unmyelinated nerve fibres

Fig. 11.5   (a) Cross-section of an intact peripheral nerve. (b, c) myelinated (b) and unmyelinated (c) nerve.

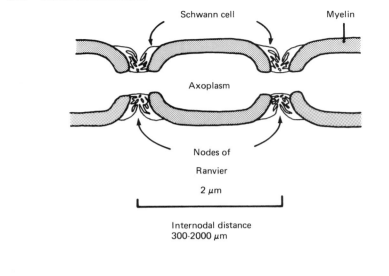

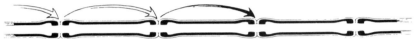

Fig. 11.6 Myelinated nerve showing nodes of Ranvier. Lower portion shows impulse propagation proceeding from one node to the next node.

adjacent to the periphery of such a bundle, circumscribing the large nucleus of the Schwann cell. The Schwann cell's plasmalemma encloses each axon separately, folding the cytoplasm of the supporting cell round most of the axon's diameter. Any one axon passes sequentially from one encasing Schwann cell to another with no apparent interruptions. The structural association between neuron and glia is maintained along the entire length of the fibre and may be functionally similar to that of the myelinated axon and its enclosing Schwann cell at each node of Ranvier.

The plasma membrane of nerve cells consists of densely staining outer surfaces, spaced 7.5–10 nm apart, which enclose a relatively electron-transparent medium. Myelinated and unmyelinated nerve fibres have the same general morphology although the membrane has characteristic features in specialized regions, such as at sensory nerve endings and at the synapses.

Morphological and electrical studies demonstrate that nerve membranes are mainly lipid bilayers encasing proteins, some of which permit ions to pass through a hydrocarbon interior of otherwise high resistance (Fig. 11.7). Both proteins and lipids in membranes are often associated with complex carbohydrate structures, located on the extracellular side of the membrane, and the proteins may also interact with the carbohydrates of the internal cytoskeleton. The emerging picture is one of a biosynthetically dynamic structure, where membrane proteins not only move about within the membrane but also are being continuously synthesized, inserted, and removed throughout the life of the neuron.

The lipid composition of the nerve membrane influences its structural and dynamic characteristics, and modulates the activities of some of the intrinsically bound enzymes. It also regulates the rate and potency of action of various drugs. The morphological and electrical properties of nerve membranes are quite similar to those of lipid bilayers which contain some protein or other ion-transporting substances. Direct structural determinations of nerve membranes by X-ray diffraction further support the bilayer model. Studies of bilayers made from lipid extracted from nerves provide data comparable with those characteristic of pure lipid bilayers.

Membranes are composed of phospholipids, cholesterol, proteins, and carbohydrates, the last of which are usually conjugated with other substances to form glycoproteins or glycolipids. Protein accounts for more than 30 per cent of non-myelinated nerve dry weight, yet most of it is localized at the membrane surface and not within the hydrocarbon region. Cholesterol is interdigitated among the phospholipids and influences their behaviour. When X-ray patterns of bilayers made only from phospholipids are compared with those made from total lipid extract, the inclusion of cholesterol appears to increase the separation of polar lipid headgroups in the bilayer to that seen in the axolemma and causes an increase in the parallel orientation of the fatty acid chains of phospholipids. The presence of cholesterol increases the degree of order in the membrane.

Despite their orderly alignment in the plane of the membrane, neural lipids behave like fluid components within the membrane interior. The fluidity in nerve membranes can be detected by electron spin resonance (ESR). 'Spin-labels' are dissolved in the hydrocarbon phase or covalently bound to molecules which become orientated in the membrane. Spin-label studies show that the hydrocarbon region of nerve membranes is very fluid at physiological

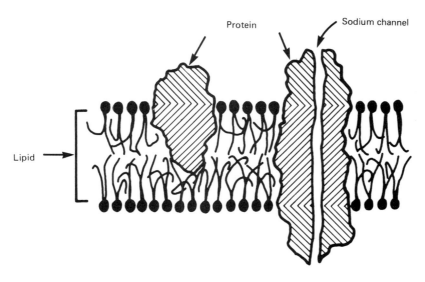

Fig. 11.7 Morphology of nerve membrane consisting of lipids and proteins with sodium channel present in the protein portion of the membrane.

temperatures. The fatty acid tails of membrane lipids are rotating and bending at frequencies up to 10^9 per second. ESR signals from long chain acids spin-labelled at different positions along the hydrocarbon chain indicate that the nerve membranes in which they are inserted are mostly fluid and have the least degree of orientation near the centre of the hydrocarbon region. The fluidity decreases while the degree of orientation increases as the label is moved closer to the polar headgroup region of the lipids. Thus, there is far more motion in the centre of a membrane than near the aqueous interface. This is of particular interest because local anaesthetics appear to distribute in lipid bilayer membranes between the fatty acid core and the phospholipid headgroup region adjacent to extracellular and cytoplasmic solutions.

Membrane surface location

About 15 per cent of the neuronal phospholipids carry net negative charges: the charged species are phosphatidylserine and phosphatidylinositol. These lipids may alter membrane excitability and also modulate the uptake of basic amine local anaesthetics. Many studies have shown that fixed charges near sodium channels in nerve can influence excitability. Such fixed charges create electric potential at the membrane surface which contribute to the electric field in the membrane, and thus influence the 'voltage sensors' which control ion permeability channels. A membrane with negative charges fixed to its surface tends to accumulate cations and repel anions in the adjacent solution. In turn, the presence of cations, particularly multivalent cations (e.g. Ca^{2+}) decreases the local surface potential due to ion accumulation and in this way can influence excitability. For example, increasing external Ca^{2+} raises the firing threshold of nerves, and this is explained by a change of the surface electric potential which in turn changes the electric field within the membrane which is detected by 'voltage sensors' of ion channels as being equivalent to a hyperpolarization of the nerve. The Ca^{2+}ions need not interact directly with the ion channels, according to this mechamism.

Negative charges fixed at membrane surfaces also attract protonated local anaesthetics and thus increase their adsorption to the membrane and so decrease the negativity of the surface of the nerve membrane. The electrostatic interactions between membrane negative charges, local anaesthetics and Ca^{2+} ions account for the binding competition observed in experimental studies. However, certain pharmacological actions cannot be explained by such electrostatic competition. For example, elevated extracellular Ca^{2+} antagonizes the inhibition from uncharged benzocaine. In addition, quaternary forms of local anaesthetics can adsorb to the outer surface of bilayer membranes, changing the potential by 10 mV, yet have no effect on nerve excitability when restricted to the extracellular solution (Frazier, Narahashi and Yamada, 1970). Therefore, local anaesthetics must exert specific effects other then those due to electrostatic interactions, but these interactions can modulate the biological effects of the anaesthetics.

Location within the nerve membrane

The highly lipid nature of the nerve membrane and the relationship between local anaesthetic potency and lipid solubility have led some investigators to conclude that the site of action of local anaesthetic agents resides within the lipid component of the nerve membrane. Seeman (1972) studied a number of different agents capable of producing conduction blockade and reported that an inverse correlation existed between the membrane/buffer partition coefficient of the agents and the concentration required in the membrane to cause conduction block.

An intramembranal site of action of local anaesthetic agents is visualized as causing some type of conformational change in the organization of the membrane. The alteration most commonly postulated is membrane expansion or change in critical volume. The membrane expansion theory of local anaesthesia is basically an extension of the Meyer–Overton law for general anaesthesia, which states that the physicochemical combination of an anaesthetic substance with cell lipids causes a change in the relationship between cell constituents which in turn leads to an inhibition of cell function. Originally the membrane expansion theory of local anaesthesia suggested a constriction of the sodium channels due to increased lateral pressure within the membrane. *In vitro* studies by Skou (1954), in which the surface pressure of monomolecular layers of lipids increased following placement of local anaesthetics into the solution below the lipid layer, served as the basis for this concept of lateral expansion within the membrane. Seeman (1972) attempted to quantify the actual change in volume of membranes during conditions of local anaesthesia. In general, membrane concentrations of 0.04 mol/kg of membrane are required for the production of conduction blockade. This concentration occupies a volume of 0.3 per cent of the membrane which results in a 2–3 per cent expansion of the membrane. The membrane expansion theory holds a certain attraction, for several reasons. It would readily explain the site and mechanisms of action of local anaesthetic agents which exist only in an uncharged form such as benzocaine and benzyl alcohol. Moreover, it would also provide a single theory for the site and mechanism of action of both general and local anaesthetic drugs. With regard to general anaesthetic agents, one of the critical experiments which has been quoted to support the concept of membrane expansion or increase in volume involves reversal of anaesthesia by exposure to elevated atmospheric pressures. This can be dramatically demonstrated in the following fashion: addition of general anaesthetics to a bath containing tadpoles abolishes the spontaneous swimming of the tadpoles; when the bath containing the anaesthetized tadpoles is exposed to hydrostatic pressures of 150–350 atm, swimming motion is re-established. indicating a removal of the state of anaesthesia. In addition, emulsions of general anaesthetics can produce conduction block in a variety of peripheral nerves, which can then be antagonized by an increase in atmospheric pressure. Similar studies with local anaesthetic agents are limited and contradictory in nature. Roth, Smith and Paton (1976) reported that high pressure could reverse the depression of action potential amplitude in frog sciatic nerves produced by chloroform, diethyl ether and halothane. However, no pressure-induced antagonism of action potential depression due to procaine or cinchocaine was observed. Similar studies were conducted by Kendig and Cohen (1977) utilizing the preganglionic sympathetic nerve of the superior cervical ganglion of the rat. Depression of action potential amplitude was induced following exposure to the general anaesthetics, halothane and methoxyflurane; the local anaesthetics, lignocaine, procaine and benzocaine; the biotoxin, tetrodotoxin; a quaternary amine analog of lignocaine, QX–572, and the spin-label molecule, TEMPO. Subsequent exposure of the blocked nerves to high pressure helium resulted in partial, but significant, antagonism of the action potential depression induced by halothane, methoxyflurane, benzocaine, lignocaine or TEMPO. However, no pressure reversal of procaine, QX–572 or tetrodotoxin induced depression was observed.

These findings are constistent with the hypothesis that conduction blockade may be related, in part, to membrane expansion following penetration of the uncharged form of local anaesthetic into the interior of the cell membrane. Since QX–572 and tetrodotoxin exist only in a charged form, these agents presumably are incapable of membrane expansion. The absence of pressure antagonism to procaine is probably related to the high pK_a of this agent, which means that at a pH of 7.4 less than 5 per cent of procaine exists in an uncharged form. These findings by Kendig and Cohen (1977) differ from the results of Boggs et al. (1976). The latter investigators utilized the rat phrenic nerve and desheathed frog sciatic nerve to study the interaction of high pressure and local anaesthetic blockade. The spin-label molecule TEMPO produced a 68 per cent decrease in action potential amplitude at normal atmospheric pressure. Upon application of 100 atm of helium pressure, a further reduction of 14 per cent in action potential height occurred. High pressure had no observable effect on the action potential depression produced by lignocaine and benzyl alcohol. Thus it appears that high pressure may enhance, antagonize or exert no effect on conduction blockade produced in peripheral nerves by various local anaesthetic substances.

A number of modifications of the membrane expansion theory have been proposed, all of which are based on an intramembrane site of anaesthetic action. A variety of experimental techniques such as nuclear magnetic resonance (NMR) have been employed to study changes in the fluidity of model membranes following exposure to local anaesthetic agents. Phospholipid membranes may undergo a transition from a gel crystalline to a liquid crystalline state. Various clinically useful local anaesthetics such as procaine, lignocaine, tetracaine and bupivacaine have been shown to increase the fluidity of these phospholipid membranes. This increase in the freedom of movement of lipid molecules within the membrane may occur with or without a concomitant increase in the volume of the membrane. For example, the increase in fluidity or disorder of the lipid molecules may result in conformational changes in the membrane proteins which are closely associated with the lipids. The concept of increased fluidity of lipid molecules resulting either in an expansion of the membrane or in a conformational change in membrane proteins is consistent with the fluid mosaic membrane model proposed by Singer and Nicholson (1972).

Irrespective of the precise membrane perturbation produced by local anaesthetics, the common feature of these various theories involves a decrease in the diameter of the sodium channel or a prevention of sodium channel opening upon membrane activation. Therefore the local anaesthetics are perceived as penetrating the interior of the cell membrane, producing a conformational change in the membrane which maintains the sodium channels in a closed state, resulting in decreased sodium permeability and ultimately conduction blockade. Although the site of local anaesthetic action within the nerve membrane is attractive from a theoretical point of view, it is difficult to prove experimentally that membrane conformational changes can produce conduction blockade. In addition, although the evidence strongly suggests that uncharged forms of local anaesthetics may act from within the cell membrane, the data are not equally strong regarding charged local anaesthetics. Finally, some data exist which indicate that local anaesthetics stabilize and inhibit conformational changes in certain membranes (rat liver mitochondria) rather than inducing alterations in membrane configuration.

Specific receptor sites within the sodium channel

The third and most common site proposed for the action of local anaesthetic agents involves specific receptors within the sodium channel. The concept of a specific receptor site for local anaesthetic activity is based on the following information: (1) *in vitro* biochemical evidence that local anaesthetic agents can bind to phospholipids and/or proteins; (2) specificity of optical isomers of local anaesthetic drugs; (3) selectivity of binding of the biotoxins tetrodotoxin and saxitoxin; and (4) modulation of local anaesthesia by the frequency of nerve stimulation.

In vitro binding studies

It has been demonstrated that local anaesthetic agents are capable of binding both to phospholipids and proteins. Feinstein (1964) suggested that one local anaesthetic molecule may serve as an electrostatic bond between the negatively charged phosphate groups of two phospholipid molecules. In addition, evidence exists for the formation of hydrogen bonds between local anaesthetics and phospholipids. Protein binding of local anaesthetics has also been well documented. Studies on nerve homogenates revealed that approximately 75 per cent of tetracaine is bound to proteins as compared to 6 per cent for procaine. Subsequent studies with plasma proteins have shown that all amide-type local anaesthetics are capable of binding to protein, but to varying degrees. A direct correlation exists between the degree of protein binding and the duration of conduction blockade. For example, action potentials recorded from the surface of an isolated frog sciatic nerve are depressed by 50 per cent following exposure to 20 mmol/l of lignocaine but return to their control height within 30 minutes following removal of lignocaine from the bathing solution. Similar experiments with bupivacaine or etidocaine show that approximately 2 hours is required for complete reversal of conduction blockade. In terms of protein binding, lignocaine is 55 per cent bound to plasma protein. It is acknowledged that these studies do not prove that local anaesthetics combine with a specific receptor in the membrane. Nevertheless, the fact that these agents can bind to lipoproteins, the lipoprotein composition of the nerve membrane and the relationship betweeen protein binding and anaesthetic activity are certainly suggestive of a local anaesthetic-lipoprotein receptor interaction.

Specificity of optical isomers of local anaesthetics

Akerman (1973) studied the optical isomers of a series of different local anaesthetics including certain agents which are employed clinically (e.g. prilocaine, mepivacaine and bupivacaine). For example, the levo form of prilocaine was twice as potent as the dextro form in terms of producing corneal anaesthesia in rabbits and cutaneous anaesthesia in guinea-pigs. Studies on the isolated sheathed and desheathed frog sciatic nerve showed as much as a fivefold difference in conduction blocking activity betweeen the isomers of different local anaesthetics; for example, l-bupivacaine was approximately four times more potent than d-bupivacaine. The most detailed study concerning site and mechanism of action of optical isomers was carried out with an experimental compound, RAC 109. This local anaesthetic substance is a succinimide derivative, in contrast to an agent such as lignocaine which is an anilide derivative. The enantiomers of RAC 109 were designated simply RAC 109 I and RAC 109 II. Although the absolute configuration of these two isomers is not known, they do possess opposite steric configurations. Measurements of the maximum rate of rise of the action potential of the squid axon revealed that 1.0 mmol/l of RAC 109 I caused an 88 per cent reduction in the maximum rate of depolarization following internal perfusion, whilst the same concentration of RAC 109 II produced only a 53 per cent decrease in the maximum rate of depolarization. Subsequent voltage clamp studies on the frog sciatic nerve demonstrated a 76 per cent reduction in sodium conductance following application of 0.28 mmol/l of RAC 109 I, but only a 42–57 per cent decrease in sodium permeability when RAC 109 II was used. Thus, RAC 109 II was approximately 20–60 per cent more active than RAC 109 I in terms of decreasing the rate of depolarization and sodium conductance. In addition, the minimum concentration (C_m) of RAC 109 II required for conduction blockade in sheathed frog sciatic nerve was five times less than that of RAC 109 I. In the desheathed preparation a threefold difference in C_m existed between the two isomers. Although these results are suggestive of a stereospecific local anaesthetic receptor, the possibility remained that the difference in activity between isomers might be related to differential uptake and penetration of the membrane. This possibility was evaluated by Akerman (1973) in several ways. The uptake of radioactive RAC 109 I and II by both sheathed and desheathed frog sciatic nerves was measured and no difference was observed in the uptake of the two isomers by the isolated sciatic nerve. Additional studies also failed to reveal any difference between the uptake and binding of radioactive RAC 109 I and II to erythrocyte and synaptosome membranes or to the phospholipid phosphatidylserine, which is known to be a component of nerve membrane. Since the isomers of RAC 109 penetrate membranes to the same extent and possess similar physicochemical properties and similar proportions of charged and uncharged form, their differential anaesthetic potencies would be difficult to explain in terms of the surface charge theory or the change in membrane volume or configuration hypothesis. The action of the optical isomers of RAC 109 is consistent with the concept of differential binding to sterospecific receptors located at the opening of the sodium channel on the inner surface of the nerve membrane.

Selectivity of binding of biotoxin tetrodotoxin and saxitoxin

Other agents exist which are capable of causing conduction blockade and which may act at specific receptor sites other than that described for the conventional type of local anaesthetic drug. Specifically, several naturally occurring biotoxins (e.g. saxitoxin and tetrodotoxin) exist which are capable of producing profound conduction blockade in isolated nerves but appear to act at the external surface of the nerve membrane rather than the internal surface. These substances are unique biologically, since they act specifically on the sodium channel to inhibit sodium conductance. Their site of action appears to be located on the external surface of the sodium channel, since internal and external perfusion of the giant squid axon with solutions of tetrodotoxin (TTX) revealed that external perfusion with 1×10^{-7} mol/l resulted in inhibition of a propagated action potential within 3–6 minutes (Narahashi, Anderson and Moore, 1967). On the other hand, axoplasmic perfusion with 1×10^{-6} mol/l and 1×10^{-5} mol/l TTX for as long as 17–37 minutes had no effect on the maximum rate of rise of the action potential. Moreover, Colquhoun and Ritchie (1972) and Henderson, Ritchie and Strichartz (1973) showed that conventional local anaesthetics such as lignocaine, which act at the internal surface of the nerve membrane, do not alter the binding of the biotoxins to the membrane.

A competitive antagonism does exist between TTX and saxitoxin (STX). Henderson, Ritchie and Strichartz (1973) demonstrated that the specific binding of 4 nmol/l of STX to frog myelinated fibres was reduced by 95 per cent when 500 nmol/l of TTX was added to the perfusion medium. Divalent ions such as calcium which are believed to act at the external surface of the nerve membrane also are capable of displacing TTX and STX from membrane-binding sites. For example, in the absence of calcium, 100 per cent of TTX and STX is bound to solubilized garfish membrane preparations. In the presence of 50 mmol/l of calcium, only 28 per cent of TTX and 34 per cent STX was bound to the garfish membrane preparation.

The binding of the biotoxins to the external opening of the sodium channel is so specific that these agents have been utilized to determine the size and number of sodium channels in various nerve preparations. Hille (1971) calculated that the external opening of the sodium channel is a space 30 nm wide by 50 nm long lined by six oxygen atoms. One molecule of TTX or STX will occupy one sodium channel opening. On the basis of the studies with TTX and STX, it was concluded that approximately 30 sodium channels/cm^2 exist in the rabbit vagus nerve, whereas in the unmyelinated fibres of the garfish olfactory nerve there are only six sodium channels/cm^2. However, studies utilizing an improved method for labelling STX indicated a significantly greater density of sodium channels. Data presented by Ritchie, Roghart and Strichartz (1976) based on STX-binding sites calculated 110 sodium channels/cm^2 in garfish nerves.

In summary, the investigations with the biotoxins provide additional evidence that the basic mechanism of local anaesthesia involves combination with a specific membrane receptor which is located at the sodium channel. The only difference between the biotoxins and the conventional local anaesthetics such as lignocaine is the receptor site location. The biotoxin receptor apparently is located at the external opening of the sodium channel whilst the receptor for the conventional local anaesthetics is present at the internal opening of the sodium channel.

Modulation of local anaesthesia by frequency of nerve stimulation

A number of studies have been conducted which show that the effect of local anaesthetics on the sodium conductance and action potential of nerves is influenced by the rate of stimulation of a nerve at the time of local anaesthetic application (Fig. 11.8). Strichartz (1973) demonstrated that the quaternary derivative of lignocaine, QX–314, could inhibit sodium currents by more than 90 per cent following axoplasmic perfusion of the frog sciatic nerve. Application of depolarizing pulses of 5 milliseconds' duration at 1–second intervals enhanced the rate and degree of sodium permeability inhibition produced by QX–314. This phenomenon has been referred to as 'use-dependent inhibition'. An increase in frequency of stimulation without a local anaesthetic does not affect the sodium currents. In the absence of depolarizing pulses, QX–314 requires 20–30 minutes to produce maximum inhibition of sodium permeability. A combination of internal perfusion of the membrane with QX–314 and application of 20 depolarizing pulses caused maximal inhibition of sodium permeability within 5 minutes. In addition, a direct correlation exists between the frequency of nerve stimulation and the degree of sodium conductance blockade.

Similar studies were conducted by Courtney (1975) with tertiary-amine-type

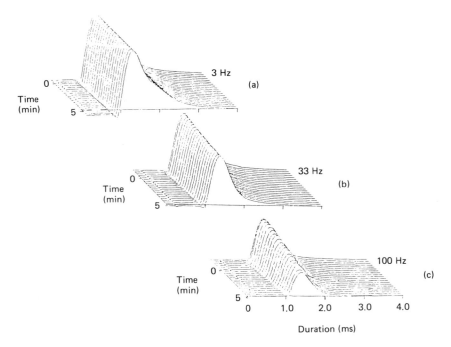

Fig. 11.8   Reduction in height of nerve action potential as a function of frequency of stimulation in the presence of lignocaine: (a) decrease in action potential amplitude at 3 Hz; (b) decrease in amplitude of action potential at 33 Hz; (c) decrease in height of action potential at 100 Hz.

of local anaesthetic agents. Most of the experiments were performed with an experimental tertiary amine compound, GEA 968, which is structurally related to lignocaine. Again, a direct correlation was found between the frequency of stimulation and the degree of inhibition of inward sodium currents in myelinated frog nerves. In the presence of 0.5 mmol/l of GEA 968, repetitive depolarization at the rate of 2 pulses per second resulted in a progressive decrease in sodium conductance, such that inward sodium current was decreased by 76 per cent after 25 pulses. Similar frequency-dependent inhibition of sodium permeability was observed with procaine and lignocaine, although frequencies of at least 2 pulses per second were required to clearly demonstrate this relationship with lignocaine.

Following maximal depression of sodium permeability and a period of rest, the inhibitory effect of both tertiary amine and quaternary-type local anaesthetics can be reversed by an increase in the frequency of nerve stimulation. Under conditions in which a large hyperpolarizing prepulse is applied to the nerve followed by a series of depolarizing pulses, the rate of reversal of local anaesthetic activity is directly related to the frequency of stimulation.

This phenomenon of use or frequency-dependent inhibition has been interpreted in the following manner. At rest, sodium channels are closed, which prevents sodium flux across the membrane. During nerve stimulation, the sodium channels open to allow the influx of sodium ions which is essential for membrane depolarization. An increase in the frequency of stimulation will permit the sodium channels to remain in an open state for a longer period of time. In addition, the degree of depolarization pulses will determine the number of channels that are open. The size and number of depolarizing pulses basically affect the phase of sodium activation. Application of a hyperpolarizing prepulse to the membrane is believed to prevent the phase of sodium inactivation. thus the combination of a hyperpolarizing prepulse and a series of depolarizing pulses of optimal size will maximize the number and duration of sodium channels opened. Both tertiary and quaternary local anaesthetic activity are enhanced. The onset of conduction block is decreased and the duration of blockade is shortened when the gates of the sodium channels are open. This strongly supports the concept that a specific local anaesthetic receptor is located within the sodium channel which is readily accessible when sodium channels are in the open position.

Multiple vs. single site of anaesthetic action

On the basis of studies with various substances which can produce conduction blockade in peripheral nerve, two theories have evolved concerning the site of action of local anaesthetic agents. One theory suggests that various sites of action exist for conduction-blocking agents of different chemical types. The following classification summarizes the different sites of action which may exist in the nerve membrane.

1.   External surface of the sodium channel. The biotoxin substances tetrodotoxin and saxitoxin are believed to act at this location.
2.   The axoplasmic side of the sodium channel. The quaternary derivatives of lignocaine such as QX–314, QX–572 and QX–222 act at this site.

3.   Within the nerve membrane, causing an expansion of the membrane or a change in membrane configuration. Agents such as benzocaine, *n*-butanol and benzyl alcohol (i.e. the neutral type of local anaesthetic drugs) are believed to cause conduction block in this fashion.

4.   Site of action both at the axoplasmic side of the sodium channel and within the membrane. Most of the clinically useful local anaesthetic agents, since they exist both in charged and uncharged form (e.g. procaine, amethocaine, lignocaine, mepivacaine, prilocaine, bupivacaine and etidocaine) are believed to act at these sites. The cationic form of these drugs would interact with a specific receptor in the axoplasmic portion of the sodium channel whilst the uncharged base form would act by a physicochemical mechanism within the membrane. Narahashi and Frazier (1975) have suggested that approximately 90 per cent of the blocking action of an agent such as lignocaine is referable to its cationic form and 10 per cent is due to the base form.

In the second, Hille (1984) has attempted to provide a unified theory for the site of action of both charged and uncharged forms of local anaesthetic drugs. He employed a voltage clamp technique to study the action of tertiary amine, quaternary amine and neutral type local anaesthetics on sodium conductance in myelinated fibres of the isolated frog sciatic nerve. Hille's theory was based on a re-evaluation of the relationship between lipid solubility, pH, voltage and frequency-dependent modulation and the rate, degree and reversal of local anaesthetic depression of sodium permeability. The time required to block half of the sodium currents varied as a function of the pK_a, the lipid solubility of the compounds and the pH of the bathing solution. In general, low pK_a, high lipid solubility and high pH enhance the onset of blockade. The results again demonstrated that the onset of action of neutral and charged agents is pH independent and the quaternary amine agents which exist only in the charged

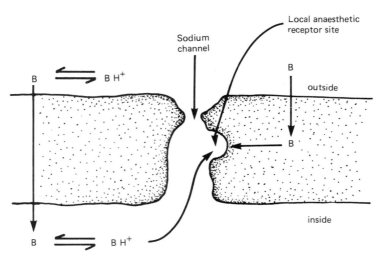

Fig. 11.9   Diagram of sodium channel in nerve membrane, depicting pathways by which local anaesthetics may reach the receptor site according to the hypothesis of Hille.

form are relatively inactive when applied to the external surface of the nerve. In addition, tertiary amine and quaternary amine molecules demonstrate voltage- and frequency-dependent inhibition, but the neutral agent benzocaine did not show a similar effect.

The model proposed by Hille (1984) involves a single receptor in the sodium channel for neutral, tertiary and quaternary types of local anaesthetics. However, differences do exist in the pathways which these various substances use to reach the receptor site. The hydrophilic quaternary amine compounds such as QX–314 are unable to penetrate the lipid-rich membrane. Thus these agents can reach the receptor site only from the internal aqueous medium when the sodium channels are open. The neutral lipophilic agents such as benzocaine penetrate into the core of the lipid membrane and use a hydrophobic pathway to reach the receptor site even when sodium channels are in the closed or inactive state (Fig. 11.9). Since tertiary amines such as procaine and lignocaine exist both in a charged hydrophilic and an uncharged lipophilic form, they may reach the receptor site by both the hydrophilic and hydrophobic pathways. The uncharged base utilizes the hydrophobic path and so can reach the receptor site while the sodium channel is in the closed or inactivated state. The cationic form must use the hydrophilic pathway and so can reach the receptor only when the sodium channels are open (Fig. 11.9). Hille's hypothesis does not account for the action of the biotoxins at the external surface of the sodium channel. However, the chemical configuration of the biotoxins is sufficiently different from other types of local anaesthetic agents that they may be unable to enter the inner aperture of the sodium channel even when the gates are open, but may be able to reach the local anaesthetic receptor from the external surface of the sodium channel.

Active form of conventional local anaesthetics

In solution, the clinically useful local anaesthetic agents exist both in the form of uncharged molecules (B) and as positively charged cations (BH$^+$). The relative proportion between the uncharged base (B) and the charged cation (BH$^+$) is dependent on the pH of the solution and the pK_a of the specific chemical compound, and can be determined by the Henderson–Hasselbalch equation:

$$pH = pK_a - \log (B)/(BH^+)$$

Since pK_a is constant for any specific compound the relative proportion of free base and charged cation in a local anaesthetic solution is basically dependent on the pH of the solution. As the pH of the solution is decreased and hydrogen ion concentration is increased, more of the local anaesthetic will exist in the charged cationic form. Conversely, an increase in pH and decrease in hydrogen ions will result in the formation of relatively greater amounts of the free base form. Ritchie, Ritchie and Greengard (1965a, b) conducted a series of experiments which evaluated the relationship between the pH of solutions of lignocaine and dibucaine and local anaesthetic activity in isolated sheath and desheathed nerves. When isolated nerves possessing an intact sheath were used, it was found that as the pH of the bathing solution containing either lignocaine or dibucaine was raised from 7.2 to 9.2, the rate of reduction in the height of the surface action potential was markedly increased. Thus, alkaline solutions containing relatively greater amounts of the uncharged base (B) were more active in supressing electrical activity of the sheath nerve. However, when the experiments were repeated with a desheathed nerve preparation, the results differed. At a pH of 7.2, dibucaine (10 μmol/l) produced a 90 per cent reduction in spike potential amplitude, whereas only a 10 per cent depression in spike potential occurred when the pH was elevated to 9.2. Similarly, 300 μmol/l of lignocaine produced almost complete abolition of the spike potential at a pH of 7.2. In an alkaline solution (pH 9.2–10.7), the same concentration of lignocaine resulted in only a 50 per cent decrease in action potential amplitude. Under these experimental conditions, the less alkaline local anaesthetic solution, which would contain a relatively greater amount of the charged cation (BH^+), was more active in terms of conduction blockade. Additional evidence favouring the cationic moiety as the active form of local anaesthetics was forthcoming from experiments by Narahashi and colleagues (Narahashi, Yamada and Frazier, 1969; Narahashi, Frazier and Yamada, 1970), who studied the conduction-blocking properties of two tertiary and two quaternary derivatives of lignocaine. The tertiary amine derivatives can exist in a partially charged/uncharged form, whereas the quaternary compounds possess only a charged configuration. When the tertiary amine compounds were applied to the external surface of the axon, a 13 per cent decrease in the maximum rate of rise of the action potential (dV/dt) was observed. Increasing the pH from 7.0 to 9.0 did not affect the degree of reduction in dV/dt. Internal perfusion of the tertiary amine at a pH of 7.0 caused a 57 per cent decrease in dV/dt. However, only a 20 per cent reduction in dV/dt occurred when the pH of the internal perfusion medium was elevated to 8.0. Since the increase in pH would tend to lower the relative concentration of the cationic form of the local anaesthetic, these results again demonstrate that the charged moiety is primarily responsible for conduction blockade. However, tertiary amines are capable of diffusing across membranes, so they are effective conduction blockers ·following either external or internal application. In order to overcome the problem of diffusion, quaternary derivatives of lignocaine were utilized. These compounds exist only as cations, which do not diffuse readily across membranes. External application of 10 mmol/l of the quaternary compound QX–314 produced less than a 10 per cent decrease in dV/dt in the squid axon. Internal perfusion of 1 mmol/l of QX–314 caused a mean reduction of 67 per cent in dV/dt. Strichartz (1973) extended these studies by determining the effects of the quaternary derivatives of lignocaine on sodium permeability of the frog sciatic nerve. External application of 5 mmol/l of QX–314 decreased the amplitude of the inward sodium currents by 7 per cent. By contrast, internal application of only 0.5 mmol/l of QX–314 diminished the sodium currents by almost 90 per cent. Since all the above studies were carried out with lignocaine and its derivatives, Narahashi, Frazier and Yamada (1970) investigated the effects of internal and external perfusion of procaine at different pH levels on the sodium permeability of the squid axon. The results demonstrated that procaine also acts primarily in the cationic form at the internal opening of the sodium channel.

On the basis of these observations, it has been postulated that the uncharged base of local anaesthetics is responsible for optimal diffusion through the nerve sheath. After penetration of the nerve sheath and the nerve membrane, re-equilibrium occurs between the base and cationic forms in the axoplasm and the charged cationic form of the drug then diffuses to the receptor site within the sodium channel. The attachment of the cationic form of the local anaesthetic to the receptor in the sodium channel results in a decrease in sodium conductance which, in turn, causes conduction blockade.

Differential nerve blockade

Classically, the susceptibility of nerves to conduction blockade was considered to be related to the fibre size; that is, a greater concentration of local anaesthetic agent is required to block nerves of large diameter. This relationship between fibre size and anaesthetic sensitivity in myelinated nerves may be a function of the length of nerve fibre and number of nodes exposed to the local anaesthetic solution. Exposure of 4 mm of myelinated nerves to 0.2 per cent procaine results in complete blockade of all fibres, However, reduction in the length of fibre exposure to 2 mm causes blockade of the A δ fibres, but not the A α fibres. Since the number of nodes of Ranvier is inversely proportional to the diameter size of the fibre, more nodes would be exposed to local anaesthetic solution per millimetre of fibre length in the A δ fibres as compared to the A α fibres. If a critical number of nodes must be blocked to insure complete inhibition of a propagated action potential, the conduction in the smaller A δ fibres will be blocked at a lower minimal anaesthetic concentration (C_m) than the larger myelinated fibres.

Although a relationship between fibre size and anaesthetic sensitivity may exist within fibres of the same classification, data have been presented which indicate that a similar relationship may not exist between fibres of different types. For example, C fibres may continue to transmit impulses when conduction blockade by a local anaesthetic is complete in A α and A δ fibres. In addition, the C_m of myelinated B fibres was found to be significantly lower than the C_m for unmyelinated C fibres. In fact, the C_m for 50 per cent suppression of action potential amplitude of B fibres was only 25–30 per cent of that required for C fibres; for example, C_m for tetracaine and prilocaine for B fibres was 5 and 10 μmol/l respectively, compared to concentrations of 20 and 300 μmol/l for C fibres. Condouris, Goebel and Brady (1976) used a computer simulation of local anaesthetic blockade to study the characteristics of blockade produced by TTX and lignocaine. The computer model indicated that myelinated nerves were more susceptible to local anaesthetic blockade than were unmyelinated nerve fibres.

Gissen, Covino and Gregus (1980, 1982a, b) re-evaluated the C_m of various local anaesthetics in mammalian A, B and C fibres. The C_m of lignocaine, amethocaine, etidocaine and bupivacaine required to produce a 50 per cent decrease in the amplitude of the action potential of A and B fibres from the desheathed rabbit vagus nerve was significantly less than the C_m required for unmyelinated C fibres (Table 11.1). These in vitro results appear to differ from in vivo clinical studies in which differential nerve blockade may be achieved

Table 11.1   Minimum blocking concentration (mmol/l) of various local anaesthetic agents on A, B, and C fibres of rabbit vagus or sciatic nerve

Drug	Fibre type		
	A	B	C
Lignocaine	0.12	0.44	0.55
Amethocaine	0.009	0.014	0.024
Etidocaine	0.047	0.073	0.145
Bupivacaine	0.083	0.126	0.159

by alterations in the concentration of local anaesthetic injected. For example, low concentration of procaine administered intrathecally is associated with sensory blockade. As the concentration of procaine is increased, sympathetic block (inhibition of B fibres) and finally motor blockade (inhibition of A fibres) can be achieved. Gissen, Covino and Gregus (1982a, b) have attempted to explain these apparently conflicting results as follows: in isolated nerves exposed to low concentrations of local anaesthetics, a reduction in the action potential amplitude of C fibres is initially observed. With time, the action potential of A fibres begins to show suppression and ultimately the degree of A fibre action potential depression exceeeds that of the C fibres, indicating that at equilibrium the C_m for A fibres is less than that for C fibres. *In vitro*, however, the isolated nerve is devoid of circulation such that the local anaesthetic remains in continuous contact with the nerve fibres. *In vivo* with intact circulation, some of the local anaesthetic injected in the region of a peripheral nerve will diffuse to the nerve membrane whilst some of the local anaesthetic will be absorbed by the vascular system and carried away from the site of injection. Thus, following injection of a low concentration of local anaesthetic in an intact animal a sufficient amount of drug may penetrate to the non-myelinated C fibres which do not have many diffusion barriers and cause conduction block of these sensory fibres. However, the large myelinated fibres are protected by diffusion barriers such that, as the local anaesthetic slowly penetrates to the nerve membrane of the A fibres, it is also being absorbed by the vascular system, resulting in a significant decrease in the amount of drug which ultimately will reach the receptor site at the nerve membrane. If the absorption of local anaesthetic is sufficient to reduce the concentration of drug arriving at the nerve membrane of the A fibre to below the C_m for that particular fibre, conduction block will not occur. Under these conditions it is possible to achieve differential sensory block without significant motor blockade.

A comparison of *in vitro* and *in vivo* studies with etidocaine and bupivacaine would tend to support this hypothesis. The physicochemical properties of bupivacaine tend to favour a slow diffusion of this agent to the site of action on the nerve membrane. Thus, *in vitro* studies show an initial onset of C fibre block with bupivacaine followed at some later time by a more intense block of A fibres. Clinically, the slow diffusional properties of bupivacaine result in essentially sensory anaesthesia without motor block when low concentrations of this agent are employed. On the other hand, etidocaine possesses physicochemical properties which result in rapid diffusion to the nerve membrane. *In vitro*, little difference in the onset of C and A fibre block is seen with this agent and A fibre sensitivity is considerably greater than C fibre sensitivity. *In vivo*, little or no separation between sensory anaesthesia and motor block is observed with etidocaine. In fact, it is not uncommon in certain situations for the degree of motor blockade to exceed the degree of sensory anaesthesia.

In summary, recent neurophysiological studies indicate that the safety margin for conduction blockade is less in large A fibres than in small C fibres following exposure of isolated nerves to local anaesthetics. However, differential sensory/motor blockade is still possible in clinical situations due to differences in the diffusional barriers surrounding A and C fibres and the absorption of injected local anaesthetics by the vascular system.

Relationship between mechanism of action of local anaesthetics and the clinical profile of local anaesthetics

Compounds which demonstrate clinical utility as local anaesthetic agents possess the following chemical arrangement:

Aromatic portion—Intermediate chain—Amine portion

The aromatic portion of the molecule is believed responsible for the lipophilic properties, whereas the amine end is associated with hydrophilicity. Alterations in the aromatic portion, amine portion or intermediate chain of a specific chemical compound will modify its anaesthetic activity (Table 11.2). For example, an increase in molecule weight within a homologous series of compounds, achieved by lengthening the intermediate chain or by the addition of carbon atoms to either the aromatic or the amine portion of the molecule, will tend to increase intrinsic anaesthetic potency up to a maximum, beyond which a further increase in molecular weight results in a decrease in anaesthetic activity. Changes in the aromatic or amine portion of a local anaesthetic substance will alter its lipid/water distribution coefficient and its protein-binding characteristics, which in turn will markedly alter the anaesthetic profile within a series of homologous compounds. A comparison between procaine and amethocaine, which are both ester derivatives of *p*-aminobenzoic acid, reveals that the addition of a butyl group to the aromatic end of the procaine molecule produces a greater than 100-fold increase in lipid solubility and a tenfold increase in protein binding. Such changes in physicochemical properties are reflected in marked alterations in biological activity. For example, the intrinsic anaesthetic potency of amethocaine as determined on an isolated nerve is approximately 16 times greater than that of procaine, whereas the duration of its anaesthetic activity as determined *in vivo* in the rat sciatic nerve preparation is approximately four times longer than that of procaine. Similar relationships exist in the amide series of compounds. The addition of a butyl group to the amine end of mepivacaine, forming bupivacaine, results in a 35-fold increase in partition coefficient and a significantly greater degree of protein binding as compared to mepivacaine. The chemical alterations of mepivacaine to bupivacaine and the subsequent

Table 11.2 Properties of local anaesthetics

Agent	Chemical configuration			Physicochemical properties				Pharmacological properties		
	Aromatic lipophilic	Intermediate chain	Amine hydrophilic	Molecular weight (base)	pKa (25°C)	Partition coefficient	Protein binding (%)	Onset	Relative potency	Duration
Esters										
Procaine	$H-N$, H (benzene ring)	$COOCH_2CH_2-N$	C_2H_5 / C_2H_5	236	8.9	0.02	6	Slow	1	Short
Tetracaine	H_9C_4N, H (benzene ring)	$COOCH_2CH_2-N$	CH_3 / CH_3	264	8.5	4.1	76	Slow	8	Long
Chloroprocaine	H_2N, Cl (benzene ring)	$COOCH_2CH_2-N$	C_2H_5 / C_2H_5	271	8.7	0.14	–	Fast	1	Short
Amides										
Prilocaine	CH_3 (benzene ring)	$NHCOCH$, CH_3	$-N$, H / C_3H_7	220	7.9	0.9	55	Fast	2	Moderate

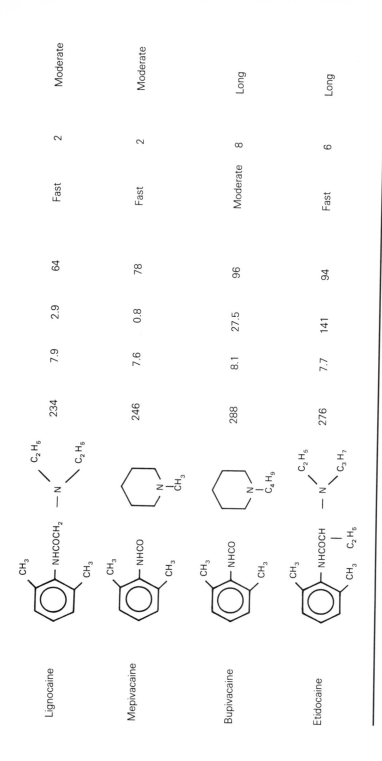

Name	Structure						
Lignocaine		234	7.9	2.9	64	Fast	2	Moderate
Mepivacaine		246	7.6	0.8	78	Fast	2	Moderate
Bupivacaine		288	8.1	27.5	96	Moderate	8	Long
Etidocaine		276	7.7	141	94	Fast	6	Long

modification of physicochemical properties result in a four-fold increase in intrinsic anaesthetic activity and a significant prolongation of anaesthetic duration.

Another example of the relationship between modification of chemical structure and biological activity is found in the comparison of lignocaine and etidocaine. Substitution in the lignocaine molecule of a propyl for an ethyl group at the amine end and the addition of an ethyl group at the α-carbon in the intermediate chain yields etidocaine. These chemical changes in structure produce an increase in partition coefficient of approximately 50-fold and a significant increase in protein binding. As in the previous examples, these alterations in chemical structure and physicochemical properties are reflected in significant changes in biological activity, such that etidocaine possesses an intrinsic anaesthetic potency four times greater than that of lignocaine and a duration of anaesthetic action approximately twice that of lignocaine.

One of the important clinical parameters in regional anaesthesia is the rapidity with which conduction blockade occurs. This pharmacological property of local anaesthetic agents can be evaluated quite accurately in an isolated nerve preparation. Onset time is probably related to the physicochemical properties of these various local anaesthetic agents (e.g. pK_a and lipid solubility). For example, a comparison of agents with similar pK_a values such as lignocaine, prilocaine and etidocaine reveals that the most lipid-soluble drug, etidocaine, demonstrates the most rapid onset of action whereas the least lipid-soluble agent, prilocaine, has the longest latency. Lignocaine occupies an intermediate position in terms of both lipid solubility and onset time. A comparison of highly lipid-soluble compounds with varying pK_a values (e.g. etidocaine, bupivacaine and amethocaine) indicates that etidocaine, which possesses the lowest pK_a, has the most rapid onset of action whereas amethocaine possesses the highest pK_a value and the slowest onset time. The pK_a and latency values for bupivacaine lie between the two extremes. These observations concerning onset time are consistent with the known relationships between pH, pK_a and relative proportion of analgesic agents in the base and cationic forms. The relationship between lipid solubility, protein binding and intrinsic anaesthetic potency and duration are also consistent with the morphology and physiology of the nerve membrane.

On the basis of the physicochemical properties of the various local anaesthetics and their mechanisms of action, it is possible to divide the clinically useful agents into three groups.

1.   Agents of intrinsically low anaesthetic potency and short duration of action (e.g. procaine and chloroprocaine). The low degree of lipid solubility and protein binding of these agents is responsible for their inherently weak anaesthetic activity and short duration of action.

2.   Agents of intermediate anaesthetic potency and duration of action (e.g. lignocaine, mepivacaine and prilocaine). These agents are more lipid soluble and more highly protein bound than the group 1 agents, which results in enhanced anaesthetic activity and longer durations of action.

3.   Agents of high anaesthetic potency and long duration of action (e.g. amethocaine, bupivacaine and etidocaine). These agents are extremely lipid soluble and highly protein bound which renders them the most potent anaesthetics with the longest durations of action.

In terms of onset time, a correlation exists between the pK_a of the various drugs and the onset of conduction blockade. Lignocaine, mepivacaine, prilocaine and etidocaine have pK_as of 7.6–7.9 and demonstrate a rapid onset of action. Procaine possesses a pK_a of 8.9 and shows the slowest onset of conduction block. Although chloroprocaine has a high pK_a and a relatively rapid onset of action clinically, this may simply be related to the ability to use large amounts of this agent clinically due to its relatively low potential for systemic toxicity.

Summary

The concepts regarding the action of local anaesthetic agents have undergone considerable changes, based in part on a greater knowledge of the morphology and physiology of the nerve membrane and the development of more refined experimental techniques to study membrane excitability. Peripheral nerves are enclosed in connective tissue sheaths, the endoneurium, perineurium and epineurium, which essentially act as barriers through which local anaesthetic agents must diffuse. In addition, certain nerve fibres contain a highly lipid myelin sheath and the cell membrane itself is composed primarily of lipids and proteins. Pores are also believed to exist in the lipoprotein axonal membrane through which cations such as sodium may pass. The cell membrane is also believed to undergo conformational changes between the resting and active state. No longer is the cell membrane considered to be a static structure. At rest, an electrical potential difference of approximately -60 to -90 mv exists across the cell membrane, due primarily to the excess concentration of potassium ions within the axoplasm. Application of a threshold stimulus to the nerve membrane results in conformational changes which allow channels in the membrane to change from a closed resting state to an open active state. Sodium ions can then pass through the membrane along its concentration gradient to cause depolarization. In turn, the membrane is repolarized by closure of the sodium channels and by the passive flow of potassium ions out of the cell to the extracellular space.

Local anaesthetic agents inhibit neural excitation by decreasing the permeability of the cell membrane to sodium ions, which prevents depolarization of the cell membrane. The sodium channel is believed to be the site at which the local anaesthetics exert their inhibitory effect on sodium permeability. Local anaesthetics such as lignocaine are believed to combine with a specific receptor within the sodium channel to inhibit sodium conductance and cause conduction blockade. The sequence by which local anaesthetic agents produce inhibition of neural conduction is as follows.

1. The clinically useful local anaesthetic agents exist in solution in both a charged and an uncharged base form. The relative proportion of the charged and uncharged form is dependent upon the pH of the anaesthetic solution, the pH at the site of injection and the specific pK_a of the chemical substance employed.

2. The uncharged base form diffuses through neural sheaths and across the axonal membrane to reach the axoplasmic surface of the sodium channel.

3. In the axoplasm the base form combines with hydrogen ions to yield the

charged cationic form of the local anaesthetic agent, which enters the open sodium channel and attaches to a receptor site inside the internal opening of the sodium channel.

4.   The local anaesthetic drug–receptor interaction results in a decrease in the permeability of the cell membrane to sodium ions.

5.   The decrease in sodium conductance prevents depolarization of the cell membrane, such that it is not possible to decrease the membrane potential to the threshold or firing level.

6.   Failure to achieve the threshold potential level results in a non-propagated action potential and conduction blockade.

References

Aceves, J. and Machne, X. (1963) The action of calcium and local anesthetics on nerve cells and their interaction during excitation. *Journal of Pharmacology and Experimental Therapeutics* **140**, 138–148

Akerman, B. (1973) *Studies on the relative pharmacological effects of enantiomers of local anesthetics with special regard to block of nervous excitation*. Doctoral Dissertation. Uppsala: Sweden.

Boggs, J.M., Roth, S.H., Young, T., Wong, E. and Hsia, J.C. (1976) Site and mechanism of anaesthetic action. II. Pressure effect on the nerve conduction-blocking activity of a spin-label anaesthetic. *Molecular Pharmacology* **12**, 136–143

Chiu, S.Y. and Ritchie, J.M. (1980) Potassium channels in nodal and internodal axonal membrane of mammalian myelinated fibres. *Nature* **284**, 170–171

Colquhoun, D. and Ritchie, J.M. (1972) The interaction at equilibration between tetrodotoxin and mammalian non-myelinated nerve fibres. *Journal of Physiology* **221**, 533–553

Condouris, G.A. (1961) A study of the mechanism of action of cocaine on amphibian peripheral nerve. *Journal of Pharmacology and Experimental Therapeutics* **131**, 243–249

Condouris, G.A., Goebel, R.H. and Brady, T. (1976) Computer simulation of local anesthetic effects using a mathematical model of myelinated nerve. *Journal of Pharmacology and Experimental Therapeutics* **196**, 737–745

Courtney, K.R. (1975) Mechanisms of frequency-dependent inhibition of sodium currents in frog myelinated nerve by the lidocaine derivative GEA 968. *Journal of Pharmacology and Experimental Therapeutics* **195**, 225–236

Frazier, D.T., Narahashi, T. and Yamada, M. (1970) The site of action and active form of local anesthetics. II. Experiments with quaternary compounds. *Journal of Pharmacology and Experimental Therapeutics* **171**, 45–51

Feinstein, M.B. (1964) Reaction of local anesthetics with phospholipids. A possible chemical basis of anesthesia. *Journal of General Physiology* **48**, 357–374

Gissen, A.J., Covino, B.G. and Gregus, J. (1980) Differential sensitivities of mammalian nerve fibers to local anesthetic agents. *Anesthesiology* **53**, 467–474

Gissen, A.J., Covino, B.G. and Gregus, J. (1982a) Differential sensitivity of fast and slow fibers in mammalian nerve. II. Margin of safety for nerve transmission. *Anesthesia and Analgesia* **61**, 561–569

Gissen, A.J., Covino, B.G. and Gregus, J. (1982b) Differential sensitivity of fast and slow fibers in mammalian nerve. III. Effect of etidocaine and bupivacaine on fast and slow fibers. *Anesthesia and Analgesia* **61**, 570–575

Henderson, R., Ritchie, J.M. and Strichartz, G.R. (1973) The binding of labelled saxitoxin to the sodium channels in nerve membranes. *Journal of Physiology* **235**, 783–804

Hille, B. (1966) The common mode of action of three agents that decrease the transient charge in sodium permeability in nerves. *Nature* **210**, 1220–1222

Hille, B. (1968) Pharmacological modifications of the sodium channels of frog nerve. *Journal of General Physiology* **51**, 199–219

Hille, B. (1971) The permeability of the sodium channel to organic cations in myelinated nerve. *Journal of General Physiology* **58**, 599–619

Hille, B. (1984) *Ionic Channels of Excitable Membranes.* Sinauer Associates: Sunderland, MA

Kendig, J.J. and Cohen, E.N. (1977) Pressure antagonism to nerve conduction block by anesthetic agents. *Anesthesiology* **47**, 6–10

Narahashi, T. and Frazier, D.T. (1975) Site of action and active form of procaine in squid giant axons. *Journal of Pharmacology and Therapeutics* **194**, 506–513

Narahashi, T., Anderson, N.C. and Moore, J.W. (1967) Comparison of tetrodotoxin and procaine in internally perfused squid giant axons. *Journal of General Physiology* **50**, 1413–1428

Narahashi, T., Yamada, M. and Frazier, D.T. (1969) Cationic forms of local anaesthetics block action potentials from inside the nerve membrane. *Nature* **223**, 748–749

Narahashi, T., Frazier, D. and Yamada, M. (1970) The site of action and active form of local anesthetics. I. Theory and pH experiments with tertiary compounds. *Journal of Pharmacology and Experimental Therapeutics* **171**, 32–44

Ritchie, J.M, Ritchie, B. and Greengard, P. (1965a) The active structure of local anesthetics. *Journal of Pharmacology and Experimental Therapeutics* **150**, 152–159

Ritchie, J.M., Ritchie, B. and Greengard, P. (1965b) The effect of the nerve sheath on the action of local anesthetics. *Journal of Pharmacology and Experimental Therapeutics* **150**, 160–164

Ritchie, J.M., Rogart, R.B. and Strichartz, G.R. (1976) A new method for labelling saxitoxin and its binding to non-myelinated fibres of the rabbit vagus, lobster walking leg and garfish olfactory nerves. *Journal of Physiology* **261**, 477–494

Roth, S.H., Smith, R.A. and Paton, D.M. (1976) Pressure antagonism of anaesthesia-induced conduction failure in frog peripheral nerve. *British Journal of Anaesthesia* **48**, 621–628

Seeman, P. (1972) The membrane action of anesthetics and tranquilizers. *Pharmacological Reviews* **24**, 583–655

Shanes, A.M., Freygang, W.H., Grundgest, H. and Amatneik, E. (1959) Anesthetic and calcium action in the voltage clamped squid giant axon. *Journal of General Physiology* **42**, 793–802

Singer, S.J. and Nicholson, G.L. (1972) The fluid mosaic model of the structure of cell membranes. *Science* **175**, 720–731

Skou, J.C. (1954) Local anaesthetics. VI. Relation between blocking potency and penetration of a monomolecular layer of lipoids from nerves. *Acta Pharmacologica et Toxicologica* **10**, 325–337

Strichartz, G.R. (1973) The inhibition of sodium currents in myelinated nerve by quaternary derivatives of lidocaine. *Journal of General Physiology* **62**, 37–57

Strichartz, G. (1975) Inhibition of ionic currents in myelinated nerves by quaternary derivatives of lidocaine. *Molecular Mechanisms of Anesthesia*, vol. 1, (Ed. Fink, B.R.), pp. 1–11. Raven Press: New York

Taylor, R.E. (1959) Effect of procaine on electrical properties of squid axon membrane. *American Journal of Physiology* **196**, 1071–1079

12

Opiates and potent analgesics

T.W. Smith and D.J. Chapple

Opiates are now established analgesic and anaesthetic agents. For decades opiates have been synonymous with analgesia, but in the 1970s the prototypic opiate, morphine, also became a popular anaesthetic following an important report by Lowenstein *et al.* (1969) on the use of intravenous morphine in patients with cardiovascular disease. Prior to this, around the turn of the century, morphine had been used as an anaesthetic agent, particularly in combination with scopolamine, but had fallen subsequently from popular use (see review by Bovill, Sebel and Stanley, 1984). With the re-emergence of morphine as an anaesthetic agent, new opiates were researched and developed primarily for use in anaesthesia, these developments leading to the introduction of fentanyl and, more recently, congeners such as alfentanil.

The use of opiates as anaesthetic agents, in either primary or 'balanced' anaesthesia may be based on the specificity of opiates for receptors distributed heterogeneously in the central nervous system (CNS) and their ability in sufficient dosage to induce analgesia and anaesthesia (Stanley, 1982). Receptors specific for opiates were demonstrated in the CNS and led to a search for endogenous opiate-like materials. The isolation and identification of methionine- and leucine-enkephalin as such endogenous opioid ligands (Hughes *et al.*, 1975) and the subsequent demonstrations of families of opioid peptides provided a great boost to opioid research and major advances to our understanding of analgesic mechanisms.

Opioid receptors

Endogenous ligands

Studies of opiates on isolated tissues *in vitro*, particularly the guinea-pig ileum and mouse vas deferens, provided an index of analgesic activity and important information about the structural requirements of opiates for interaction with opioid receptors, particularly of stereospecific requirements (Kosterlitz and Waterfield, 1975). The marked stereospecifity of opiates indicated that these drugs had an affinity for a receptor of correspondingly specific characteristics and was an important factor leading to the concept of selective opioid receptors in the brain. With the advent of tritium-labelled opiates of high specific activity, binding and autoradiographic studies enabled the presence of opioid receptors in the brain to be confirmed (Pert and Snyder, 1973). From these studies, opioid receptors were found to be distributed widely, but heterogeneously throughout the CNS. Among the regions of the brain rich in opioid receptors were areas associated closely with analgesia (e.g. periaqueductal grey). The demonstration of endogenous opioid-specific receptors in the brain led to speculation that an endogenous ligand for these receptors may exist, speculation which culminated in the isolation and identification of the pentapeptides methionine (met)- and leucine (leu)-enkephalin (Hughes *et al.*, 1975). These peptides were clearly opioid in nature and interacted selectively with opioid receptors *in vitro*. The distribution of met- and leu-enkephalin showed a close correlation with the distribution of opioid receptors in the brain, their locations thereby including sites of analgesic importance. *In vivo*, enkephalins were shown to be analgesic on intracere-broventricular administration, although the effects were brief due to rapid metabolism (Belluzzi *et al.*, 1976). A close relationship developed, therefore, between enkephalins and analgesia. More recently this relationship has been extended as evidence has mounted that morphine, enkephalins and stimulation-produced analgesia from electrical, environmental or other stimuli may all share a common physiological substrate. This relationship will be explored in more detail in a later section.

The enkephalins, however, are by no means the only endogenous opioid peptides. Soon after its discovery, the amino acid sequence of met-enkephalin was recognized to be contained within the hormone β-lipotrophin and the fragment of the hormone beginning with the met-enkephalin sequence, β-endorphin, was demonstrated to be a potent opioid peptide producing long-lasting analgesia (see Holaday and Loh, 1981). Dynorphin, a peptide commencing with the leu-enkephalin sequence, is also now recognized as an endogenous opioid peptide of possible major importance. Besides these examples, however, a bewildering array of opioid peptides has now been described, including various extensions of both the met- and the leu-enkephalin sequences, and some examples are shown in Table 12.1. Fortunately, however, recent advances in recombinant genetic cloning techniques have enabled the various opioid peptides to be categorized into three distinct families, dependent upon their precursor molecules (Table 12.2). Thus pro-opiomelanocortin, pro-enkephalin and pro-dynorphin may now be considered as precursors of all the opioid peptides, with β-endorphin, met- and leu-enkephalins and dynorphin possibly representing the most important

Table 12.1   Structure of met- and leu-enkephalin and C-terminal extensions

Met-enkephalin	H.Tyr.Gly.Gly.Phe.Met.OH
Heptapeptide	H.Tyr.Gly.Gly.Phe.Met.Arg.Phe.OH
Octapeptide	H.Tyr.Gly.Gly.Phe.Met.Arg.Gly.Leu.OH
β-Endorphin*	H.Tyr.Gly.Gly.Phe.Met.Thr.Ser.Glu.Lys.Ser...
Leu-enkephalin	H.Tyr.Gly.Gly.Phe.Leu.OH
α-Neo-endorphin	H.Tyr.Gly.Gly.Phe.Leu.Arg.Lys.Tyr.Pro.Lys.OH
Dynorphin (1–17)*	H.Tyr.Gly.Gly.Phe.Leu.Arg.Arg.Ile.Arg.Pro....

*Only partial structures are shown.

Table 12.2   Precursors containing opioid fragments

Precursor	Opioid fragments
Pro-opiomelanocortin	β-Endorphin
Pro-enkephalin	Met-enkephalin (multiple copies)
	Leu-enkephalin
	Met-enkephalin.Arg^6.Phe^7
	Met-enkephalin.Arg^6.Gly^7.Leu^8
Pro-dynorphin	Dynorphin A (1–17)
	Dynorphin B
	α-Neo-endorphin

products of the precursors. Within a precursor molecule, the biologically active opioid fragments are contained between paired basic amino acid residues. In adrenal pro-enkephalin, for example, four copies of met-enkephalin, one of leu-enkephalin and two met-enkephalin C-terminal extensions, met-enkephalin-Arg^6-Phe^7 and met-enkephalin-Arg^6-Gly^7-Leu^8 are bound by pairings of arginine and/or lysine, except the last which is present at the C-terminus of pro-enkephalin (Gubler *et al.*, 1982; Noda *et al.*, 1982).

Multiple opioid receptors

In addition to the large number of endogenous peptides which may interact with opioid receptors, there appears to be more than one type of opioid receptor itself. The concept of opioid receptor subtypes stemmed originally from observations in the chronic spinal dog and led to the proposal of two types of opioid receptor, designated μ and ×-receptors, the prototype ligands being morphine and ketocyclazocine, respectively (Martin, 1967). A third receptor type, the σ-receptor with *N*-allyl normetazocine as prototype, was also described although this receptor may not be opioid in nature.

The multiple opioid receptor concept was substantiated by the use of parallel *in vitro* assays such as the guinea-pig ileum and the mouse vas deferens, and displacement studies of [^{3}H][Leu]enkephalin and [^{3}H]naloxone in homogenates of guinea-pig brain. With these techniques, another subtype, the δ-receptor, was described with leu-enkephalin as the prototype ligand (Lord *et al.*, 1977). The three proposed opioid receptor subtypes μ, × and δ, may be differentiated on isolated tissues, for example, by their relative sensitivity to antagonists such as naloxone, as shown in Table 12.3.

Table 12.3   Opioid receptor classification by naloxone antagonism

Agonist	Naloxone K_e (nmol/l)			
	Guinea-pig ileum	Receptor type	Mouse vas deferens	Receptor type
Normorphine	2.64	μ	1.84	μ
Met-enkephalin	2.45	μ	22.6	δ
Ethylketocyclazocine	14.9	×	11.0	×

K_e is the equilibrium dissociation constant.

Table 12.4 Possible major pharmacological effects mediated by opioid receptor subtypes

Opioid receptor subtype	Typical ligand	Possible effects
μ-Receptor	Morphine Fentanyl	Analgesia Respiratory depression Addictive liability Miosis Muscle rigidity
ϰ-Receptor	Ethylketocyclazocine Dynorphin	Analgesia sedation/dysphoria Miosis
δ-Receptor	Enkephalin	Analgesia(?) Epileptogenesis Behavioural effects

What, then, is the regional distribution of the opioid receptor subtypes? The distribution of total opioid receptors may be achieved using a ligand of high affinity to μ-, ϰ- and δ-sites, and has been described extensively with the use of diprenorphine (Atweh and Kuhar, 1977). To study distribution of individual subtypes, however, one major limitation is the lack of total specificity to the receptor types by the common ligands. In studies using low concentrations of [^{3}H]morphine and [^{3}H][D.Ala^2,D.Leu^5] enkephalin as ligands for μ- and δ-binding sites respectively, however, ratios of μ-selective to δ-selective sites were heterogeneous throughout the CNS, and in the areas associated with analgesic actions, periaqueductal grey, the raphe nuclei and the dorsal horn of the spinal cord, a high predominance of μ-receptors was described (Ninkovic *et al.*, 1981). It has been difficult to associate definitively pharmacological effects mediated by stimulation of the various opioid receptor subtypes in the CNS. This difficulty has arisen primarily due to the lack of selective agonists or antagonists for an individual receptor subtype with little or no affinity for the remaining subtypes. Studies with series of closely related opioid analogues and with ligands of improved specificity, however, have enabled some tentative relationships to be established, as shown in Table 12.4. The common dual effects of opiates used in anaesthetic practice, namely analgesia and respiratory depression, are associated in general with stimulation of μ-receptors although a further subdivision of this receptor type differentiating these two effects has been postulated recently (Ling *et al.*, 1985). Although the use of opioids in anaesthesia is restricted entirely at present to opiates such as morphine and fentanyl, it is interesting to note that at least one short opioid peptide, Tyr-D-Ala-Gly-Phe-D.Leu-NHEt, has been reported to induce anaesthesia (Miller, Saunders and Wheatley, 1980).

Analgesia

The profound analgesia associated with opiates results from interaction with specific opioid receptors distributed heterogeneously throughout the CNS. Over the last two decades, the increasing knowledge of relationships between exogenous opiates, endogenous opioid peptide and analgesia has enabled clear advances to be made in mechanistic approaches to the analgesic action of opioids. Of prime importance in this respect has been the identification of inhibitory neuronal systems arising at supraspinal sites and descending in the spinal column, together with the recognition of the role of the dorsal horn of the spinal cord in analgesic mechanisms.

Descending inhibitory pathways

Opiates

Direct evidence that morphine effects may be elicited by interaction with supraspinal sites was first provided by Tsou and Jang (1964), who demonstrated that analgesia was evoked by injection of morphine into the periaqueductal grey (PAG). Microinjection of opiates into periaqueductal–periventricular regions, resulting in behavioural analgesia, is now well documented. In addition, on local injection into these midbrain loci, naloxone has been shown to reverse morphine-induced analgesia, stereospecificity of the response demonstrated with optical isomers of opiates and local anaesthetics shown to be inactive (see Mayer and Price, 1976). Activation of opioid receptors in the PAG area, therefore, results in analgesia. The analgesic effects initiated by opiates in the PAG, however, may be mediated at the level of the dorsal horn of the spinal cord. Thus, morphine microinjection into the PAG inhibits activity of neurons within the dorsal horn which respond selectively to noxious stimulation. Dorsal horn neuronal activity elicited by non-noxious stimuli is unaffected by such morphine microinjection. Neuronal activity at the spinal cord level resulting from administration of morphine to the PAG must require a neuronal projection from the supraspinal to spinal sites. Such a projection appears to be in part through the dorsal part of the lateral funiculus since opiate responses are attenuated by subtotal lesions of the spinal cord (Basbaum et al., 1977). There are few spinal projections from the PAG to relevant areas of the dorsal horn, however, and the connection includes an important medullary relay, particularly at the nucleus raphe magnus (NRM). There are ample neuronal connections from the PAG to the NRM (and adjacent areas), and terminals of NRM projections may be located in the dorsal horn laminae (Fig. 12.1). Disruption of the NRM–spinal cord projections by lesions of the dorsolateral funiculus inhibits analgesia induced by microinjection of morphine into the NRM.

The importance of the PAG–NRM–spinal cord descending inhibitory system may apply not only to analgesia resulting from direct injections of morphine supraspinally but also to that related to the more widespread use of morphine. Analgesia evoked by systemic administration of morphine has been shown to be reduced or abolished by various manipulations of the descending inhibitory system, including microinjection of naloxone to the NRM, lesions of the NRM and bilateral lesions of the dorsolateral funiculus. Considerable evidence has accumulated, therefore, to suggest that morphine-induced analgesia may result, at least in part, from an increase in descending inhibitions of brainstem origin which control the transmission of pain information at the level of the dorsal horn of the spinal cord.

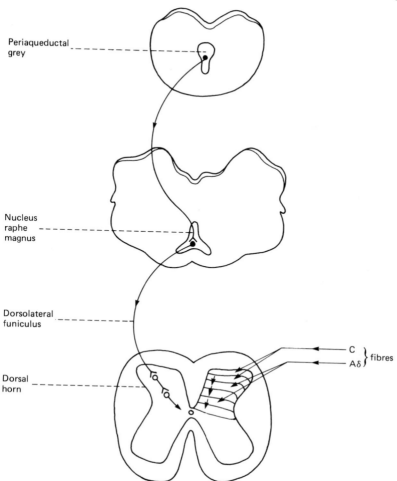

Periaqueductal grey

Nucleus raphe magnus

Dorsolateral funiculus

Dorsal horn

C } fibres
Aδ

Fig. 12.1   The dorsal horn of the spinal cord receiving input from sensory fibres (C and Aδ) and descending projections from supraspinal sites. The descending inhibitory pathways are shown schematically to originate in the periaqueductal grey, relay through the nucleus raphe magnus, descend in the dorsolateral funiculus and terminate at interneurons in the dorsal horn.

This hypothesis, however, remains controversial. One point of issue, for example, is whether morphine-induced analgesia leads to *activation* of descending inhibitory systems. Evidence supporting morphine-induced activation may be exemplified by the studies of Oleson, Twombly and Liebeskind (1978) and Mohrland and Gebhart (1981). In the former study, spontaneous multiple unit activity was recorded at various dorsal raphe nuclei and significantly increased activity was elicited by intravenous morphine administration, particularly in the nucleus raphe magnus. In the latter study, microinjections of morphine in the PAG excited firing in approximately half the neurons examined. In both studies, the doses of morphine used induced analgesia. Electrophysiological studies which do not support brainstem activation, however, include microelectrophoretic application of morphine near the PAG and NRM, producing depression of neuronal firing as the major effect, and intravenous administration of morphine, producing multifarious effects on firing rates of NRM neurons. These and many other studies of the electrophysiological effects of morphine in the brainstem have been reviewed extensively by Duggan and North (1984), who present a critical appraisal of the concept of brainstem activation by morphine. Perhaps of particular importance are those studies where attempts to measure directly descending inhibition of spinal neurons have also failed to show activation; thus Jurna and Grossman (1976) and Duggan, Griersmith and North (1980) observed reduced descending inhibition in animal models after intravenous morphine. These experiments, therefore, argue against morphine-induced activation of descending inhibiting systems, but do not exclude the possibility of morphine-induced analgesia resulting from a reduction of a tonically active descending inhibitory system (Duggan and North, 1984).

Independent of these arguments, an alternative major site for morphine-induced analgesia may be considered, namely direct effects at the level of the dorsal horn of the spinal cord. Before considering this alternative site, however, the clear demonstrations of morphine-induced analgesia arising from application of the opiate to specific supraspinal sites and the involvement of a descending inhibitory system in the expression of this analgesia have important parallels in analgesia elicited not by opiates but by focal electrical stimulation of such supraspinal sites. This in turn has led to promulgation of endogenous opioid and non-opioid *endogenous* analgesic mechanisms, which will now be considered briefly.

Stimulation-induced analgesia
Electrical stimulation at specific brain loci produces analgesia (stimulation-produced analgesia, SPA). This phenomenon was first demonstrated by Reynolds (1969), who showed that electrical stimulation near the border between the PAG and the midbrain reticular formation in rats produced profound analgesia, sufficient to enable surgical procedures to be carried out. Although within the PAG the best sites for SPA do not correspond precisely to the most effective sites for microinjection of morphine (Lewis and Gebhart, 1977), the general level of overlap is striking and the concept that SPA and morphine may share supraspinal sites is an important one. More than this, however, the similarity between the effects of morphine and SPA have led to the proposal that these two stimuli share a common mechanism of action, namely via activation of the PAG–NRM–spinal cord descending inhibitory system (see Mayer and Price, 1976). The close parallelism of SPA and morphine-induced analgesia in this respect may be easily illustrated. Electrical stimulation of the PAG causes excitation of many neurons within the NRM, and stimulation in the PAG or NRM is also attenuated by lesions of the dorsolateral funiculus. The relationship between morphine-induced analgesia and SPA, however, may be identified even more closely. Tolerance, a property invariably associated with repeated administration of opiates, has been observed to the analgesic effects of SPA on repeated stimulation, as has cross-tolerance between SPA and opiates (Mayer and Hayes, 1975). SPA may also

be at least partially antagonized by naloxone, and, following SPA, an enkephalin-like material has been reported to be present in the cerebrospinal fluid of man (Akil, Richardson and Barchas, 1979).

Thus the important concept which has emerged from analgesic studies with exogenously administered opiates and focal electrical stimulation of the brain is that both stimuli may share an endogenous, opioid-mediated, analgesic mechanism utilizing descending inhibitory systems. The ramifications of this endogenous opioid analgesic system extend to other stimuli. Mayer, Price and Rafii (1977) first showed that analgesia produced by acupuncture could be reversed completely by naloxone. These investigators used needling of the ho-ku points in the hands to induce analgesia determined as an increase in the pain threshold to electrical stimulation of the teeth. Other investigators, however, have shown much less dramatic evidence of sensitivity of stimulation techniques to naloxone. Chapman and Benedetti (1977), for example, demonstrated with naloxone only a partial reversal of analgesia obtained with transcutaneous electrical stimulation at facial acupuncture sites. The naloxone-resistant portion of the analgesic response, therefore, arises presumably from stimulation of non-opioid endogenous mechanisms. A clear demonstration that both opioid and non-opioid pathways may be stimulated to produce analgesia in man was described by Sjolund and Eriksson (1979).

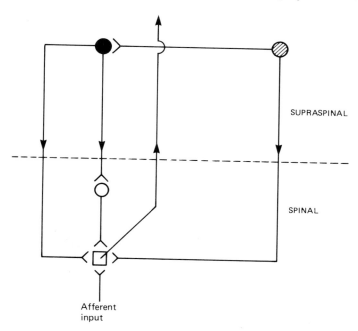

Fig. 12.2 A schematic representation of descending inhibitory systems arising supraspinally and terminating in the dorsal horn of the spinal cord. One descending pathway is suggested to contain 5HT (●) and to exert inhibitory actions directly on dorsal horn cells or through activation of enkephalin-containing neurons (O). A non-opioid-dependent descending inhibitory system (⊘), possibly catecholamine containing, is also shown, modifying afferent inputs of a noxious nature to dorsal horn cells. (Adapted, with permission, from Basbaum *et al.*, 1983.)

In this study, analgesia was elicited by both high-frequency low-intensity and low-frequency high-intensity stimulation, but only that resulting from the latter stimulus parameters could be antagonized by naloxone. Opioid-containing neuronal systems, therefore, may run parallel with non-opioid analgesic pathways; for example, catecholamine-containing pathways (Fig. 12.2) (see Basbaum, Moss and Glazer, 1983).

For any given stimulus or combination of stimuli, the relative degree of involvement of the opioid and non-opioid pathways may be controlled by many factors and a fine balance exists between the systems. In rats, inescapable electric footshock applied at constant intensity can elicit equipotent, but qualitatively different, analgesic responses depending upon the temporal parameters of its application (see Lewis et al., 1984). Exposure to prolonged, intermittent footshock for 20–30 minutes or brief, continuous footshock for 1–2 minutes will produce analgesia which may be antagonized by naloxone or naltrexone. In contrast, rats exposed to brief continuous footshock for 4–5 minutes display an analgesic response equipotent to that derived by the former stimuli, but completely insensitive to opiate antagonists. The respective opioid and non-opioid nature of these responses may be further illustrated. Analgesia elicited by 1 minute of continuous or 20 minutes of intermittent footshock demonstrates tolerance on multiple exposure and cross-tolerance with each other and with morphine, and hence appears to be mediated by opioid mechanisms. The analgesic response to 4 minutes of continuous footshock, however, does not develop tolerance or cross-tolerance with morphine with 1 minute of continuous or 20 minutes of intermittent forms of stress-induced analgesia. Presumably, therefore, it is mediated by non-opioid mechanisms.

Spinal mechanisms

Although opiates applied directly to relevant supraspinal sites such as PAG produce analgesia, these are not the only sites at which opiate-induced analgesia may be initiated. An alternative major site to be considered is the dorsal horn of the spinal cord. Noxious stimuli activate 'pain receptors', and transmission of nociceptive information passes via small-diameter unmyelinated (C) or thinly myelinated (Aδ) fibres which terminate in the discrete laminae of the dorsal horn (Table 12.5). Morphine administered

Table 12.5   Properties of nociceptive afferent fibres

Nociceptor	Stimulus	Nerve type	Properties	Major terminations
High threshold mechanoreceptor	Intense mechanical	Aδ		
			Thiny myelinated conduction	Laminae I, II–inner, III, V
Heat nociceptor	Intense thermal and mechanical	Aδ	2.5–36 m/sec	
C polymodal nociceptor	Noxious, thermal, mechanical and chemical	C	Unmyelinated conduction 0.7–1.5 m/sec	Laminae I, II–outer, V

intrathecally produces analgesia and depresses spontaneous firing. Excitation of dorsal horn neurons elicited by stimulation of unmyelinated fibres or application of a noxious stimulus is also reduced. These morphine-induced effects are generally reversed by opiate antagonists. Intrathecal administration of enkephalins also depresses neuronal excitability of dorsal horn cells, and met-enkephalin-containing cell bodies, axons and nerve terminals have been described within the dorsal horn. The enkephalin content of these neurons is unaffected by rhizotomy or sectioning of the cord, suggesting their nature as local interneurons.

At least part of the descending inhibitory systems arising in the PAG and NRM terminate in the dorsal horn with an opioid synapse. Thus Levine *et al.* (1982) demonstrated that the analgesic effects of morphine administered to the fourth ventricle were completely blocked by intrathecal naloxone. As suggested in Fig. 12.2, this final opioid link in the descending inhibitory system is probably expressed by an opioid-containing interneuron. The enkephalin-containing interneurons described in the dorsal horn, therefore, at least in part, may represent the terminations of a descending inhibitory system, and the analgesia following intrathecal injection of morphine may represent a mimicry of the effects of naturally occurring opioid peptide release from such interneurons.

Opioids generally depress neuronal excitability and enkephalins inhibit both spontaneous and evoked discharges of single neurons. In the spinal cord, two sites of action of enkephalins to depress neuronal excitability have been postulated: presynaptic actions on excitatory neurons or postsynaptic actions directly on cell membranes.

A presynaptic action of opioids has been suggested from studies with cultured spinal neurons; opiate-induced depression of transmitter release from cultured dorsal root ganglion cells, for example, has been demonstrated (Macdonald and Nelson, 1978). This has been supported by demonstrations *in vitro* and *in vivo* of opioid-induced inhibition of release of the putative excitatory transmitter substance P from spinal cord neurons. Information about noxious stimuli is carried to the spinal cord by small diameter fibres which terminate in the superficial layers of the spinal grey matter, namely the marginal layer (lamina I) and the substantia gelatinosa (laminae II–III). Particularly from the substantia gelatinosa, information is relayed to deeper laminae and thence passed via ascending neurons to the brain. Opioid administration to the substantia gelatinosa inhibits the excitation of deeper neurons. Substance P has been postulated as an excitatory transmitter in small diameter nociceptive fibres terminating in the substantia gelatinosa, although this role of substance P is by no means certain (Wall and Fitzgerald, 1982). Jessell and Iversen (1977) demonstrated that potassium-evoked release of substance P from slices of rat spinal trigeminal nucleus was inhibited by opioids in a stereospecific and naloxone-sensitive manner. *In vivo*, morphine has been shown to inhibit substance P release on intrathecal superfusion of the cat spinal cord (Jessell, 1982). From the original *in vitro* observations, a model was proposed whereby enkephalin-containing interneurons found locally in regions of primary afferent synapses provided axo-axonic terminals on substance-P-containing small diameter afferents and hence provided an inhibitory system for selective blockade of nociceptive information by opioids.

Evidence for the existence of such axo-axonic synapses, however, has not been forthcoming and the precise mechanism of opioid inhibition of substance P release remains unclear (Jessell, 1982).

Effective modulation of the transmission of pain information could equally well result from reduction in the effectiveness of released excitatory transmitter as from a reduction in the amount of transmitter released. Evidence for such an effect has been obtained in spinal cord neurons with l-glutamate where the depolarization induced by this excitatory amino acid is reduced by opioids (Zieglgansberger and Tulloch, 1979). The relevance of this finding is obscure, but such an inhibitory effect of opioids may occur by modulation of ion fluxes through a chemically excitable sodium ion channel. Alternatively, opioids may increase potassium ion conductance to produce hyperpolarization of cell membranes. This mechanism has been shown in a number of opioid-sensitive tissues, and rat substantia gelatinosa neurons display hyperpolarization to opioid peptides in a dose-dependent, naloxone-reversible manner. Direct hyperpolarization of a population of substantia gelatinosa cells which are excited by noxious stimuli and may be interneurons in a pain pathway, therefore, could underlie the analgesic effects of opiates at the level of the dorsal horn of the spinal cord (Yoshimura and North, 1983).

Opiates in anaesthesia

Development

Opiates, particularly in high doses, exhibit not only analgesia but also a wide variety of side effects, perhaps the most well known being respiratory depression and tolerance/dependence. One important reason for the reintroduction of morphine–oxygen anaesthesia, however, was the benign

Table 12.6   Advantages and disadvantages of narcotic–oxygen anaesthesia*

Advantages	Disadvantages
Little effect on myocardial mechanics or cardiovascular dynamics	Prolonged postoperative respiratory depression
Increased circulating catecholamines	Chest wall rigidity
Depressed laryngeal and tracheal reflexes	Induction of bradycardia and hypotension
High oxygen levels may be administered	Insufficient dosage leads to inadequate anaesthesia
Blockade of some stress-induced hormonal changes	Return of narcotic effects after antagonists
Little pro-arrhythmic activity	Nitrous oxide-induced cardiovascular depression
Non-toxic and non-allergenic metabolites	

*Compiled from Stanley (1982).

effects of this technique on cardiovascular dynamics; indeed, the report of Lowenstein *et al.* (1969) described the use of morphine in patients with severe aortic valvular disease. The criteria for satisfactory opiate-induced anaesthesia is the production of deep, complete anaesthesia without significant alteration of myocardial mechanics or cardiovascular or respiratory dynamics. A profile of the advantages and disadvantages of narcotic–oxygen anaesthesia is shown in Table 12.6 (Stanley, 1982).

For many years, morphine represented the template on which chemical and pharmacological research on opiates was based. With the potential which opiate-induced anaesthesia appeared to offer, parallel lines of development were opened to find analgesics suitable primarily for use in anaesthesia. Such developments enabled less concern to be placed on abuse and dependence potential and more emphasis to centre on opiate-induced cardiovascular and respiratory effects. The most significant development of this type led to the 4-anilinopiperidine series of opiate agonists and the introduction of fentanyl into clinical practice in the 1960s. More recently, pharmacokinetic consideration has led to the introduction of shorter acting alternatives such as alfentanil.

Cardiovascular effects

The opiates have a wide range of cardiovascular effects depending upon route and rate of administration. The classic opiate, morphine, not only causes its effects by central mechanisms but peripheral mechanisms such as histamine release may also be involved.

Morphine in doses ranging from 0.15 to 3 mg/kv i.v. causes hypotension which can be severe. Although morphine causes histamine release, as evidenced by the triple response seen when injected intradermally, the actual cause of this hypotension is unclear. However, a number of different mechanisms have been postulated in animals and in man. In spinalized cats, morphine will produce hypotension which can be reversed by a H_1-receptor antagonist (Evans, Nasmyth and Stewart, 1952), and recent clinical evidence has shown that after morphine administration plasma histamine levels increase, leading to hypotension. In patients pretreated with a histamine H_1-receptor antagonist together with a histamine H_2-receptor antagonist the hypotensive effects of morphine are reduced (Philbin *et al.*, 1981). Recent *in vitro* studies have demonstrated that the histamine release by morphine is probably not dependent on opiate receptor activity (Hermens *et al.*, 1985). Other mechanisms which may contribute to morphine-induced hypotension include changes in regional blood flow distribution (Priano and Vatner, 1981), reduction in venous and arterial tone (Zelis *et al.*, 1974) and decreases in venous return to the heart (Stanley *et al.*, 1973).

Concurrently with the hypotension, a bradycardia occurs in both humans and animals after morphine administration. Premedication with atropine can minimize the bradycardia induced by morphine (Stanley, 1981) and vagotomy has been found to abolish both the morphine-induced hypotension and the bradycardia in rats and dogs. A central site for these actions has been postulated since injections of morphine into the nucleus ambiguus will cause hypotension and bradycardia (Laubie, Schmitt and Vincent, 1979). Another mechanism for the morphine-induced bradycardia, however, may be an effect on the sinoauricular node, although this is very species dependent (Kosterlitz and Taylor, 1959).

Morphine will also produce hypertension (Stoelting and Gibbs, 1973). As before, the mechanism is unclear but a variety of hypotheses have been put forward. In dogs, morphine has been demonstrated to cause an increase in plasma noradrenaline/adrenaline levels, due probably to release from the adrenal medulla (Kayaalp and Kaymakcalan, 1968) and possibly noradrenaline release from sympathetic nerve endings (Klingman and Maynert, 1962). There is also a possibility that the hypertension is due to reflex mechanisms after hypotension.

Studies with high doses of fentanyl and alfentanil have demonstrated that cardiovascular effects similar to those of morphine may be observed (Liu et al., 1976; Rucquoi and Camu, 1983), although generally (e.g. with alfentanil) blood pressure and heart rate remain stable during anaesthesia irrespective of the type of surgery. Unlike morphine, fentanyl and its analogues do not cause histamine release (Rosow et al., 1984; Hermens et al., 1985).

Pethidine, unlike the other opiate analgesics, causes tachycardia and depresses myocardial contractility together with hypotension (Bovill, Sebel and Stanley, 1984). The tachycardia appears due to atropine-like activity which results in cardiac vagal blockade (Gourlay and Cousins, 1984).

Muscle rigidity

One of the disadvantages of morphine–oxygen anaesthesia is chest wall muscle rigidity (see Table 12.6). Chest wall rigidity (and abdominal wall, face, neck and upper limb rigidity) is also a potential problem with fentanyl and alfentanil (Askgaard et al., 1977; Nauta et al., 1982), at its most severe rendering a patient unable to be ventilated, and less severe as a sensation of stiffness. The high incidence of chest wall rigidity requires the use of benzodiazepine premedication and/or a non-depolarizing skeletal muscle relaxant (Nauta et al., 1982).

Muscle rigidity may result from depression of spinal and monosynaptic reflexes (Sugai, Maruyama and Goto, 1982), and many opiates may interact with nitrous oxide in this effect (Gillman and Lichtigfield, 1983).

Respiratory depression

A common feature of opiate agonists is their ability to produce dose-dependent respiratory depression. In terms of respiration dynamics, low doses of opiates such as morphine and fentanyl reduce respiration rate whilst maintaining or increasing tidal volume to produce a satisfactory minute ventilation (Swerdlow, Foldes and Siker, 1955). Higher doses of opiates depress both respiration rate and tidal volume, the resulting reduction in minute ventilation being lethal. Opiate-induced respiratory changes are accompanied generally by an increase in CO_2 levels, as the responsiveness of those brain centres usually stimulated by CO_2 is reduced. The activity of the reticular formation at the lower brainstem level appears to be of major importance in respiratory control. Opiates, like many other centrally acting drugs, reduce reticular activity and thus CO_2-mediated homoeostatic mechanisms. Opiate effects on respiratory centres, however, are opioid-receptor mediated, probably primarily by μ-receptors, and a close correlation may exist between analgesic potency and respiratory depression. α-agonists are believed not to exhibit such marked respiratory depression.

With the strong relationship between respiratory depression and opiates, the use of opiates in anaesthesia has always been limited by the possibility of respiratory depression outlasting the duration of the operation – a problem potentiated in the postoperative period since opiate-induced respiratory depression may be exacerbated by sleep. The development of opiates for use in anaesthesia, therefore, has favoured short-acting compounds and resulted in the introduction of compounds such as fentanyl and, more recently, alfentanil. Alfentanil (10 μg/kg), for example, reduced minute volume in conscious rabbits for only 5 minutes, peak effects occurring at 1–2 minutes, whereas an equiactive analgesic dose of fentanyl significantly depressed respiration for 15 minutes (Brown, Pleuvry and Kay, 1980). Short-acting opioid agents, therefore, offer the possibility of adapting the dosage to the expected length of the surgical procedures, thereby minimizing postoperative respiratory depression.

References

Akil, H., Richardson, D.E. and Barchas, J.D. (1979) Pain control by focal brain stimulation in man: relationship to enkephalins and endorphins. In: *Mechanism of Pain and Analgesic Compounds* (Eds. Beers, R.F. Jr and Bassett, E.G.), pp. 239–248. Raven Press: New York

Askgaard, B., Nilsson, T., Ibler, M., Jansen, E. and Hansen, J.B. (1977) Muscle-tone under fentanyl–nitrous oxide anaesthesia measured with a transducer apparatus in cholecystectomy incisions. *Acta Anaesthesiologica Scandinavica* 21, 1–4

Atweh, S.F. and Kuhar, M.J. (1977) Autoradiographic localisation of opiate receptors in rat brain. II. The brain stem. *Brain Research* 129, 1–12

Basbaum, A.I., Moss, M.S. and Glazer, E.J. (1983) Opiate and stimulus-produced analgesia: the contribution of monoamines. *Advances in Pain Research and Therapy* 5, 323–339

Basbaum, A.I., Marley, N., O'Keefe, J. and Clanton, C.H. (1977) Reversal of morphine and stimulus produced analgesia by subtotal spinal cord lesions. *Pain* 3, 43–56

Belluzzi, J.D., Grant, N., Garsky, V., Sarantakis, D., Wise, C.D. and Stein, L. (1976) Analgesia induced *in vivo* by central administration of enkephalin in rat. *Nature* 260, 625–626

Bovill, J.G., Sebel, P.S. and Stanley, T.H. (1984) Opioid analgesics in anesthesia: with special reference to their use in cardiovascular anesthesia. *Anesthesiology* 61, 731–755

Brown, J.H., Pleuvry, B.J. and Kay, B. (1980) Respiratory effects of a new opiate analgesic, R39,209, in the rabbit; comparison with fentanyl. *British Journal of Anaesthesia* 52, 1101–1106

Chapman, C.R. and Benedetti, C. (1977) Analgesia following transcutaneous electrical stimulation and its partial reversal by a narcotic antagonist. *Life Sciences* 21, 1645–1648

Duggan, A.W. and North, R.A. (1984) Electrophysiology of opioids. *Pharmacological Reviews* 35, 219–281

Duggan, A.W., Griersmith, B.T. and North, R.A. (1980) Morphine and supraspinal inhibition of spinal neurons: evidence that morphine decreases tonic descending inhibition in the anaesthetised cat. *British Journal of Pharmacology* **69**, 461–466

Evans, A.G.J., Nasmyth, P.A. and Stewart, H.C. (1952) The fall of blood pressure caused by intravenous morphine in the rat and the cat. *British Journal of Pharmacology* **7**, 542–555

Gillman, M.A. and Lichtigfeld, F.J. (1983) Nitrous oxide interacts with opioid receptors: more evidence. *Anesthesiology* **58**, 483–484

Gourlay, G.K. and Cousins, M.J. (1984) Strong analgesics in severe pain. *Drugs* **28**, 79–91

Gubler, U., Seeburg, P., Hoffman, B.J., Gage, L.P. and Udenfriend, S. (1982) Molecular cloning establishes proenkephalin as precursor of enkephalin-containing peptides. *Nature* **295**, 206–208

Hermens, J.M., Ebertz, J.M., Hanifin, J.M. and Hirshman, C.A. (1985) Comparison of histamine release in human skin mast cells induced by morphine, fentanyl and oxymorphone. *Anesthsiology* **62**, 124–129

Holaday, J.M. and Loh, H.H. (1981) Neurobiology of β-endorphin and related peptides. *Hormonal Proteins and Peptides* **10**, 203–291

Hughes, J., Smith, T.W., Kosterlitz, H.W., Fothergill, L.A., Morgan, B.A. and Morris, H.R. (1975) Identification of two related peptapeptides from the brain with potent opiate agonist activity. *Nature* **258**, 577–579

Jessell, T.M. (1982) Substance P in nociceptive sensory neurons. In: *Substance P in the Nervous System*, Ciba Foundation Symposium 91 (Eds. Porter, R. and O'Connor, M.), pp. 225–248. Pitman: London

Jessell, T.M. and Iversen, L.L. (1977) Opiate analgesics inhibit substance P release from rat trigeminal nucleus. *Nature* **268**, 549–551

Jurna, I. and Grossman, W. (1976) The effect of morphine on the activity evoked in ventrolateral tract axons of the cat spinal cord. *Experimental Brain Research* **24**, 473–483

Kayaalp, S.O. and Kaymakcalan, S. (1968) Studies on the morphine-induced release of catecholamines from the adrenal glands in the dog. *Archives Internationales de Pharmacodynamie et de Therapie* **172**, 139–147

Klingman, G.I. and Maynert, E.W. (1962) Tolerance to morphine. III. Effects of catecholamines in the heart, intestine and spleen. *Journal of Pharmacology and Experimental Therapeutics* **135**, 300–305

Kosterlitz, H.W. and Taylor, D.W. (1959) The effect of morphine on vagal inhibition of the heart. *British Journal of Pharmacology* **14**, 209–214

Kosterlitz, H.W. and Waterfield, A.A. (1975) *In vitro* models in the study of structure–activity relationships of narotic analgesics. *Annual Review of Pharmacology* **15**, 29–47

Laubie, M., Schmitt, H. and Vincent, M. (1979) Vagal bradycardia produced by microinjections of morphine-like drugs into the nucleus ambiguus in anaesthetised dogs. *European Journal of Pharmacology* **59**, 287–291

Levine, J.D., Lane, S.R., Gordon, N.C. and Fields, H.L. (1982) A spinal opioid synapse mediates the interaction of spinal and brainstem sites in morphine analgesia. *Brain Research* **236**, 85–91

Lewis, V.A. and Gebhart, G.F. (1977) Evaluation of the periaqueductal central gray (PAG) as a morphine-specific locus of action and examination of morphine-induced and stimulation-produced analgesia at coincident PAG loci. *Brain Research* **124**, 283–303

Lewis, J.M., Terman, G.W., Shavit, Y., Nelson, L.R. and Liebeskind, J.C. (1984) Neural, neurochemical and hormonal bases of stress-induced analgesia. *Advances in Pain Research and Therapy* **6**, 277–288

Ling, G.S.F., Spiegal, K., Lockhart, S.W. and Pasternak, G.W. (1985) Separation of opioid analgesia from respiratory depression: evidence for different receptor mechanisms. *Journal of Pharmacology and Experimental Therapeutics* **232**, 149–155

Liu, W.S., Bidwai, A.V., Stanley, T.H. and Isern-Amaral, J. (1976) Cardiovascular dynamics after large doses of fentanyl and fentanyl plus N_2O in the dog. *Anesthesia and Analgesia* **55**, 168–172

Lord, J.A.H., Waterfield, A.A., Hughes, J. and Kosterlitz, H.W. (1977) Endogenous opioid peptides: multiple agonists and receptors. *Nature* **267**, 495–499

Lowenstein, E., Hallowell, P., Levine, F.H., Daggett, W.M., Austen, W.G. and Laver, M.B. (1969) Cardiovascular response to large doses of intravenous morphine in man. *New England Journal of Medicine* **281**, 1389–1393

Macdonald, R.L. and Nelson, P.G. (1978) Specific opiate-induced depression of transmitter release from dorsal horn ganglion cells in culture. *Science* **199**, 1449–1451

Martin, W.R. (1967) Opioid antagonists. *Pharmacological Reviews* **19**, 463–521

Mayer, D.J. and Hayes, R. (1975) Stimulation-produced analgesia: development of tolerance and cross-tolerance to morphine. *Science* **188**, 941–943

Mayer, D.J. and Price, D.D. (1976) Central nervous system mechanisms of analgesia. *Pain* **2**, 379–404

Mayer, D.J., Price, D.D. and Rafii, A. (1977) Antagonism of acupuncture analgesia in man by the narcotic antagonist naloxone. *Brain Research* **121**, 368–372

Miller, A.A., Saunders, I.A. and Wheatley, P.L. (1980) Behavioural and EEG studies on an anaesthetic enkephalin peptide. *British Journal of Pharmacology* **68**, 159–160P

Mohrland, J.S. and Gebhart, G.F. (1981) Effect of morphine administered in the periaqueductal gray and at the recording locus on nociresponsive neurons in the medullary reticular formation. *Brain Research* **225**, 401–412

Nauta, J., de Lange, S., Koopman, D., Spierdijk, R., van Kleef, J. and Stanley, T.H. (1982) Anesthetic induction with alfentanil; a new short acting narcotic analgesic. *Anesthesia and Analgesia* **61**, 267–272

Ninkovic, M., Hunt, S.P., Emson, P.C. and Iverson, L.L. (1981) The distribution of multiple opiate receptors in bovine brain. *Brain Research* **214**, 163–167

Noda, M., Furutani, Y., Takahashi, H. *et al.* (1982) Cloning and sequence analysis of cDNA for bovine adrenal preproenkephalin. *Nature* **295**, 202–206

Oleson, T.D., Twombly, D.A. and Liebeskind, J.C. (1978) Effects of pain attenuating brain and morphine on electrical activity in the raphe nuclei of the awake rat. *Pain* **4**, 211–230

Pert, C.B. and Snyder, S.H. (1973) Opiate receptors: demonstration in nervous tissue. *Science* **179**, 1011–1014

Philbin, D.M., Moss, J., Akins, C.W. *et al.* (1981) The use of H_1 and H_2 histamine antagonists with morphine anaesthesia: a double-blind study. *Anesthesiology* **55**, 292–296

Priano, L.L. and Vatner, S.F. (1981) Morphine effects on cardiac output and regional blood flow distribution in conscious dogs. *Anesthesiology* **55**, 236–243

Reynolds, D.V. (1969) Surgery in the rat during electrical analgesia induced by focal brain stimulation. *Science* **164**, 444–445

Rosow, C.E., Philbin, D.M., Keegan, C.R. and Moss, J. (1984) Hemodynamics and histamine release during induction with sufentanil or fentanyl. *Anesthesiology* **60**, 489–491

Rucquoi, M. and Camu, F. (1983) Cardiovascular responses to large doses of alfentanil and fentanyl. *British Journal of Anaesthesia* **55**, 223–230S

Sjolund, B.H. and Eriksson, M.B.E. (1979) The influence of naloxone and analgesia produced by peripheral conditioning stimulation. *Brain Research* **173**, 295–302

Stanley, T.H. (1981) The pharmacology of intravenous narcotic anaesthetics. In: *Anesthesia* (Ed. Miller, R.D.), pp. 425–449. Churchill Livingstone: New York

Stanley, T.H. (1982) High-dose narcotic anaesthesia. *Seminars in Anaesthesia* **1**, 21–32

Stanley, T.H., Gray, N.H., Stanford, W. and Armstrong, R. (1973) The effect of high dose morphine on fluid and blood requirements in open-heart operations. *Anesthesiology* **38**, 536–541

Stoelting, R.K. and Gibbs, P.S. (1973) Hemodynamic effects of morphine and morphine–nitrous oxide in valvular heart disease and coronary heart disease. *Anesthesiology* **38**, 45–52

Sugai, N., Maruyama, H. and Goto, K. (1982) Effect of nitrous oxide alone and its combination with fentanyl on spinal reflexes in cats. *British Journal of Anaesthesia* **54**, 567–570

Swerdlow, M., Foldes, F.F. and Siker, E.S. (1955) The effects of nisentil HCl (alphaprodine HCl) and levallorphan tartrate on respiration. *American Journal of Medical Science* **230**, 237–250

Tsou, K. and Jang, C.S. (1964) Studies on the site of analgesic action of morphine by intracerebral microinjection. *Scientia Sinica* **13**, 1099–1109

Wall, P.D. and Fitzgerald, M. (1982) If substance P fails to fulfil the criteria as a neurotransmitter in somatosensory afferents, what might be its function? In: *Substance P in the Nervous System*, Ciba Foundation Symposium 91 (Eds. Porter, R. and O'Connor, M.), pp. 249–266. Pitman: London

Yoshimura, M. and North, R.A. (1983) Substantia gelatinosa neurones hyperpolarized *in vitro* by enkephalin. *Nature* **305**, 529–530

Zelis, R., Mansour, E.J., Capone, R.J. and Mason, D.T. (1974) The cardiovascular effect of morphine: the peripheral capacitance and resistance vessels in human subjects. *Journal of Clinical Investigation* **54**, 1247–1258

Zieglgansberger, W. and Tulloch, I.F. (1979) The effects of methionine and leucine enkephalin on spinal neurones of the cat. *Brain Research* **167**, 53–64

13

Non-opiate analgesics and prostaglandins

H. Mattie

Until recently any chapter on non-opiate analgesics in pharmacology textbooks contained descriptions of many apparently unrelated effects of these drugs in the body. One could only speculate that these effects seemed to result from interference with the inflammatory reaction mechanisms of the body. All this has changed with the growing appreciation that this group of aspirin-like drugs interferes with prostaglandin production. Therefore, before discussion of the non-opiate analgesics, it is necessary that the properties of these so-called autacoids be presented.

Prostaglandins

Prostaglandin was the name given by one of the discoverers to a substance isolated from semen (Von Euler, 1936). At that time only a few functions for this substance could be detected; one was that it stimulates uterine movements. The rediscovery of prostaglandins and their physiological importance has stimulated interest in this field as well as in the mode of action of analgesics which affect their behaviour. At present the name prostaglandin is given to a class of endogenous substances (autacoids) which are derived from arachidonic acid specifically through modification by cyclo-oxygenases. All prostaglandins are related structurally but not functionally. Their structural relationship is such that they may be regarded as analogues of prostanoic acid, a substance which does not occur in nature. Hence the collective name of prostanoids for the group of substances that is formed from arachidonic acid by cyclo-oxygenation (Granström, 1983).

Although different prostaglandins may have different effects, they have a common origin. Arachidonic acid is released rapidly from phospholipids in cell membranes whenever local damage occurs. In addition to local trauma other stimuli (e.g. neuronal or hormonal) can precipitate this initial step, which occurs in virtually all kinds of structures and tissues. From there on, two major pathways of chemical transformation are known: one by cyclo-oxygenation leading to the formation of prostanoids, and one by lipo-oxygenation leading to the formation of leukotrienes. Arachidonic acid itself has no physiological effects, but its addition to *in vitro* systems gives rise to the formation of prostanoids and leukotrienes, and its administration to animals produces the effects of prostanoids and leukotrienes in various organs. Apparently cyclo-oxygenase exists as many isoenzymes. Further enzymatic and non-enzymatic steps lead to the formation of different prostaglandins in different tissues, and also to two other kinds of substances: prostacyclin (also called prostaglandin I_2) and thromboxane A_2. For example, thromboxane A_2 is formed from platelets (Longenecker, 1982) and prostacyclin is readily formed from blood vessel walls (Moncada, Higgs and Vane, 1977). In some tissues prostaglandins are produced very rapidly, whilst in others their production is a slow process. As a broad generalization, it appears that the production of prostanoids and leukotrienes may be regarded principally as a local reaction to injury or related stimuli. In this respect they are not unique, because other substances, such as bradykinin, are also regarded as the product of local response (Higgs and Moncada, 1983). However, the arachidonic acid pathway seems to lead to the most widely differentiated and organ-specific responses.

In order to act locally rather than systemically the prostanoids should not be able to reach other organs in significant concentrations, and indeed most of any drug released into the blood is inactivated in the lungs (Moncada, Flower and Vane, 1980). The discovery that the analgesics act on this system in the body by inhibiting cyclo-oxygenation, but not lipo-oxygenation, of arachidonic acid has been of the utmost importance in allowing an understanding of their mechanism of action. The various effects of prostanoids are therefore discussed here in order to appreciate the manner in which analgesics cause their pharmacological effect.

Effects of prostaglandins

The classic effects of aspirin-like drugs are anti-inflammatory, analgesic and antipyretic. The role of prostanoids in inflammation, pain and fever will therefore be discussed.

Inflammation

Inflammation is one of the most important and vital reaction mechanisms of the body. It leads ultimately to the elimination of noxious agents and to tissue repair after damage. Totally effective suppression of all inflammatory responses would make the body defenceless against otherwise relatively harmless infections. Prostanoids play an important role in the acute inflammatory process, although this is of less importance in long-standing inflammation. They are relatively more important in acute inflammation of many tissues such as soft tissue, joints, skin and gastrointestinal epithelium. Leukotrienes also play a role in some inflammatory reactions (Granström, 1983), but this is secondary to the role of the prostaglandins.

Pain

Pain, although often regarded as a nuisance, is essentially a useful sensation, leading to behavioural response to avoid or minimize exposure to noxious stimuli. Patients without pain sensation are often crippled by the sequelae of all kinds of damage. The mechanism of pain is possibly more complex than that of inflammation itself, but the inflammatory process is often an essential part of the genesis of pain. In many acute inflammations, pain is strongly correlated with the degree of inflammation, and probably both are produced by the same prostaglandins. Prostaglandins applied locally cause signs of inflammation as well as a burning pain sensation. The role of prostaglandins in the central pathways of pain is less well documented. However, it is possible that prostaglandins may play a role, together with many other substances, in the central aspects of pain. Brain tissue is certainly able to form prostaglandins (Curro, Greenberg and Gardier, 1982).

Fever

Fever is part of the inflammatory process; it is most often due to infection, and it improves in some way the chance of survival – hence its ubiquitous occurrence in the animal kingdom (Kluger, 1979). Prostaglandins seem to play no role in the regulation of normal body temperature but they do in fever. It is proposed that exogenous pyrogens (e.g. those of bacterial origin) do not cause fever directly but induce the generation of the endogenous pyrogen interleukin-1 (Dinarello, 1984). This in turn promotes prostaglandin synthesis in the central nervous system, and may be responsible for the febrile response.

Other effects of prostanoids

The effects of prostaglandins on various organ systems are still incompletely understood. They are difficult to interpret because many actions are interdependent. For example, the effect on the vascular smooth musculature may differ, depending upon the organs studied. Moreover, apart from a direct action on vascular musculature there may also be an effect of noradrenergic transmission to the vessel wall (Greenberg, 1982). However, in the uterus, endogenous prostaglandins cause relaxation of vascular smooth muscle and they also depress responsiveness to noradrenaline (Clark and Brody, 1982), whilst in other vascular beds the reverse situation may exist and prostaglandin release itself may be under neurogenic control.

Experimental data on the effects of exogenous administration of various prostaglandins do not always reflect the physiological role of endogenous prostaglandins. Sometimes experiments in which arachidonic acid is administered are more easily understood because it stimulates the formation of endogenous prostaglandins. However, they do not throw much light on the circumstances under which the tissue itself is normally induced to liberate arachidonic acid (James and Church, 1978).

In the rest of this section, possible physiological roles of prostaglandins in various organs will be discussed in the light of what is known about their pharmacological effects in experimental conditions.

Platelets and blood vessels
The interaction of different prostanoids with platelets and blood vessels is a good example of the difficulty in understanding the possible physiological role of these substances (Moncada and Vane, 1979). Platelets can produce only

thromboxane A_2 in significant amounts. Apparently this substance is one of those involved in the aggregation of platelets, although it is by no means the only substance released during platelet aggregation and clotting. By producing thromboxane, platelets are able to induce their own stickiness where and when it is necessary. At the same time a similar injury will cause the vascular epithelium to form prostacyclin, which is an inhibitor of platelet aggregation (Longenecker, 1982). It is possible that the way these prostanoids interact is such to produce a balance: aggregation occurs where it is needed and is inhibited where it might be harmful.

Kidney

The autoregulation of renal function is still incompletely understood, but it seems probable that prostaglandins play an important role under some circumstances (Venuto and Ferris, 1982). It is known that the kidney is able to maintain its functions, to a large extent, independent of physiological changes in the rest of the body. Renal perfusion is of primary importance in renal function, and changes in the circulation which reduce renal perfusion have to be counteracted by intrarenal mechanisms. Prostaglandins may play a part in this mechanism, as they may increase renal blood flow and produce a diuresis. However, it is probable that in most conditions other systems such as the renin–angiotensin system are more important. Both positive and negative interactions occur between the various systems which regulate renal function. One result of those interactions is found in Bartter's syndrome, in which increased renal prostaglandin production is associated with insensitivity to angiotensin (Editorial, 1976). What induces the increase in prostaglandin production is poorly understood, but inhibiting it restores sensitivity to angiotensin.

Gastrointestinal tract

Prostaglandins play a role in the production of secretions in the gastrointestinal tract (Rask-Madsen and Bukhave, 1981). This is important in the stomach in maintaining the mucosal resistance to the peptic effect of gastric juice, and possibly also in maintaining the mucosal integrity in the gut. In many forms of diarrhoea, increased production of intestinal secretion due to prostaglandin is involved. It is tempting to speculate that prostaglandins thus play a phylogenetic role in eliminating noxious substances. It is possible that a direct action of prostaglandins on intestinal musculature contributes to the increased motility of the gut (Sanders, 1984).

Lungs

Various prostaglandins affect the bronchial smooth musculature: either constrictory or dilatory (Editorial, 1981). It is tempting to suggest that it may be physiologically desirable to control the ventilation of sections of the bronchial tree in order to regulate ventilation and perfusion in response to various local stimuli, but experimental data are inconclusive. It has also been suggested that the overall preponderance of constrictor effects of prostaglandins may play a role in asthma. Leukotrienes are also thought to play a role in causing bronchoconstriction in chronic obstructive lung disease.

Uterus

The uterus is able to function independently of the nervous system. Although hormonal influences are very important, uterine blood flow and motility are modified by endogenous prostaglandins. They play an especially important part during the menstrual cycle as well as in parturition.

The interaction of prostaglandins and endorphins

Because endorphins play an important role in regulating pain sensations, many studies have examined whether there are interactions between prostaglandins and endorphins (Higgs and Moncada, 1983). In the pain process the endorphins seem to act to inhibit vital reactions, which often have been initiated by prostaglandins. In this respect endorphins (and the opiates) can be regarded as natural prostaglandin antagonists. This antagonism is not limited to the central nervous system but is found also in various other organs such as the intestines. It is therefore no longer tenable to regard the non-opiate analgesics as having a purely 'peripheral' action (Ferreira, 1983).

Conclusion

From what is known of the effects of prostaglandins it seems that their main function is a local mechanism to enable organs and tissues to react appropriately to local conditions, more or less independently of systemic influences and without themselves influencing the functioning of the organism as a whole.

Analgesic drugs

The category of drugs known as non-opiate analgesics nowadays could more appropriately be renamed 'prostaglandin synthesis inhibitors'. Most drugs in this category also have anti-inflammatory properties and therefore are commonly called non-steroidal anti-inflammatory drugs (NSAIDs). Before it was known how these drugs worked it was apparently easier to classify them as what they are *not* than as what they are. Not all the drugs which have analgesic effects due to prostaglandin synthesis inhibition have anti-inflammatory properties, but most of them are antipyretic as well, hence the alternative name 'antipyretic analgesics'. In this section the analgesic property will be regarded as the desired effect, and all others as side effects although they are not always fully undesired. There has been some debate as to whether these drugs exert their analgesic effect mainly through inhibition of inflammation or whether they also have a specific independent analgesic effect. This is not merely a semantic question: although many painful conditions are the result of inflammatory processes, certainly not all of them are. It was argued by proponents of the mainly anti-inflammatory action, for instance, that visceral pain did not respond well to this kind of drug, although there was not much experimental proof for this thesis. Now that we know that prostaglandins may play a role in some painful visceral conditions, opinions are changing although convincing experimental evidence is lacking.

The ideal pure analgesic would be a drug which would combat pain without having any other effect. However, it has been suggested that this is likely to be virtually unattainable because inhibition of prostaglandin synthesis would automatically influence the reactions of many physiological systems. On the other hand, it is at least theoretically possible that there are more selective inhibitors of pain. It is known that all analgesics with anti-inflammatory properties studied so far are unselective cyclo-oxygenase inhibitors. Because of this they inhibit formation of all prostaglandins, prostacyclin and thromboxane. None of them inhibits lipo-oxygenase, by which leukotrienes are formed. Because the latter also play a role in some inflammatory processes, anti-inflammatory analgesics are incomplete in their effect. Corticosteroids do not exhibit this shortcoming and have a much wider spectrum of effects. Moreover, since one of the first steps in the formation of prostanoids is the release of arachidonic acid, inhibition of cyclo-oxygenase may leave more arachidonic acid for conversion into leukotrienes. One of the practical consequences of this is the well-documented risk of provoking an asthma attack in some patients by the use of NSAIDs (Editorial, 1981). Obviously leukotrienes are important mediators in some forms of asthma. Patients in whom one anti-inflammatory analgesic drug produces an asthmatic attack often respond in the same way to all others, even if they are structurally unrelated. This rules out cross-hypersensitivity on an immunological basis as a mechanism for producing these attacks. The widely used analgesic paracetamol and its predecessor phenacetin have virtually no anti-inflammatory effects. In itself this would not be a particular advantage of these drugs, but it has been shown that paracetamol also lacks effects on many other systems where prostanoids play a role – although, interestingly, it is effective in combating fever. The antipyretic effect of these drugs is probably the result of a direct action on the central nervous system. This corresponds with the experimental finding that paracetamol *in vitro* inhibits prostaglandin synthesis in brain homogenates but not in spleen homogenates (Curro, Greenberg and Gardier, 1982). This strongly suggests that the antipyretic effect of other analgesics is also a central effect (Dinarello and Wolff, 1978). It may be argued that the analgesic effect of paracetamol may also be a central effect. However, the fact that paracetamol has no effect on inflammation at the site of inflammation does not rule out the probability that it has an analgesic effect by virtue of an action at the site of a painful condition, whilst it is possible that the analgesic effect of anti-inflammatory analgesics is also mainly central. There are a few observations which corroborate this hypothesis. For example, it has been shown that zomepirac exerts a central analgesic effect (Schady and Torebjörk, 1984). Aspirin, probably the most extensively investigated analgesic both experimentally and clinically, exerts its analgesic effect at much lower doses than its anti-inflammatory effect. This might well be due to differences in affinity for different cyclo-oxygenases or it might result from different sites of action. From these and other findings it seems that there are different cyclo-oxygenases in different organs. Paracetamol appears to be unique in that it inhibits only certain cyclo-oxygenases, whilst most other analgesics inhibit all kinds of cyclo-oxygenases. However, it cannot be ruled out that the differences between paracetamol and many other analgesic drugs are at least partly due to different pharmacokinetic parameters rather than to differences in sensitivity of end-organs.

The possible consequences of the growing knowledge of the mechanism of action of analgesics have not yet been fully explored. It is important to keep all possible effects in mind when using these drugs.

Paracetamol

At present paracetamol forms an exception to the rule, as it may be regarded as a drug with only analgesic and antipyretic properties and devoid of anti-inflammatory action in clinical doses.

Although it is commonly used for its analgesic properties, these have not been fully explored; for example, the dose–effect range for analgesia in man is not known. However, clinical experience suggests that a maximal effect is reached with about 1 g (Ameer and Greenblatt, 1977). The frequency of administration is essentially determined by pharmacokinetic and pharmacodynamic properties. The half-life of paracetamol is about 2 hours but this gives no indication of the optimal dosing interval. No firm data have been established on the relation between concentration and analgesic effect. Moreover, it is not known whether the effect is rapidly reversible or whether cyclo-oxygenase is inhibited for some time after the drug has been eliminated from the plasma. From clinical experience it appears that the duration of the analgesic effect is considerably longer than the relatively short plasma half-life would lead one to expect. Many other analgesics have been found to be more potent than paracetamol. However, it is very doubtful whether the maximal analgesic effect of any of the other non-opiate analgesics is greater than that of paracetamol. When inflammation is an important factor in the genesis of pain, it is possible that alternative, anti-inflammatory, analgesics will act better. In general, however, the latter are more toxic.

The antipyretic effect of paracetamol is most probably an effect on central nervous system temperature regulation. It is devoid of effects on the effector organs of temperature regulation (e.g. sweat glands and skin vasculature). All analgesic antipyretic drugs act by normalizing the set point for body temperature. It is not known whether the dose–effect range for this effect is identical to that for the analgesic effect. However, in many patients the maximal antipyretic effect (i.e. the dose required for complete normalization of the body temperature) is attained at high dosages, at least higher than those regarded as maximal for analgesia. Clinical observation may be a more reliable guide with respect to temperature regulation than to pain. The antipyretic response may vary considerably between patients and is probably related to the different origins of the fever. In some patients with bacterial infections a dose of 500 mg may have a profound and long-lasting effect. A rapid and powerful effect is not always desirable because of the limited capacity to dissipate body heat, in the order of magnitude of 1°C per 30 minutes. This may produce profuse sweating and skin vasolidation, which are not without danger as hypothermia and circulatory insufficiently may develop, especially in children and old people.

Paracetamol lacks most effects of other analgesics on prostaglandin synthesis. This makes it one of the safest, if not the safest, pure analgesic. However, two toxicological aspects must be mentioned: acute toxicity to the liver and chronic toxicity to the kidney.

Acute toxicity of paracetamol to the liver is unique in so far as it is totally unrelated to the analgesic effect. It is solely the result of the metabolism of paracetamol (Davis, Labadarios and Williams, 1976). After oral administration the liver is exposed to a relatively high concentration of paracetamol, which it rapidly converts to intermediate metabolites, which in turn are converted to stable, inactive metabolites. The result is that inside the liver cell a concentration of intermediate metabolites develops, and it is these metabolites that are actively cytotoxic. However, the liver cell is protected against this activity by the antioxidant activity of glutathione. Therefore, in normal liver cells at therapeutic dosage levels toxicity is nil. Toxicity occurs whenever there is a discrepancy between the formation of intermediary metabolites and the amount of glutathione present. This is what happens after a large overdose of paracetamol. It is remarkable that phenacetin is devoid of this kind of toxicity. Phenacetin is largely transformed to paracetamol, which causes its analgesic effect, but the rate at which this occurs is slow enough to prevent rapid accumulation of toxic intermediary metabolites. Logically, treatment of paracetamol overdose consists in administration of drugs which are able to reactivate glutathione or to bind the intermediary metabolites.

The chronic toxicity of paracetamol for the kidney is a matter of debate. Phenacetin has been replaced by paracetamol in nearly all commercially available analgesic preparations, explicitly because of its supposed lesser renal toxicity (Ameer and Greenblatt, 1977).

The causative relationship between phenacetin and renal damage is still not understood, although there is no doubt about the association between long-standing abuse of phenacetin with renal papillary necrosis. Experimental and epidemiological data indicate that many analgesics share the ability to induce renal damage after long-term use. An effect on renal prostaglandin synthesis has been suggested. However, even patients with rheumatoid arthritis who have been using analgesic drugs extensively all their life may show renal damage at autopsy without having suffered from severe renal insufficiency, which is the characteristic complaint of analgesic abusers. What is remarkable in the histories of analgesic abusers with renal insufficiency is that they have taken amounts of the drug which go far beyond those that induce a maximal analgesic effect. It might be possible that renal damage depends not on the drug's potential to cause damage but on its potential to cause abuse. Admittedly, there are as yet no clear-cut data to solve this riddle. However, as long as these analgesics are prescribed only for painful conditions there seems to be no real danger to the patient.

Glafenine and floctafenine

The pharmacology of glafenine and floctafenine has not been investigated as thoroughly as that of other analgesics. They seem to be pure analgesics, devoid not only of an anti-inflammatory effect but also of significant antipyretic properties (Peterfalvi and Deraedt, 1975; Deraedt et al., 1976). Because of this apparently unique specificity it is remarkable that these drugs have been neglected by pharmacologists. In practice, however, using them as analgesics seems not to offer an advantage over paracetamol, unless one wishes to avoid the antipyretic effect of the latter.

Salicylates

In many textbooks salicylates are treated as a group of drugs. This obscures the fact that there are only a very few of these drugs, with important differences between them in pharmacological properties and therapeutic applications (Atkinson and Collier, 1980).

Salicylate is the anion of salicylic acid. It has been widely used as an antirheumatic drug, but as such it has been superseded by more modern anti-inflammatory agents and also by acetylsalicylic acid, or aspirin. Aspirin had been used for decades as a readily available analgesic before its adverse effects became clear. It may still be regarded as an effective and mostly innocuous analgesic, although it has been replaced in many countries by paracetamol, which is equally effective. As mentioned previously, the analgesic effect of aspirin is reached at relatively low dosages – not more than 2–3 g daily. At that dose it has, in the experience of rheumatologists, no important anti-inflammatory effect in rheumatic disease. The antipyretic effect is also present at these dosages; in this respect it resembles paracetamol. To treat inflammatory disease, higher dosages are needed – up to 6 g daily. Because acetylsalicylic acid is rapidly hydrolysed in the body into salicylate, the long-term anti-inflammatory effect is ascribed to the salicylate. However, salicylate itself has no remarkable analgesic effect in low doses. Therefore it is reasonable to regard the analgesic effect of aspirin as a specific effect. The importance of this observation is that, because the undesired effects of many analgesics are associated with their anti-inflammatory properties, if a non-opiate analgesic is to be an effective anti-inflammatory drug, most, if not all, will have the unwanted effects of inhibition of prostaglandin synthesis in the body. The most serious side effect in this respect is the potential to cause gastric ulcers and to inhibit platelet function. Whether other effects of minor importance have gone unrecognized so far is difficult to tell. It should be borne in mind that the potential of aspirin to cause gastric haemorrhage went undetected for many decades in which hundreds of thousands of subjects had been exposed. Some of these other effects will be discussed later.

Aspirin has a place of its own as far as gastric haemorrhage and other bleeding tendencies are concered. It shares with other anti-inflammatory drugs the potential to cause gastric ulcers by diminishing resistance of the gastric epithelium to the peptic effect of the gastric juice. Moreover, by inhibiting platelet function it may increase a bleeding tendency, like other anti-inflammatory drugs. However, the effect of aspirin on platelets is long-standing because its acetyl group binds to the platelet membrane (Cronberg, Wallmark and Söderberg, 1984). As a result, the platelets remain less effective even after the drug itself has been cleared from the blood. The prolongation of bleeding time by an analgesic dose of aspirin is very modest in most instances, to about 5–6 minutes. This does not itself explain profuse bleeding. Moreover, the usual occurrence in patients who present with massive gastric bleeding after just one tablet of aspirin is that they do not have an ulcer but that blood oozes from many small erosions in the gastric mucosa. Often these patients have a greatly prolonged bleeding time – up to 15 minutes or more. Further investigation has revealed that a very small proportion of the population is indeed very sensitive to this effect of aspirin. The clinical picture can thus be explained by many erosions which are caused by local effects of high concentrations of aspirin in the stomach; these bleed profusely because of the greatly increased bleeding tendency in those patients; sensitive patients should never again use aspirin, although it is not at all clear whether they are also equally at risk with other anti-inflammatory drugs.

This effect has been reported to cause prolonged bleeding after tooth extraction, tonsillectomy and during menstruation. The use of aspirin should be discouraged in situations where bleeding might be a potential risk. Although aspirin is in itself an effective analgesic in postoperative pain, to know for certain whether a particular patient is at risk would demand a preoperative aspirin tolerance test.

Other analgesics

Most other non-opiate analgesics are used mainly in rheumatoid disease. One of the best known of these is indomethacin. Its clinical and pharmacological effects have been widely investigated, and it has become one of the most valuable pharmacological tools in the study of the effects of prostaglandins. It is widely used where the aim is to inhibit prostaglandin synthesis other than for analgesic or anti-inflammatory ends. For example, it has been used in the treatment of Bartter's syndrome (Gill et al., 1976) and in the treatment of enteritis due to irradiation. It also enhances closing of the ductus arteriosus, which may be a desired effect in some cases (Halliday, Hirata and Brady, 1979). Although it has a measurable effect on renal function, this seems to be insignificant in most instances. However, under circumstances of restricted renal perfusion it may contribute to oliguria or anuria. Although the subclinical effect on blood pressure is not important under normal circumstances, it is as yet not certain that it never is significant (Negus, Tannen and Dunn, 1976; Gerber, 1983).

Indomethacin is also often used as an antipyretic, partly because it can be administered easily as a suppository. However, the standard dose of this drug is intended to be used in inflammatory disease. The antipyretic effect of these dosages is often much greater than needed, and may cause undesired effects, such as hypothermia by profuse sweating and postural hypotension due to maximal skin vasodilation.

There is no good reason to assume that other anti-inflammatory analgesics differ much from indomethacin with respect to undesired inhibition of prostaglandin synthesis. Some of them have undesired effects which seem to be unrelated to the inhibition of prostaglandin synthesis. The most important, because they are potentially more serious, are the haematological side effects. The class of pyrazolone derivatives are the most dangerous in this respect, but it is not unequivocally certain whether this is due to the great popularity of these drugs for the treatment of minor ailments such as low back pain, or whether the relative frequency of these effects is indeed higher. There are many indications that the latter explanation is likely. Because blood abnormalities are most often due to immunological phenomena, cross-hypersensitivity exists for other drugs of the same class. Because of these side effects there should be very good reasons for using strong anti-inflammatory drugs as analgesics, as safer drugs are available with more specific analgesic properties.

References

Ameer, B, and Greenblatt, D.J. (1977) Acetaminophen. *Annals of Internal Medicine* **87**, 202

Atkinson, D.C. and Collier, H.O.C. (1980) Salicylates: molecular mechanism of therapeutic action. *Advances in Pharmacology and Chemotherapy* **17**, 233

Clark, K.E. and Brody, M.J. (1982) Prostaglandins and uterine blood flow. In: *Prostaglandins Organ- and Tissue-specific Actions* (Eds. Greenberg, S., Kadowitz, Ph.J. and Burks, Th.F.), p. 107. Marcel Dekker: New York, Basel

Cronberg, S., Wallmark, E. and Söderberg, I. (1984) Effect on platelet aggregation of oral administration of 10 non-steroidal analgesics to humans. *Scandinavian Journal of Haematology* **33**, 155

Curro, F.A., Greenberg, S. and Gardier, R.W. (1982) Effects of prostaglandins on central nervous system function. In: *Prostaglandins. Organ- and Tissue-specific Actions* (Eds. Greenberg, S., Kadowitz, Ph.J. and Burks, Th.F.), p. 367. Marcel Dekker: New York, Basel

Davis, M., Labadarios, D. and Williams, R.S. (1976) Metabolism of paracetamol after therapeutic and hepatotoxic doses in man. *Journal of International Medical Research* **4**, suppl. 4, 40

Deraedt, R., Jouquey, S., Benzoni, J. *et al.* (1976) Inhibition of prostaglandin biosynthesis by non-narcotic analgesic drugs. *Archives Internationales de Pharmacodynamie et de Thérapie* **224**, 30

Dinarello, C.A. (1984) Interleukin-1 and the pathogenesis of the acute-phase response. *New England Journal of Medicine* **311**, 1413

Dinarello, C.A. and Wolff, S.M. (1978) Pathogenesis of fever in man. *New England Journal of Medicine* **298**, 607

Editorial (1976) Bartter's syndrome. *Lancet* **2**, 721

Editorial (1981) Arachidonic acid, analgesics, and asthma. *Lancet* **2**, 1266

Ferreira, S.H. (1983) Prostaglandins: peripheral and central analgesia. *Advances in Pain Research and Therapy* **5**, 627

Gerber, J.G. (1983) Indomethacin-induced rises in blood pressure. *Annals of Internal Medicine* **99**, 555

Gill, J.R. Jr, Frolich, J.C., Bowden, R.E. *et al.* (1976) Bartter's syndrome: a disorder characterized by high urinary prostaglandins and a dependence of hyperreninemia on prostaglandin synthesis. *American Journal of Medicine* **61**, 43

Granström, E. (1983) Biochemistry of the prostaglandins, thromboxanes, and leukotrienes. *Advances in Pain Research and Therapy* **5**, 605

Greenberg, S. (1982) Prostaglandins and vascular smooth muscle in hypertension. In: *Prostaglandins. Organ- and Tissue-specific Actions* (Eds. Greenberg, S., Kadowitz, Ph.J. and Burks, Th.F.), p. 25, Marcel Dekker: New York, Basel

Halliday, H.L., Hirata, T. and Brady, J.P. (1979) Indomethacin therapy for large patent ductus arteriosus in the very low birth weight infant: results and complications. *Pediatrics* **64**, 154

Higgs, G.A. and Moncada, S. (1983) Interactions of arachidonate products with other pain mediators. *Advances in Pain Research and Therapy* **5**, 617

James, G.W.L. and Church, M.K. (1978) Hyperalgesia after treatment of mice with prostaglandins and arachidonic acid and its antagonism by anti-inflammatory–analgesic compounds. *Arzneimittel-Forschung/Drug Research* **28**, 804

Kluger, M.J. (1979) *Fever. Its biology, evolution and function.* Princeton University Press: Princeton, NJ

Longenecker, G.L. (1982) Prostaglandins and the platelet prostanoid compounds. In: *Prostaglandins. Organ- and Tissue-specific Actions* (Eds. Greenberg, S., Kadowitz, Ph.J. and Burks, Th.F.) p.255. Marcel Dekker: New York, Basel

Moncada, S. and Vane, J.R. (1979) Arachidonic acid metabolites and the interaction between platelets and blood-vessel walls. *New England Journal of Medicine* **300**, 1142

Moncada, S., Flower, R.J. and Vane, J.R. (1980) Prostaglandins, prostacyclin, and thromboxane A$_2$. In: *The Pharmacological Basis of Therapeutics*, 5th edn. (Eds. Goodman, L.S. and Gilman, A.) p. 668. Macmillan: New York

Moncada, S., Higgs, E.A. and Vane, J.R. (1977) Human arterial and venous tissues generate prostacyclin (prostaglandin X), a potent inhibitor of platelet aggregation. *Lancet* **1**, 18

Negus, P., Tannen, R.L. and Dunn, M.J. (1976) Indomethacin potentiates the vasoconstrictor actions of angiotensin II in normal man. *Prostaglandins* **12**, 175

Peterfalvi, M. and Deraedt, R. (1975) Floctafenine, a new non-narcotic analgesic. *Archives Internationales de Pharmacodynamie et de Thérapie* **216**, 97

Rask-Madsen, J. and Bukhave, K. (1981) The role of prostaglandins in diarrhoea. *Clinical Research Reviews* 1, suppl. 1, 33

Sanders, K.M. (1984) Role of prostaglandins in regulating gastric motility. *American Journal of Physiology* **247**, G117

Schady, W. and Torebjörk H.E. (1984) Central effects of zomepirac on pain evoked by intraneuronal stimulation in man. *Journal of Clinical Pharmacology* **24**, 429

Venuto, R.C. and Ferris, T.F. (1982) Prostaglandins and renal function. In: *Prostaglandins. Organ- and Tissue-specific Actions* (Eds. Greenberg, S., Kadowitz, Ph.J. and Burks, Th.F.), p. 131. Marcel Dekker: New York, Basel

Von Euler, U.S. (1936) On the specific vaso-dilating and plain muscle stimulating substances from accessory genital glands in man and certain animals (prostaglandin and vesiglandin). *Journal of Physiology* **88**, 213

14

Antihistamine drugs

P.K. Barnes

The pharmacology of histamine and histamine antagonists has considerable relevance to anaesthetists. This is particularly true now because adverse reactions to anaesthetic drugs, mediated by histamine, are frequently reported, and there has been an increase in the usage of the H_2-receptor antagonists to reduce the volume of acidic stomach contents prior to anaesthesia.

Introduction

'Benadryl and related compounds, completely annul the vasodilator effects of the minimal doses of histamine which produce maximal vasodilation. The effect of large doses of histamine, five times greater than the minimum dose and upwards, depending on the basic sensitivity to histamine, is not annulled or even diminished by any amounts of antagonistic drug'.

'It is suggested that there are two types of receptors sensitive to histamine, only one of which can be blocked by benadryl and related compounds.'

These two conclusions appear in the summary of a paper on observations on reactive hyperaemia by Folkow, Haeger and Kahlson (1948). They had studied the depressor and vasodilator responses to moderate doses of histamine in the cat and dog, and found that these responses to histamine could be blocked by diphenhydramine (H_1-receptor antagonist) but when larger doses of histamine were used the response could not be blocked. Confirmatory evidence that histamine exerts its pharmacological effect by interaction with two types of receptor was produced 18 years later. In 1966, Ash and Schild compared the characteristics of a typical antihistamine receptor in guinea-pig ileum with the histamine receptors in rat uterus and stomach. A limited number of histamine analogues were examined and their relative activity supported the differentiation of histamine receptors into at least two subtypes. The antagonism of some actions of histamine by low concentrations of antihistamine drugs characterized one type of histamine receptor, for which they suggested the symbol H_1.

In 1972, Black and colleagues discovered that the actions of histamine which could not be blocked by H_1-receptor antagonists were mediated by a second

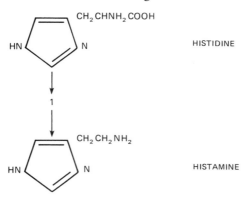

Fig. 14.1   Synthesis of histamine. 1 = L-histidine decarboxylase.

histamine receptor, which they designated H_2. This was the culmination of work begun eight years previously, of an examination of 700 compounds which differed slightly from histamine, and resulted in the production of an H_2-receptor antagonist called burimamide.

Pharmacology of histamine

Histamine is formed in the body by the decarboxylation of histidine within the lumen of the intestine and in many different types of cell (Fig. 14.1). Histamine is stored in the body in three sites.

1. *Granules of mast cells and basophils.* Here histamine is bound with heparin. It can be released by antigen–antibody complexes and also by histamine-releasing chemicals. Anaesthetic induction agents, with the exception of etomidate, and neuromuscular blocking agents, with the exception of vecuronium, have the capability to release histamine from this site, as have a range of other drugs used by anaesthetists.

2. *The mucosal layer of gastrointestinal tract.*

3. *Brain.* Large amounts of histamine are present in the anterior and posterior pituitary and the adjacent median eminence of the hypothalamus. Most of the histamine in the posterior pituitary is in mast cells but it is not contained within the mast cells in other areas. In other parts of the brain the histamine levels are low but various parts of the brain contain histamine-activated adenyl cyclase. The histamine content of the brain is increased by chlorpromazine and mescaline, and is depleted by reserpine.

Once released, histamine is rapidly broken down (Fig. 14.2). Histamine produces its pharmacological effect by interaction with two types of receptor, presumed to be a component of the cell surface and named H_1 and H_2. These receptors have different structural requirements for both binding and activation. The understanding of the pharmacological effects of histamine has been extended considerably since the discovery of specific agonists (Fig. 14.3)

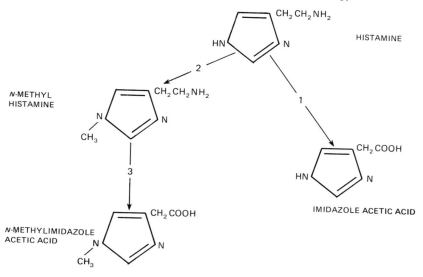

Fig. 14.2   Metabolism of histamine. 1 = diamine oxidase; 2 = histamine N-methyl transferase; 3 = monoamine oxidase.

and antagonists. The pharmacological effects of histamine have been classically described as:

1. Relaxation of vascular smooth muscle.
2. Contraction of some non-vascular smooth muscle.
3. Stimulation of glands.

Relaxation of vascular smooth muscle

Peripheral vasculature

The effect of histamine on the peripheral vasculature differs according to the species examined. In man H_1 and H_2 receptors are believed to be involved in

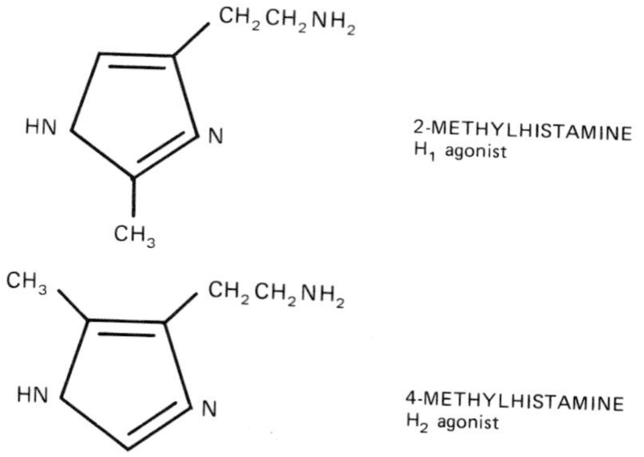

2-METHYLHISTAMINE
H_1 agonist

4-METHYLHISTAMINE
H_2 agonist

Fig. 14.3   Histamine receptor agonists.

the direct inhibition of vascular smooth muscle in arterioles, metarterioles and precapillary sphincters. This results in a fall in peripheral vascular resistance and a decrease in blood pressure. Flushing of the skin occurs, which is characteristically pronounced on the upper trunk and the face. The action of histamine on small venules is to cause contraction. This has the effect of increasing capillary pressure and increasing the porosity of the adjacent endothelium, with resultant increase in vascular permeability. These effects are mediated by H_1 receptors. The H_1 and H_2 receptors involved in these responses produce the classic itching of the skin and the 'triple response' to histamine released in the skin. They also produce the state of circulatory collapse with loss of intravascular volume in response to anaphylactic or anaphylactoid reactions.

Pulmonary vasculature
Experiments in animal tissues have suggested that H_1 receptors produce a vasoconstriction and H_2 receptors vasodilation. Similarly, in man H_2 receptors have been found to be associated with vasodilation both *in vitro* and *in vivo*. Braude and co-workers (1984) examined the effect of inhaled histamine on lung epithelial permeability. They found that permeability was increased and that this effect could be blocked by pretreatment with an H_2-receptor antagonist, ranitidine. They postulated that the increase in permeability was produced by increase in pulmonary blood flow.

Coronary vessels
Vasoconstriction and vasodilatation of the coronary vessels is also mediated by H_1 and H_2 receptors. Ginsberg *et al.* (1980) investigated the histamine receptor subtypes in an *in vitro* preparation of isolated coronary arteries in man. They found that the H_1 receptor mediates contraction in coronary vascular smooth muscle and that the H_2 receptor mediates relaxation.

Non-vascular smooth muscle

H_1 and H_2 receptors are widely scattered in the intestine, the gall bladder and in the smooth muscle of the bronchi and the genitourinary system. In general, H_1 receptors cause contraction and H_2 receptors relaxation.

Stimulation of glands

Stomach
Histamine, gastrin and direct vagal stimulation act on the gastric parietal cells to promote the secretion of hydrogen ions, pepsin and intrinsic factor. If the cholinergic input is blocked either by section of the vagus or by atropinization, the effect of histamine on the output of hydrogen ions from the parietal cells is diminished. Histamine is present in high concentrations in the gastric mucosa, where it is formed from histidine. The effects of histamine on the parietal cells are mediated by H_2 receptors. The action of histamine in promoting oxygen uptake by the parietal cells can also be blocked by an H_2-receptor antagonist (Soll and Walsh, 1979). Quite apart from its effect on the

regulation of gastric secretion, histamine also controls the microcirculation in the stomach and increases blood flow by activation of H_1 and H_2 receptors.

Other pharmacological effects

Heart

Histamine produces positive inotropic and chronotropic effects in many species. In human right atrial specimens *in vitro*, the chronotropic effect may be demonstrated, and is abolished by the use of an H_2-receptor antagonist, cimetidine (Gristwood, Lincoln and Owen, 1980). The chronotropic effect of histamine is produced by an increased rate of firing of the sinotrial node by enhancement of phase 4 of depolarization (Levy and Pappano, 1978). Histamine has other effects on cardiac rhythm and may cause dysrhythmias by causing varying degrees of atrioventricular block (H_1) or enhancing automaticity (H_2). The positive inotropic effect of histamine has been demonstrated in both human atrial and ventricular myocardium *in vitro*, and is mediated by H_2 receptors (Ginsberg *et al.*, 1980).

Brain

Histamine almost certainly has a neurotransmitter role in the brain, where H_1 and H_2 receptors have been widely demonstrated.

Nerve endings

Stimulation of nerve endings in the skin results in itching and contributes to the 'triple response'.

Mechanism of action of histamine

Adenylate cyclase is a particulate enzyme localized to the plasma membrane of the cell surface. It activates adenosine triphosphate (ATP), to form cyclic adenosine monophosphate (cAMP). Stimulation of adenylate cyclase or elevated levels of cAMP have been demonstrated in various tissues, both in animals and in human lymphocytes and leucoctyes exposed to histamine (Lichtenstein and Gillespie, 1975; Busse and Sosman, 1977). The effect in human white cells can be blocked by the use of H_2- but not H_1-receptor antagonists. The implication of this is that the response to the combination of histamine and H_2 receptor is to stimulate adenylate cyclase to produce an increase in cAMP, which may be the method in which histamine's effect is accomplished. For example, the combination of histamine with its receptor in the gastric parietal cell may trigger the release of cAMP as the first step in the production of hydrogen ions by the parietal cell. There is also evidence for the importance of calcium in the initiation of the inotropic effects of histamine in the heart. The association of histamine and its receptor may initiate changes in membrane permeability to ions such as calcium, and Bertaccini, Coruzzi and Vitali (1978) have demonstrated that the calcium channel blocker verapamil can block the inotropic effect of histamine on guinea-pig papillary muscle.

Cyclic guanosine-3',5'-monophosphate (cGMP) is also responsible for a

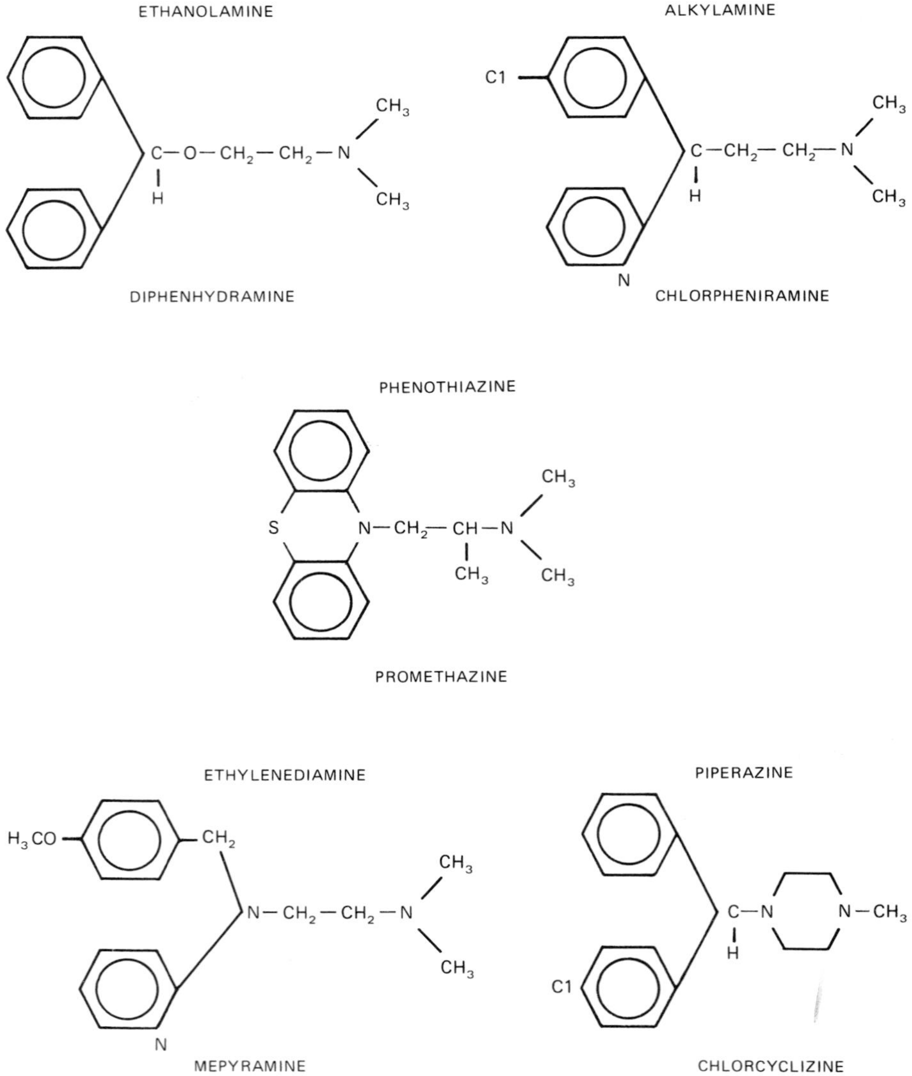

ETHANOLAMINE

DIPHENHYDRAMINE

ALKYLAMINE

CHLORPHENIRAMINE

PHENOTHIAZINE

PROMETHAZINE

ETHYLENEDIAMINE

MEPYRAMINE

PIPERAZINE

CHLORCYCLIZINE

Fig. 14.4 H_1-receptor antagonists.

variety of intracellular responses. It is activated by guanylate cyclase, which is bound to cell membranes. Elevation in cGMP has been found in smooth muscle contracting through H_1 stimulation, and following H_2 stimulation in mouse neuroblastoma cells (Richelson, 1978) and the bovine superior cervical ganglion (Study and Greengard, 1978). In the mouse neuroblastoma cells the effect was reduced by the use of H_1 antagonists. It is possible that H_1-mediated effects may utilize cGMP as an intermediary between receptor and effector tissue.

Histamine antagonists

H₁-receptor-blocking drugs

Bovet and Staub (1937) were the first to report the discovery of specific antihistamine drugs. Since then, a large number of drugs with varying specificity have been discovered. They belong to different chemical groups (Fig. 14.4) and have in common a large blocking group linked by a chain of suitable length to a tertiary amine group:

Aromatic groups –C–C– tertiary amino group

The antihistamines, parasympatholytics and antipsychotic agents have a similar configuration and show some of the same pharmacological properties. The antihistamines are drugs with a specific effect at the H_1 receptor, but possess weak atropine-like and tranquillizing side effects. They are all lipophilic and act by competitive inhibition. A new potent H_1 receptor antagonist SK&F 93944 has recently been described (Durant et al., 1984). It differs from those currently used as it is not a tertiary amine. It does not cross the blood–brain barrier and has insignificant antimuscarinic activity in animal tissues.

H₂-receptor antagonists

Burimamide was the first H_2-receptor antagonist to be used experimentally (Black et al., 1972). Since then, research has produced two compounds, cimetidine and ranitidine, which have gained widespread acceptance in clinical practice. The H_2-receptor antagonists differ from the H_1-receptor-blocking drugs in that they are quite dissimilar in structure and are hydrophilic. They are similar in structure to histamine (Fig. 14.5).

Ranitidine possesses a furan ring rather than an imidazole ring, so this does not appear to be essential for receptor recognition. Unlike histamine, the H_2-receptor antagonists have longer side chains. Modifying and lengthening the side chains increases potency and selectivity. Ranitidine is four to six times more potent than cimetidine. Unlike cimetidine, ranitidine does not bind to testosterone receptors (Pearce and Funder, 1980), inhibit cytochrome P450 in the liver (Henry et al., 1980) or release prolactin (Nelis and Van der Meene, 1980).

Cimetidine and ranitidine are both well absorbed when given orally. Peak plasma concentration of ranitidine occurs 2 hours after ingestion, that of cimetidine is half that time although it is delayed in non-fasting subjects. Bioavailability of the oral dose is approximately 70 per cent for cimetidine and 50 per cent for ranitidine; both drugs are subject to first-pass metabolism in the liver. The elimination half-life of cimetidine is 2 hours, most of the drug being excreted unchanged in the urine although a sulphoxide metabolite is formed in the liver and subsequently excreted in urine. The elimination half-life of ranitidine is 2–3 hours, with about 70 per cent excreted unchanged through the kidney after intravenous administration. In patients with impaired renal function the elimination half-life of ranitidine is prolonged (McGonigle

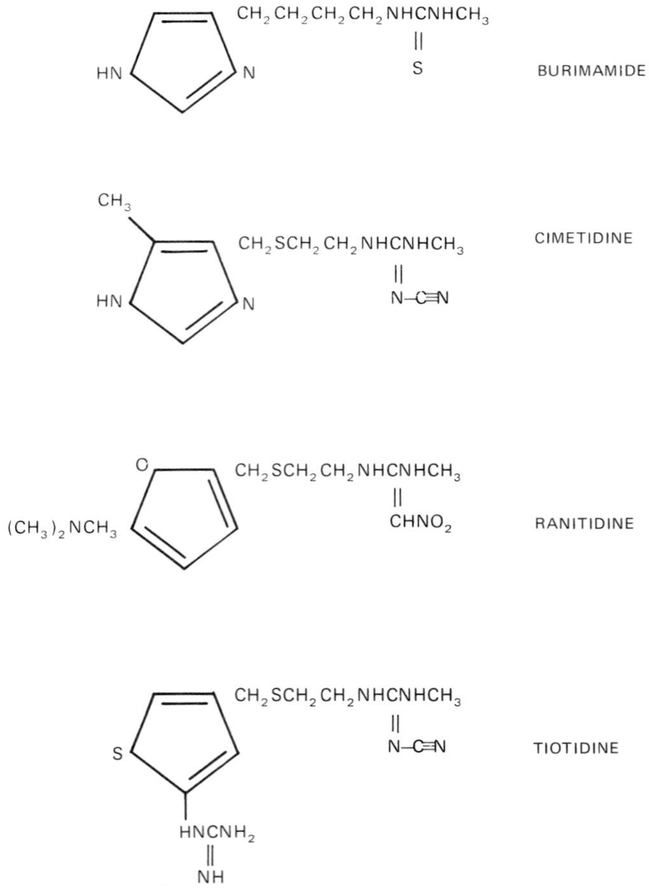

Fig. 14.5 H$_2$-receptor antagonists.

et al., 1982), and the rate of excretion of cimetidine is reduced (Caravan and Briggs, 1977).

H$_1$- and H$_2$-receptor antagonists

The difference in structure of the H$_1$- and H$_2$-receptor antagonists has suggested that the receptors are quite distinct. However, a preliminary report has described the compound SK&F 93319 as possessing the ability to block both types of receptor in animal tissue *in vitro* (Blakemore *et al.*, 1983). Such a compound would enable the cardiovascular effects of histamine to be attenuated using a single compound, and this has been demonstrated successfully in the cat (Harvey and Owen, 1984). This compound differs from the other H$_2$-receptors in that it does not possess an imidazole or furan ring which is replaced by a 3-methoxypyridine ring (Fig. 14.6).

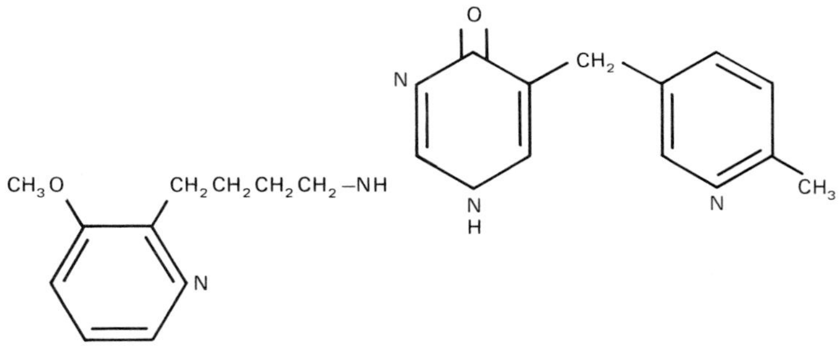

SK&F 93319

Fig. 14.6   Histamine H_1- and H_2-receptor antagonist.

Summary

The discovery of a drug with the potential to block both types of histamine receptors will undoubtedly lead to a further surge in interest in the pharmacology of histamine, as did the discovery of the H_2-receptor blockers. It is quite possible that more receptor subtypes will be defined, and drugs produced which will further simplify the treatment of histamine-related pathological states.

References

Ash, A.S.F. and Schild, H.O. (1966) Receptors mediating some actions of histamine. *British Journal of Pharmacology and Chemotherapy* **27**, 427–439

Bertaccini, G., Coruzzi, G. and Vitali, T. (1978) Effect of histamine and related compounds on the papillary muscle in the guinea pig. *Pharmacological Research Communications* **10**, 747

Black, J.W., Duncan, W.A.M., Durant, C.J., Ganellin, C.P. and Parsons, E.M. (1972) Definition and antagonism of histamine H_2 receptors. *Nature* **236**, 385–390

Blakemore, R.C., Brown, T.H., Cooper, D.G. *et al.* (1983) SK&F 93319– a specific antagonist of histamine H_1 and H_2 receptors. *British Journal of Pharmacology* **80**, Proceedings suppl., 437P

Bovet, D. and Staub, A. (1937) Action protectrice des ethers phenoliques au cours de l'intoxication histaminique. *Comptes rendus des seances de la Societe de Biologie et de ses Filiales* **124**, 547–549

Braude, S., Royston, B., Coe, C. and Barnes, P.J. (1984) Histamine increases lung permeability by an H_2 receptor mechanism. *Lancet* **2**, 372

Busse, W.W. and Sosman, J. (1977) Decreased H_2 histamine response of granulocytes of asthmatic patients. *Journal of Clinical Investigation* **59**, 1080

Caravan, J.S.F. and Briggs, J.D. (1977) Cimetidine clearance in renal failure. In: *Cimetidine: Proceedings of the Second International Symposium on Histamine H_2 Antagonists* (Eds. Burland, W.L. and Simkins, M.A.), pp. 75–80. Excerpta Medica: Amsterdam

Durant, G.J., Ganellin, G.R., Griffith, R. *et al.* (1984) SK&F 93944. Potent H_1

receptor histamine antagonist with negligible ability to penetrate the CNS. *British Journal of Pharmacology* **83**, 232P

Folkow, B., Haeger, K. and Kahlson, G. (1948) Observations of reactive hyperaemia as related to histamine, on drugs antagonising vasodilation induced by histamine on vasodilator properties and adenosinetriphosphate. *Acta Anaesthesiologica Scandinavica* **15**, 264–278

Ginsberg, R., Bristow, M.R., Stinson, E.B. and Harrison, D.C. (1980) Histamine receptors in the human heart. *Life Sciences* **26**, 2245

Gristwood, R.W., Lincoln, J.C.R. and Owen, D.A.A. (1980) Effect of histamine on human isolated heart muscle: comparison with effect of noradrenaline. *Journal of Pharmacy and Pharmacology* **32**, 145–146

Harvey, C.A. and Owen, D.A.A. (1984) Cardiovascular studies with SK&F 93319 an antagonist of histamine at both H_1 and H_2 receptors. *British Journal of Pharmacology* **83**, 427

Henry, D.A., MacDonald, I.A., Kitchingman, G., Bell, G.D. and Langman, M.J.S. (1980) Cimetidine and ranitidine: comparison of effects on hepatic drug metabolism. *British Medical Journal* **281**, 775

Levi, R. and Pappano, A.J. (1978) Modification of the effects of histamine and norepinephrine on the sinoatrial node pacemaker by potassium and calcium. *Journal of Pharmacology and Experimental Therapeutics* **204**, 625

Lichtenstein, L.M. and Gillespie, E. (1975) The effects of the H_1 and H_2 antihistamines on allergic histamine release and its inhibition by histamine. *Journal of Pharmacology and Experimental Therapeutics* **192**, 441

McGonigle, R.J.S., Williams, I.C., Amphlett, G.E., England, R.J. and Parsons, V. (1982) The pharmacokinetics of ranitidine in renal disease. In: *The Clinical Use of Ranitidine* (Eds. Misiewicz, J.J. and Wormsley, K.G.), Medicine Publishing Foundation series 5, pp. 41–46. Medicine Publishing: Oxford

Nelis, G.F. and Van der Meene, J.G.C. (1980) Comparative effects of cimetidine and ranitidine on prolactin secretion. *Postgraduate Medical Journal* **56**, 478

Pearce, P. and Funder, J.W. (1980) Histamine H_2 receptor antagonist radioreceptor assay for antiandrogenic side effects. *Clinical and Experimental Pharmacology and Physiology* **7**, 442

Richelson, E. (1978) Histamine H_1 receptors mediated guanosine $3',5'$-monophosphate formation by cultured mouse neuroblastoma cells. *Science* **201**, 69

Soll, A. and Walsh, J.H. (1979) Regulation of gastric acid secretion. *Annual Review of Physiology* **41**, 35

Study, R.E. and Greengard, P. (1978) Regulation by histamine of cyclic nucleotide levels in sympmathetic ganglia. *Journal of Pharmacology and Experimental Therapeutics* **207**, 767

15

Hypotensive agents

Valerie A. Goat

Arterial blood pressure varies in healthy subjects, generally, increasing with age and showing diurnal fluctuations. However, large increases in blood flow can occur without producing changes in mean arterial blood pressure. Blood flow is mainly determined by the metabolic requirement of the tissues, increased flow being accommodated by an expansion in the capacity of the intravascular bed. The increased venous return stretches the fibres of the normal myocardium, which responds by the Frank–Starling mechanism causing increased cardiac output. In order to enable each tissue to control its own flow, a sufficient head of pressure must be supplied – the mean arterial pressure. This is determined in part by the intravascular volume which is regulated by the renin–angiotensin–aldosterone axis. Rapid changes in vascular tone are effected via the autonomic nervous system, which adjusts the distribution of the intravascular volume in order to meet the changing needs of the body, both physiological and pathological.

The sympathetic nervous system is part of the autonomic system and is concerned with both the regulation of homoeostasis and the vegetative functions of the body. The central component of the sympathetic nervous system is located in the hypothalamus and the medulla oblongata. The peripheral part consists of pressor detectors located in the major blood vessels, and the sympathetic nerves which increase vasomotor tone by producing vasoconstriction. There are a number of pressor receptors, each responding to changes in blood pressure within a limited range; thus the effective range of control is increased. Some vessels are richly supplied by sympathetic vasoconstrictor fibres; for instance, blood vessels supplying the skin, muscle and abdominal viscera. Blood vessels to vital organs such as the brain and kidney have fewer sympathetic fibres, so blood flow to these organs is maintained at the expense of other tissues during periods of increased sympathetic activity. Capacitance and resistance vessels both have sympathetic innervation, the former responding to a lower frequency of sympathetic stimulation (Mellander and Johanssan, 1968). Venoconstriction can compensate for circulatory changes induced by posture, but arteriolar constriction is required to compensate for further stress. Neural vasodilatation plays a minor role; some blood vessels respond to adrenergic stimulation by dilatation. Flow to some muscles is increased by sympathetic cholinergic fibres which cause vasodilatation.

The heart has both sympathetic and parasympathetic innervation; the latter is normally dominant. An increase in sympathetic activity produces both positive inotropic and chronotropic changes with dilation of the coronary vessels.

Hypotensive drugs may be classified according to their site of action. Those listed in *italic* will be dealt with specifically in this chapter; some of the other agents are dealt with in greater detail in other chapters.

1. Adrenergic blockers
   (a) Central

   Clonidine
   Methyldopa
   Reserpine

   (b) Ganglion blockers

   Hexamethonium
   Pentolinium
   Trimetaphan

   (c) Inhibitors of noradrenaline synthesis, release or reuptake

   Reserpine
   Guanethidine
   Bethanidine

   (d) α–Blockers

   Phenoxybenzamine
   Phentolamine

   (e) β–Blockers

   Propranolol
   Practolol
   Labetalol (+ α–blockade)

2. Directly acting vasodilators
   arterial

   Calcium channel blockers
   Hydralazine
   Diazoxide
   Adenosine triphosphate
   Sodium nitroprusside
   Nitroglycerin

   venous

3. Myocardial depressants

   Volatile anaesthetics
   Calcium channel blockers

4. Inhibitors of the renin–angiotensin system

   Saralasin
   Captopril

Adrenergic blockade

Central

Inhibition of sympathetic activity can occur centrally, by depression of the medullary centres. This occurs with most general anaesthetic agents, and also with some specific vasomotor depressants, clonidine, methyldopa, reserpine and possibly β–blockers.

Clonidine

Clonidine (Fig. 15.1) is chemically related to tolazoline, an α–blocking drug, and was initially used to produce topical vasoconstriction. However, the

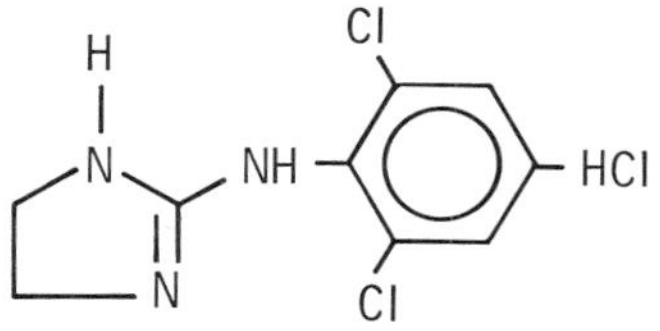

Fig. 15.1   Clonidine hydrochloride.

pressor response to an intravenous injection of the drug is followed by hypotension and bradycardia. Clonidine appears to act as a partial agonist, stimulating peripheral receptor sites before causing a block in transmission.

Clonidine stimulates central α–adrenergic receptors in the medulla oblongata to produce hypotension and bradycardia. This reduces sympathetic activity and increases vagal tone. In experimental animals the central hypotensive action of clonidine can be blocked by α–adrenergic blocking agents.

Clonidine does not interfere with the homoeostatic control of blood pressure. Acute withdrawal may produce a hypertensive crisis which is best managed either with clonidine or with α– plus β–blockade.

Ganglion blockers

The anatomical division of the autonomic nervous system into sympathetic and parasympathetic systems was largely the work of Gaskell (1916).

The sympathetic efferent nerves emerge from the lateral grey horn of the spinal cord in the thoracic and lumbar regions. The preganglionic fibres are short; they synapse with postganglionic neurons in a discrete chain of ganglia which can be found on the vertebral bodies. The postsynaptic neuron has a long axon which travels along with somatic nerves to reach its target organ.

There are two distinct parasympathetic outflows from the spinal cord, the cranial and the sacral. The preganglionic fibres of the parasympathetic division are long, the synapses occurring within ganglia which can be found within the tissue of the organ supplied.

Some organs of the body receive both sympathetic and parasympathetic innervation, their actions being antagonistic. Other tissues receive fibres from one division only.

Acetylcholine (ACh) is the transmitter involved in ganglionic transmission. It is also found at parasympathetic and a few sympathetic nerve endings. Noradrenaline, and to a lesser extent adrenaline, is the transmitter liberated from sympathetic nerve endings.

It has been postulated that other neurohumoral transmitters may be involved in transmission within the autonomic nervous system. These include dopamine, 5–hydroxytryptamine (5HT), the adenyl nucleotides and prostaglandins.

It is now realized that ganglionic transmission within the autonomic nervous system is complex and involves several different pathways. The primary route is mediated by ACh acting as a nicotinic agonist. An early excitatory postsynaptic potential (EPSP) results from the combination of transmitter with the nicotinic cholinoceptor. If this is of a sufficient magnitude, it will produce an action potential in the postsynaptic neuron, and transmission will occur. *In vivo* it may be necessary for more than one synapse to be activated before transmission results. This primary pathway is the classic one blocked by the ganglion–blocking drugs.

A secondary pathway also involves ACh as the transmitter. This produces a late excitatory postsynaptic potential. This potential can be blocked by atropine and stimulated by muscarinic agonist drugs, so muscarinic cholinoceptors appear to be involved. It may be that the secondary pathway facilitates transmission through the primary one.

An inhibitory postsynaptic potential (IPSP) is also seen. This is blocked by the administration of both α–adrenergic blocking drugs and atropine, but is not affected by classic ganglionic-blocking agents. Catecholamine-containing cells are present within the ganglia and it may be that these act as interneurons, activated by ACh to release dopamine which is responsible for the inhibition of transmission (Eränko, 1978).Thus the autonomic ganglion contains a heterogeneous population of receptors, with the secondary synaptic events serving to modulate the initial EPSP.

Ganglion-blocking drugs block nicotinic cholinoceptors. This cholinoceptor is a relatively simple one: it has only one major point for attachment of the neurotransmitter, so the structural requirements for antagonist drugs are minimal. As a result, a whole range of chemically unrelated compounds are able to block ganglionic transmission. These include some quaternary ammonium compounds and secondary and tertiary amines.

The discovery of specific ganglion-blocking drugs resulted from experiments on drugs with neuromuscular-blocking properties (Paton and Zaimis, 1948), hexamethonium being one of the earliest used in clinical practice. The ganglion-blocking drugs are perhaps best classified according to their mode of action

1. *Depolarizing drugs*, which initially stimulate before blocking transmission (e.g. nicotine). Some workers consider these agents as partial agonists.

2. *Non-depolarizing drugs*, which block transmission without stimulation. The agents which are clinically useful fall within this group and tend to produce a competitive type of blockade (e.g. hexamethonium, trimetaphan, pentolinium). These drugs have a high affinity for the nicotinic receptor within the ganglion, but do not have intrinsic cholinergic activity. Competitive blockade is never totally complete, but in clinical practice a virtual total block can occur since the amount of transmitter which can be produced is finite.

The cardiovascular effects of ganglionic blockade are variable and unpredictable, depending upon the level of pre-existing sympathetic activity. The capacitance vessels respond to lower frequencies of sympathetic activity and will be the first to dilate following ganglionic blockade. Thus the ability to respond to changes in posture will be abolished, and postural hypotension will ensue (Organe, Paton and Zaimis, 1949). Sympathetic activity produces constriction of resistance vessels as well, and this will also be prevented by ganglionic blockade. Ganglion-blocking agents are relatively ineffective in reducing the blood pressure of normovolaemic, supine conscious patients, but their effects can be enhanced by changes in posture and by general anaesthesia.

The predominant cardiac vagal tone is reduced, resulting in a tachycardia; cardiac output normally falls, but again will reflect pre-existing sympathetic activity. The reduction in preload may benefit patients in heart failure and cardiac output may increase. Rowe, Alfonse and Lugas (1964) reported a precipitous fall in coronary blood flow in the dog, associated with the reduction in sympathetic activity. The combination of the reduction in mean arterial pressure with vasoconstriction of coronary vessels resulted in inadequate coronary blood flow in these experimental animals.

Cerebral blood flow remains unchanged in conscious normotensive subjects until the mean arterial pressure is reduced to below 50–60 mmHg. In hypertensive subjects the margin of safety is unpredictably reduced (Finnerty, Witkin and Fazekas, 1954). The cerebral blood vessels are largely unaffected by sympathetic stimulation; thus sympathetic blockade will produce minimal cerebral vasodilation with only marginal improvement in cerebral blood flow. This is in marked contrast to the effect of the directly acting vasodilating agents (Michenfelder and Theye, 1977).

Renal blood flow is decreased, although it usually remains adequate to meet metabolic requirements. Glomerular filtration may temporarily cease.

Ganglion-blocking drugs affect all autonomic ganglia; thus their action depends upon the predominant autonomic tone. There are many unwanted side effects, including cycloplegia, mydriasis, abolition of sweating, and atony of the bladder and the gastrointestinal tract. Some drugs have actions outside the autonomic ganglion. Trimetaphan causes histamine release (Larson, 1963) and may stabilize the postsynaptic membrane (Wang, Liu and Katz, 1977). Both these properties contribute to vasodilation and hypotension.

The oral absorption of the quaternary ammonium compounds is unpredictable and they are no longer used in the management of hypertension. The major use of these drugs is to produce hypotension for surgery, using posture and general anaesthetic agents to assist in this technique of 'controlled circulation' (Enderby, 1954). They have also been used in the management of autonomic hyper-reflexia (Basta, Niejadlik and Pallares, 1977). One advantage in clinical practice of drugs acting on the autonomic ganglia is that their action can be overcome by vasoconstrictors acting peripherally.

Hexamethonium

This bisquaternary ammonium compound (Fig. 15.2) was the first competitive blocker to achieve wide clinical use. The two quaternary nitrogen groups are linked by a methylene bridge. Autonomic blockade reaches a maximum when this bridge contains six carbon atoms (Kharkevich, 1967). Increasing the length of the methylene bridge produces drugs with neuromuscular-blocking properties.

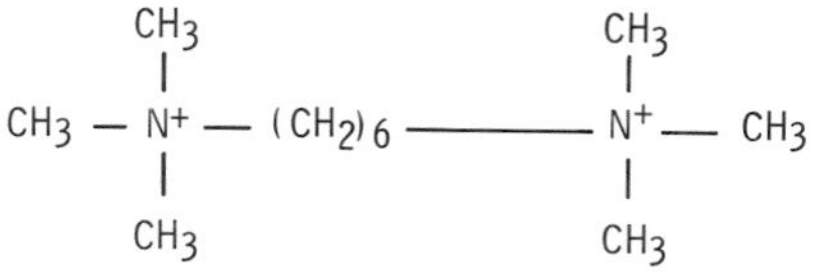

$$CH_3 - \overset{\overset{\displaystyle CH_3}{|}}{N^+} - (CH_2)_6 \longrightarrow \overset{\overset{\displaystyle CH_3}{|}}{\underset{\underset{\displaystyle CH_3}{|}}{N^+}} - CH_3$$

Fig. 15.2 Hexamethonium (C6).

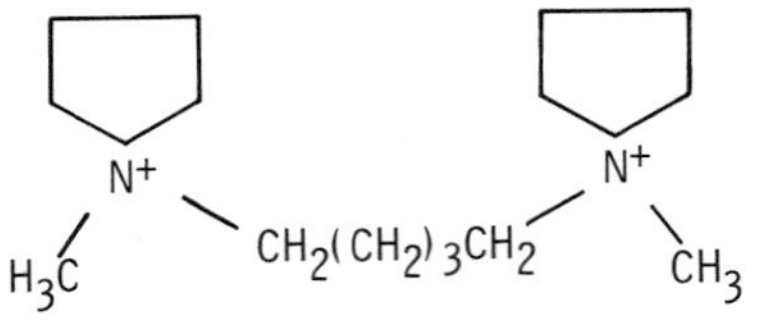

Fig. 15.3 Pentolinium.

Hexamethonium is a specific ganglion blocker, acting only at nicotinic cholinoceptors. Tachyphylaxis develops rapidly, and is thought to be related to increased dominance of the secondary pathways once the primary one has been blocked. There is considerable variation in the sensitivity of different ganglia to hexamethonium, the superior cervical ganglion being most sensitive, the visceral and cardiac vagal ones the least.

Pentolinium
Pentolinium (Fig. 15.3) is a bisquaternary competitive ganglion-blocking agent. It is more potent than hexamethonium and has a longer duration of action. It has been claimed that, of the ganglion-blocking drugs, pentolinium is one which causes less tachycardia (Enderby, 1954) although the reason for this remains uncertain.

Pentolinium has been used in the treatment of hypertension resistant to sodium nitroprusside (Jones, Hartler and Knight, 1981). It reduces sympathetic activity and would also appear to decrease plasma renin activity. It produces a pharmacological sympathectomy which will reduce the normal response of the body to stress. Fahmy and Battit (1975) observed that blood glucose levels did not rise during surgery when pentolinium was employed to induce hypotension. Pentolinium has also been used as an alternative to spinal anaesthesia to control the autonomic hyper-reflexia associated with spinal cord injury (Basta, Niejadlik and Pallares, 1977).

Trimetaphan
Trimetaphan (Fig. 15.4) can be regarded as a monoquaternary compound, the sulphur atom functioning as a quaternary nitrogen group. Following intravenous injection, trimetaphan rapidly produces ganglionic blockade.

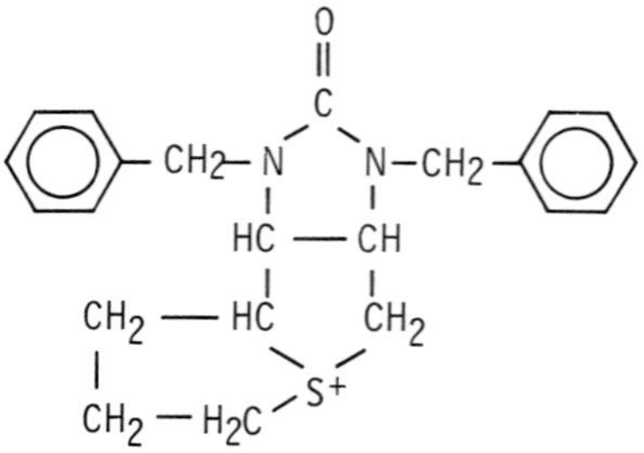

Fig. 15.4 Trimetaphan.

There is a reduction in both peripheral resistance and venous return, resulting in a fall in mean arterial pressure. A reduction in cardiac output occurs when anaesthetized patients are placed in the head-up position; this is not seen when the subjects remain supine (Scott *et al.*, 1972). The cardiovascular effects of trimetaphan last for 10–30 minutes following discontinuation of the infusion. In clinical concentrations trimetaphan behaves as a competitive antagonist of ACh, blocking nicotinic cholinoceptors. However, trimetaphan has a direct vasodilating action upon canine blood vessels (Harioka *et al.*, 1984), and histamine release may contribute to its hypotensive action. Tewfik (1957) suggested that trimetaphan is metabolized by pseudocholinesterase, but no metabolites have been isolated to date.

Recently there has been interest in the use of a mixture of trimetaphan and sodium nitroprusside (Wildsmith *et al.*, 1983). The drugs are chemically compatible and appear to have synergistic actions, thus allowing the total dose of both agents to be reduced. The synergism seen may be due to the inhibition of plasma renin activity already mentioned.

Directly acting vasodilators

Contraction of vascular smooth muscle is dependent upon two main mechanisms (Robinson, 1981). There is a phasic mechanism which relies upon the intrinsic activity of the vascular smooth muscle, and is seen predominantly in resistance vessels. Sustained contraction of vessels results from the combination of agonist (noradrenaline) and receptor, and occurs mainly in capacitance vessels.

Directly acting vasodilators act upon the smooth muscle in the vessel wall, preventing vasoconstriction. Their mode of action may vary but it is likely that the final common pathway of all these drugs is a reduction in the level of intracellular calcium, since a minimum concentration is required for the initiation of contraction. Some vasodilators act mainly upon resistance vessels; others upon capacitance.

Hydralazine
Hydralazine (Fig. 15.5) is a directly acting dilator, acting predominantly on arterioles. It has very little effect upon capacitance vessels. The mechanism of action is unknown but may be related to the ability of hydralazine to chelate trace metals involved in smooth muscle contraction (Albrecht, *el al.*, 1978).

Since the homoeostatic mechanisms for circulatory control remain unaffected by hydralazine, the reduction in peripheral resistance results in

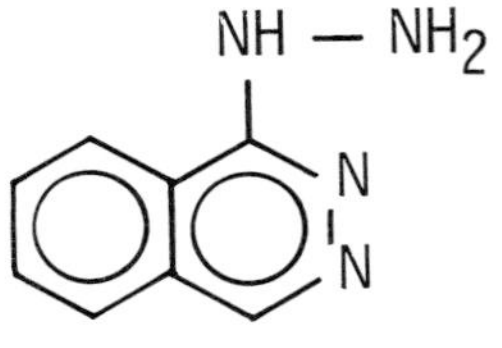

Fig. 15.5   Hydralazine.

increased sympathetic activity, with an increase in heart rate, and myocardial contractility. Thus the mean arterial blood pressure returns to control levels and myocardial oxygen consumption increases. These compensatory mechanisms can be prevented by the addition of β–blocking drugs, allowing the blood pressure to fall. An increase in plasma renin activity also occurs; this, too, can be prevented by β–blockade (Koch-Wesser, 1976).

Hydralazine can be given orally, intramuscularly or intravenously. The bioavailability of the orally administered drug is genetically determined; some individuals are able to acetylate hydralazine quickly, resulting in a rapid clearance of the drug from the plasma. The duration of action of an intravenous injection of hydralazine lasts from 15 minutes to 3–4 hours. After acetylation, hydralazine is conjugated with glucuronic acid and excreted by the kidneys.

Diazoxide

Diazoxide (Fig. 15.6) is a vascular dilator related to the thiazide diuretics. It acts predominantly on resistance vessels, having little effect upon veins. Again, the mechanism of action of diazoxide is obscure, but it may act by preventing the entry of calcium into vascular smooth muscle, thus blocking the initiation of contraction, It has also been suggested that diazoxide may compete with calcium for specific receptors on the vascular smooth muscle membrane. Diazoxide is an inhibitor of phosphodiesterase, an enzyme involved in the breakdown of cyclic adenosine monophosphate (cAMP); thus increased levels of AMP may be responsible for its hypotensive action.

Diazoxide has no effect upon autonomic reflexes, so its use is accompanied by tachycardia and an increase in stroke volume, which maintains or even increases cardiac output. This can be prevented by the use of β–blocking agents. There is also an increase in the level of circulating catecholamines and in plasma renin activity. Diazoxide has a long half-life; this is related to extensive protein binding, which delays renal excretion. Hyperglycaemia is frequently seen and is probably related to a decrease in the release of insulin. It has limited use in man, and will reduce blood pressure only to normal levels. It has been used in the management of eclampsia and hypertensive encephalopathy.

Adenosine triphosphate

Adenosine triphosphate (ATP) and adenosine are naturally occurring purines and are potent vasodilators. It is thought that, physiologically, they are involved in the regulation of local blood flow (Olsson, 1981). Recent concern about the toxicity of sodium nitroprusside has led to an increased interest in these rapidly acting agents.

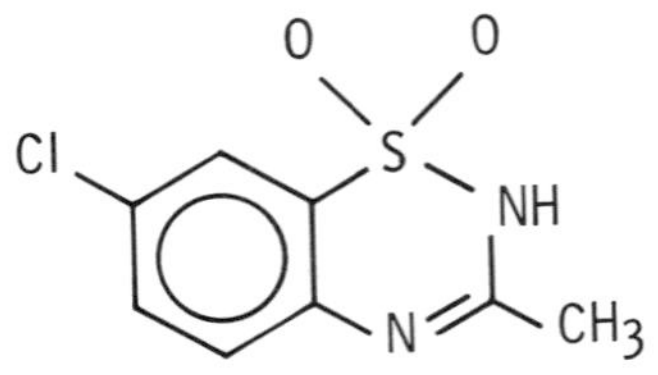

Fig. 15.6   Diazoxide.

Adenosine triphosphate produces hypotension in experimental animals (Van Aken *et al.*, 1984b) and in man (Fukunaga *et al.*, 1983). Its mechanism of action is uncertain but it would appear to be a directly acting vasodilator, with a predominant effect upon resistance vessels.

Hypotension is produced rapidly, within 30 seconds from the start of an infusion; the blood pressure remains stable during administration of the drug, and recovery also is rapid (Fukunaga *et al.*, 1983). There is a significant reduction in both systemic and pulmonary vascular resistance; this appears to be dose dependent (Van Aken *et al.*, 1984b). Cardiac output and stroke volume are unchanged or may slightly increase. Tachycardia is rarely seen but bradycardia has been reported by some workers. This latter may result from a reduction in the rate of discharge of the pacemaker cells within the heart (Rall, 1980). A small decrease in left ventricular stroke work is seen (Ma *et al.*, 1982), which suggests that cardiac depression may occur. Coronary sinus blood flow increases in the dog, as the vessels dilate (Bloor *et al.*, 1982) and myocardial oxygen consumption falls.

Cerebral blood flow increases initially with dilatation of cerebral vessels (Van Aken *et al.*, 1984a). Intracranial pressure increases at this time, and these changes are magnified when there is intracranial hypertension. As the mean arterial pressure falls, cerebral blood flow returns to control values, and then falls *pari passu* with the reduction in mean arterial pressure. In the baboon, loss of autoregulation occurred when the mean arterial pressure was reduced to 60 per cent of control (Van Aken *et al.*, 1984b). Despite this, no evidence of brain ischaemia could be detected following the reduction of the cerebral perfusion pressure to 30 mmHg in these animals. In the cat, the integrity of the membrane of cortical brain cells is lost at a higher mean pressure when hypotension induced with ATP is compared with that from sodium nitroprusside (Heuser *et al.*, 1984). This suggests that brain ischaemia is more likely during hypotension produced with ATP.

Rebound hypertension is not seen, and there is no increase in plasma catecholamines (Bloor *et al.*, 1982) or in plasma renin activity (Lagerkranser *et al.*, 1983). The blood pressure in experimental animals receiving ATP was further reduced by controlled haemorrhage. These animals failed to produce the normal increase in plasma renin activity, and it has been suggested that ATP may produce a presynaptic blockade of sympathetic transmission.

Adenosine triphosphate is rapidly hydrolysed to adenosine by a 5'–nucleotidase present in serum, red blood cells and myocardial cells. This hydrolysis occurs during one passage through the pulmonary vascular bed and it would appear that the hypotensive action of ATP is due to its metabolite, adenosine. Sollevi and his co-workers (1984) have shown that the level of blood pressure is directly related to the concentration of adenosine in the arterial blood. Adenosine could be used as the hypotensive agent but, unfortunately, it is unstable, thus making storage difficult. Adenosine is inactivated and eventually converted to uric acid with the liberation of phosphate. Man is unable to metabolize uric acid, and this results in an increase in its concentration in the plasma. This has been seen in the experimental animal (Van Aken *et al.*, 1984b). Dendrick and his co-workers (1982) infused conscious rats with ATP, 10 mg/kg per minute. Several animals died from pulmonary oedema, which occurred soon after the infusion was begun. All animals developed serious cardiac dysrhythmias, including multifocal ventricular ectopics and bigeminy. The authors suggested that the problems were related to the high level of phosphate which occurred during metabolism of the drug, causing chelation of either calcium or magnesium. However, it must be stressed that the dose used was greatly in excess of that employed in man, in whom infusions of 0.2–0.6 mg/kg per minute are sufficient for clinical use.

The amount of ATP (or adenosine) required can be reduced by the addition of an adenosine inhibitor, dipyridamole (Persantin).

Sodium nitroprusside
Sodium nitroprusside (SNP) is a powerful vasodilator. It was first synthesized by Playfair in 1849, and has been used sporadically in medicine ever since. In the early 1950s it became an accepted treatment in the management of hypertensive crises, and later its evanescent action proved useful in the induction of hypotension during general anaesthesia. Since its initial enthusiastic introduction into clinical practice, reports of toxicity have tempered its use, although it still remains a valuable hypotensive agent.

Five cyanide groups and a nitroso radical surround a central iron atom (Fig. 15.7). SNP is a potent vasodilator, mainly acting upon small arterioles (Longnecker, Creasy and Ross, 1979) although dilation of capacitance vessels also occurs (Wildsmith et al., 1973). It is thought to act directly upon blood vessels, since its action is not prevented by α– or β–adrenergic-blocking drugs, or by muscarinic cholinergic blockade. However, autonomic transmission may be indirectly affected since SNP depletes the neuronal stores of noradrenaline. Little is known about the cellular pharmacology of SNP. In 1929, Johnson suggested that the nitroso group was the active component; some years later, Page (1955) and his co-workers suggested that SNP interacted with sulphydryl groups in the cell membrane. This theory was supported by work carried out by Needleman and his colleagues (1973) who demonstrated that, in isolated aortic strips, pretreatment with ethacrynic acid (which alkylates sulphydryl groups) blocks the vasodilating action of SNP. It has been further proposed that the interaction between SNP and membrane suphydryl groups, stabilizes the cell membrane, thus preventing the ionic flux of calcium which is necessary for the initiation of contraction.

Other workers have suggested that SNP may act via the cyclic nucleotides. The evidence so far is conflicting, although changes in nucleotide concentration have been measured following the administration of SNP.

Arteriolar and venodilatation occur approximately 90 seconds after an

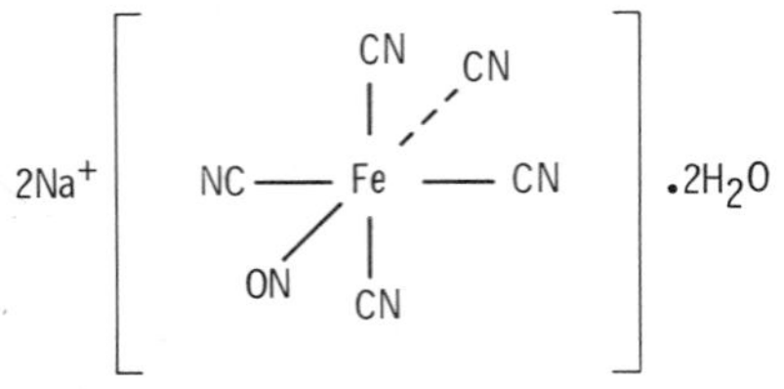

Fig. 15.7   Sodium nitroprusside.

intravenous injection of SNP. Thus both peripheral resistance and venous return are reduced, resulting in a profound fall in systemic blood pressure. This activates the baroreceptors, causing a compensatory tachycardia which may be particularly troublesome in young healthy adults.

There may be no change in cardiac output (Styles, Coleman and Leary, 1973) or the cardiac output may increase (Wildsmith *et al.*, 1973). The latter is mainly seen in anaesthetized patients and in patients in whom a reduction in afterload may be beneficial (Franciosa *et al.*, 1972). SNP has no direct effect on the heart, contractility remains unchanged (Adams *et al* ., 1974). When injected directly into the coronary circulation of dogs SNP dilates coronary blood vessels (Wang, Liu and Katz, 1977), producing an increase in coronary blood flow. However, the metabolic requirements of the myocardium are reduced during hypotension with SNP, since arteriolar dilatation significantly reduces cardiac work. This could explain the unchanged or reduced coronary blood flow recorded by the same workers following intravenous administration of the drug. When SNP was used to reduce the systolic blood pressure to 50 mmHg in anaesthetized healthy patients, some ischaemic changes on the ECG were seen, but these did not persist (Simpson, Bellamy and Cole, 1976). However, in the presence of severe coronary artery disease, dilation of normal coronary vessels may further impair flow through diseased vasospastic ones, reducing the oxygen supply to compromised areas of myocardium (Chiariello *et al.*, 1976).

Autoregulation of cerebral blood flow allows fluctuation in mean arterial blood pressure to occur without producing major changes in cerebral blood flow. There is sympathetic innervation of the pial arteries, but maximum sympathetic stimulation results only in a 20 per cent reduction of cerebral blood flow. Thus sympathetic-blocking drugs have a marginal effect upon cerebral blood flow. SNP directly dilates cerebral blood vessels, increasing cerebral blood flow, and allowing lower levels of mean arterial pressure to be safely achieved. This shift in autoregulation of cerebral blood flow to the left has been demonstrated both in man and in experimental animals (Griffiths *et al.*, 1974; Stoyka and Schutz, 1975; Michenfelder and Theye, 1977; Maekawa, McDowall and Okuda, 1979).

However, dilation of cerebral vessels may not always be beneficial; intracranial pressure will increase because of the increase in blood volume, and this may reduce cerebral perfusion since the cerebral perfusion pressure reflects the difference between the mean arterial and the intracranial pressures. Turner and his co-workers (1977) reported a rise in intracranial pressure occurring during the adminstration of SNP. This intracranial hypertension persisted until the mean blood pressure had been reduced to 70 per cent of control. In the presence of an intracranial mass lesion, the additional rise in intracranial pressure may produce signs of global ischaemia (Marsh *et al*, 1979). Dilatation of normal cerebral blood vessels may result in a 'steal' effect, diverting blood away from areas of focal ischaemia, supplied by vasospastic vessels. This could increase the risk of infarction or ischaemic damage.

SNP appears to reduce the integrity of the blood–brain barrier in the dog (Ishikawa *et al.*, 1983), and increases in the concentration of cyanide in the cerebrospinal fluid have been reported in man (Casthely *et al.*, 1981).

Arterial oxygen tension falls during hypotension with SNP. The action of nitroprusside upon normal pulmonary vessels remains uncertain but the normal vasoconstrictor response to hypoxia is attenuated (D'Oliveira *et al.*, 1981). This increases blood flow to underventilated areas of lung. Khambatta, Stone and Matteo (1982) failed to demonstrate an increase in physiological dead space during hypotension produced with SNP and concluded that the changes in VD/VT reported by other workers were due to relative hypovolaemia.

In the dog, autoregulation of renal blood flow is maintained to a mean arterial pressure of 60 mmHg during the administration of SNP. It has been shown by Maseda and his colleagues (1981) that renal blood flow and urine production improved in post cardiac surgical patients when low concentrations of SNP were used to prevent hypertension.

Rebound hypertension has been a persistent problem, occurring when the infusion of SNP is stopped (Miller *et al.*, 1977; Khambatta, Stone and Khan, 1979). This is caused by stimulation of the renin–angiotensin axis and can be prevented by β–blocking drugs (Marshall *et al.*, 1981), ganglionic blockers (Jones, Hartler and Knight, 1981) and angiotensin inhibitors (Delaney and Miller, 1980).

Sodium nitroprusside is soluble in water; it forms a brown solution which turns blue on exposure to light, due to reduction of the ferric iron to ferrous. Solutions of SNP should be freshly prepared before use and protected from light at all times.

SNP is broken down in the blood stream – some slowly in the plasma by the sulphydryl groups present in amino acids, and some more rapidly by an non-enzymatic process within the red blood cell (Smith and Kruszyna, 1976). An electron is donated from oxyhaemoglobin to produce an unstable nitroprusside radical which rapidly decomposes, liberating five cyanide ions from each molecule of sodium nitroprusside. One of the cyanide ions is taken up by the methaemoglobin formed; the others enter the plasma. It is thought that rapid hydrolysis of SNP by the erythrocyte occurs only when the plasma concentrations of SNP are high; otherwise, the breakdown of SNP occurs more slowly in the plasma (Ivankovich, Miletich and Tinker, 1978).

Within the plasma, about 80 per cent of the free cyanide is converted to thiocyanate; this requires thiosulphate as the substrate and rhodanase enzyme. Thiocyanate is a weak vasodilator and is excreted unchanged in the urine. A small amount may be oxidized back to cyanide. Plasma thiocyanate levels correlate poorly with plasma cyanide and cyanide toxicity. Alternative pathways exist for the elimination of cyanide but play a relatively unimportant role. They include the combination of cyanide with hydroxycobalamin to form cyanocobalamin which is then excreted by the kidneys.

If the rate of breakdown of SNP to cyanide exceeds the clearance of cyanide from the plasma, cyanide toxicity occurs. Cyanide reacts with cytochrome in the mitochondria, preventing cellular respiration. Thus histotoxic hypoxia occurs with a progressive metabolic acidosis and, ultimately, death. Michenfelder (1977) demonstrated that, in the experimental animal, the rate of infusion of SNP is the most important factor in producing cyanide toxicity. If too much is given, the enzyme system responsible for its detoxification is overloaded and the concentration of cyanide within the plasma reaches toxic levels.

In man, all the reported fatal cases of cyanide toxicity associated with the use of nitroprusside have involved the use of large amounts of drug. McDowall and colleagues (1974) looked at the action of SNP in the baboon and found that those animals which failed to recover had received at least four times the dose used in the group of surviving animals. Apparent resistance to the hypotensive action of SNP has been noted, and this tachyphylaxis precedes the severe metabolic disturbances. Grayling, Miller and Peach (1978) demonstrated that the sensitivity of isolated aortic strips to SNP could be reduced by the addition of cyanide to the perfusate. This may explain the development of resistance to SNP, although these results are a little surprising since cyanide itself reduces vascular tone.

Various guidelines have been suggested to ensure the safe use of SNP, of which the most important is to limit the dose. Vesey, Cole and Simpson (1976) recommended that the total dose of SNP should not exceed 1.5 mg/kg when the drug is used 'acutely', and that the plasma cyanide concentration should not exceed 300 nmol/l. For 'chronic' use the rate of infusion of SNP should not exceed $4\mu g$/kg per minute. β–Blockers or alternative drugs should be given to limit the amount of SNP required. To this end, mixtures of SNP and trimetaphan have been used, in the ratio $1:10$ (Wildsmith et al., 1983). The hypotensive action of these two drugs, acting at different sites, appears to be synergistic, thus allowing the total dose of both drugs to be reduced. SNP should be avoided in patients in whom it is anticipated that its metabolism and excretion is impaired. These include hypothermic subjects and patients suffering from malnutrition, vitamin B_{12} deficiency, severe liver disease or renal failure.

Pretreatment with hydroxocobalamin (Ivankovich et al., 1980), sodium thiosulphate and methaemoglobin-producing compounds (Michenfelder and Tinker, 1977) has been used to reduce the incidence of cyanide toxicity. Methylene blue and nitrites have been employed in the treatment of established cyanide poisoning but have been largely superseded by cobalt edetate. However, cyanide toxicity is best prevented by limiting the amount of nitroprusside used.

The degradation of SNP to cyanide has been questioned by Bissett and his co-workers (1981). They claim that the high plasma levels of cyanide measured in many studies result from the breakdown of SNP during the colorimetric method used for its analysis, and that its breakdown does not occur in the blood stream. It is the firm opinion of these authors that cyanide toxicity is always associated with photodegradation of SNP before the administration of the drug. However, this theory is not accepted by other authorities (Vesey, Cole and Simpson, 1982; Arnold, Longnecker and Epstein, 1984) and it would seem prudent at present to limit the dose of SNP.

Nitroglycerin (glyceryl trinitrate)
Nitroglycerin (Fig. 15.8) has been used in the treatment of angina for over a century. It is effective when given by all routes except the oral one since rapid first-pass metabolism terminates its action.

Nitroglycerin is a direct vasodilator. The actual mechanism of action remains uncertain but, like other nitrates, it is thought to react with sulphydryl groups within the vessel wall. It is rapidly metabolized in the liver to glyceryl dinitrate,

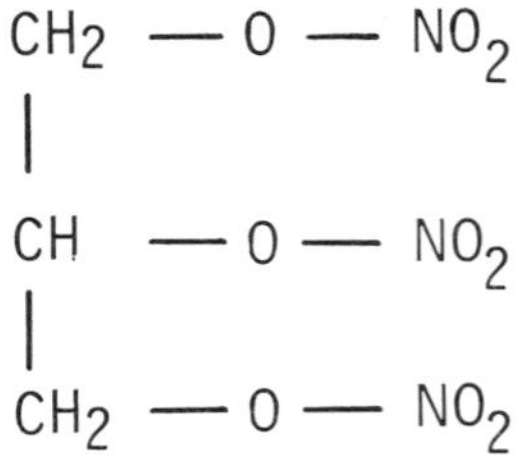

$$CH_2 - O - NO_2$$
$$|$$
$$CH - O - NO_2$$
$$|$$
$$CH_2 - O - NO_2$$

Fig. 15.8 Nitroglycerin.

glyceryl mononitrate and inorganic nitrite, all of which are weak vasodilators. Inorganic nitrite converts oxyhaemoglobin to methaemoglobin, and increased levels have been reported (Aveling and Verner, 1981). However, Hussum, Lindeburg and Jacobsen, 1982), using a massive infusion of nitroglycerin for 24 hours, for the treatment of ergotamine poisoning, failed to show any significant methaemoglobinaemia.

Capacitance vessels are preferentially dilated by nitroglycerin, resulting in venodilation with a reduction in cardiac filling. The left ventricular end-diastolic pressure falls, with an improvement in subendocardial perfusion (Bale, Powles and Wyatt, 1982). When low concentrations are used, cardiac output and pulse rate remain unchanged although some increase in pulse rate accompanies systemic hypotension. Fahmy (1978) compared the cardiovascular effects of nitroglycerin to equipotent doses of SNP. The systolic blood pressure was reduced to comparable levels, but the diastolic and mean blood pressures were consistently higher with nitroglycerin.

The mechanism by which nitroglycerin reduces cardiac pain has been a subject of some controversy since its introduction into clinical practice. Nitroglycerin directly dilates coronary vessels in the animal model, and it would appear to improve blood flow through both normal and vasospastic vessels. Improvement in the depression of the ST segment has been reported by several workers (Kaplan, Dunbar and Jones, 1976; Tobias, 1981) during nitroglycerin administration in patients undergoing coronary artery surgery. The endocardial viability ratio is improved and appears to correlate well with subendocardial perfusion (Bale, Powles and Wyatt, 1982). Myocardial oxygen consumption is also decreased (Sethna et al., 1982).

The reduction in venous return may be a problem in the failing heart, reducing myocardial contractility even further, and may require the concurrent use of inotropes.

Pulmonary blood vessels dilate, causing a reduction in pulmonary vascular resistance (Tobias, 1981). The vasoconstrictor response to hypoxia is reduced (Colley, Cheney and Hlastala, 1981; D'Oliveira et al., 1981) and may result in an increase in shunt.

Intracranial pressure rises as cerebral veins dilate (Rogers et al., 1979; Morris, Todd and Philbin, 1982); the increases are greater in the presence of intracranial hypertension. Burt, Verniquet and Homi (1982) showed that when mean arterial pressure is reduced to 75 per cent of control, intracranial pressure returns to normal and then falls as the blood pressure is further decreased. Again care must be exercised with the use of nitroglycerin in subjects with an intracranial mass lesion.

The onset of action of nitroglycerin is rapid but not so fast as nitroprusside; it is also less potent. The rate of infusion of drug must be titrated against its effect. An intravenous preparation is now commercially available and is usually diluted to produce a 0.01 per cent solution. Tachyphylaxis is not a problem; neither is rebound hypertension although an increase in plasma renin activity has been reported (Guggiari *et al.*, 1985). The hepatic metabolism of nitroglycerin results in the production of water-soluble metabolites which are readily excreted by the kidney. Nitroglycerin is adsorbed onto polyvinylchloride infusion sets, with a consequent reduction in its activity. To prevent this problem it is recommended that glass or rigid plastic syringes be used in combination with polyethylene tubing.

Nitroglycerin is used in the treatment of angina, to reduce pain and to improve coronary perfusion when there is critical ischaemia. It has been used during coronary artery surgery (Viljoen, 1968; Kaplan, Dunbar and Jones, 1976) to control episodes of hypertension. Its use as a hypotensive agent for general surgery remains limited, although it has been used to attenuate the pressor response to laryngoscopy and intubation (Fasoulaki and Kaniaras, 1983).

Myocardial depressants

The volatile anaesthetic agents halothane and enflurane produce hypotension by depressing myocardial contractility. Another group of myocardial depressant drugs which have been used to lower the blood pressure are the calcium–channel–blocking agents verapamil, nifedipine, perhexiline and prenylamine. These agents inhibit the entry of calcium into both myocardial cells and vascular smooth muscle; thus vasodilation accompaines myocardial depression. Verapamil is used as an antiarrhythmic agent as it prevents calcium entry in atrioventricular nodal cells.

Halothane
Halothane produces arterial hypotension. Many theories have been postulated to explain this, and it is now generally accepted that halothane directly depresses myocardial contractility and that this is a dose-related phenomenon(Eger *et al.*, 1970; Prys-Roberts *et al.*, 1972). There is a reduction in stroke volume and cardiac output, right atrial pressure rises, and the pulse rate and systemic vascular resistance remain unchanged (Prys-Roberts *et al.*, 1972). This agrees with work carried out by Brown and Crout (1971) on the isolated paced papillary muscle of the cat. Early workers suggested that halothane produced its circulatory changes secondarily to a reduction in peripheral resistance (Morrow and Morrow, 1961; Deutsch *et al.*, 1962). Vasodilation of some vessels does occur (those supplying the skin, brain and splanchnic beds) but this is offset by vasoconstriction of renal and muscle vasculature, so there is no net change (Adams, 1980).

As the cardiac output falls, total body oxygen consumption decreases; but with further depression of myocardial function, desaturation of mixed venous blood is seen. Bland and Lowenstein (1976) observed that, in the non-failing canine heart, halothane appeared to reduce the area of infarction induced experimentally by occlusion of a coronary vessel supplying a small area of myocardium. However, if larger areas of the heart were rendered ischaemic before halothane was administered, the subsequent administration of halothane resulted in severe irreversible changes in the ischaemic myocardium (Francis et al., 1982). Halothane depresses the sensitivity of the baroreceptors; there is no tachycardia in response to the reduced arterial pressure (Bristow et al., 1969).

The effect of halothane on the circulation is partly dependent upon the mode of ventilation and the level of the arterial carbon dioxide tension. Respiration is depressed with halothane, so during spontaneous ventilation the resultant hypercarbia produces a sympathetic response which partially counteracts the depressant effects of the anaesthetic (Bahlman et al., 1972). A return towards control values has been observed by several workers (Deutsch et al., 1962; Eger et al., 1970) following prolonged administration of halothane.

Halothane is a cerebral vasodilator and is often used in combination with other agents to produce hypotension during neurosurgical procedures, its effect on intracranial pressure being modifed by moderate hyperventilation. Michenfelder and Theye (1977) showed that, during profound hypotension in the dog, the hypotensive technique used did not affect the outcome; however, when the arterial pressure was reduced so that the cerebral perfusion pressure was marginal, halothane and sodium nitroprusside produced fewer episodes of cerebral ischaemia than did either haemorrhagic hypotension or ganglionic blockade.

Enflurane
This halogenated ether has very similar effects on the cardiovascular system as halothane. There is a reduction in cardiac output, stroke volume and mean arterial pressure, with a slight reduction in systemic peripheral resistance and heart rate (Calverley et al., 1978). β–Blockade and enflurane anaesthesia would appear to be a lethal combination in dogs during haemorrhage (Horan et al., 1977).

Isoflurane
Isoflurane is a halogenated methyl-ethyl ether, an isomer of enflurane. Isoflurane produces a reduction in blood pressure with a decrease in stroke volume. Total peripheral resistance falls but cardiac output is maintained by an increase in heart rate (Stevens et al., 1971). Isoflurane would appear to be unique among the volatile anaesthetic agents in that it produces an overall decrease in peripheral vascular resistance.

Isoflurane dilates coronary blood vessels, but this may lead to regional areas of ischaemia since blood is diverted from diseased vasospastic coronaries (Reiz et al., 1983). It has been used to produce hypotension for neurosurgical procedures (Lam and Gelb, 1983), and it is claimed that there is no increase in intracranial pressure when used in anaesthetic concentrations during controlled ventilation; thus the cerebral perfusion pressure is maintained. Autoregulation of cerebral blood flow occurs with concentrations up to 1.5 MAC, and the vascular response to changes in arterial carbon dioxide tension appears to be retained (Frost, 1984). Cerebral oxygen consumption is reduced along with cerebral blood flow when the blood pressure is lowered, and some workers suggest that isoflurane may have a protective role. Newberg, Milde and Michenfelder (1984) reduced the blood pressure of dogs to a mean arterial pressure of 40 mmHg and maintained this for 1 hour using isoflurane. The cerebral activity of these experimental animals remained normal throughout the experiment.

Inhibitors of the renin – angiotensin system

The release of renin from the juxtaglomerular apparatus of the kidneys is stimulated by a reduction in blood volume, or by a decrease in the perfusion of the kidneys or by a reduction in the concentration of sodium in the plasma. Renin acts on a plasma protein precursor to produce angiotensin I. This is a relatively inert substance which is converted to angiotensin II by peptidyl dipeptidases. Angiotensin II is a potent pressor agent causing vasoconstriction, and also stimulates the release of catecholamines and aldosterone from the adrenal gland. In addition, angiotensin II increases the release of noradrenaline from postganglionic sympathetic nerves. A negative feedback regulates further renin production.

There are two major types of antagonists: (1) angiotensin II antagonists (e.g. saralasin); and (2) inhibitors of peptidyl dipeptidases (e.g. captopril).

Saralasin

Saralasin acts by blocking specific receptors for angiotensin II. It should be regarded as a partial agonist since stimulation does occur, resulting in an initial pressor response. It has an extremely short half-life of 4 minutes, and needs to be given as an intravenous infusion. It has been used in experimental animals and in man, and would appear to be more effective in reducing the blood pressure of hypertensive subjects.

Captopril

Captopril is an inhibitor of peptidyl dipeptidases. Thus both the conversion of angiotensin I to angiotensin II and the destruction of bradykinin are reduced. This results in a decrease in vasoconstrictor agents with a concomitant increase in potent vasodilators. There is a decrease in the level of circulating catecholamines, and plasma aldosterone concentrations fall. Plasma renin activity will actually be increased because of the reduced levels of angiotensin II.

Captopril is used in the treatment of malignant hypertension and for renovascular emergencies. It has recently been used to prevent rebound hypertension following the use of ultra-short-acting vasodilators (Fahmy, 1984; Pasch et al., 1984). Oral pretreatment is effective, and also reduces the amount of hypotensive agent required, thus decreasing the likelihood of toxicity.

348   Hypotensive agents

References

Adams, A.P. (1980) Drugs in elective hypotension. In: *The Circulation in Anaesthesia* (Ed. Prys-Roberts, C.), pp. 491–508. Blackwell Scientific: Oxford

Adams, A.P., Clark, T.N.S., Edmonds-Seal, J., Foex, P., Prys-Roberts, C. and Roberts, J. (1974) The effect of sodium nitroprusside on myocardial contractility and haemodynamics. *British Journal of Anaesthesia* 46, 807–817

Albrecht, R.F., Toyooka, E.T., Polk, S.L.H. and Zahed, B. (1978) Hydralazine therapy for hypertension during the anaesthetic and post anaesthetic periods. In: *International Anesthesiology Clinics. Nitroprusside and other short acting hypotensive agents*, pp. 299–312. Little, Brown: Boston, MA

Arnold, W.P., Longnecker, D.E. and Epstein, R.H. (1984) Photodegradation of sodium nitroprusside: biologic activity and cyanide release. *Anesthesiology* 61, 254–260

Aveling, W. and Verner, I.R. (1981) Profound hypotension with intravenous nitroglycerine. In: *International Symposium on the Clinical Use of Tridil. Intravenous Nitroglycerin* (Eds. Robinson, B.F. and Kaplan, J.A.). Medicine Publishing Foundation: Oxford

Bahlman, S.H., Eger, E., Halsey, M.J. *et al.* (1972) The cardiovascular effects of halothane in man during spontaneous ventilation. *Anesthesiology* 36, 494–501

Bale, R., Powles, A. and Wyatt, R. (1982) IV Glyceryl trinitrate: haemodynamic effects and clinical use in cardiac surgery. *British Journal of Anaesthesia* 54, 297–301

Basta, J.A., Niejadlik, K, and Pallares, V. (1977) Autonomic hyperreflexia: intraoperative control with pentolinium tartrate. *British Journal of Anaesthesia* 49, 1087–1091

Bisset, W.I.K., Butler, A.R., Glidewell, C. and Reglinski, J. (1981) Sodium nitroprusside and cyanide release: reasons for reappraisal. *British Journal of Anaesthesia* 51, 1015–1018

Bland, J.H.L. and Lowenstein, E. (1976) Halothane-induced decrease in experimental myocardial ischemia in the non-failing canine heart. *Anesthesiology* 45, 287–293

Bloor, B.D., Fukunaga, A.F., Flacke, W. *et al.* (1982) Coronary sinus blood flow during hypotension induced by sodium nitroprusside or adenosine triphosphate infusions. *Anesthesiology* 57S, A51

Bristow, J.P., Prys-Roberts, C., Fisher, A., Pickering. J.G. and Sleight, P. (1969) Effects of anesthesia on baroreflex control of heart rate in man. *Anesthesiology* 31, 422–428

Brown, B.R. and Crout, J.R. (1971) A comparative study of the effect of five general anesthetics on myocardial contractility. *Anesthesiology* 34, 236–245

Burt, D.E.R., Verniquet, A.J.W. and Homi, J. (1982) The response of canine intracranial pressure to systemic hypotension induced with nitroglycerine. *British Journal of Anaesthesia* 54, 665–672

Calverley, R.K., Smith, N.T., Prys-Roberts, C., Eger, E. I. and Jones, C.W. (1978) Cardiovascular effects of enflurane anesthesia during controlled ventilation in man. *Anesthesia and Analgesia* 57, 619–628

Casthely, P.A., Cottrell, J.E., Patel, K.P., Marlin, A. and Turndorf, H. (1981) Cerebrospinal fluid cyanide after nitroprusside infusion in man. *Canadian Anaesthetists' Society Journal* 28, 228–231

Chiariello, M., Gold, H.K., Leinbach, R.C., Davis, M.A. and Maroko, P.R. (1976) Comparison between the effects of nitroglycerin and nitroprusside on ischemic injury during acute myocardial infarction. *Circulation* 54, 766–773

Colley, P.S., Cheney, F.W. and Hlastala, M.P. (1981) Pulmonary gas exchange effects of nitroglycerine in canine edematous lungs. *Anesthesiology* 55, 114–119

Delaney, T.J. and Miller, E.D. (1980) Rebound hypertension after sodium nitroprusside prevented by Saralasin in rats. *Anesthesiology* 52, 154–156

Dendrick, D.E., Mans, A.M., Campbell, P.A., Hawkins, R.A. and Biebuyck, J.F. (1982) Does ATP-induced hypotension cause potentially serious metabolic complications. *Anesthesiology* **57**, 66

Deutsch, S., Linde, H.W., Dripps, R.D. and Price, H.L. (1962) Circulatory and respiratory actions of halothane in normal man. *Anesthesiology* **23**, 631–638

D'Oliveira, M., Sykes, M.K., Chakrabarti, M.K., Orchard, C. and Keslin, J. (1981) Depression of hypoxic pulmonary vasoconstriction by sodium nitroprusside and nitroglycerine. *British Journal of Anaesthesia* **53**, 11–18

Eger, E.I. II, Smith, N.T., Stoelting, R.K., Cullen, D.J., Kadis, L.B. and Whitcher, C.E. (1970) Cardiovascular effects of halothane in man. *Anesthesiology* **32**, 396–409

Enderby, G.E.H. (1954) Pentolinium tartrate in controlled hypotension. *Lancet* **ii**, 1097–1098

Eränko, O. (1978) Small intenselv fluorescent (SIF) cells and nervous transmission in sympathetic ganglia. *Annual Review of Pharmacology and Toxicology* **18**, 417–430

Fahmy, N.R. (1978) Nitroglycerin as a hypotensive drug during general anesthesia. *Anesthesiology* **49**, 17–20

Fahmy, N.R. (1984) Impact of oral captopril or propranolol on nitroprusside induced hypotension. *Anesthesiology* **61**, 41

Fahmy, N.R. and Battit, G.E. (1975) Effects of pentolinium on blood sugar and serum potassium concentrations during anaesthesia and surgery. *British Journal of Anaesthesia* **47**, 1309–1314

Fasoulaki, A. and Kaniaris, P. (1983) Intranasal administration of nitroglycerin attenuates the pressor response to laryngoscopy and intubation of the trachea. *British Journal of Anaesthesia* **55**, 49–52

Finnerty, F.A., Witkin, L. and Fazekas, J.F. (1954) Cerebral hemodynamics during cerebral ischemia induced by acute hypotension. *Journal of Clinical Investigation* **33**, 1227–1232

Franciosa, J.A., Guiha, N.H., Limas, C.J., Rodriguera, E. and Cohn, J.N. (1972) Improved left ventricular function during nitroprusside infusion in acute myocardial infarction. *Lancet* **i**, 650–654

Francis, C.M., Foex, P., Lowenstein, E. *et al.* (1982) Interaction between regional myocardial ischaemia and left ventricular performance under halothane anaesthesia. *British Journal of Anaesthesia* **54**, 965–980

Frost, E.A.M. (1984) Inhalation anaesthetic agents in neurosurgery. *British Journal of Anaesthesia* **56**, 475–565

Fukunaga, A.F., Sodeyama, O., Matsuzaki, Y., Ikeda, K., Matsuda, I. and Sato, K. (1983) Hemodynamic and metabolic changes of ATP induced hypotension during surgery. *Anesthesiology* **59**, A12

Fukunaga, A.F., Ito, H., Jinno, S. and Kubota, Y. (1984) Dipyridamole potentiates the hypotensive action of ATP. *Anesthesiology* **61**, A39

Gaskell, W.H. (1916) *The Involuntary Nervous System*. Longmans Green: London

Grayling, G.W., Miller, E.D. and Peach, M.J. (1978) Sodium cyanide antagonism of the vasodilator action of sodium nitroprusside in the isolated rabbit aortic strip. *Anesthesiology* **49**, 21–25

Griffiths, D.P.G., Cummins, B.H., Greenbaum, R. *et al.* (1974) Cerebral blood flow and metabolism during hypotension induced with sodium nitroprusside. *British Journal of Anaesthesia* **46**, 671–679

Guggiari, M., Dagneou, F., Lienhart, A. *et al.* (1985) Use of nitroglycerine to produce controlled decreases in mean arterial pressure to less than 50 mmHg. *British Journal of Anaesthesia* **57**, 142–147

Harioka, T., Hatano, Y., Mori, K. and Toda, N. (1984) Trimetaphan is a direct arterial vasodilator and an α–adrenegic antagonist. *Anesthesia and Analgesia* **63**, 290–296

Heuser, D., Guggenberger, H, and Morris, P.J. (1984) ATP or SNP for intraoperative controlled hypotension. An experimental study on CBF and extracellular ion homoeostasis. *British Journal of Anaesthesia* **56**, 1296P

Horan, B.F., Prys-Roberts, C., Hamilton, W.K. and Roberts, J.G. (1977) Haemodynamic responses to enflurane anaesthesia and hypovolaemia in the dog and their modification by propranolol. *British Journal of Anaesthesia* **49**, 1189–1197

Hussum, B., Lindeburg, T. and Jacobsen, E. (1982) Methaemoglobin formation after nitroglycerin infusion. *British Journal of Anaesthesia* **54**, 571

Ishikawa, T., Funatsu, N., Okamoto, K., Takeshita, H. and McDowall, D.G. (1983) Blood-brain barrier function following drug induced hypotension in the dog. *Anesthesiology* **59**, 526–531

Ivankovich, A.D., Miletich, D.J. and Tinker, T.H. (1978) Sodium nitroprusside: metabolism and general considerations. In: *Nitroprusside and Other Short-acting Hypotensive Agents,* International Anesthesiology Clinics (Ed. Ivankovich, A.D.), pp. 1–29. Little, Brown: Boston, MA

Ivankovich, A.D., Braverman, B., Kanuara, R.P., Heyman, H.J. and Paulissan, R. (1980) Cyanide antidotes and methods of their administration in dogs. *Anesthesiology* **52**, 210–216

Johnson, C.C. (1929) The actions and toxicity of sodium nitroprusside. *Archives Internationals de Pharmacodynamie et de Thérapie* **35**, 480–496

Jones, R.M., Hartler, C.B. and Knight, P.R. (1981) Use of pentolinium in postoperative hypertension resistant to sodium nitroprusside. *British Journal of Anaesthesia* **53**, 1151–1154

Kaplan, N., Dunbar, R.W. and Jones, E.L. (1976) Nitroglycerin infusion during coronary artery surgery. *Anesthesiology* **45**, 14–21

Khambatta, H.J., Stone, J.G. and Khan, E. (1979) Hypertension during anesthesia on discontinuation of sodium nitroprusside induced hypotension. *Anesthesiology* **51**, 127–130

Khambatta, H.J., Stone, J.G. and Matteo, R.S. (1982) Effect of sodium nitroprusside and induced hypotension on pulmonary dead space. *British Journal of Anaesthesia* **54**, 1197–1200

Kharkevich, D.A. (1967) *Ganglion-blocking and Ganglion-stimulating Agents.* Pergamon: New York

Koch-Weser, J. (1976) Hydralazine. *New England Journal of Medicine* **295**, 320–323

Lagerkranser, M., Andreen, M., Irestedt, L., Sollevi, A. and Tidgren, B. (1983) Adenosine inhibits renin release during controlled hypotension and hemorrhagic shock in the dog. *Anesthesiology* **59**, 13

Lam, A.M. and Gelb, A.W. (1983) Cardiovascular effect of isoflurane-induced hypotension for cerebral aneurysm surgery. *Anesthesia and Analgesia* **62**, 742–748

Larson, A.G. (1963) A new technique for inducing controlled hypotension. *Lancet* **i**, 128–131

Longnecker, D.E., Creasy, R.R. and Ross, D.C. (1979) A microvascular site of action of sodium nitroprusside in striated muscle of the rat. *Anesthesiology* **50**, 111–117

Ma, C.C., Fukunaga, A.F., Flacke, W.E. and Oleivine, S.K. (1982) Comparison of hemodynamic responses during hypotension induced by halothane and adenosine triphosphate. *Anesthesiology* **57**, A67

Maekawa, T., McDowall, D.G. and Okuda, Y. (1979) Brain surface oxygen tension and cerebral cortical blood flow during hemorrhagic and drug-induced hypotension in the cat. *Anesthesiology* **51**, 313–320

Marsh, M.A., Shapiro, H.M., Smith, R.W. and Marshall, L.F. (1979) Changes in neurological status and intracranial pressure associated with sodium nitroprusside administration. *Anesthesiology* **51**, 336–338

Marshall, W.K., Bedford, R.F., Arnold, W.P. *et al.* (1981) Effects of propranolol on the cardiovascular and renin–angiotensin systems during hypotension produced by sodium nitroprusside in humans. *Anesthesiology* **55**, 277–280

Maseda, J., Hilberman, M., Derby, G.C., Spencer, R.J., Stinson, E.B. and Myers,

B.D. (1981) The renal effects of sodium nitroprusside in postoperative cardiac surgical patients. *Anesthesiology* **54**, 284–288

McDowall, D.G., Keaney, N.P., Turner, J.M., Lane, J.R. and Okuda, Y. (1974) The toxicity of sodium nitroprusside. *British Journal of Anaesthesia* **46**, 327–332

Mellander, S. and Johanssan, B. (1968) Control of resistance, exchange and capacitance functions in the peripheral circulation. *Pharmacological Reviews* **20**, 117–195

Michenfelder, J.D. (1977) Cyanide release from sodium nitroprusside in the dog. *Anesthesiology* **46**, 196–201

Michenfelder, J.D. and Theye, R.A. (1977) Canine systemic and cerebral effects of hypotension induced by hemorrhage, trimetaphan, halothane or nitroprusside. *Anesthesiology* **46**, 188–195

Michenfelder, J.D. and Tinker, J.H. (1977) Cyanide toxicity and thiosulfate protection during chronic administration of sodium nitroprusside in the dog. *Anesthesiology* **47**, 441–448

Miller, E.D., Ackerley. J.A., Vaughan, E.D., Peach, M.J. and Epstein, R.M. (1977) The renin angiotensin system during controlled hypotension with sodium nitroprusside. *Anesthesiology* **47**, 257–262

Morris, P.J., Todd, M. and Philbin, D. (1982) Changes in canine intracranial pressure in response to infusions of sodium nitroprusside and trinitroglycerin. *British Journal of Anaesthesia* **54**, 991–995

Morrow, D.H. and Morrow, A.G. (1961) The effect of halothane on myocardial force and vascular resistance. *Anesthesiology* **22**, 537–541

Needlemann, P., Jakschik, B. and Johnson, E.M. (1973) Sulfhydryl requirement for relaxation of vascular smooth muscle. *Journal of Pharmacology and Experimental Therapeutics* **187**, 324–331

Newberg, L.A., Milde, J.H. and Michenfelder, J.D. (1984) Systemic and cerebral effects of isoflurane-induced hypotension in dogs. *Anesthesiology* **60**, 541–546

Olsson, R.A. (1981) Local factors regulating cardiac and skeletal muscle blood flow. *Annual Review of Physiology* **43**, 385–395

Organe, G., Paton, W.D.M. and Zaimis, E.J. (1949) Preliminary trials of bistrimethyl ammonium decane and pentane diiodide (C10 and C5) in man. *Lancet* **i**, 21–23

Page, I.H., Corcoran, A.C., Dunstan, H.P. and Koppanyi, T. (1955) Cardiovascular actions of sodium nitroprusside in animals and hypertensive patients. *Circulation* **11**, 187–198

Pasch, T., Pinchl, J., Kleierl-Lindner, C. and Gotz, H. (1984) Hypertensive reactions following vasodilator-induced hypotension and their prevention by captopril. *British Journal of Anaesthesia* **56**, 1296P

Prys-Roberts, C., Gersh, B.J., Baker, A.B. and Reuben, S.R. (1972) The effects of halothane on the intereactions between myocardial contractility, aortic impedence and L.V. performance. I. Theoretical considerations and results. *British Journal of Anaesthesia* **44**, 634–649

Rall, T.W. (1980) Central nervous stimulants. In: *Goodman and Gilman's Pharmacological Basis of Theurapeutics* 6th edn (Eds. Goodman, L.S. and Gilman, A.). MacMillan: New York

Reiz, S., Balfors, E., Sørenson, M.B., Ariola, S., Freidman, A. and Truedssson, H. (1983) Isoflurane: a powerful coronary vasodilator in patients with coronary artery disease. *Anesthesiology* **59**, 91–97

Robinson, B.F. (1981) Pharmacology of vasodilators. In: *The International Symposium on the Clinical Use of Tridil. Intravenous Nitroglycerin* (Eds. Robinson, B.F. and Kaplan, J.A.). Medicine Publishing Foundation: Oxford

Rogers, M.C., Hamburger, C., Owen, K. and Epstein, M.H. (1979) Intracranial pressure in the cat during nitroglycerin-induced hypotension. *Anesthesiology* **51**, 227–229

Rowe, G.G., Alfonse, S. and Lugas, J.E. (1964) Systemic and coronary hemodynamic effects of trimetaphan camphorsulphonate (Arfonad) in the dog. *Anesthesiology* **25**, 156–160

Scott, D.B., Stephen, G.W., Marshall, R.L., Jenkinson, J.L. and MacRae, W.R. (1972) Circulatory effects of controlled arterial hypotension during nitrous oxide/ halothane anaesthesia. *British Journal of Anaesthesia* **44**, 523–527

Sethna, D.H., Moffett, E.A., Bussell, J.A., Raymond, M.J., Matloft, J.M.. and Gray, R.J. (1982) Intravenous nitroglycerin and myocardial metabolism during anesthesia in patients undergoing myocardial revascularization. *Anesthesia and Analgesia* **61**, 828–833

Simpson, P., Bellamy, D. and Cole, P. (1976) Electrocardiographic studies during hypotensive anaesthesia using sodium nitroprusside. *Anaesthesia* **31**, 1172–1178

Smith, P.R. and Kruszyna, H. (1976) Nitroprusside and cyanide. *British Journal of Anaesthesia* **48**, 396

Sollevi, A., Lagerkranser, M., Irestedt, L. Gordon, E. and Lindquist, C. (1984) Controlled hypotension with adenosine in cerebral aneurysm surgery. *Anesthesiology* **61**, 400–405

Stevens, W.C., Cromwell, T.H., Halsey, M.J., Eger, E.I., Shakespeare, T.F. and Bahlman, S.H. (1971) The cardiovascular effects of a new inhalational anesthetic, Forane, in human volunteers at constant arterial carbon dioxide tension. *Anesthesiology* **35**, 8–16

Stoyka, W.W. and Schutz, H. (1975) The cerebral response to sodium nitroprusside and trimetaphan controlled hypotension. *Canadian Anaesthetists' Society Journal* **22**, 275–283

Styles, M., Coleman, A.J. and Leary, W.P. (1973) Some hemodynamic effects of sodium nitroprusside. *Anesthesiology* **38**, 173–176

Tewfik, G. (1957) Trimetaphan: its effects on the pseudocholinesterase level of man. *Anaesthesia* **12**, 326–329

Tobias, M.A. (1981) Comparison of nitroprusside and nitroglycerine for controlling hypertension during coronary artery surgery. *British Journal of Anaesthesia* **53**, 891–896

Turner, J.M., Powell, D., Gibson, R.M. and McDowall, D.G. (1977) Intracranial pressure changes in neurosurgical patients during hypotension induced with sodium nitroprusside or trimetaphan. *British Journal of Anaesthesia* **49**, 419–428

Van Aken, H., Puchstein, C., Anger, C., Hanecke, A. and Lawin, P. (1984a) Changes in intracranial pressure and compliance during adenosine triphosphate hypotension in dogs. *Anesthesia and Analgesia* **63**, 381–388

Van Aken, H., Puchstein, C., Fitch, W. and Graham, D.I. (1984b) Haemodynamic and cerebral effects of ATP-induced hypotension. *British Journal of Anaesthesia* **56**, 1409–1416

Vesey, C.J., Cole, P.V. and Simpson, P.J. (1976) Cyanide and thiocyanate concentrations following sodium nitroprusside infusion in man. *British Journal of Anaesthesia* **48**, 651–660

Vesey, C.J., Cole, P.V. and Simpson, P.J. (1982) Sodium nitroprusside and cyanide release. *British Journal of Anaesthesia* **54**, 791–792

Viljoen, J.F. (1968) Anaesthesia for internal mammary implant surgery. *Anaesthesia* **23**, 515–520

Wang, H.H., Liu, L.M.P. and Katz, R.L. (1977) A comparison of the cardiovascular effects of sodium nitroprusside and trimetaphan. *Anesthesiology* **46**, 40–48

Wildsmith, J.A.W., Marshall, R.L., Jenkinson, J.L., MacRae, W.R. and Scott, D.B. (1973) Haemodynamic effects of sodium nitroprusside during nitrous oxide/ halothane anaesthesia. *British Journal of Anaesthesia* **45**, 71–74

Wildsmith, J.A.W., Sinclair, C.J., Thorn, J., MacRae, W.R., Fagan, D, and Scott, D.B. (1983) Haemodynamic effects of induced hypotension with a nitroprusside–trimethaphan mixture. *British Journal of Anaesthesia* **55**, 381–389

16

Channel blockers

P. Foëx

Regulation of cell function relies on two messengers, calcium ions (Ca^{2+}) and cyclic AMP (cAMP), which ensure the coupling of stimuli and physiological responses. Ca^{2+} and cAMP nearly always function together even though the Ca^{2+} messenger system is more complicated than the cAMP messenger (Rasmussen and Barrett, 1984). Calcium ions play a decisive role in the electrical activity of the heart, in the excitation–contraction coupling of skeletal, cardiac and vascular smooth muscle, and in the release of neurotransmitters at the presynaptic junctions. The plasma membrane is relatively impermeable to Ca^{2+} so the intracellular concentration of Ca^{2+} is very low (0.1 μmol/l) whilst the extracellular is very high (approximately 1000 μmol/l). Active mechanisms pump Ca^{2+} out of the cell so that the low concentration can be maintained in the face of a 10^4 concentration gradient. However, in order for Ca^{2+} to act as a messenger, it is necessary for calcium fluxes to occur across the plasma membrane. This is possible through three major types of ion channels: (1) voltage-dependent calcium channels; (2) receptor-operated calcium channels; and (3) sodium channels, which may also allow the transfer of some Ca^{2+}. The role of calcium ions, the physiology of calcium channel blockade will be discussed together with their implications for anaesthesia.

Role of calcium ions

Electrophysiology

Electrical impulses in nerve and muscle are generated by local changes in the permeabilities of these cells to certain ions (Hodgkin and Huxley, 1952). These changes in permeabilities regulate the electrical potential differences across the cell membranes. The local changes in membrane potential cause voltage gradients which in turn force the movement of intra- and extracellular ions. These ionic movements constitute local circuits which spread the impulse from active to passive regions (i.e. impulse propagation).

In active regions, positively charged ions move through open channels (inward current) and depolarize the cell membrane. This excitatory inward current is carried by sodium and calcium ions. Because of localized

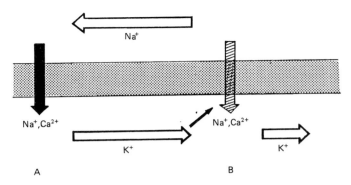

Fig. 16.1 In the active regions (A), positively charged ions add positive charges to the inner surface of the cell membrane. A longitudinal voltage difference is established between the active (A) and passive (B) regions. This voltage difference forces K^+ ions to flow towards the passive region. The change in charges causes ion channels to open (arrow) so that the passive region becomes active. The local current loop is completed by the flow of Na^+ from passive to active region.

depolarization, an intracellular longitudinal voltage difference is established. This voltage difference forces potassium ions to move from active to passive areas. This flow of positively charged ions causes, in turn, some local depolarization of the passive region (current leak) which increases membrane permeabilities to sodium and calcium ions so that the passive regions become active. The current loop is completed by an extracellular movement of sodium and chloride ions from the passive to the active region (Fig. 16.1). During repolarization the direction of the local current loop is reversed, with outward flow across the membrane in the active region.

Mathematical models of impulse conduction show that the total transmembrane current consists of ionic and capacity currents. These models predict that conduction velocity is proportional to fibre radius and to the magnitude of the ionic current.

Ions move across membranes through channels which possess ion selectivity (i.e. discriminate between charge carriers). The electrical potential difference across the membrane can modify the conductance of the ion-selective channels (Reuter, 1979, 1984). Some channels open in response to depolarization. The mechanism of the change in conductance resides in the movement of charged particles (gating particles) in the cell membrane. If the gating particle is removed, the channel opens and ions start to flow.

It is because of differences in the morphology of the action potential of ventricular muscle and sinoatrial or atrioventricular node, as well as differences of threshold potential, that the existence of two distinct inward currents has been postulated (Fig. 16.2). One current, carried by sodium ions, is responsible for the rapid upstroke and fast impulse conduction which characterize atrial, ventricular and His–Purkinje fibres (Colatsky and Tsien, 1979). The other, carried by calcium ions, is responsible for the slower upstroke and slow conduction seen in sinoatrial and atrioventricular nodes (Cranefield, 1977).

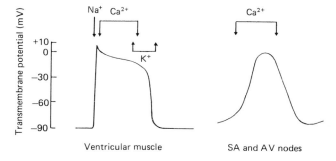

Fig. 16.2 While in the ventricular muscle, most of the acute depolarization is due to an influx of Na^+ ions; in sinoatrial (SA) and atrioventricular (AV) nodes, depolarization is due mostly to influx of Ca^{2+} ions.

Sodium current

The inward sodium current (I_{Na}), also called 'fast' current, is initiated when the membrane is depolarized beyond $-65mV$. During the plateau phase of depolarization, most sodium channels are closed. The slow removal of inactivation (phase 4 of the cardiac action potential) increases the number of channels available for the flow of sodium ions and, therefore, for the development of an action potential. Local anaesthetics displace the inactivation curve of the sodium channels so that stronger depolarization is needed to initiate impulses. Tetrodotoxin also blocks the sodium channels. The sodium channel density per surface area ranges from about 1–2 channels μm^{-2} in cultured cardiac cells to about 16 channels μm^{-2} in isolated cells from adult rat hearts (Cachelin *et al.*, 1983).

Calcium current

Voltage-clamp studies have shown the existence of a slow (calcium) inward current (I_{si}), enhanced by catecholamines and blocked by Mn^{2+}, which is distinct from the sodium current (Reuter, 1967; Reuter and Scholtz, 1977; Tsien, 1984). This current underlies impulse conduction in nodal tissue and is responsible for the plateau phase of the action potential. Sodium and potassium ions can move through the calcium channels but to a very much smaller extent (approximately 1/100) than calcium itself. The slow inward current (I_{si}) is increased by adrenergic agonists, either because of an increase in the number of channels or by an increase in their conductance. Ischaemia and hypoxia also increase the slow inward current.

The calcium channels seem to have two separate gating mechanisms (Fig. 16.3). One, located on the extracellular side of the sarcolemmal membrane, is voltage dependent. The other, located on the cytoplasmic side of the channel, is less voltage dependent and appears to be regulated by cyclic nucleotides such as cAMP and cGMP. Voltage dependence means that when the cell is depolarized the gate is open, and when the cell is repolarized the gate is closed. Nucleotide dependence means that a critical phosphorylation reaction at the inner gate of the Ca^{2+} channel determines the state of the gate

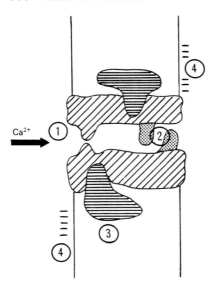

Fig. 16.3 Schematic representation of a calcium channel. The channel is represented as a pore with a 'selectivity filter' (1), and channel gates (2). Voltage sensors (3) confer voltage-dependence to the channel. Binding of cations at the surface of the membrane (4) may modulate the transmembrane voltage potential. (After Triggle, 1982; reproduced with permission.)

(Reuter and Scholtz, 1977; Tsien, 1984). The calcium channels are blocked by Mn^{2+}, Co^{2+}, Ni^{2+}, La^{2+} and by organic calcium blockers (Dhalla *et al.*, 1982).

The slow inward current plays an important role in the development of arrhythmias. In the case of ischaemia, sodium channels are inactivated and electrical activation is initiated by the calcium inward current. This causes delay in impulse propagation which facilitates re-entry, a frequent cause of arrhythmias.

Excitation–contraction coupling in cardiac muscle and vascular smooth muscle

Cardiac muscle

The contractile apparatus of the myocardial cells consists of the proteins actin and myosin which slide past one another. This process is ATP dependent and the interaction between actin and myosin is inhibited by the regulatory proteins troponin and tropomyosin. The increase in myoplasmic Ca^{2+} concentration from 10^{-7} to 10^{-5} mol/l which occurs with depolarization of the myocardial cell permits the binding of Ca^{2+} to troponin (Sperelakis and Schneider, 1976; Fabiato and Fabiato, 1979). This releases the troponin inhibition of the interaction between actin and myosin so that contraction may occur. The transmembrane Ca^{2+} influx during the action potential is too small to raise the myoplasmic concentration of Ca^{2+} to initiate contraction, but it triggers the release of Ca^{2+} from intracellular stores (Ca^{2+}-triggered Ca^{2+} release). Drugs

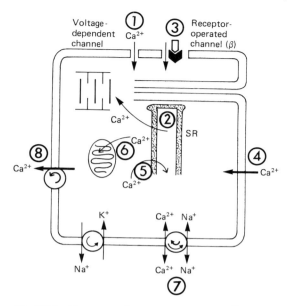

Fig. 16.4 Diagrammatic representation of Ca^{2+} ion fluxes in cardiac muscle. Ca^{2+} ions enter the cell during the plateau phase of action potential (1), through voltage-dependent channels. This triggers the release of Ca^{2+} (2) from the sarcoplasmic reticulum (SR). Ca^{2+} also penetrates the cell through receptor-operated channels (3) and by passive diffusion (4). In order for relaxation to occur, myoplasmic Ca^{2+} concentration must decrease. This is possible because of Ca^{2+} sequestration in the SR (5) and mitochondria (6). Extrusion of Ca^{2+} from the cell is possible through $Ca^{2+} - Na^{+}$ exchange (7) and an ATP-dependent Ca^{2+} pump (8). (After Braunwald, 1982; reproduced with permission.)

which increase the inotropic state of the myocardium, such as the β-adrenoceptor agonists, increase the influx of calcium through the slow channels during depolarization, enhance the release of Ca^{2+} from the intracellular stores and also increase the sensitivity of the contractile system to calcium ions (Braunwald, Sonnenblick and Ross, 1980).

Relaxation of the cardiac fibre occurs when the inflow of Ca^{2+} ceases and the intracellular concentration of Ca^{2+} is lowered by at least three mechanisms: (1) the Ca^{2+}-stimulated Mg^{2+}-dependent ATPase which transfers Ca^{2+} from the myoplasm into the sarcoplasmic reticulum; (2) the extrusion of Ca^{2+} from the cell by $Na^{+}-Ca^{2+}$ exchange (ATP dependent); and (3) the transfer of Ca^{2+} into the mitochondria. With the lowering of the myoplasmic Ca^{2+} concentration, calcium is released from the troponin and this allows troponin to inhibit the interaction between actin and myosin (Dhalla *et al.*, 1982). The mechanisms and channels involved in the control of myoplasmic Ca^{2+} are summarized in Fig. 16.4.

Vascular smooth muscle

Contraction of vascular smooth muscle requires the interaction between actin and myosin. Whilst tropomyosin is present in the contractile apparatus, its function is unknown. The other regulatory protein, troponin, is replaced by

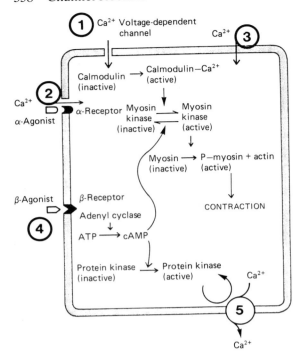

Fig. 16.5 Diagrammatic representation of the calcium ion fluxes in vascular smooth muscle. Ca^{2+} enters the cell through voltage-dependent channels (1), receptor-operated channels (2) and by diffusion (3). The increase in myoplasmic Ca^{2+} is necessary for the activation of calmodulin and myosin kinase. Note that β-adrenoceptor stimulation (4) facilitates Ca^{2+} extrusion (5) through a protein kinase dependent Ca^{2+} pump. (After Braunwald, 1982; reproduced with permission.)

another protein, calmodulin. The chain of reaction leading to contraction starts with the rise in Ca^{2+} concentration to 10^{-6} mol/l (Fig. 16.5). Ca^{2+} then binds to calmodulin, which activates the enzyme myosin kinase. This enzyme phosphorylates the light chains of myosin. Once phosphorylation has occurred, myosin interacts with actin and vasoconstriction occurs (Adelstein and Eisenberg, 1980). The intracellular Ca^{2+} concentration may be linked to the transmembrane Na^+ gradient via the Na^+–Ca^{2+} exchange mechanism. An increase in myoplasmic Na^+ may cause sufficient influx of Ca^{2+} to permit sustained vasoconstriction. Stimulation of the α-adrenoceptors increases Ca^{2+} fluxes into the vascular smooth muscle, thus causing vasoconstriction. This receptor-mediated mechanism is the primary mechanism for increasing calcium fluxes and initiates vasoconstriction. The more sustained tonic contraction depends upon trans-sarcolemmal calcium influx through both voltage-dependent and receptor-operated channels (Zelis and Flaim, 1981). Conversely, β-adrenoceptor stimulation causes vasodilation by: (1) activation of a cAMP-dependent protein kinase which accelerates the efflux of Ca^{2+} from smooth muscle cells; and (2) inactivation of the myosin kinase by a separate cAMP-mediated enzyme system.

Neuromuscular transmission

Calcium ions play an important role in synaptic and neuromuscular transmission. The release of the neurotransmitter acetylcholine (ACh) from the presynaptic cell is triggered by Ca^{2+} which enters the presynaptic membrane. Inside the cell, Ca^{2+} binds to calmodulin which, once activated, initiates a chain of reactions leading to the release of the neurotransmitter in the synaptic cleft. Calcium influx blockers may decrease the calcium conductance of the presynaptic membrane, thereby reducing the release of ACh. They may also decrease the intracellular presynaptic calcium pool and possibly decrease the sensitivity of the muscle end-plate to ACh (Durant *et al.*, 1982).

Specific blockade of the slow channels

In 1963, Fleckenstein observed that two newly synthesized coronary vasodilators, prenylamine and an unnamed substance later to be known as verapamil, mimicked the cardiac effects of Ca^{2+} withdrawal. Both inhibited the excitation–contraction coupling, diminishing the contractile force without a major change in the action potential (Fleckenstein, 1964). Several years later, Fleckenstein and his colleagues demonstrated that verapamil and nifedipine selectively depress the slow transmembrane Ca^{2+} current (Kohlhardt *et al.*, 1972; Kohlhardt and Fleckenstein, 1977).

A number of agents which inhibit the slow inward current are available. Verapamil, nifedipine and diltiazem are the most commonly used. These agents, often termed 'calcium antagonists', are also referred to as slow channel blockers, calcium channel blockers, calcium entry blockers or calcium blockers. As pointed out by Fleckenstin, complete blockade of transmembrane Ca^{2+} entry is incompatible with life and therefore the term 'calcium blockade' should be avoided (Fleckenstein, 1983). However, the term 'calcium antagonist' implies that calcium and its 'antagonists' interact at specific receptors. This is probably not the case. Their predominant action is to reduce Ca^{2+} fluxes at specific sites, including the cell membrane. They vary in their chemical structure, may exhibit selectivity between cardiac and smooth muscle Ca^{2+} channels (Triggle and Swamy, 1983) and their effects are not always completely reversed by calcium ions. In this respect they cannot be considered as specific competitive Ca^{2+} antagonists. Moreover, the electrophysiological effects may not be limited to the slow inward current. Diltiazem at high concentrations inhibits both slow and fast inward currents. Verapamil is capable of blocking an outward current carried by K^+ which occurs during repolarization. Verapamil appears to modify the kinetics of the slow channel (i.e. activation and recovery from activation), whilst nifedipine simply reduces the number of available channels. Thus there are at least two groups of calcium channel blockers: those which prevent the activation of the slow channels and those which alter their kinetics (Triggle, 1982; Reuter, 1984).

A striking feature of the calcium antagonists is their chemical heterogeneity, which suggests that they act at different receptor sites. Molecular studies of receptor recognition sites for calcium antagonists have focused on the recognition of sites for the dihydropyridines (nifedipine, nimodipine as antagonists, Bay K8644 as agonist) using [^{3}H]nitrendepine (Murphy *et al.*, 1983). All dihydropyridines compete for a single binding site. However, the binding pattern for verapamil is different: even at maximal concentrations of the drug only 30–40 per cent of [^{3}H]nitrendepine binding is blocked. It is therefore likely that a distinct verapamil receptor is linked 'allosterically' to the dihydropyridine receptor. Diltiazem, unlike verapamil, increases [^{3}H]nitrendepine binding; this suggests the existence of yet another distinct diltiazem receptor also 'allosterically' linked to the dihydropyridine receptor and capable of enhancing its binding characteristics. Calcium antagonists such as lidoflazine, flunarizine and cinnarizine act at the site of verapamil receptors. The three types of receptors are associated with the voltage-dependent calcium channels. Recently, an agonist dihydropyridine (Bay K8644) has been identified. It stimulates cardiac and smooth muscle contraction and enhances the calcium flux into depolarized cells by stabilizing the voltage-dependent channels in the open mode (Hess, Lansman and Tsien, 1984). The identification of an agonist dihydropyridine suggests that the calcium antagonist receptors are physiologically meaningful. The calcium antagonist drugs do not plug the calcium channels but bind to receptors functionally linked with the calcium channels. The discovery of an agonist at these receptors completes the analogy with a neurotransmitter agonist which can be blocked by exogenous compounds.

Pharmacokinetics

Only the three calcium influx blockers most commonly used will be discussed in detail. Their structure is shown in Fig. 16.6.

Verapamil

Verapamil is a synthetic papaverine derivative which is well absorbed after oral administration. Its (−) isomer is very specific for slow channel blockade while its (+) isomer is much less potent and also blocks the fast inward current. The commercial preparation is a racemic mixture. Despite almost complete absorption, bioavailability after oral administration ranges from 10 to 20 per cent because of first-pass metabolism in the liver. It has been suggested that the more active (−) isomer is eliminated by the liver to a greater extent than the (+) isomer (Eichelbaum *et al.*, 1980), resulting in the cumulation of the less active isomer. This would explain why much higher plasma levels of verapamil are required to produce specific effects after oral rather than intravenous administration (McAllister, 1982). Biotransformation in the liver consists in *N*-alkylation. The metabolites of verapamil may be active, but their contribution to the overall therapeutic effect of the drug is unknown. Elimination is essentially renal (70 per cent) with some elimination via the gastrointestinal tract. Ninety per cent of verapamil in the serum is protein bound and its free fraction is increased if other highly protein bound drugs are administered simultaneously (Singh, Ellrodt and Peter, 1978; Dominic *et al.*, 1981). The drug exhibits a bi-exponential decline with a distribution phase (alpha half-time) ranging from 2 to 35 minutes and a slower elimination phase (beta half-time) ranging between 1.8 and 13.6 hours (Schomerus *et al.*, 1976).

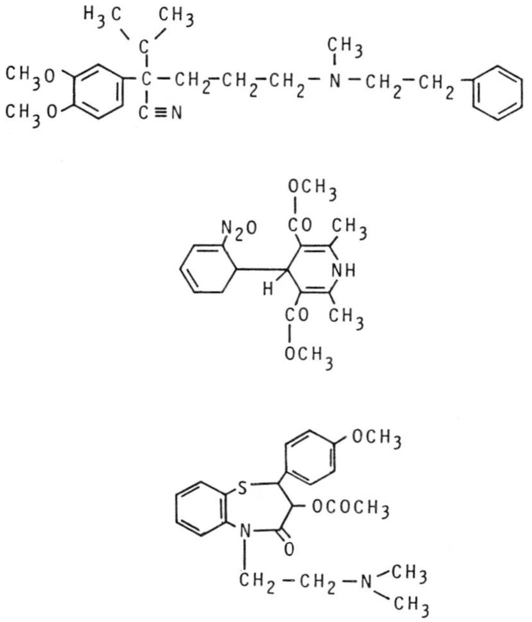

Fig. 16.6   Structure of verapamil, nifedipine and diltiazem.

The elimination is slowest in patients with liver disease. After intravenous administration the onset of action is within 1–2 minutes with a fairly short-lived hypotensive action (dissipated after 20 minutes) and a more prolonged chronotropic effect still detectable after a few hours. Because the duration of atrioventricular node depression exceeds that of other haemodynamic effects, it has been suggested that verapamil binds preferentially to the atrioventricular nodal tissue (Singh, Collet and Chew, 1980). The oral dose of verapamil is 80–160 mg 8-hourly, and the intravenous dose 75–150 µg/kg.

Nifedipine
Nifedipine is a dihydropyridine which, like verapamil, is well absorbed after oral administration. Its bioavailability is much greater than that of verapamil and attains 65–70 per cent of the oral dose. Biotransformation in the liver is by oxidation to a free acid or lactate, both of which are inactive. Approximately 75 per cent of the metabolized drug is eliminated by the kidneys and 15 per cent by the gastrointestinal tract (Stone *et al.*, 1980; McAllister, 1982). Like verapamil, nifedipine is 90 per cent protein bound. The alpha half-time is of the order of 2.5–3 hours and the beta half-time is about 4–5 hours. Nifedipine can be given sublingually and intranasally as well as orally. The oral dose is of the order of 10–20 mg 4- to 8-hourly.

Diltiazem
Diltiazem is a benzothiazepine which is rapidly and almost completely absorbed by the gastrointestinal tract. Its first-pass effect is similar to that of

verapamil and its plasma half-life is approximately 5–7 hours (Kinney, Moskowitz and Zelis, 1981; Zelis and Kinney, 1982). It is 80 per cent protein bound in the plasma. However, only 50 per cent is bound to plasma albumin, so there is little interaction with other albumin-bound drugs (i.e. warfarin, phenytoin, indomethacin). About 60 per cent of the drug is metabolized by the liver and about 40 per cent is eliminated by the kidneys. (Kohno *et al.*, 1977; Rovei *et al.*, 1980; Britt, 1985). Desacetyl diltiazem is the only active metabolite. The oral dose is 60–90 mg 8-hourly, and the intravenous dose 75–150 μg/kg.

Cardiovascular effects of calcium influx blockers

The selective inhibition of transmembrane influx of Ca^{2+} (and of other movements of Ca^{2+} in the cells) is responsible for the depression of sinus automaticity, atrioventricular conductivity, negative inotropy and vasodilation caused by the calcium influx blockers. Their effects on the circulation and their therapeutic uses have been extensively reviewed (Antman *et al.*, 1980; Stone *et al.*, 1980; Merin, 1981; Braunwald, 1982; Reves *et al.*, 1982; Reves, 1984; Jones, 1984, 1985).

Chronotropic and dromotropic effects

The rate of sinus node discharge is depressed and conduction velocity through the atrioventricular node is decreased; however, the relative potencies of negative chronotropic and dromotropic properties of the calcium influx blockers differ substantially. In isolated sinoatrial and atrioventricular blood-perfused preparations verapamil and nifedipine cause equal decrements in automaticity whilst nifedipine is twice as effective in reducing atrioventricular conduction. Diltiazem is much less potent than either verapamil or nifedipine. However, in the intact organism verapamil and not nifedipine decreases sinus node activity and atrioventricular conduction. This difference may be explained by the greater vasodilation elicited by nifedipine, which in turn causes sympathetic stimulation. β-adrenergic stimulation is known to reverse the chronotropic and dromotropic effects of the calcium influx blockers.

In patients with sinus node dysfunction verapamil may worsen function, and in all patients in sinus rhythm verapamil increases the atrioventricular conduction time. Similarly, diltiazem prolongs the atrio–His bundle interval whilst nifedipine does not.

Verapamil can slow the atrial rate in sinus tachycardia and is most effective in terminating re-entrant paroxysmal supraventricular tachycardia. It is much more effective than β-adrenoceptor antagonists. Verapamil slows the ventricular rate in atrial fibrillation and increases the atrioventricular block in atrial flutter with conversion to sinus rhythm in some patients. Verapamil is not very effective in the treatment of ventricular arrhythmias.

Negative inotropy

Calcium influx blockers decrease myocardial contractility in a dose-dependent fashion. In isolated heart muscle preparations, depression is greater for nifedipine than verapamil and diltiazem (Henry, 1980). This effect on contractility is not associated with changes in the resting potential or in the upstroke of the action potential (i.e. it does not depend on membrane stabilization by non-selective blockade of sodium channels) and is purely due to blockade of the slow inward current. The negative inotropy of verapamil and nifedipine is enhanced by acidosis (Briscoe and Smith, 1982).

Vasodilatation

Vascular smooth muscle in the arteriolar bed is much more sensitive to the action of Ca^{2+} channel blockers than is venous smooth muscle (Braunwald, 1982). Arteriolar vasodilatation is widespread, so systemic vascular resistance is reduced. Splanchnic and cerebral vasodilation occur. Renal vascular resistance is reduced and, with nifedipine, renal autoregulation appears to be abolished. The calcium influx blockers also decrease smooth muscle tone in the coronary arteries so that coronary vascular resistance decreases (Millard et al., 1983) and coronary blood flow may increase (Stone, Stephens and Banim, 1983). This effect is observed with doses which are three to ten times smaller than those causing depression of contractility. Nifedipine appears to be the most potent coronary vasodilator, being approximately 30 times more powerful than verapamil and diltiazem and at least 1000 times more powerful than papaverine. Diltiazem reduces coronary vascular resistance more than cerebral or renal resistance.

The calcium channel blockers decrease the vascular responsiveness to α- and β-adrenoceptor antagonists and also to angiotensin. This effect is not influenced by β-adrenergic blockade, catecholamine depletion or vagotomy. The vasodilatation can be blunted or abolished only by increasing the extracellular Ca^{2+} concentration. Experimental studies have shown that collateral coronary blood flow distal to a ligated coronary artery is augmented by calcium blockers (Henry et al., 1979).

Global haemodynamic effects

The overall effect of the calcium influx blockers depends upon their relative inhibiting potencies on excitation–contraction coupling in cardiac muscle and vascular smooth muscle. In the intact circulation the direct negative inotropy may be masked by baroreceptor-mediated reflex-positive inotropic and chronotropic responses. If substantial peripheral vasodilation occurs, reflex-induced β-adrenoceptor stimulation will offset the direct myocardial effects. Because nifedipine is a more potent vasodilator than verapamil and diltiazem, it causes more reflex-induced β-adrenoceptor stimulation (Nakaya, Schwartz and Millar, 1983). Its overall effects are coronary vasodilatation, reduced myocardial oxygen consumption (reduced afterload), and little change in inotropy, chronotropy and atrioventricular conduction. This makes nifedipine an effective drug in the treatment of coronary artery disease, particularly when coronary artery spasm plays an important role, and in the treatment of arterial hypertension. Verapamil is much less powerful a vasodilator than nifedipine and therefore causes much less reflex increase in β-adrenoceptor activity. Negative chronotropy and prolongation of atrioventricular conduction are more prominent with verapamil than with nifedipine. Diltiazem causes even less vasodilatation than verapamil and, therefore, less reflex increase in β-adrenoceptor activity. Thus, its negative chronotropy and dromotropy are little influenced by β-adrenoceptor blockade. However, cardiac depression is small because diltiazem depresses inotropy less than do nifedipine and verapamil. Because of these differences, verapamil and diltiazem are more effective antiarrhythmic agents than nifedipine. Conversely, they are less effective in the treatment of arterial hypertension but play an important role in promoting coronary vasodilatation.

Effect on the ischaemic myocardium

Protection of the ischaemic myocardium may be considered in terms of balance between oxygen demand and supply, prevention of coronary spasm, coronary vasodilatation and cellular protection. Calcium blockers may reduce heart rate and contractility while inducing vasodilatation, all of which decrease oxygen consumption. At the same time, they decrease coronary vascular resistance and thus facilitate oxygen supply. Moreover, calcium blockers prevent coronary spasm. However, there may be situations where vasodilatation promotes coronary steal. Such a steal is known to occur with some coronary vasodilators such as dipyridamole. It is also important to remember that the effects of calcium influx blockade depend upon the quality of the myocardium. Because of afterload reduction, cardiac output may increase in patients with normal or moderately reduced ejection fractions (Singh and Roche, 1977). However, in patients with severely reduced ejection fractions, calcium influx blockade may substantially reduce cardiac output and may increase the pulmonary capillary wedge pressure (Chew et al., 1981). Moreover, calcium influx blockade may cause regional cardiac dysfunction. Serruys and his colleagues have shown that intracoronary nifedipine may delay the onset of contraction and relaxation in the apical region of the left ventricle of patients with coronary artery disease. This asynchrony of contraction may contribute to the overall depression which may attend calcium influx blockade (Serruys et al., 1983).

In acute myocardial ischaemia, calcium overload plays an important role and contributes to permanent damage in the ischaemic muscle. Pretreatment with calcium influx blockers minimizes the damage caused by total ischaemia (Smith et al., 1975). This may be explained by selective depression of the myocardium since ischaemic injury can be decreased by reducing contractility (Smith et al., 1976). The recovery of active tension after ischaemia is enhanced by calcium influx blockade. Similarly, the energy-rich phosphate reserves are better preserved during ischaemia and after reperfusion. Mitochondrial respiration and the ATP-generating capacity are maintained. Calcium influx blockade prevents the ischaemic swelling of the mitochondria and allows the myofibrils to maintain their normal ultrastructure (Nayler, 1980; Nayler, Mas-Oliva and Williams, 1980; Bush et al., 1981).

Prevention of calcium overload is important to maintain diastolic function. In the ischaemic myocardium, reduction of available ATP decreases the extrusion of calcium from the cell. Whilst elevated calcium concentration exerts a positive inotropic effect, this is not the case when oxygen supply is inadequate and so systolic function is depressed. However, during diastole it is essential for the myoplasmic Ca^{2+} concentration to decrease. This is an energy-requiring process which is inhibited in ischaemic conditions. If the myoplasmic Ca^{2+} concentration remains high, relaxation is incomplete and this, in turn, will cause increases in diastolic wall tension which contribute to

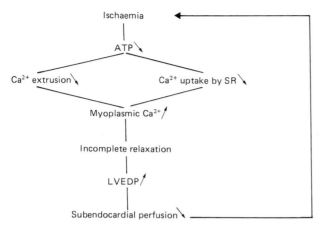

Fig. 16.7 Diagrammatic representation of the effect of calcium overload in ischaemia. Because of the reduction of available ATP, Ca^{2+} extrusion and reuptake by the sarcoplasmic reticulum (SR) are reduced. The abnormally high myoplasmic Ca^{2+} hinders relaxation and worsens subendocardial perfusion so that a vicious circle develops. LVEDP = left ventricular end-diastolic pressure.

poorer coronary perfusion (Fig. 16.7). Calcium influx blockers prevent the reduction in ventricular compliance which attends calcium overload. However, in the absence of calcium overload, calcium influx blockade exerts an antirelaxant effect on the normal heart (Gelpi *et al.*, 1983).

Therapeutic indications

Myocardial ischaemia

The potency of the calcium influx blockers as coronary dilators is of greatest benefit in the treatment of vasospastic angina. All three well-tried calcium influx blockers have been shown to be effective in the treatment of Prinzmetal angina. Attacks of angina at rest are markedly reduced in frequency, and ventricular tachyarrhythmias are often eliminated. Successful control of unstable angina and of effort-induced angina has been reported, as well as control of angina shortly after myocardial infarction (Braunwald, 1982). Whenever coronary artery spasm is concerned, the efficacy of the calcium influx blockers can be easily attributed to coronary dilatation. In effort-induced angina other factors such as reduced oxygen demand may also play a role. However, in effort-induced angina, acute coronary vasoconstriction may also occur. The constrictor response to the cold pressure test may cause myocardial lactate production and is abolished by nifedipine. Besides protection against coronary vasospasm, important beneficial effects of calcium influx blockade are reduction of arterial pressure and stability of the rate–pressure product. The association of calcium influx blockers and β-adrenoceptor blockers or nitrates makes it possible to use smaller doses of these drugs and, thus, to minimize their side effects. The best combinations are verapamil–nitrates or nifedipine–β-adrenoceptor blockers. The association nitrate–nifedipine is likely to cause exaggerated vasodilatation (Stone *et al.*, 1980). The association of verapamil and β-adrenoceptor blockers may potentiate negative inotropy, chronotropy and dromotropy.

In experimental myocardial infarction, calcium influx blockers seem to reduce the size of infarction, because of improved collateral blood supply and reduced oxygen demand. There is some suggestion that verapamil may also reduce the size of infarction in man. In experimental studies of acute ischaemia followed by reperfusion – a situation analogous to cardiac surgery – ischaemic contracture is minimized, function is better preserved after reperfusion and ultrastructure is maintained (Nayler, 1980).

Arrhythmias

The most important effect of slow channel blockade is depression of the atrioventricular node. Because of prolonged atrioventricular node refractoriness, nodal re-entrant supraventricular tachycardias are abolished and the ventricular responses in atrial fibrillation and flutter are controlled (Singh, Collet and Chew, 1980). Although nifedipine has the same electrophysiological effect as verapamil, its potency as a vasodilator is such that the doses required to treat arrhythmias are not achieved in clinical practice and verapamil or diltiazem must be used. Although not usually recommended for the treatment of ventricular arrhythmias, verapamil may be effective to treat refractory ventricular arrhythmias after cardiopulmonary bypass (Kapur *et al.*, 1984c), in keeping with its known efficacy to attenuate ischaemic ventricular arrhythmias (Brooks, Verrier and Lown, 1980).

Arterial hypertension

Calcium influx blockers reduce arterial pressure in direct proportion to the degree of hypertension. At variance with other arteriolar dilators, they induce coronary vasodilation and improve left ventricular relaxation and subendocardial perfusion. This is an important advantage in view of the risk of worsening of myocardial ischaemia which attends peripheral vasodilatation with drugs such as hydralazine (Klein *et al.*, 1983). Nifedipine is effective in the treatment of malignant hypertension complicated by encephalopathy and left ventricular failure (Stone *et al.*, 1980; Bertel *et al.*, 1983).

Pulmonary hypertension

Calcium influx blockers may be effective in treating pulmonary hypertension but only in a minority of patients (Kambara *et al.*, 1981). When pulmonary hypertension is caused by hypoxia, pulmonary artery pressure and resistance can be substantially decreased by calcium influx blockade. Similarly, calcium blockers may be effective in relieving pulmonary congestion in patients with mitral valve disease, especially when it has been initiated by supraventricular tachycardia (Kopman, 1983). However, calcium influx blockers do not decrease normal pulmonary vascular resistance.

Congestive heart failure

Afterload reduction by calcium influx blockade is proportional to the basal level of resistance and will facilitate ejection. Moreover, improvement of subendocardial perfusion is likely to enhance ventricular performance. This is combined with better left ventricular relaxation, so that both systolic and diastolic function are improved (Klugmann, Salvi and Camerini, 1980).

Hypertrophic cardiomyopathy
The major effect of calcium influx blockade is to improve relaxation so that the relationships between pressure and volume during diastole become more normal (Lorell *et al.*, 1982).

Cerebral artery vasospasm
Vasospasm is commonly associated with subarachnoid haemorrhage and trauma. Nifedipine and verapamil are effective in blocking experimental vasospasm. However, there is the possibility of further increases in intracranial pressure when calcium influx blockers are administered to treat vasospasm after head injuries (Lynch and Bedford, 1983). After neurosurgical procedures, calcium influx blockers can be used to reduce blood pressure and to reduce vasospasm (Reves *et al.*, 1982). This is particularly important because hypertension is associated with a significantly greater mortality than is normotension (McKay *et al.*, 1981).

Cardioplegia
Protection of the ischaemic myocardium during cardiopulmonary bypass is achieved by the use of a variety of 'cardioplegic' solutions, local myocardial cooling and whole-body hypothermia. Hypothermic potassium cardioplegic solutions have been established experimentally and clinically as providing excellent myocardial protection during ischaemic cardiac arrest. However, when the ischaemic interval is prolonged, the concentration of adenosine triphosphate (ATP) may fall substantially and may be further reduced after restoration of coronary blood flow. The reperfusion injury is initiated by increased calcium fluxes into the ischaemic myocardium. Calcium overload in the presence of reduced ATP stores causes myocardial rigor, intracellular oedema and disrupts the mitochrondrial membranes. Calcium influx blockers could be expected to protect the heart against these complications. Indeed, calcium channel blockade with verapamil or diltiazem has been shown experimentally to protect the stores of high energy phosphates and to allow the myocardium to exhibit more normal function after cardiac arrest (Vouhe, Helias and Grondin, 1983; Yamamoto *et al.*, 1983; Balderman, Chan and Gage, 1984). Some studies suggest that calcium channel blockade associated with hypothermia is more effective than either alone (Port, Jones and Stanley, 1983). However, the need for inotropic support appears to be greater when verapamil is added to a cardioplegic solution (Kaplan *et al.*, 1984).

Hypotensive anaesthesia
Verapamil has been used to electively decrease arterial pressure during neurolept anaesthesia (Zimpfer, Fitzal and Tonczar, 1981), and although effective, it caused an increase in the PR interval. It has been suggested that an advantage of deliberate hypotension with verapamil is that tachycardia is minimized while coronary and cerebral vasodilatation maximize blood flow despite the lowered perfusion pressure (Reves *et al.*, 1982). Moreover, in experimental animals, substantial arterial hypotension can be obtained with

Table 16.1   Relative potencies of nifedipine, verapamil and diltiazem in the intact circulation

	Vasodilatation	Negative inotropy	Negative dromotropy	Positive chronotropy
Nifedipine	+++	+	+	+++
Verapamil	+	+++	+++	++
Diltiazem	+	+++	+++	+

The positive chronotropy is elicited by baroreceptor stimulation and is not a direct effect of calcium channel blockade.

verapamil and diltiazem without reduction of renal blood flow (Hantler *et al.*, 1983b; Hung *et al.*, 1983).

Selectivity
Studies of the effects of nifedipine, verapamil and diltiazem show that the ranking potencies for vasodilatation and reflexly mediated tachycardia are almost opposite to the ranking potencies for negative inotropy and dromotropy (Table 16.1). These ranking potencies are influenced by the administration of other drugs, such as the β-adrenoceptor antagonists (see 'Myocardial ischaemia', above), and explain the differences in clinical uses between these agents as well as some of the differences in their interactions with anaesthesia.

Interactions with anaesthesia

Cardiovascular interactions

Because of the growing use of calcium influx blockers in the treatment of supraventricular arrhythmias, coronary heart disease and arterial hypertension, an increasing number of patients presenting for elective or emergency surgery are taking these drugs. Many recent studies have investigated the interactions between calcium influx blockade and anaesthesia. Most studies have examined the effect of acute administration of calcium influx blockers during steady state anaesthesia, but recently the effects of anaesthesia in the presence of calcium influx blockade have been reported.

Interactions with verapamil and diltiazem
One of the earliest studies is that of Brichard and Zimmerman, who used verapamil for the treatment of supraventricular and ventricular arrhythmias during light halothane anaesthesia. They observed reductions of systolic and diastolic arterial pressure after verapamil 20 mg i.v. which they attributed to vasodilatation. However, cardiac output was not measured in these patients and the hypotension may have been caused by potentiated cardiac depression (Brichard and Zimmerman, 1970). Verapamil has also been used in a study of the mechanisms of ketamine-induced hypertension. Intravenous verapamil caused immediate reductions in systolic pressure and decreased the amplitude of the finger and muscle plethysmograms. More recently, Zimpfer and his colleagues have reported transient reductions in arterial pressure and systemic vascular resistance accompanied by small increases in cardiac output, in

patients given verapamil (0.07 mg/kg) under neurolept anaesthesia. After between 5 and 10 minutes the haemodynamic values had essentially returned to their control levels. However, atrioventricular conduction remained significantly prolonged even after 20 minutes (Zimpfer, Fitzal and Tonczar, 1981).

The modern volatile anaesthetics, halothane, enflurane and isoflurane, all cause dose-dependent depression of contractile performance, may modify atrioventricular conduction and may cause peripheral vasodilatation. The last is particularly important with the administration of isoflurane. Additive effects or potentiation of cardiac depression, vasodilatation and slowing of conduction may be expected to occur when these volatile agents are administered together with calcium influx blockers (Merin, 1981; Reves et al., 1982; Reves, 1984). Indeed, experimental studies of the effects of verapamil under halothane, enflurane or isoflurane anaesthesia have shown that contractility is depressed beyond what can be expected from anaesthesia alone (Kapur and Flacke, 1981; Kates et al., 1983; Kapur et al., 1984a; Kates et al., 1984). Substantial depression of mean arterial pressure, cardiac output and left ventricular performance, proportional to the plasma verapamil concentration, have been reported with isoflurane and enflurane anaesthesia. Under isoflurane anaesthesia, systemic vascular resistance did not change, whereas under enflurane anaesthesia it was reduced. Higher plasma levels of verapamil were tolerated during isoflurane anaesthesia than during enflurane or halothane anaesthesia, possibly because of higher baseline sympathetic tone.

In an experimental model involving right heart bypass preparation, isoflurane caused concentration-dependent depression of left ventricular function, indicated by reductions in left ventricular $dPdt_{max}$ and systolic shortening at constant filling pressure. This depression was enhanced by verapamil in a concentration-dependent manner so that, at any isoflurane concentration, performance was halved when a plasma concentration of verapamil of 70 ng/ml had been obtained (Kates et al., 1983).

These additive effects are not unexpected. Myocardial depression and vasodilatation observed during the administration of modern inhalational anaesthetics are at least in part related to modifications of movements of Ca^{2+} across the cell membrane and within the cells themselves (Altura et al., 1980; Price and Ohnishi, 1980; Blanck and Thompson, 1982; Lynch, 1984). The negative inotropy of halothane appears to be caused by changes in intracellular calcium kinetics (Blanck and Thompson, 1981; Blanck et al., 1984), including decreased sensitivity of myofibrillar ATPase to Ca^+ (Pask, England and Prys-Roberts, 1981). Thus it is not surprising that calcium channel blockade with verapamil potentiates the negative inotropy of halothane. In this respect it must be noted that halothane is almost as effective as verapamil in preventing reperfusion arrhythmias (Kroll and Knight, 1984). This suggests a common mechanism of action which involves calcium blockade.

Of considerable clinical importance is the potential for severe impairment of atrioventricular conduction which may not respond to administration of calcium; thus close monitoring of the PR interval is essential. Sinus node and atrioventricular function are substantially depressed by verapamil and diltiazem in the presence of voltatile anaesthetics (Hantler et al., 1983a; Kapur and Tippit, 1984). This is not surprising because the prolongation of the atrioventricular conduction time by halothane is attributed to calcium channel blockade. Disorders of atrioventricular conduction have been reported with other inhalational anaesthetics, including isoflurane. The association of diltiazem with isoflurane has been shown to cause sinoatrial arrest in experimental animals (Skarvan, Priebe and Gale, 1984). Against this background of adverse interactions between calcium influx blockade and anaesthesia, it must be remembered that verapamil protects against adrenaline-induced ventricular arrhythmias (Kapur and Flacke, 1981). Unlike the haemodynamic effects of verapamil which parallel its plasma concentration, the protective effect against these arrhythmias may persist when plasma levels are very low (Kapur and Flacke, 1982).

Verapamil has been shown to cause additional depression of cardiac contractility in patients undergoing coronary artery surgery who were on chronic β-blocker therapy and were anaesthetized with halothane. Significant vasodilatation occurred and mean arterial pressure was further reduced by verapamil while left ventricular end-diastolic pressure increased (Schulte-Sasse et al., 1984). This seemingly adverse effect of verapamil during halothane anaesthesia is at variance with the lack of alteration of the pulmonary capillary wedge pressure observed when verapamil is administered during morphine anaesthesia, when the main effect of verapamil is vasodilatation and the left ventricular filling pressure remains unchanged (Kates and Kaplan, 1983). In association with high dose fentanyl, verapamil causes marked vasodilatation with little change in cardiac output (Kapur et al., 1984b).

Nifedipine

Nifedipine causes peripheral vasodilatation and could be expected to increase cardiac output. Indeed, clinical studies have shown that nifedipine is effective in the treatment of postoperative hypertension (Sodoyama et al., 1983). The reduction of arterial pressure is accompanied by an increase in cardiac output in the awake patient. During high dose fentanyl anaesthesia, nifepidine increases cardiac output but the associated vasodilatation causes substantial hypotension (Griffin et al., 1984). However, during anaesthesia with halothane or enflurane, left ventricular performance decreases with the administration of nifedipine and cardiac output may be reduced. Experimentally, the association of nifepidine and high concentrations of halothane causes substantial vasodilatation accompanied by hypotension (Tosone et al., 1983), whilst the association of nifedipine with isoflurane appears to be better tolerated (DeWolf et al., 1984).

Several reports of the effects of anaesthesia in patients treated with nifepidine have been published. In patients receiving nifepidine and propranolol, anaesthesia with fentanyl caused marked hypotension which required the administration of volume expanders and of a vasopressor (Freis and Lappas, 1982). It must be noted that muscle relaxation was obtained with metocurine. An interaction between nifedipine and metocurine may have played a role since no exaggerated hypotension was observed in patients receiving nifepidine, anaesthetized with fentanyl, and in whom muscle relaxation was obtained with pancuronium (Nussmeier et al., 1983). It must be stressed that interactions between narcotics and calcium blockers appear to be variable. In patients with coronary artery disease, the haemodynamic values before induction, at intubation, during anaesthesia and at the time of sternotomy were essentially the same in patients taking nifedipine, or nifedipine and a β-blocker, or β-blockers alone. The only significant difference was that under steady state anaesthesia, arterial pressure was lower in those patients taking nifedipine or nifedipine and a β-blocker (Skarvan, 1983). However, in patients receiving nifedipine and propranolol, anaesthesia with halothane caused hypotension and depressed left ventricular function (Fahmy and Lappas, 1983). In contrast, anaesthesia with enflurane supplementing nitrous oxide did not cause undue hypotension in patients taking nifedipine but no β-adrenoceptor antagonist (Reves, Barker and Smith, 1983).

Another calcium influx blocker, nicardipine, which appears to have much more vascular than cardiac effects, has been advocated for the treatment of hypertension in anaesthetized patients. Nicardipine 1 μg i.v. decreased systolic and diastolic pressures by about 35 per cent in patients anaesthetized with nitrous oxide supplemented by fentanyl and diazepam. The marked reduction in systemic vascular resistance was accompanied by an increase in cardiac output (Kishi, Okumura and Furuya, 1984).

Besides the possibility of cardiac depression, one of the major concerns about calcium influx blockade in anaesthesia is the risk of severe conduction disorders. In practice, the greatest reductions of heart rate and the highest incidence of first degree heart block after cardiopulmonary bypass are observed in groups of patients treated with β-blockers rather than calcium blockers (Henling et al., 1984). However, the possibility of disorders of conduction exists, and careful monitoring of the ECG is essential, particularly when halothane and enflurane are used, because they, by themselves, modify the atroventricular conduction.

Other interactions relevant to anaesthesia

Reduced minimum alveolar concentration (MAC)
Verapamil causes some blockade of the sodium channels and therefore could be expected to reduce the anaesthetic requirement for inhalational anaesthetics as do the local anaesthetics (Himes, DiFazio and Burney, 1977). Maze and his colleagues have shown that, in dogs, MAC for halothane is reduced by about 25 per cent after administration of therapeutic doses of verapamil (Maze, Mason and Kates, 1983). These authors suggest that the inspired concentration of halothane should be deliberately reduced in the presence of verapamil because of the lower anaesthetic requirement and in order to minimize cardiovascular depression.

Exaggerated neuromuscular blockade
Calcium influx blockers in high concentrations may decrease the amplitude of muscle twitch in isolated frog nerve–muscle preparation (Lawson, Kraynack and Gintautas, 1983). This effect may be mediated by a reduction in calcium and/or sodium conductance of the presynaptic membrane. It could also be postulated that verapamil decreases the sensitivity of the muscle end-plate to ACh (Durant et al., 1982). The potential exists for synergy between calcium influx blockers, neuromuscular blocking drugs and some antibiotics which also

appear to act on presynaptic terminals (Pollard and Jones, 1983). Indeed, verapamil and nifedipine have been shown to increase the potency of neuromuscular-blocking agents (Bikhazi, Leung and Foldes, 1982, 1983). Even in the absence of muscle relaxants, the neuromuscular blockade which attends the administration of inhalational anaesthetics such as enflurane, may be potentiated by verapamil (Williams *et al.*, 1983).

Exaggerated hyperkalaemia
Acute hyperkalaemia is known to cause intraventricular conduction defects and, more exceptionally, second or even third degree heart block (Bashour *et al.*, 1975). Calcium is the initial treatment of choice for hyperkalaemia because it restores the membrane excitability (Kunis and Lowenstein, 1977). Calcium influx blockade may be expected to increase the sensitivity of the myocardium to hyperkalaemia. Indeed, Nugent and his co-workers have shown that after therapeutic doses of verapamil, intravenous potassium caused atrioventricular block and depressed cardiac function in dogs (Nugent, Tinker and Moyer, 1984). Moreover, much smaller doses of potassium were required to produce the effects of severe hyperkalaemia in animals treated with verapamil than in control animals. The adverse effects of hyperkalaemia were only partly reversed by calcium. The authors suggest that transfusion of stored blood may cause more severe hyperkalaemia and more cardiovascular depression (accompanied by conduction disorders) in patients treated with verapamil than in other subjects.

Reversal of calcium blockade by intravenous calcium
In animal studies, the reversibility of the haemodynamic and electrophysiological effects of calcium influx blockade have been found to be incomplete. Whilst the negative inotropy of verapamil was abolished by calcium, the prolongation of the atrio–His bundle interval was not and heart rate remained slow (Hariman *et al.*, 1979). Similarly, the circulatory depression caused by nifedipine and β-adrenoceptor blockade was only partially reversed by calcium chloride (DeWolf *et al.*, 1984), and the cardiovascular effects of hyperkalaemia (followed by calcium influx blockade) were also only partially reversed by calcium chloride (Nugent, Tinker and Moyer, 1984).

Abrupt withdrawal of calcium blockade
Adverse effects of the abrupt withdrawal of β-adrenoceptor blockade have been reported, and the danger of withdrawing β-blockers during the perioperative period are well known. Less is known about the risk of adverse cardiovascular events in the case of untimely withdrawal of calcium influx blockade. Using ambulatory monitoring of the ECG, Subramanian and colleagues (1983) have shown that ischaemic changes may develop shortly after discontinuation of verapamil and diltiazem. Moreover, there may be recurrence of angina.

Conclusion

Calcium ions play a key role in the electrophysiology of the heart, the excitatation–contraction coupling in cardiac muscle and in vascular smooth muscle. Calcium influx blockers modify the action potential and its transmission (negative chronotropy and dromotropy), the strength of contraction (negative inotropy) and vascular tone (vasodilatation, prevention of vascular spasm). Their main uses are in the treatment of coronary heart disease, arterial hypertension, supraventricular arrhythmias and vascular spasm (Prinzmetal angina). Some of their direct effects may be masked by an increase in sympathetic activity mediated by the arterial baroreceptors. Their effects on the circulation are potentiated by inhalational anaesthetics (negative inotropy and chronotropy) and by narcotics (exaggerated vasodilatation). Whilst withdrawal of calcium influx blockers before elective surgery is not advocated, the interactions with anaesthesia must be borne in mind and the doses and concentrations of anaesthetic agents must be closely monitored.

References

Adelstein, R.S. and Eisenberg, E. (1980) Regulation and kinetics of actin–myosin–ATP interaction. *Annual Review of Biochemistry* **49**, 921–956

Altura, B.M., Altura, B.T., Carella, A., Turlapaty, P.D.M.V. and Weinberg, J. (1980) Vascular smooth muscle and general anaesthetics. *Federation Proceedings* **39**, 1584–1591

Antman, E.M., Stone, P.H., Muller, J.E. and Braunwald, E. (1980) Calcium channel blocking agents in the treatment of cardiovascular disorders. I. Basic and clinical electrophysiologic effects. *Annals of Internal Medicine* **93**, 875–885

Balderman, S.C., Chan, A.K. and Gage, A.A. (1984) Verapamil cardioplegia: improved myocardial preservation during global ischemia. *Journal of Thoracic and Cardiovascular Surgery* **88**, 57–66

Bashour, T., Hsu, I., Gorfinkel, J.H., Wickramesekaran, R. and Rios, J.C. (1975) Atrioventricular and intraventricular conduction in hyperkalemia. *American Journal of Cardiology* **35**, 199–203

Bertel, O., Conen, D., Radu, E.W., Muller, J., Lang, C. and Dubach, U.C. (1983) Nifedipine in hypertensive emergencies. *British Medical Journal* **286**, 19–21.

Bikhazi, G.B., Leung, I. and Foldes, F.F. (1982) Interaction of neuromuscular blocking agents with calcium channel blockers. *Anesthesiology* **57**, A268

Bikhazi, G.B., Leung, I. and Foldes, F.F. (1983) Ca-channel blockers increase potency of neuromuscular blocking agents *in vivo*. *Anesthesiology* **59**, A269

Blanck, T.J.J., Stevenson, R.L., Im, K. and Fisher, Y.I. (1984) Halothane decreases specific binding of calcium channel blocker to cardiac membranes. *Anesthesiology* **61**, A16

Blanck, T.J.J. and Thompson, M. (1981) Calcium transport by cardiac sarcoplasmic reticulum: modulation of halothane action by substrate concentration and pH. *Anesthesia and Analgesia* **60**, 390–394

Blanck, T.J.J. and Thompson, M. (1982) Enflurane and isoflurane stimulate calcium transport by cardiac sarcoplasmic reticulum. *Anesthesia and Analgesia* **61**, 142–145

Braunwald, E. (1982) Mechanisms of action of calcium-channel-blocking agents. *New England Journal of Medicine* **307**, 1618–1627

Braunwald, E., Sonnenblick, E.H. and Ross, J. Jr (1980) Contraction of the normal heart. In: *Heart Disease* (Ed. Braunwald, E.), pp. 413–452. W.B. Saunders: Philadelphia, PA

Brichard, G. and Zimmerman, P.E. (1970) Verapamil in cardiac dysrhythmias during anaesthesia. *British Journal of Anaesthesia* **42**, 1005–1072

Briscoe, M.G. and Smith, H.J. (1982) Sensitivity of cat papillary muscles to verapamil and nifedipine: enhanced effects in acidosis. *Cardiovascular Research* **16**, 173–177

Britt, B.A. (1985) Diltiazem. *Canadian Anaesthetists' Society Journal* **32**, 30–40

Brooks, W.W., Verrier, R.L. and Lown, B. (1980) Protective effect of verapamil on vulnerability to ventricular fibrillation during myocardial ischaemia and reperfusion. *Cardiovascular Research* **14**, 295–302

Bush, L.R., Li, Y.P., Shlafer, M., Jolly S.R. and Lucchesi, B.R. (1981) Protective effects of diltiazem during myocardial ischaemia in isolated cat hearts. *Journal of Pharmacology and Experimental Therapeutics* **218**, 653–661

Cachelin, A.B., De Peyer, J.E., Kakubun, S. and Reuter, H. (1983) Sodium channels in cultured cardiac cells. *Journal of Physiology* **340**, 389–401

Chew, C.Y.C., Hecht, H.S., Collett, J.T., McAllister, R.G. and Singh, B.N. (1981) Influence of severity of ventricular dysfunction on hemodynamic responses to intravenously administered verapamil in ischemic heart disease. *American Journal of Cardiology* **47**, 917–922

Colatsky, T.J. and Tsien, R.W. (1979) Sodium channels in rabbit cardiac Purkinje fibres. *Nature* **278**, 265–268

Cranefield, P.F. (1977) Action potentials, afterpotentials and arrhythmias. *Circulation Research* **41**, 415–423

DeWolf, A., Marquez, J., Nemoto, E., Waterman, P., Kang, Y. and Bleyaert, A. (1984) Cardiovascular effects of isoflurane, enflurane and halothane anesthesia with calcium and beta blockade in monkeys. *Anesthesiology* **61**, A13

Dhalla, N.S., Pierce, G.N., Panagia, V., Singal, P.K. and Beamish, R.E. (1982) Calcium movements in relation to heart function. *Basic Research in Cardiology* **77**, 117–139

Dominic, J.A., Bourne, D.W.A., Tan, T.G., Kirsten, E.B. and McAllister, R.G. Jr (1981) The pharmacology of verapamil. III. Pharmacokinetics in normal subjects after intravenous drug administration. *Journal of Cardiovascular Pharmacology* **3**, 25–38

Durant, N.N., Nguyen, N., Briscoe, J.R. and Katz, R.L. (1982) Potentiation of pancuronium and succinylcholine by verapamil. *Anesthesiology* **57**, A267.

Eichelbaum, M., Birkel, P., Grube, E., Gutgemann, U. and Somogyi, A. (1980) Effects of verapamil on P–R intervals in relation to verapamil plasma levels following single i.v. and oral administration and during chronic treatment. *Klinische Wochenschrift* **58**, 919–925

Fabiato, A. and Fabiato, F. (1979) Calcium and cardiac excitation–contraction coupling. *Annual Review of Physiology* **41**, 473–484

Fahmy, N.R. and Lappas, D.G. (1983) Interaction of nifedipine, propranolol and halothane in humans. *Anesthesiology* **59**, A39

Fleckenstein, A. (1964) Die Bedeutung der energiereichen Phosphate fur Kontraktilitat und Tonus des Myokards. *Verhandlung der Deutschen Gesselschaft für Innere Medizin* **70**, 81–90

Fleckenstein, A. (1983) History of calcium antagonists. *Circulation Research* **52**, suppl. 1, 3–16

Freis, E.S. and Lappas, D.G. (1982) Chronic administration of calcium entry blockers and the cardiovascular responses to high doses of fentanyl in man. *Anesthesiology* **57**, A295

Gelpi, R.J., Mosca, S.M., Rinaldi, G.J., Kosoglov, A. and Cingolani, H.E. (1983) Effect of calcium antagonism on contractile behavior of canine hearts. *American Journal of Physiology* **244**, H378–H386

Griffin, R.M., Dimich, I., Jurado, R., Pratilas, V., Kaplan, J.A. and Fagerstrom, R. (1984) Cardiovascular effects of nifedipine infusion during fentanyl anesthesia. *Anesthesiology* **61**, A10

Hantler, C.B., Felbeck, P.G., Kroll, D.A. and Knight, P.R. (1983a) Effects of verapamil on sinus and av nodal function in the presence of volatile anesthetics. *Anesthesiology* **59**, A38

Hantler, C.B., Felbeck, P.G., Tait, A.R. and Knight, P.R. (1983b) Renal vascular interactions between halothane and verapamil. *Anesthesiology* **59**, A45

Hariman, R.J., Mangiardi, L.M., McAllister, R.G. Jr, Surawicz, B., Shabetai, R. and Kishida, H. (1979) Reversal of the cardiovascular effects of verapamil by calcium and sodium: differences between electrophysiologic and hemodynamic responses. *Circulation* **59**, 797–804

Henling, C.E., Slogoff, S., Kodali, S.V. and Arlund, C. (1984) Heart block after coronary artery bypass. Effects of chronic administration of calcium-entry blockers and β-blockers. *Anesthesia and Analgesia* **63**, 515–520

Henry, P.D. (1980) Comparative pharmacology of calcium antagonists: nifedipine, verapamil, and diltiazem. *American Journal of Cardiology* **46**, 1047–1058

Henry, P.D., Shuchleib, R., Clark, R.E. and Perez, J.E. (1979) Effect of nifedipine on myocardial ischemia: analysis of collateral blood flow, pulsatile heat and regional muscle shortening. *American Journal of Cardiology* **44**, 817–824

Hess, P., Lansman, J.B. and Tsien, R.W. (1984) Different modes of Ca channel gating behaviour favoured by dihydropyridine Ca agonists and antagonists. *Nature* **311**, 538–544

Himes, R.S., DiFazio, C.A. and Burney, R.G. (1977) Effects of lidocaine on the anesthetic requirement for nitrous oxide and halothane. *Anesthesiology* **47**, 437–440

Hodgkin, A.L. and Huxley, A.F. (1952) A quantitative description of membrane current and its application to conduction and excitation in nerve. *Journal of Physiology* **117**, 500–544

Hung, J.H., Fukunaga, A.F., Olewine, S.K. and Van Etten, A. (1983) Hemodynamic, metabolic, and hormonal changes following diltiazem-induced hypotension. *Anesthesiology* **59**, A20

Jones, R.M. (1984) Calcium antagonists. *Anaesthesia* **39**, 747–749

Jones, R.M. (1985) Calcium antagonists. In: *Recent Advances in Anaesthesia and Analgesia* (Eds. Atkinson, R.S. and Adams, A.P.), pp. 89–106. Churchill Livingstone: London

Kambara, H., Fujimoto, K., Wakabayashi, A. and Kawai, C. (1981) Primary pulmonary hypertension: beneficial therapy with diltiazem. *American Heart Journal* **101**, 230–231

Kaplan, J.A., Guffin, A.V., Jones, E.L., Kates, R.A. and Holbrook, G.W. (1984) Verapamil and myocardial preservation in patients undergoing coronary artery bypass surgery. *Anesthesia and Analgesia* **63**, 230

Kapur, P.A., Bloor, B.C., Flacke, W.E. and Olewine, S.K. (1984a) Comparison of cardiovascular responses to verapamil during enflurane, isoflurane, or halothane anesthesia in dog. *Anesthesiology* **61**, 156–160

Kapur, P.A. and Flacke, W.E. (1981) Epinephrine-induced arrhythmias and cardiovascular function after verapamil during halothane anesthesia in the dog. *Anesthesiology* **55**, 218–225

Kapur, P.A. and Flacke, W.E. (1982) Lack of correlation of verapamil plasma level with cumulative protective effects against halothane–epinephrine ventricular arrhythmias. *Journal of Cardiovascular Pharmacology* **4**, 652–657

Kapur, P.A., Norel, E.J., Cohen, G.R. and Dajee, H. (1984b) Verapamil administration after high dose fentanyl with or without chronic nifedipine therapy in man. *Anesthesia and Analgesia* **63**, 231

Kapur, P.A., Norel, E., Dajee, H. and Cimochowski, G. (1984c) Verapamil treatment of intractable ventricular arrhythmias after cardiopulmonary bypass. *Anesthesia and Analgesia* **63**, 460–463

Kapur, P.A. and Tippit, S.E. (1984) Correlation of cardiovascular effects with plasma levels of diltiazem during isoflurane anesthesia. *Anesthesiology* **61**, A12

Kates, R.A. and Kaplan, J.A. (1983) Cardiovascular responses to verapamil during coronary artery bypass graft surgery. *Anesthesia and Analgesia* **62**, 821–826

Kates, R.A., Kaplan, J.A., Guyton, R.A., Dorsey, L., Hug, C.C. and Hatcher, C.R. (1983) Hemodynamic interactions of verapamil and isoflurane. *Anesthesiology* **59**, 132–138

Kates, R.A., Zaggy, A.P., Norfleet, E.A. and Heath, K.R. (1984) Comparative cardiovascular effects of verapamil, nifedipine, and diltiazem during halothane anesthesia in swine. *Anesthesiology* **61**, 10–18

Kinney, E.L., Moskowitz, R.M. and Zelis, R.F. (1981) The pharmacokinetics and pharmacology of oral diltiazem in normal volunteers. *Journal of Clinical Pharmacology* **21**, 337–342

Kishi, T., Okumura, F. and Furuya, H. (1984) Haemodynamic effects of nicardepine hydrochloride. *British Journal of Anaesthesia* **56**, 1003–1007

Klein, W., Brandt, D., Vrecko, K. and Harringer, M. (1983) Role of calcium antagonists in the treatment of essential hypertension. *Circulation Research* **52**, suppl. 1, 174–181

Klugmann, S., Salvi, A. and Camerini, F. (1980) Haemodynamic effects of nifedipine in heart failure. *British Heart Journal* **43**, 440–446

Kohlhardt, M. and Fleckenstein, A. (1977) Inhibition of the slow inward current by nifedipine in mammalian ventricular myocardium. *Nauyn-Schmiedeberg's Archives of Pharmacology* **298**, 267–272

Kohlhardt, M., Bauer, B., Krause, H. and Fleckenstein, A. (1972) Differentiation of the transmembrane Na and Ca channel in mammalian cardiac fibres by the use of specific inhibitors. *Pflügers Archiv* **335**, 309–332

Kohno, K., Takenchi, Y., Etoh, A. and Noda, K. (1977) Pharmacokinetics and bioavailability of diltiazem (CRD-401) in dog. *Arzneimittel-Forschung* **27**, 1424–1428

Kopman, E.A. (1983) Intravenous verapamil to relieve pulmonary congestion in patients with mitral valve disease. *Anesthesiology* **58**, 374–376

Kroll, D.A. and Knight, P.R. (1984) Antifibrillatory effects of volatile anesthetics in acute occlusion/reperfusion arrhythmias. *Anesthesiology* **61**, 657–661

Kunis, C.L. and Lowenstein, J. (1977) The emergency treatment of hyperkalemia. *Medical Clinics of North America* **65**, 165–176

Lawson, N.W., Kraynack, B.J. and Gintautas, J. (1983) Neuromuscular and electrocardiographic responses to verapamil in dogs. *Anesthesia and Analgesia* **62**, 50–54

Lorell, B.H., Paulus, W.J., Grossman, W., Wynne, J. and Cohn, P.F. (1982) Modification of abnormal left ventricular diastolic properties by nifedipine in patients with hypertrophic cardiomyopathy. *Circulation* **65**, 499–507

Lynch, C. (1984) Are volatile anesthetics really calcium entry blockers? *Anesthesiology* **61**, 644–646

Lynch, C. and Bedford, R.F. (1983) Adverse effect of verapamil on ICP in patients with brain tumours. *Anesthesiology* **59**, A392

McAllister, R.G. (1982) Clinical pharmacokinetics of calcium channel antagonists. *Journal of Cardiovascular Pharmacology* **4**, S340–S345

McKay, R.D., Newfield, P., Reves, J.G., Brummett, C. and Morawetz, R.B. (1981) Hypertension and mortality in neuro ICU patients. *Anesthesiology* **55**, A101

Maze, M., Mason, D.M. and Kates, R.E. (1983) Verapamil decreases MAC for halothane in dogs. *Anesthesiology* **59**, 327–329

Merin, R.G. (1981) Slow channel inhibitors, anesthetics, and cardiovascular function. *Anesthesiology* **55**, 198–200

Millard, R.W., Grupp, G., Grupp, I.L., DiSalvo, J., DePover, A. and Schwartz, A. (1983) Chronotropic, inotropic, and vasodilator action of diltiazem, nifedipine and verapamil. *Circulation Research* **52**, suppl. 1, 29–39

Murphy, K.M.M., Gould, R.J., Largent, B.L. and Snyder, S.H. (1983) A unitary mechanism of calcium antagonist drug action. *Proceedings of the National Academy of Sciences of the USA* **80**, 860–864

Nakaya, H., Schwartz, A. and Millar, R.W. (1983) Reflex chronotropic and inotropic effects of calcium channel-blocking agents in conscious dogs. Diltiazem, verapamil and nifedipine compared. *Circulation Research* **52**, 302–311

Nayler, W.G. (1980) Cardioprotective effects of calcium ion antagonists in myocardial ischaemia. *Clinical and Investigative Medicine* **3**, 91–99

Nayler, W.G., Mas-Oliva, J. and Williams, A.J. (1980) Cardiovascular receptors and calcium. *Circulation Research* **46**, suppl. 1, 161–166

Nugent, M., Tinker, J.H. and Moyer, T.P. (1984) Verapamil worsens rate of development and hemodynamic effects of acute hyperkalemia in halothane–anesthetized dogs: effects of calcium therapy. *Anesthesiology* **60**, 435–439

Nussmeier, N.A., Curling, P.E., Murphy, D.A. *et al.* (1983) Nifedipine: cardiovascular effects after sublingual administration during fentanyl–pancuronium anesthesia in man. *Anesthesiology* **59**, A34

Pask, H.L., England, P.J. and Prys-Roberts, C. (1981) Effects of volatile inhalational anaesthetic agents on isolated bovine cardiac myofibrillar ATPase. *Journal of Molecular and Cellular Cardiology* **13**, 293–301

Pollard, B.J. and Jones, R.M. (1983) Interactions between tubocurarine, pancuronium and alcuronium demonstrated in the rat phrenic nerve hemidiaphragm preparation. *British Journal of Anaesthesia* **55**, 1127–1131

Port, J.D., Jones, R.L. and Stanley, T.H. (1983) Protection of the ischemic myocardium during cardiopulmonary bypass: Ca^{++} blockers vs. hypothermia. *Anesthesiology* **59**, A42

Price, H.L. and Ohnishi, S.T. (1980) Effects of anesthetics on the heart. *Federation Proceedings* **39**, 1575–1579

Rasmussen, H. and Barrett, P.Q. (1984) Calcium messenger system: an integrated view. *Physiological Reviews* **64**, 938–984

Reuter, H. (1967) The dependence of slow inward current in Purkinje fibres on the extra-cellular concentration. *Journal of Physiology* **192**, 479–492

Reuter, H. (1979) Properties of two inward membrane currents in the heart. *Annual Review of Physiology* **45**, 413–424

Reuter, H. (1984) Ion channels in cardiac cell membranes. *Annual Review of Physiology* **41**, 473–484

Reuter, H. and Scholtz, H. (1977) The regulation of the Ca^{++} conductance of cardiac muscle by adrenaline. *Journal of Physiology* **264**, 49–62

Reves, J.G. (1984) The relative hemodynamic effects of Ca^{++} entry blockers. *Anesthesiology* **61**, 3–5

Reves, J.G., Barker, S. and Smith, L.R. (1983) Significance of nifedipine plasma levels and hemodynamic changes during anesthesia induction. *Anesthesiology* **59**, A41

Reves, J.G., Kissin, I., Lell, W.A. and Tosone, S. (1982) Calcium entry blockers: uses and implications for anesthesiologists. *Anesthesiology* **57**, 504–518

Rovei, V., Gomeni, R., Mitchard, M. *et al.* (1980) Pharmacokinetics and metabolism of diltiazem in man. *Acta Cardiologica* **35**, 35–45

Schomerus, M., Spiegelhalder, B., Stieren, B. and Eichelbaum, M. (1976) Physiological disposition of verapamil in man. *Cardiovascular Research* **10**, 605–612

Schulte-Sasse, U., Hess, W., Markschies-Hornung, A. and Tarnow, J. (1984) Combined effect of halothane anesthesia and verapamil on systemic and left ventricular myocardial contractility in patients with ischemic heart disease. *Anesthesia and Analgesia* **63**, 791–798

Serruys, P.W., Hooghoudt, T.E.H., Reiber, J.H.C., Slager, G., Brower, R.W. and Hugenholtz, P.G. (1983) Influence of intracoronary nifedipine on left ventricular function, coronary vasomotility, and myocardial oxygen consumption. *British Heart Journal* **49**, 427–441

Singh, B.N. and Roche, A.H.G. (1977) Effects of verapamil on hemodynamics in patients with heart disease. *American Heart Journal* **94**, 593–599

Singh, B.H., Collet, J.T. and Chew, C.Y.C. (1980) New perspectives in the pharmacologic therapy of cardiac arrhythmias. *Progress in Cardiovascular Diseases* **22**, 243–301

Singh, B.N., Ellrodt, G. and Peter, C.T. (1978) Verapamil: a review of its pharmacological properties and therapeutic uses. *Drugs* **15**, 169–197

Skarvan, K. (1983) Preoperative nifedipine treatment and anesthesia in patients with coronary heart disease. *Anesthesiology* **59**, 362–363

Skarvan, K., Priebe, H.-J. and Gale, J. (1984) Effects of diltiazem and isoflurane on cardiovascular function and coronary hemodynamics in dogs. *Anesthesiology* **61**, A9

Smith, H.J., Singh, B.N., Nisbet, H.D. and Norris, R.M. (1975) The effect of verapamil on infarct size following coronary artery occlusion. *Cardiovascular Research* **9**, 569–578

Smith, H.J., Goldstein, R.A., Griffith, J.M., Kent, K.M. and Epstein, S.E. (1976) Regional contractility. Selective depression of ischemic myocardium by verapamil. *Circulation* **54**, 629–635

Sodoyama, O., Ikeda, K., Matsuda, I., Fukunaga, A.F. and Bishay, E.G. (1983) Nifedipine for control of postoperative hypertension. *Anesthesiology* **59**, A18

Sperelakis, N. and Schneider, J.A. (1976) A metabolic control mechanism for calcium ion influx that may protect the ventricular myocardial cell. *American Journal of Cardiology* **37**, 1079–1085

Stone, D.L., Stephens, J.D. and Banim, S.O. (1983) Coronary haemodynamic effects of nifedipine. Comparison with glyceryl trinitrate. *British Heart Journal* **49**, 442–446

Stone, P.H., Antman, E.M., Muller, J.E. and Braunwald, E. (1980) Calcium channel blocking agents in the treatment of cardiovascular disorders. II. Hemodynamic effects and clinical applications. *Annals of Internal Medicine* **93**, 886–904

Subramanian, V.B., Bowles, M.J., Khurmi, M.S., Davies, A.B., O'Hara, M.J. and Raftery, E.B. (1983) Calcium antagonist withdrawl syndrome: objective demonstration with frequency-modulated ambulatory ST-segment monitoring. *British Medical Journal* **286**, 520–521

Tosone, S.R., Reves, J.G., Kissin, I., Smith, L.R. and Fournier, S.E. (1983) Hemodynamic responses to nifedipine in dogs anesthetized with halothane. *Anesthesia and Analgesia: Current Researches* **62**, 903–908

Triggle, D.J. (1982) Biochemical pharmacology of calcium blockers. In: *Calcium Blockers. Mechanisms of Action and Clinical Applications* (Eds. Flaim S.F. and Zelis, R.). Urban and Schwartzenberg: Baltimore, Munich

Triggle, D.J. and Swamy, V.C. (1983) Calcium antagonists. Some chemical–pharmacologic aspects. *Circulation Research* **52**, suppl. 1, 17–18

Tsien, R.W. (1984) Calcium channels in excitable membranes. *Annual Review of Physiology* **45**, 341–358

Vouhe, P.R., Helias, J. and Grondin, C.M. (1980) Myocardial protection through cold cardioplegia using diltiazem, a calcium channel blocker. *Annals of Thoracic Surgery* **30**, 342–347

Williams, J.P., Broadbent, M.P., Pearce, A.C. and Jones, R.M. (1983) Verapamil potentiates the neuromuscular blocking effects of enflurane *in vitro*. *Anesthesiology* **59**, A276

Yamamoto, F., Manning, A.S., Baimbridge, M.V. and Hearse, D.J. (1983) Cardioplegia and slow calcium-channel blockers. *Journal of Thoracic and Cardiovascular Surgery* **86**, 252–261

Zelis, R. and Flaim, S.F. (1981) 'Calcium influx blockers' and vascular smooth muscle: do we really understand the mechanisms? *Annals of Internal Medicine* **94**, 124–126

Zelis, R.F. and Kinney, E.L. (1982) The pharmacokinetics of diltiazem in healthy American men. *American Journal of Cardiology* **49**, 529–532

Zimpfer, M., Fitzal, S. and Tonczar, L. (1981) Verapamil as a hypotensive agent during neurolept anaesthesia. *British Journal of Anaesthesia* **53**, 885–889

Part three
Appendices

Appendix 1
Toxicity

Jeffrey M. Baden*

Toxicity is defined as any harmful effect of a chemical or drug on a target organism, and is usually divided into three types: acute, subchronic and chronic. Acute toxicity is an adverse effect occurring within a short time of administration of a single dose of a chemical or multiple doses given within 24 hours. Subchronic and chronic toxicities are adverse effects occurring from repeated daily dosing of a chemical for days to months and months to years, respectively. Surgical patients who generally are exposed to high doses of anaesthetics over a period of hours are most likely to suffer acute toxic reactions. On the other hand, operating room personnel who are exposed to trace concentrations of inhaled anaesthetics for months or years are most likely to suffer chronic toxic reactions.

Toxic effects of drugs used in anaesthesia occur by a number of mechanisms. They may merely be an extension of the normal pharmacological action of the drug, as exemplified by respiratory and cardiac arrest caused by direct effects of high concentrations of inhaled anaesthetics on the central nervous system and myocardium. These unwanted or side effects are important and must be recognized and properly treated by the anaesthetist. They are discussed elsewhere or can be inferred from the general properties of individual drugs. Mechanisms of toxicity which will be discussed in this chapter are those related to metabolism. In addition, mention will be made of the physicochemical reaction of N_2O with vitamin B_{12}, and the inhibition of adrenal steroidogenesis by the intravenous anaesthetic etomidate.

Metabolism and toxicity

Most toxic reactions associated with drugs used in anaesthesia are due not to the parent compounds, which are seldom reactive, but rather to their metabolites. This is particularly true of the volatile anaesthetics which are highly lipid soluble rather than capable of strong covalent binding to tissues. Several mechanisms of toxicity are recognized.

* Supported in part by the Veterans Administration

Metabolic end-products

Accumulation of a metabolic end-product to a concentration above a toxic threshold is an occasional cause of toxicity. The metabolite may directly inhibit or modify enzymatic or structural systems necessary for maintaining cellular integrity. Alternatively, it may indirectly damage a target cell by initiating an unwanted pharmacological action such as vasoconstriction, which may itself lead to tissue hypoxia and cell necrosis. The reason that toxic effects occur only above a threshold tissue concentration probably relates in part to the decreased availability of protective endogenous substances such as glutathione.

The classic example of a toxic end-product in anaesthetic practice is the production of high levels of inorganic fluoride (F^-) sufficient to cause polyuric renal failure. The syndrome was first reported in 13 of 41 patients receiving methoxyflurane anaesthesia for abdominal surgery (Crandell, Pappas and MacDonald, 1966). The causative agent was later shown to be F^-, an end-product of methoxyflurane's biotransformation as shown in Fig. A1.1.

This conclusion is based on the observation that serum F^- levels following methoxyflurane administration in man are positively correlated with degree of renal dysfunction (Mazze, Shue and Jackson, 1971). In addition, a renal insufficiency syndrome similar to that seen in man and rats after prolonged methoxyflurane anaesthesia can be easily elicited in Fischer 344 rats injected with sodium fluoride (Mazze, Cousins and Kosek, 1972). The exact site and mechanism whereby F^- produces the acute renal lesion are unclear. Inorganic fluoride is, however, a potent inhibitor of the enzyme Na,K-ATPase and of the chloride pump in the ascending limb of the loop of Henle (Wiseman, 1970). Furthermore, high concentrations of F^- may interfere with iso-osmotic reabsorption of proximal tubular fluid, may render the collecting ducts insensitive to ADH and may cause renal medullary vasodilatation sufficient to interfere with counter-current exchange (Mazze, 1983).

Other examples of toxic metabolic end-products of anaesthetic drugs include the renal and hepatic toxin, trifluoroethanol, produced in certain animals from fluroxene (Blake et al., 1967) and the methaemoglobin-inducing agent, 6-hydroxytoluidine, produced in man from prilocaine (Kiese, 1965).

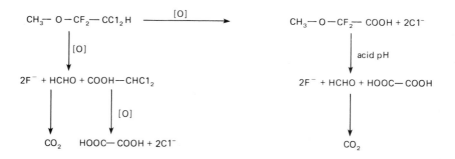

Fig. A1.1   Biotransformation of methoxyflurane. The molecule can be oxygenated either at the methyl carbon or at the dichloromethyl carbon.

Reactive intermediates

Perhaps the most important mechanism of toxicity is the production of reactive intermediate metabolites which are the ultimate toxicants and which combine covalently with various tissue macromolecules or initiate destructive chain reactions. When these intermediates bind covalently to protein, lipid, DNA, RNA or other macromolecules they form alkylated or arylated derivatives. Whilst most investigators agree that the derivatives are important for toxicity, the processes leading to cellular damage are, with few exceptions, unknown. Presumably the derivatives alter the normal function of organelles such as the endoplasmic reticulum, mitochrondria, lysosomes or nucleus and thereby disrupt normal cellular homeostasis. As with toxicity produced by metabolic end-products, toxicity produced by reactive intermediates is likely to involve depletion of certain intracellular compounds such as glutathione and other sulphydryl-containing compounds. These antioxidants normally protect the cell from damage by preferentially binding to the toxicant but they can be overwhelmed if the toxicant is present in high enough concentration. In many cases the ultimate toxicant cannot easily be identified because cellular damage is not correlated with the pharmacokinetics of the parent compound or even with its major metabolites. The reason may be that the ultimate toxicant, although highly reactive, is only a quantitatively minor metabolite or that the specific covalent binding which leads to cellular damage is only a small fraction of the total binding.

Free radicals constitute the most important group of reactive intermediates and are thought to be involved in the majority of toxic drug effects. Most drugs are stable compounds with paired electrons of opposite spin in their outer molecular orbital. During metabolism, intermediates known as free radicals with unpaired electrons in their outer orbitals may be produced. They are highly reactive and generally do not escape from the tissues where they are formed. In addition to binding to cellular constituents, they are capable of initiating destructive chain reactions which occur in three phases. The first is the initiation phase during which free radicals are generated by a single or series of reactions. The second is the propagation phase during which a sequence of cellular interactions occur and the number of free radicals is conserved or increased. Finally, there is the termination phase during which the free radicals are destroyed. The chain reactions occurring during free radical formation include polymerization or cross-linking of enzymes and other proteins (Tappel, 1973) and destructive changes in nucleic acids such as main chain breaks and degradation of purine acid pyrimidine rings (Weinstein, Yamaguchi and Gebert, 1975). Perhaps the most ubiquitous chain reaction, however, and the one which has the greatest implication for drug toxicity is lipoperoxidation (auto-oxidation of lipids) within organelle membranes. Lipoperoxidation has also been implicated as an important process in ageing, mutagenesis, carcinogenesis and oxygen toxicity, among others (Recknagel *et al.*, 1982). It occurs when the relatively unstable α-methylene hydrogens of unsaturated lipids are subject to hydrogen extraction by free radicals (Demopoulos, 1973; Tappel, 1973).

The result, as seen in Fig. A1.2 is the formation of an organic radical and a rearrangement of double bonds to form a relatively stable conjugated diene. Subsequent attack by molecular oxygen results in cleavage of the radical with

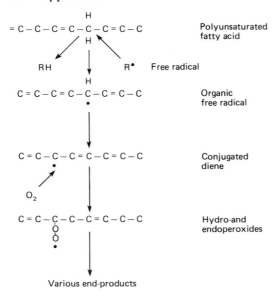

Fig. A1.2   Lipoperoxidation initiated by free radicals.

formation of a number of stable end-products, including hydroxylcarbonyl compounds, malonic dialdehyde, ethane and pentane. During the course of the reaction, further free radicals are formed which perpetuate the process. The sequence of events leading from lipoperoxidation to cellular damage and death is unknown.

Many other classes of reactive intermediates exist. They generally consist of unstable molecules which are capable of directly alkylating or arylating tissue macromolecules. For example, ethyleneimines and epoxides (Fig. A1.3) have strained ring structures which can easily be broken. They are typical alkylating agents. Whilst quantitatively less important than free radicals, compounds such as epoxides are thought to be involved in many toxic reactions, most notably mutagenesis and carcinogenesis.

The volatile anaesthetic, halothane, is an excellent example of a drug which is metabolized to reactive intermediates which covalently bind to tissue

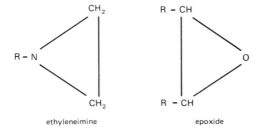

Fig. A1.3   Examples of 'strained-ring' reactive intermediates.

macromolecules. The production of these reactive intermediates, some of which are free radicals, has important implications for the hepatotoxicity associated with halothane. Like other volatile anaesthetics, halothane undergoes metabolism catalysed by the cytochrome P450 or mixed function oxidase system. Stier and colleagues (Stier 1964; Stier *et al.*, 1964) demonstrated that major metabolites of halothane are bromide and trifluoroacetic acid. Van Dyke, Chenoweth and Van-Poznak (1964) found that 2.9 per cent of an injected dose of [^{36}Cl]halothane appeared as ^{36}Cl in the urine. From these early studies, it was concluded that halothane undergoes mainly oxidative metabolism as follows:

$$CF_3–CHClBr \xrightarrow{[O]} [CF_3–COCl] + Br^- \xrightarrow{[HOH]} CF_3–COOH + Cl^-$$

Rehder *et al.* (1967) established that about 20 per cent of halothane taken up by the body is metabolized. Neither of the end-products, trifluoroacetic acid or bromide, is thought to be associated with clinical toxicity. Trifluoroacetic acid which is completely ionized at body pH is relatively innocuous, and bromide levels seldom reach 3 mEq/l in man even after prolonged exposure to halothane; levels of 6–10 mEq/l are required to produce early signs of bromism.

The finding that trifluoroacetylethanolamide was also present in the urine of human volunteers administered halothane was of great interest (Cohen, 1971). It implied that a halothane metabolite, probably the postulated intermediate of oxidative metabolism, trifluoroacetyl chloride, was capable of binding covalently to phosphatidylethanolamine in the membrane of hepatic endoplasmic reticulum.

Later, a second pathway of halothane metabolism, which operates under conditions of low oxygen tension, was found to exist. Whilst quantitatively less important than oxidative metabolism, reductive metabolism of halothane has important implications for toxicity. The reaction probably proceeds via cytochrome P450 catalysed one- or two-electron reduction of halothane as follows (Sipes, Gandolfi and Brown, 1981):

$$CF_3CHClBr \xrightarrow{e^-} CF_3CHBrCl^- \longrightarrow Br^- + CF_3CHCl \xrightarrow{e^-} \begin{cases} CF_2CHCl + F^- & (CDE) \\ CF_3CH + Cl^- & (TFMC) \\ CF_3CH_2Cl & (CTE) \end{cases}$$

Some details of this pathway, including the exact nature of the intermediate metabolites, are unknown. Trifluoromethyl carbene (TFMC) remains a postulated end-product (Mansuy, Nastainczyk and Ullrich, 1974). Inorganic fluoride, however, has been definitely identified (Van Dyke and Gandolfi, 1976), as have the two volatile end-products, chlorodifluoroethylene (CDE) and chlorotrifluoroethane (CTE) (Mukai *et al.*, 1977; Sharp, Trudell and Cohen, 1979). In addition, Cohen *et al.* (1975) reported the presence of ^{14}C-labelled ethanolamide and cysteine conjugates in the urine of heart transplant donors administered [^{14}C]halothane. They postulated that these were degradation products of hepatic lipids and proteins which had combined covalently with reactive intermediates of halothane metabolism. Free radicals have also been detected during the metabolism of halothane by several investigators (Poyer *et al.*, 1981; Fujii *et al.*, 1982; Plummer *et al.*, 1982). For example, Plummer *et al.* (1982) used α-phenyl-*t*-butyl nitrone (PBN) to spin trap free radicals in rats administered halothane, enflurane or isoflurane. Only halothane was converted to free radicals.

Many investigators have suggested that the reductive pathway of halothane metabolism is more likely than the oxidative pathway to be associated with hepatotoxicity. Widger, Gandolfi and Van Dyke (1976) and many others have found that covalent binding of halothane metabolites to lipids and proteins is greatly increased under hypoxic conditions. Furthermore, models of halothane hepatitis have been developed in which rats whose enzymes are induced with phenobarbitone are exposed to halothane at low oxygen concentrations (Sipes and Brown, 1976). The extent to which liver necrosis occurs can be correlated with the degree of reductive metabolism. Rats exposed to halothane under conditions of hypoxia or enzyme induction alone show little evidence of liver necrosis (Cousins *et al.*, 1979). The role of lipoperoxidation, if any, in the production of hepatic necrosis remains in doubt; whilst small increases in conjugated dienes have been observed after halothane exposure, they have not been sufficient to account for cellular damage. Over all, the hypothesis that the reductive metabolism of halothane is responsible for hepatotoxicity is an attractive one, but the evidence for it remains circumstantial because no ultimate toxicant has yet been identified.

Halothane is not the only volatile anaesthetic associated with hepatotoxicity and the binding of metabolites to hepatic proteins and lipids. Chloroform and trichlorethylene are known to be hepatotoxic under certain conditions and are metabolized to compounds which bind strongly to liver tissue. Enflurane has occasionally been linked to hepatotoxicity in man (Lewis *et al.*, 1983). However, the argument for a causal relationship is not strong. About 2–3 per cent of enflurane taken up by the body is metabolized under aerobic but not anaerobic conditions; binding of metabolites is minimal (Van Dyke, 1982). The most recently introduced volatile anaesthetic, isoflurane, is even less likely than enflurane to produce serious liver injury. Only about 0.2 per cent of the amount taken up by the body is metabolized under aerobic conditions. Production of reactive intermediates is thought unlikely, and a reductive pathway of metabolism has not been found (Van Dyke, 1982).

In addition to producing such reactions as acute toxicity, reactive intermediates are the most likely candidates for producing chronic toxicity such as mutagenicity and carcinogenecity. Many studies have been performed to determine whether inhaled anaesthetics are chemical mutagens; that is, agents capable of producing heritable changes in genetic information. The reason for such interest is twofold. First, mutations are almost always deleterious and interfere with the normal function of our most precious resource, the human genome. Secondly, finding that a particular drug is a mutagen often implies that it is a reactive chemical which can initiate other toxicity such as carcinogenicity and teratogenicity. Several reviews of the mutagenicity of inhaled anaesthetics have been published (Baden and Simmon, 1980; Baden, 1983). In general, findings from numerous studies indicate that modern inhaled anaesthetics have little or no mutagenic potential whereas several older anaesthetics such as divinyl ether ($CH_2=CH-O-CH=CH_2$), trichloroethylene ($CHCl=CCl_2$) and fluroxene ($CF_3-CH_2-O-CH=CH_2$) are chemical mutagens. These mutagenic anaesthetics have a double-bonded structure and probably are metabolized to epoxide intermediates which combine covalently and alkylate DNA bases. Subsequent misreading of the altered DNA leads to mutation. Findings from animal studies of the carcinogenic potential of inhaled anaesthetics closely parallel those of the mutagenicity studies. Trichlorethylene is weakly carcinogenic whereas the modern inhaled anaesthetics halothane, enflurane and isoflurane administered for prolonged periods do not increase the incidence of tumours (Baden, 1983). The role of reactive intermediates in producing teratogenic changes is a complicated one because mutations, toxic reactions early in development and numerous other mechanisms may be involved. In any case, with the exception of nitrous oxide, which will be discussed later, inhaled anaesthetics and other drugs used in anaesthetic practice do not appear to be teratogenic themselves, although the severe maternal physiological changes which they occasionally produce may lead to congenital anomalies (Baden, 1983).

Immunological reactions

There has been increasing awareness in recent years that immunological mechanisms play an important role in the toxicity of some drugs and chemicals. The basic immunological processes which lead to such toxicity constitute a vast and complex subject which has been partly reviewed in several excellent publications (Mathieu and Kahan, 1975; Luster, Dean and Moore, 1982; Walton, 1982). Only a brief summary of the salient features will be presented here.

'Non-specific immunity' refers to a battery of general host defence mechanisms which protect the organism against foreign substances. It includes phagocytosis by polymorphonuclear leucocytes and macrophages, and a variety of bactericidins and microbial inhibitors such as gastric acid, acids in sweat, lysozymes and interferon. In addition, the important complement system which enhances many immune responses, including phagocytosis, is part of the non-specific immune system (Walton, 1982).

'Specific immunity' refers to the mechanism whereby lymphocytes recognize and respond to specific antigens. Part of the response is establishment of long-term memory of the specific antigen by long-lived lymphocytes so that an enhanced immunological response may be mounted upon subsequent exposure. Specific immunity may be either humoral mediated or cell mediated.

B-cells (B-lymphocytes) which are formed in the haemopoietic organs are responsible for humoral-mediated immunity. When an antigen is introduced into the body, it interacts with a specific B-cell which then proliferates into a clone of cells. Some of these differentiate and divide to produce a population of specific antibody-secreting plasma cells. Various classes of antibodies, including IgM, IgG, IgA, IgD and IgE, are produced by plasma cells. They are antigenically and functionally distinct. For example, IgM which is produced early in response to infection is a potent agglutinin and cytolytic and is found in the blood, whereas IgG which is produced during a secondary immune response is able to neutralize bacterial toxin and is found in extravascular tissues. Other cells of the clone remain as antigen-sensitive memory cells, ready to respond to a new challenge by the same antigen.

T-cells (T-lymphocytes) or thymus-derived cells are responsible for cell-mediated immunity. As for B-cells, a specific T-cell is activated by a specific antigen and then undergoes cell division to form a clone of sensitized cells. Some of these cells are cytotoxic and attack target cells such as those in allografts. Other cells are capable of suppressing or amplifying antibody responses of B-cells and also releasing active substances (lymphokines) while yet others act as memory cells.

Immunological hypersensitivity (allergy) accounts for a large number of toxic reactions to drugs. Three types of hypersensitivity are due to B-cell activity, while a fourth type is due to T-cell activity. Type I is classic anaphylaxis and occurs when an IgE antibody in combination with an antigen triggers mast cells to release histamine and serotonin. Type II is a cytotoxic reaction and occurs when circulatory antibodies contact cell-surface antigens and cause cell damage or death. Sometimes drugs or their metabolites acting as haptens combine with proteins on the cell surface and initiate this type of hypersensitivity. Type III is a complex-mediated reaction and occurs when antibody–antigen complexes deposited in tissues cause marked inflammatory reactions and tissue damage. Type IV is cellular or delayed hypersensitivity and occurs 24 hours or more after exposure to the drug. It is mediated by T-cells and includes reactions to purified tuberculin protein derivative (PPD) and dermatitis from antibiotic and other ointments.

Hypersensitivity reactions have been reported for almost all drugs administered parenterally in anaesthetic practice. For example, adverse reactions to thiopentone occur with a frequency of about 1 in 14 000 (Evans and Keogh, 1977). Any of the four types of hypersensitivity may be responsible for a particular adverse drug reaction. Care should be taken to distinguish immunologically mediated reactions from drug intolerance and idiosyncrasy. Intolerance is a qualitatively normal but excessive response to a drug, and idiosyncrasy is a qualitatively abnormal response which has no immunological basis.

The sporadic nature of halothane-associated hepatitis, its lack of dose-response and its increased frequency on multiple exposure suggest that it may have an immunological basis. Further evidence is the observation that some patients with halothane-associated hepatitis show the clinical signs normally seen with hypersensitivity reactions. Several patients have even shown a recurrence of hepatitis after being rechallenged with halothane under controlled conditions, although such cases do not prove that an immunological mechanism is involved since the hepatitis could equally well be due to intolerance or idiosyncrasy. Autoantibodies have been reported by some investigators (Rodriguez et al., 1969) in patients with halothane-associated hepatitis, but not by others (Walton et al., 1976).

Many attempts have been made to demonstrate that cell-mediated hypersensitivity is the cause of halothane-associated hepatitis. They range from early studies with lymphocyte transformation tests to more recent studies with leucocyte migration and cytotoxicity tests. These studies, together with the whole subject on the immunological basis of halothane-associated hepatitis, have been well reviewed by Walton (1982), among others. Only a few points need emphasis. First, results of studies have been inconsistent and difficult to interpret; for example, whilst autoantibodies such as those to mitochrondria may initiate liver damage, they also appear as part of a secondary response to liver damage. Secondly, if an immunological mechanism is involved, it is more likely to be initiated by a metabolite of halothane acting as a hapten rather than by molecular halothane which is comparatively unreactive. Finally, the possibility cannot be excluded that more than one mechanism may lead to halothane-associated hepatitis.

Nitrous oxide and vitamin B$_{12}$

The serious toxicity occasionally seen following exposure to nitrous oxide (N_2O) is due to a non-enzymatic physicochemical reaction of molecular N_2O with vitamin B$_{12}$. Thus, in contrast to the toxicity associated with the fluorinated anaesthetics, toxicity associated with N_2O is unrelated to metabolism. The biochemical and toxic effects of N_2O have been reviewed extensively (Eger, 1985).

Banks, Henderson and Pratt (1968) found that N_2O irreversibly oxidized vitamin B$_{12}$ which contains the transition metal, cobalt. The non-enzymatic reactions involved are most likely as follows:

$$\text{Cob(I)alamin} + N_2O + H_2O \rightarrow \text{cob(III)alamin} + N_2 + 20H^-$$
$$\text{Cob(I)alamin} + \text{cob(III) alamin} \rightarrow 2\text{cob(II) alamin}$$

The oxidation of vitamin B$_{12}$ which occurs both *in vivo* and *in vitro* causes the inactivation of methionine synthase. This important cytosol enzyme catalyses the transmethylation reaction in which methionine is synthesized from homocysteine and methyltetrahydrofolate. Vitamin B$_{12}$ is the co-enzyme for methionine synthase and is covalently bound to its apoenzyme. Apparently, it must be in the completely reduced form for the enzyme to function normally. Inactivation of methionine synthase by N_2O is concentration and time dependent. At high concentrations, significant inactivation occurs within minutes in rats (Deacon *et al.*, 1980) and mice (Koblin *et al.*, 1981) but somewhat less rapidly in man (Koblin *et al.*, 1982). Concentrations lower than 1000 p.p.m. do not significantly inactivate methionine synthase, regardless of the time of exposure (Sharer *et al.*, 1983).

Inhibition of methionine synthase results not only in decreased methionine production but also in decreased thymidine and DNA production. Thymidine is a DNA base which is produced from deoxyuridine and 5,10-methylenetetrahydrofolate in a reaction catalysed by the enzyme thymidylate synthase. The substrate 5,10-methylenetetrahydrofolate is itself produced from tetrahydrofolate, an end-product of the transmethylation reaction catalysed by methionine synthase.

Many of the clinical consequences of the effect of N_2O on vitamin B$_{12}$ and hence on methionine and DNA production have been clearly identified. After prolonged exposure to high concentrations of N_2O, a clinical syndrome of vitamin B_{12} deficiency occurs which is akin to that seen in pernicious anaemia. The syndrome includes megaloblastic haemopoiesis together with pancytopenia as reported by Lassen et al. (1956) in six patients with severe tetanus who received 50% N_2O for 5–6 days. These effects are presumably the result of decreased DNA synthesis in rapidly dividing haemopoietic tissue. After even longer exposures, subacute combined degeneration of the spinal cord may occur (Layzer, 1978; Sahenk et al., 1978). The demyelinating neuropathy probably is due to methionine deficiency, since in monkeys it may be almost completely reversed by addition of exogenous methionine (Scott et al., 1981).

One question which remains unanswered is whether N_2O causes adverse reproductive effects in humans. In rodents, N_2O administered for long periods at critical times during gestation is weakly teratogenic (Baden, 1983). No comparable data exist for man. The mechanism for the teratogenic effects of N_2O in rodents is unknown but a reasonable hypothesis is that it is due to decreased DNA synthesis.

Etomidate and adrenal steroidogenesis

The intravenous anaesthetic etomidate recently has been found to inhibit steroid production in the adrenal cortex. Low levels of plasma cortisol were first noticed in patients receiving prolonged sedation with etomidate in an intensive care setting (Finlay and McKee, 1982; Ledingham et al., 1983). More recently, etomidate administered for short periods to surgical patients for induction and maintenance of anaesthesia has been found markedly to decrease plasma levels of cortisol and aldosterone (Fragen et al., 1984; Wagner and White, 1984; Wagner et al., 1984). The mechanism appears to be a concentration-dependent blockade by etomidate of two mitochrondrial enzymes, cholesterol-side-chain cleavage enzyme and 11β-hydroxylase (Wagner et al., 1984). The details of the reactions involved are still being elucidated. At this stage, however, the evidence indicates that the blockade is a direct effect of etomidate and is unrelated to its metabolism.

References

Baden, J.M. (1983) Chronic toxicity of inhalation anaesthetics. In: *Inhalation Anaesthesiology* (Ed. Mazze, R.I.), pp. 441–454. W.B. Saunders: London

Baden, J.M. and Simmon, V.F. (1980) Mutagenic effects of inhalational anaesthetics. *Mutation Research* 75, 196–189

Banks, R.G.S., Henderson, R.J. and Pratt, J.M. (1968) Reaction of gases in solution. III. Some reactions of nitrous oxide with transition-metal complexes. *Journal of the Chemical Society, A* 2886–2889

Blake, D.A., Rozman, R.S., Cascorbi, H.F. and Krantz, J.C. Jr (1967) Anesthesia. LXXIV: Biotransformation of fluroxene. I. Metabolism in mice and dogs *in vivo*. *Biochemical Pharmacology* 16, 1237–1248

Cohen, E.N. (1971) Metabolism of the volatile anesthetics. *Anesthesiology* 35, 193–202

Cohen, E.N., Trudell, J.R., Edmunds, H.N. and Watson, E. (1975) Urinary metabolites of halothane in man. *Anesthesiology* **43**, 392–401

Cousins, M.J., Sharp, H., Gourlay, G.K., Adams, J.F., Haynes, W.D. and Whitehead, R. (1979) Hepatoxicity and halothane metabolism in an animal model with application for human toxicity. *Anaesthesia and Intensive Care* **7**, 9–24

Crandell, W.B., Pappas, S.G. and MacDonald, A. (1966) Nephrotoxicity associated with methoxyflurane anesthesia. *Anesthesiology* **27**, 591–607

Deacon, R., Lumb, M., Perry, J. *et al.* (1980) Inactivation of methionine synthase by nitrous oxide. *European Journal of Biochemistry* **104**, 419–420

Demopoulos, H.B. (1973) Control of free radicals in biological systems. *Federation Proceedings* **32**, 1903–1908

Eger, E.I. II (Ed.) (1985) *Nitrous Oxide.* Elsevier: New York

Evans, J.M. and Keogh, J.A.M. (1977) Adverse reactions to intravenous anaesthetic agents. *British Medical Journal* **2**, 735–736

Finlay, W.E.I. and McKee, J.I. (1982) Serum cortisol levels in adversely stressed patients. *Lancet* **1**, 1414–1415

Fragen, R.J., Shanks, C.A., Molteni, A. and Avram, M.J. (1984) Effects of etomidate on hormonal responses to surgical stress. *Anesthesiology* **61**, 652–656

Fujii, K., Miki, N., Kanashiro, M. *et al.* (1982) A spin trap study on anaerobic dehalogenation of halothane by a reconstituted liver microsomal cytochrome P-450 enzyme system. *Journal of Biochemistry* **91**, 415–418

Kiese, M. (1965) Relationship of drug metabolism to methemoglobin formation. *Annals of the New York Academy of Sciences* **123**, 141–155

Koblin, D.D., Watson, J.E., Deady, J.E., Stokstad, E.L.R. and Eger, E.I. II (1981) Inactivation of methionine synthetase by nitrous oxide in mice. *Anesthesiology* **54**, 318–324

Koblin, D.D., Waskell, L., Watson, J.E., Stokstad, E.L.R. and Eger, E.I. II (1982) Nitrous oxide inactivates methionine synthetase in human livers. *Anesthesia and Analgesia* **61**, 75–78

Lassen, H.C.A., Hendriksen, E., Neukirch, F. and Kristensen, H.S. (1956) Treatment of tetanus: severe bone-marrow depression after prolonged nitrous-oxide anaesthesia. *Lancet* **1**, 527–530

Layzer, R.B. (1978) Myeloneuropathy after prolonged exposure to nitrous oxide. *Lancet* **2**, 1227–1230

Ledingham, I.M., Finlay, W.E.I., Watt, I. and McKee, J.I. (1983) Etomidate and adrenocortical function. *Lancet* **1**, 1434

Lewis, J.H., Zimmerman, H.J., Ishak, K.G. and Mulleck, F.G. (1983) Enflurane hepatotoxicity. A clinicopathologic study of 24 cases. *Annals of Internal Medicine* **98**, 984–992

Luster, M.I., Dean, J.H. and Moore, J.A. (1982) Evaluation of immune functions in toxicology. In: *Principles and Methods of Toxicology* (Ed. Hayes, A.W.), pp. 561–586. Raven Press: New York

Mansuy, D., Nastainczyk, W. and Ullrich, V. (1974) The mechanism of halothane binding to microsomal cytochrome P-450. *Nauyn-Schmiedeberg's Archives of Pharmacology* **285**, 315–324

Mathieu, A. and Kahan, B.D. (1975) *Immunologic Aspects of Anesthetic and Surgical Practice.* Grune & Stratton: New York

Mazze, R.I. (1983) Nephrotoxicity of fluorinated anaesthetic agents. In: *Inhalation Anaesthesiology* (Ed. Mazze, R.I.), pp. 474–475. W.B. Saunders: London

Mazze, R.I., Cousins, M.J. and Kozek, J.C. (1972) Dose-related methoxyflurane nephrotoxicity in rats: a biochemical and pathologic correlation. *Anesthesiology* **36**, 571–587

Mazze, R.I., Shue, G.L. and Jackson, S.H. (1971) Renal dysfunction associated with methoxyflurane anesthesia. A randomized prospective clinical evaluation. *Journal of the American Medical Association* **216**, 278–288

Mukai, S., Morio, M., Fukii, K. and Hanaki, C. (1977) Volatile metabolites of halothane in the rat. *Anesthesiology* **47**, 248–251

Plummer, J.L., Beckwith, A.L.J., Bastin, F.N., Adams, J.F., Cousins, M.J. and Hall, P. (1982) Free radical formation *in vivo* and hepatoxicity due to anesthesia with halothane. *Anesthesiology* **57**, 160–166

Poyer, J., McCay, P., Weddle, C. and Downs, P. (1981) *In vivo* spin-trapping of radicals formed during halothane metabolism. *Biochemical Pharmacology* **30**, 1517–1519

Recknagel, R.O., Glende, E.A. Jr, Waller, R.L. and Lowrey, K. (1982) Lipid peroxidation: biochemistry, measurement, and significance in liver cell injury. In: *Toxicology of the Liver* (Eds. Plaa, G.L. and Hewitt, W.R.), pp. 214–215. Raven Press: New York

Rehder, K., Forbes, J., Alter, J., Hessler, O. and Stier, A. (1967) Halothane biotransformation in man: a quantitative study. *Anesthesiology* **28**, 711–715

Rodriguez, M., Paronetti, F., Schaffner, F. and Popper, H. (1969) Antimitochondrial antibodies in jaundice following drug administration. *Journal of the American Medical Association* **208**, 148–150

Sahenk, Z., Mendell, J.R., Couri, D. and Nachtman, J. (1978) Polyneuropathy from inhalation of N_2O cartridges through a whipped-cream dispenser. *Neurology* **28**, 485–487

Scott, J.M., Dinn, J.J., Wilson, P. and Weir, D.S. (1981) Pathogenesis of subacute combined degeneration: A result of methyl group deficiency. *Lancet* **1**, 334–340

Sharer, N.M., Nunn, J.F., Royston, J.P. and Chanarin, I. (1983) Effects of chronic exposure to nitrous oxide on methionine synthase activity. *British Journal of Anaesthesia* **55**, 693–701

Sharp, J.H., Trudell, J.R. and Cohen, E.N. (1979) Volatile metabolites and decomposition products of halothane in man. *Anesthesiology* **50**, 2–8

Sipes, I.G. and Brown, B.R. Jr (1976) An animal model of hepatotoxicity associated with halothane anesthesia. *Anesthesiology* **45**, 622–628

Sipes, I.G., Gandolfi, A.J. and Brown, B.R. Jr (1981) Halothane-associated hepatitis: evidence for direct toxicity. In: *Drug Reactions and the Liver* (Ed. Davis, M.), pp. 219–231. Pitman Medical: London

Stier, A. (1964) Trifluoroacetic acid as metabolite of halothane. *Biochemical Pharmacology* **13**, 1544

Stier, A., Alter, H., Hessler, O. and Rehder, K. (1964) Urinary excretion of bromide in halothane anesthesia. *Anesthesia and Analgesia* **43**, 723–728

Tappel, A.L. (1973) Lipid peroxidation damage to cell components. *Federation Proceedings* **32**, 1870–1874

Van Dyke, R.A. (1982) Metabolism of anesthetic agents: toxic implications. *Acta Anaesthesiologica Scandinavica* **75**, 7–9

Van Dyke, R.A. and Gandolfi, A.J. (1976) Anaerobic release of fluoride from halothane. Relationship of the binding of halothane metabolites to hepatic cellular constituents. *Drug Metabolism and Disposition* **4**, 40–44

Van Dyke, R.A., Chenoweth, M.B. and Van Poznak, A. (1964) Metabolism of volatile anesthetics. I. Conversion *in vivo* of several anesthetics to $^{14}CO_2$ and chloride. *Biochemical Pharmacology* **13**, 1239–1247

Wagner, R.L. and White, P.F. (1984) Etomidate inhibits adrenocortical function in surgical patients. *Anesthesiology* **61**, 647–651

Wagner, R.L., White, P.F., Dan, P.B., Rosenthal, M.H. and Feldman, D. (1984) Inhibition of adrenal steroidogenesis by the anesthetic etomidate. *New England Journal of Medicine* **310**, 1415–1421

Walton, B. (1982) Immunological aspects of anaesthetic practice. In: *Scientific Foundations of Anaesthesia* (Ed. Scurr, C. and Feldman, S.A.), pp. 363–373.

Heinemann Medical: London

Walton, B., Simpson, B.R., Strunin, L., Doniach, D., Perrin, J. and Appleyard, A.J. (1976) Unexplained hepatitis following halothane. *British Medical Journal* **1**, 1171–1176

Weinstein, I.B., Yamaguchi, R. and Gebert, R. (1975) Use of epithelial cell cultures for studies on the mechanism of transformation by chemical carcinogens. *In Vitro* **11**, 130–135

Widger, L.A., Gandolfi, A.J. and Van Dyke, R.A. (1976) Hypoxia and halothane metabolism *in vivo*: release of inorganic fluoride and halothane metabolite binding to cellular constituents. *Anesthesiology* **44**, 197–201

Wiseman, A. (1970) Effect of inorganic fluoride in enzymes. In: *Handbook of Experimental Pharmacology: Pharmacology of Fluorides* (Ed. Smith, F.A.), pp. 48–93. Springer Verlag: New York

Appendix 2

The measurement of drugs in blood

Vincent Marks

Twenty years or so ago the measurement of drugs in blood and other biological fluids was confined almost exclusively to their use in research laboratories and, to a lesser extent, in forensic science laboratories. Nowadays, due to a growing appreciation of the clinical value of the information so obtained, it is commonplace. This has become possible largely due to developments in the technology of measurement, mostly in the fields of chromatography and immunoassay. Currently most assays are performed on serum or plasma or – where partitioning is predictable – on saliva, although in the case of volatile agents such as alcohol, halothane, etc. respiratory gases can be used to advantage. The last-named type of methodology will be dealt with separately at the end of this Appendix. Here it will be possible to do no more than mention briefly some of the more widely used methods for making drug measurements on body fluids, with references, where appropriate, to sources of more detailed information.

General

The choice of analytical procedure for a given drug will depend upon a number of its characteristics, both chemical and physical, as well as upon its concentration in solution and the presence of potentially interfering substances in the matrix.

Most methods for measuring plasma drug levels (apart from those utilizing bio- or immunoassay procedures – and even here occasionally) depend upon an initial extraction procedure wherein the drug to be measured is separated from proteins and other substances likely to interfere in the assay. The tenacity with which many drugs bind to proteins and its variability at different drug concentrations may cause less than complete recovery, the extent of which may vary from one sample to another. For this reason it is considered important in most analytical work, where at all possible, to include an internal standard, with physicochemical properties closely similar to the drug to be measured, which is added in known amounts to the sample to be measured.

Thorough denaturation of the plasma proteins together with efficient extraction by use of the most appropriate solvents can overcome problems of incomplete recovery in many cases, but even established and well-tried procedures have sometimes been shown to yield valid information only over a limited concentration range.

Of primary importance is the end-point signal which will be measured, since all other stages of the analytical procedures are subordinate to it. Most drugs are not usually present in sufficiently high concentration or do not give a sufficiently strong physicochemical signal to enable them to be measured without undergoing some degree of processing, the exact nature of which depends both upon the individual drug and the end-point signal adopted.

Colorimetry

Apart from aspirin and paracetamol, there are few drugs of clinical importance for which colorimetry now provides an effective method of measurement, and even paracetamol is now measured more easily and precisely by a specific enzymatic procedure commercially available as a kit. This kit requires only a minimum of technical expertise and depends upon the use of a specific enzyme (a microbial aryl acylamidase) to transform paracetamol into a hydrolysis product (p-aminophenol) which reacts with o-cresol to produce a coloured compound (Brown et al., 1983). The colour so produced can be measured in a comparatively simple and cheap colorimeter to provide an accurate and clinically useful analytical result within 10 minutes of sample collection, should it be necessary, enabling treatment for overdosage to be instituted immediately, when it is most likely to be effective. Aspirin can be measured at the same time, using stable colorimetric reagents available in most laboratories and the same basic apparatus.

Spectrophotometry and fluorimetry

Although widely used in the past (Gifford, 1981), especially for the measurement of barbiturates in blood, spectrophotometry is too insensitive, non-specific and labour intensive to find any place today in the measurement of drugs in blood except when used as an elegant detection and quantification system in conjunction with high performance liquid chromatography (HPLC). This applies also to spectrofluorimetry which, although far more sensitive than spectrophotometry (Bridges, 1978), is relevant to a smaller range of compounds and is even more susceptible to interference from extraneous compounds unless these have been removed by prior extraction and separation by chromatography.

Bioassay

Bioassays of one sort or another were the principal methods for measuring antibiotics and antitumour agents in biological fluids until the advent of immunoassay techniques by which they have been largely (but not entirely) surplanted for clinical, though not necessarily for research, purposes (White and Reeves, 1981). Although sensitive and reliable when only one drug is present, bioassays are generally too labour intensive, time consuming and slow to yield clinically useful information. Their application is affected by the presence, in the sample, of substances (including other antibiotics) which possess similar biological (i.e. antibacterial) properties to the drug under investigation. This can be advantageous when, for example, the drug itself is a mixture of substances rather than a pure compound (e.g. bleomycin) or disadvantageous when, for example, only one of a couple of antibiotics is nephro- or ototoxic but both are antimicrobial in the assay system. Radioreceptor assays are a special kind of 'bioassay' which employ most of the tools and expertise of radioimmunoassay and will be considered separately later.

Flame photometry and atomic absorption

These methods are employed exclusively for the measurement of lithium (used for the treatment and prevention of psychoaffective disorders) and organometallic compounds, such as those containing gold and platinum used for the treatment of chronic inflammatory and neoplastic diseases. It is likely, however, that in the case of organometallic drugs it is the complex, as a whole rather than the metal itself, which is therapeutically relevant. Consequently, measurements made by atomic absorption which measure only the metallic moiety, in whatever form it is present, may be inconsequential – not to say misleading. They should, therefore, not be made unless this fact is taken into consideration.

Chromatography

Gas–liquid chromatography (GLC), high performance thin layer chromatography (HPTLC) and, above all, high performance liquid chromatography (HPLC) are used extensively for the measurement of drugs in biological fluids in clinical work as well as in research, where HPLC is especially valuable.

Gas–liquid chromatography (GLC)

Gas–liquid chromatography was the first of the three techniques to be widely applied to the problem of detecting and quantifying drugs in plasma and other body fluids (Chakraborty and Lynaugh, 1978; Agurell and Lindgren, 1981). It has the sensitivity necessary to make it suitable for use for measuring all but the most potent drugs provided they are volatile and stable at temperatures up to about 200°C or can be rendered so by simple pre-column or on-column derivatization. Many of the problems encountered in the early days of GLC have been surmounted by improvements in the equipment, the nature and reliability of the chromatographic columns, the detectors and the extraction procedures. The introduction of automatic sampling, temperature programming and microprocessor-controlled data handling has gone a long way towards removing the tedium formerly associated with this technique –

which is, however, still relatively capital and labour intensive. It is also relatively slow, time consuming and more suitable for batch than single sample analysis. Thus, like HPLC and HPTLC (which is still in its infancy for this application), GLC is more suited to investigative or research work involving the detection, identification and/or measurement of drugs in biological fluids in, for example toxicological screening (Jarvie and Simpson, 1984; Deutsch ad Bergert, 1985) than to therapeutic drug monitoring when simplicity, availability and speed are at a premium (Marks, 1985).

No useful purpose would be served, at this juncture, by detailing the principles of GLC which have been amply described elsewhere (Chakroborty and Lynaugh, 1978), save to emphasize that it provides an excellent tool for investigating not only the presence and concentration of native drug in a sample but also, under most circumstances, those of its major metabolites. Capillary columns which permit almost unlimited separation of individual constituents of complex mixtures of compounds are now available for use with most conventional GLC instruments; by appropriate choice of detector – for example, flame ionization (general purpose), nitrogen amplified flame ionization, electron capture and even mass spectrometry (GC-MS) – the sensitivity of GLC can be arranged so that it is capable of measuring specific compounds in solution, provided they have the correct physicochemical properties, at concentrations down to 1 nmol/l or less. Peptide and proteinacious drugs and many antibiotics which are heat labile are refractory to measurement by GLC but are amenable to measurement by HPLC.

High performance liquid chromatography (HPLC)

Originally referred to as high *pressure* liquid chromatography, indicating its unique dependence upon the application of high pressure to the solvent used to elute the compounds of interest from the chromatographic column, HPLC is nowadays a compromise between the conflicting requirements for resolution, speed, sensitivity, ease of operation, reliability and cost of equipment necessary to achieve optimum performance; in this process, pressure is only one of the many variables which need to be considered.

The theory (Koeningsberger, 1978; Drayer, 1984) underlying the principles of HPLC, like that of GLC, is complex and its exposition would be out of place in a volume devoted to its use rather than its design. In general, HPLC provides an opportunity of separating into its constituents a complex mixture of compounds on the basis of their individual physicochemical properties and measuring each one of them as they emerge from the column by one of the many techniques available. The most commonly employed detection and quantification systems at the present time include visible, ultraviolet and infrared absorptiometry, and fluorescence and electrochemical detection.

Collection of the individual fractions as they emerge from the column for subsequent analysis by immunoassay or mass spectrometry provides an opportunity for even greater specificity and sensitivity than can be achieved by virtually any other analytical technique.

In gas chromatography the mobile phase does not play an important part in effecting separation – but in HPLC it does. So-called 'normal phase' HPLC columns employing silica gel as support medium, for example, allow for early elution of the non-polar (i.e. lipid-soluble) native drug in a rapidly moving non-polar solvent system; the generally less polar metabolites elute somewhat later. By changing the nature of the support medium and/or solvent pH, temperature, etc., different patterns can be obtained and the most useful chosen for regular use depending upon the purpose for which the chromatography is being performed.

What is generally referred to as reverse phase HPLC is much more commonly used for making drug measurements than is 'normal phase' chromatography. Reverse phase HPLC depends upon the use of non-polar support columns and polar solvents (of which those containing methanol or acetonitrile are the most common) to effect elution. These columns have a high resolving power, and the weak surface energies of the non-polar support medium plus the polar nature of the mobile phase permits rapid analysis of underivatized drugs (and their metabolites).

For straightforward therapeutic drug monitoring, where interest centres entirely upon one substance, conditions which permit rapid through-put without sacrifice of sensitivity or specificity will generally be selected; if the purpose is, however, to study not only the native compound but also its metabolites and/or the presence or other compounds of interest, operating conditions will be adjusted accordingly.

The perceived advantages of HPLC over GLC are: its wider applicability to analysis whereby it can be used for compounds of almost every kind; a reduced need for prepurification and derivatization (although advantage can, where necessary or desirable, be taken of both); greater amenability to automation; and, finally, the preservation (rather than the destruction) of the specimen, permitting further identification to be carried out upon it if necessary.

The sensitivity of HPLC ultimately depends upon the quality of apparatus used – especially the pumps. The general proposition that the better the equipment the more it costs is as true of HPLC as with any other technology. Probably the most important single factor is the nature and reliability of the detector and its suitability for the drug in question. The most commonly used detectors employ visible or ultraviolet light absorption (UV detection) but greater sensitivity can often be obtained by using fluorimetric or electrochemical detection when the substances being measured have the appropriate physicochemical attributes (Moore *et al.*, 1984). By means of such instrumentation sensitivity equal to, or surpassing, that of GLC can often be obtained.

HPLC is still technically demanding, although much less so than formerly. It is comparatively robust, and new methods are generally easier to develop than with GLC or immunoassay, making it an excellent research tool for anyone wishing to study drug disposition within the body. The apparatus is necessarily large and neither it nor the methodology is well suited to decentralized clinical usage, for which immunoassay in one form or another is the method of choice.

High performance thin layer chromatography (HPTLC)

It is still too early to say what place, if any, HPTLC will play in the quantification of drugs of clinical interest now that sensitive and robust reflectance absorptiometers are available for use in conjunction with exquisitively fine, thin layer, chromatographic plates. It is unlikely, however, that HPTLC will ever become a serious rival to immunoassay or HPLC for clinical therapeutic drug monitoring although it may find a role in the detection and/or quantification of drug abuse and in polypharmacy.

Immunoassay

The introduction of immunoassay for the measurement of drugs in blood, more than anything else, made the concept of therapeutic drug monitoring a practical rather than theoretical proposition (Marks et al., 1980; Marks, 1981; Widdop, 1985). Although the original radioimmunoassay techniques have now largely given way, for clinical use, to procedures which are easier to perform but conceptually more complex (Collins, 1985), they remain the method of choice during the developmental phase of a drug assay or when very low concentrations (i.e. below 1 nmol/l) are expected to be encountered.

Few drugs are naturally immunogenic but most can be rendered so by conjugating them to proteins by any one of many different procedures, each of which has its own advantages and disadvantages (Marks, Morris and Teale, 1974). Conjugation makes it possible to produce specific drug-binding antibodies which are the most important of the three key reagents required for any immunoassay, the other two being appropriate standards and a label. The label must be capable of being measured by a physicochemical technique.

The principles of immunoassay in general, and of those used for the measurement of drugs in biological fluids in particular, have been extensively reviewed (Marks, Morris and Teale, 1974; Teale, 1978; Marks et al., 1980; Collins, 1985). Many of the newest techniques are covered by patents and are available only as kits from their manufacturers.

Of the three key reagents common to all immunoassay methods, it is the antibody that confers sensitivity and specificity; the label – which can be a radioactive isotope, an enzyme, a fluorophore, a chemi- or bioluminescent label or a drug-protein, drug-gold-sol or drug-latex particle conjugate, amongst others (Marks et al., 1980; Collins, 1985; Hemmila, 1985) – is one of the main determinants of its simplicity and type of apparatus required. Most of the drug immunoassays available commercially and many of those developed by researchers themselves (Marks et al., 1980) can be performed without pretreatment of the specimen (i.e. on unextracted samples) and are both rapid and simple to perform provided the manufacturer's instructions are followed.

Although an immunoassay can be developed from scratch for virtually any drug, this requires both knowledge and expertise as well as at least 12 months to produce a usable antibody and incorporate it into a reliable, precise and accurate method. Most clinicians and researchers are well advised to use one or other of the commercially available kits which are available for most of the commonly measured drugs, especially if their intention is to perform therapeutic drug monitoring, and when no suitable kit exists and immunoassay rather than HPLC has been decided upon, to seek advice and help from an expert immunoassayist.

Radioimmunoassay

In radioimmunoassay – the prototype from which all other types of immunoassay were developed – the drug (analyte) present in a sample at unknown concentration is allowed to compete with a known, constant amount of radiolabelled analyte for a limited number of antibody-binding sites. At equilibrium both the labelled and the unlabelled drug exist either bound to antibody or unbound (i.e. 'free'). Since binding is competitive, the amount of labelled drug bound to the antibody is inversely proportional to the amount of native (unknown) drug present. The 'bound' and 'free' labels are separated by any of a number of different techniques. The amount of drug present in the original sample can then be computed from a standard curve prepared by treating known standards in exactly the same way as the samples, using either the 'free' or the 'bound' counts – whichever is the more convenient or appropriate (Teale, 1978).

Because radioimmunoassay requires separation of the bound from the free fractions, they are often referred to as heterogeneous assays and demand considerably more expertise for their performance than so-called homogeneous assays. In these the nature of the signal emitted by the antibody-bound label is different (and can, therefore, be distinguished) from that emitted by the free label. Consequently, physical separation of the two components is not necessary and the whole reaction, from the addition of sample to the reagents to making the final physicochemical measurement, can be carried out in a single tube. In some of the latest techniques the whole reaction is carried out on a reagent-impregnated strip not very dissimilar in appearance from those used for semiquantiative urine analysis (Busch and Virgi, 1985; Rupchock *et al.*, 1985).

Homogeneous assays

The first homogeneous immunoassays to be made available commercially employed a free radical label and measurements were made by observing alterations in its electron spin resonance characteristics. This type of assay suffered from several disadvantages, chief amongst them being its relative insensitivity, non-amenability to anything more than semiquantitative measurement, and the need for sophisticated, expensive and dedicated instrumentation.

It was soon superseded by an enzyme-based homogeneous assay system developed and marketed by the SYVA company under the trade mark EMIT. This assay system, because of its simplicity, specificity and accuracy, produced a revolutionary attitude towards therapeutic drug monitoring practice which, though only recently introduced in concept, had begun to flounder for lack of suitable and practicable technology. The past five years have seen the introduction of several more homogeneous immunoassay systems suitable for the rapid, precise and accurate measurement of drugs in biological fluids under clinical conditions. These systems include the reagents necessary to perform the assay as well as the microprocessor-controlled equipment, specifically designed to work with them, which not only carries out the physicochemical measurement at completion of the reaction but also turns it into a clinically useful piece of information.

Assays can usually be performed on microsamples (100 μl or less) of unextracted plasma (or serum) and are capable of producing results within 10 minutes or less of commencing the assay. Coefficients of variation are generally within the range of 3–5 per cent and – except in very rare cases of interference from other drugs or abnormalities in the plasma matrix – the results are accurate provided the manufacturers instructions are followed faithfully.

The new analytical systems are, however, available for only the comparatively small range of drugs whose measurements are considered more or less routine. Moreover, unless an extraction and/or concentration step is first introduced, they are generally incapable of measuring drugs present in solution at concentrations below 5 nmol/l. Nevertheless, their simplicity, speed, reliability and, above all, suitability for making blood drug measurements nearer the patient, in the clinic or ward side-room, make homogeneous immunoassay procedures deservedly extremely popular for therapeutic drug monitoring. Each system has its advantages and disadvantages which are based not so much upon technical as upon financial and other considerations, including convenience, size of workload and availability of servicing support. Some of the assay systems available lend themselves to automation but, in the context of clinical use, this is a less obvious advantage than the immediate availability of results achievable by making measurements where and when available (Marks, 1985).

Plasma free drug concentrations

Many drugs are more or less tightly bound to plasma proteins *in vivo* and, according to modern theory, thereby are rendered unavailable to receptors on effector organs (Reidenberg, 1981). Some eminent investigators (though not all) believe, therefore, that measurement of the 'free' – i.e. non-protein bound, dialysable or diffusible – fraction of a drug provides a more meaningful result than a total blood drug measurement. Methods designed to measure the 'free' drug concentration in plasma have in the past relied exclusively upon use of ultrafiltration or dialysis to separate 'protein-bound' from 'free' fractions, with measurement of the latter by GLC, HPLC or immunoassay. Whilst providing invaluable information in the research context, the cumbersomeness of these techniques has prevented their widespread adoption in clinical practice. Measurements made on saliva are a poor substitute for actual plasma free drug measurements but can give useful information provided partitioning of the drug between blood and saliva can be shown not to be influenced by variables such as salivary pH, flow rate and site of collection (Scott, Chakraborty and Marks, 1984).

An alternative, but still theoretical, approach to the measurement of plasma free drug levels is by means of the analogue tracer technique. At present this patented method is available commercially for only the measurement of 'free plasma thyroxine' but could, if clinical demands dictated, be adapted for use with drugs of all descriptions.

Radioreceptor assays

If the antibody used in a competitive radioimmunoassay is replaced by drug receptors prepared from sonicated cells by centrifugation a so-called radioreceptor assay (RRA) can be developed with different specificities but similar sensitivities to those of a radioimmunoassay developed against the same drug (Tune, 1984). Radioreceptor assays utilize a radioactive – usually tritiated – preparation of the drug as tracer which competes not only with the native drug but also with its active (and possibly inactive blocking) metabolites for the limited number of binding sites provided by the receptors available. Because of the uncertainty attending the exact nature of the compounds capable of binding to drug receptors, results obtained with radioreceptor assays must be interpreted with caution. Indeed, results obtained by these methods and those using more conventional methods (e.g. GLC, HPLC and immunoassay) do not always correlate very closely. Nevertheless, used prudently, RRA is a valuable addition to the research analyst's armamentarium.

Analyses in respiratory gases

Measurement of drug concentration in the breath can be used to give a close approximation to the concentration of numerous volatile and gaseous drugs (e.g. alcohol and many anaesthetics) in blood, provided appropriate samples are analysed (Pfaffli, Nikki and Ablain, 1974; Manolis, 1983). These must be either deep alveolar or, preferably, rebreathed air which has become completely equilibrated with blood in the alveolar capillaries of the lungs (Jones, 1983). The concentration of the vapour or gas itself can be measured by a number of different techniques (Hill, 1982), of which infrared absorptiometry and GLC are the two most popular. With modern microprocessor-controlled instrumentation, operation of breath analysers can be so simplified as to be within the capability of relatively unskilled personnel given only a modicum of training.

The many factors which can influence interpretation of the results have been examined in great detail in relation to alcohol, mainly because of its medicolegal implications, but apply equally to other volatile and gaseous drugs.

Choice of methods

Which of the many methods for measuring the concentration of any particular drug in blood will be used depends upon a number of factors. For the most commonly monitored drugs – i.e. those for which an optimum therapeutic range has been established (Table A2.1) operator-friendly immunoassay systems or kits are available. These are generally capable, provided the necessary apparatus is ready to hand, of permitting measurements to be made on microsamples of blood plasma (i.e. 100–200 μl) within 10–20 minutes of sample collection. They are therefore the preferred methods for clinical use.

Table A2.1 Drugs whose measurement in blood is of proven value in monitoring treatment

Drug	Recommended assay methods	Optimum therapeutic concentration plasma	
		Mass units	SI units†
Anticonvulsants			
Carbamazepine	(1) Immunoassay (2) HPLC	Steady state 4–12 mg/l	15–46 μmol/l
Ethosuximide	(1) Immunoassay (2) HPLC	Steady state 40–100 mg/l	280–700 μmol/l
Phenytoin	(1) Immunoassay (2) HPLC	Steady state 10–20 mg/l	40–80 μmol/l
Antidepressants			
Imipramine	(1) HPLC (2) GLC	Steady state > 100 μg/l	>350 nmol/l
Lithium	Flame photometry	—	0.5–1.2 mmol/l 12 h after last dose
Nortriptyline	(1) HPLC (2) GLC	Steady state 50–150 μg/l	190–570 nmol/l
Antibiotics			
Amikacin	(1) Immunoassay (2) HPLC	Peak 15–25 mg/l; trough <4–6 mg/l	
Gentamicin	(1) Immunoassay (2) HPLC	Peak 4–12 mg/l; trough <2 mg/l	
Kanamycin	(1) Immunoassay (2) HPLC	Peak 20–25 mg/l; trough <4–6 mg/l	
Tobramycin	(1) Immunoassay (2) HPLC	Peak 4–10 mg/l; trough <2 mg/l	
Antitumour			
Methotrexate	(1) Immunoassay (2) HPLC	<4.5 mg/l 24 h after i.v. dosing	<10 μmol/l
Cardioactive			
Digitoxin	Immunoassay	Steady state 10–30 μg/l	13–40 nmol/l
Digoxin	Immunoassay	Steady state 1–2 μg/l	1.3–2.6 nmol/l
Lignocaine	(1) Immunoassay (2) HPLC	Steady state 2–5 mg/l	8–20 μmol/l
Procainamide	(1) Immunoassay (2) HPLC	Steady state 4–10 mg/l	16–40 μmol/l
Miscellaneous			
Theophylline	(1) Immunoassay (2) HPLC	Steady state 10–15 mg/l	55–84 μmol/l

* For most of the drugs for which therapeutic monitoring has been established as useful, simple-to-use homogeneous immunoassay kits are available commercially.

† The Association of Clinical Biochemists has recommended (Ratcliffe and Worth, 1986) that the SI system should, where possible, be used for reporting drug concentration in biological fluids.

For drugs for which suitable kits are not yet available, either because of their non-commercial viability or because of the novelty of the drug, it is necessary to resort to the use of HPLC or 'home-brew' immunoassays using appropriate antisera and labelled tracers produced 'in-house' or by specialist immunoreagent suppliers.

Immunoassays can generally be made more sensitive than HPLC techniques, being capable of detecting and measuring drugs in nanogram to microgram (picomolar to nanomolar) amounts per litre, whereas HPLC can seldom achieve sensitivities better than microgram (micromolar) amounts per litre which, whilst adequate for most drugs, is insufficiently sensitive for particularly potent compounds such as digoxin and some of the newer benzodiazepines. GC is the method of choice for measuring volatile drugs in biological fluids and has a sensitivity comparable with, or better than, that of HPLC but is even more technically demanding. Where interference with the results of analysis by metabolites or other substances is a problem and absolute identification as well as quantification is paramount – as in forensic cases – it may be necessary to resort to the use of a combination of techniques such as HPLC with immunoassay or GC with mass spectrometry. These 'state of the art' techniques are complex, technically demanding and expensive.

References

Agurell, S. and Lindgren, J.E. (1981) Gas chromatography – mass spectrometry in drug level analysis. In: *Therapeutic Drug Monitoring* (Eds. Richens, A. and Marks, V.), pp. 110–130. Churchill Livingstone: Edinburgh, New York

Bridges, J.W. (1978) Fluorescence and phosphorescence. In: *Scientific Foundations of Clinical Biochemistry*, vol. 1 (Eds. Williams, D.L., Nunn, R.F. and Marks, V.), pp. 72–94. Heinemann Medical: London

Brown, S.S., Campbell, R.S., Price, C.P. *et al.* (1983) Collaborative trial of an enzyme-based assay for the determination of paracetamol in plasma. *Annals of Clinical Biochemistry* **20**, 353–359

Busch, R.P. and Virgi, M.A. (1985) Serum theophylline assay by Ames Seralyzer compared with Abbott TDX in pediatric care. *Clinical Chemistry* **31**, 1247–1248

Chakraborty, J. and Lynaugh, N. (1978) Gas-liquid chromatography – mass spectrometry. In: *Scientific Foundations of Clinical Biochemistry* , vol. 1 (Eds. Williams, D.L., Nunn, R.F. and Marks, V.), pp. 144–165. Heinemann Medical: London

Collins, W.P. (1985) *Alternative Immunoassays*. John Wiley: Chichester, New York

Deutsch, D.G. and Bergert, R.J. (1985) Evaluation of a bench-top capillary gas chromatograph–mass spectrometer for clinical toxicology. *Clinical Chemistry* **31**, 741–746

Drayer, D.E. (1984) Reversed phase length performance liquid chromatography: optimizing peak resolution. In: *Proceedings of the Second World Conference on Clinical Pharmacology and Therapeutics* (Eds. Lemberger, L. and Reidenberg, M.), pp. 809–819. American Society of Pharmacology and Experimental Therapeutics: Washington DC

Gifford, L. (1981) Spectrophotometry and fluorimetry. In: *Therapeutic Drug Monitoring* (Eds. Richens, A. and Marks, V), pp. 61–84. Churchill Livingstone: Edinburgh, New York

Hemmila, I. (1985) Fluoroimmunoassays and immunofluorometric assays. *Clinical Chemistry* **31**, 359–370

Hill, D.W. (1982) Methods of analysis in the gaseous and vapour phase. In: *Scientific Foundations of Anaesthesia*, 3rd edn. (Eds. Scurr, C. and Feldman, S.A.), pp. 80–96. Heinemann Medical: London

Jarvie, D.R. and Simpson, D. (1984) Gas chromatographic screening for drugs and metabolites in plasma and urine. *Annals of Clinical Biochemistry* 21, 92–101

Jones, A.E. (1983) Role of rebreathing in determination of the blood–breath ratio of expired ethanol. *Journal of Applied Physiology (Respiratory Environmental and Exercise Physiology)* 55, 1237–1241

Koeningsberger, R. (1978) High performance chromatography. In: *Scientific Foundations of Clinical Biochemstry*, vol. 1 (Eds. Williams, D.L., Nunn, R.F. and Marks, V.), pp. 165–185. Heinemann Medical: London

Manolis, A. (1983) The diagnostic potential of breath analysis. *Clinical Chemistry* 29, 5–15

Marks, V. (1981) Immunoassay of drugs. In: *Therapeutic Drug Monitoring* (Eds. Richens, A. and Marks, V.), pp. 154–182. Churchill Livingstone: Edinburgh, New York

Marks, V. (1985) Therapeutic drug monitoring. In: *Clinical Chemistry Nearer the Patient* (Eds. Marks, V. and Alberti, K.G.M.M.), pp. 190–194. Churchill Livingstone: Edinburgh, New York

Marks, V., Morris, B.A. and Teale, J.D. (1974) Pharmacology. *British Medical Bulletin* 30, 80–85

Marks, V., Mould, G.P., O'Sullivan, M.J.O. and Teale, J.D. (1980) Monitoring of drug disposition by immunoassay. In: *Progress in Drug Metabolism*, vol. 5 (Eds. Bridges, J.W. and Chasseaud, L.F.), pp. 255–310. John Wiley: Chichester, New York

Moore, R.A., Baldwin, D., McQuay, H.J. and Bullingha, R.E.S. (1984) HPLC of morphine with electrochemical detection: analysis in human plasma. *Annals of Clinical Biochemistry* 21, 125–130

Pfaffli, P., Nikki, P. and Ablain, K. (1974) Halothane and nitrous oxide in end-tidal air and venous blood of surgical personnel. *Annals of Clinical Research* 4, 273–277

Ratcliffe, J.G. and Worth, H.G.H. (1986) Recommended units for reporting drug concentrations in biological fluids. Lancet 1, 202–203

Reidenberg, M. (1981) Is protein binding important? In: *Therapeutic Drug Monitoring* (Eds. Richens, A. and Marks, V.), pp. 23–30. Churchill Livingstone: Edinburgh, New York

Rupchock, P., Sommer, R., Greenquist, A., Tyhack, R., Walter, B. and Zipp, A. (1985) Dry reagent strips used for determination of theophylline in serum. *Clinical Chemistry* 31, 737–748

Scott, N.R., Chakraborty, J. and Marks, V. (1984) Determination of caffeine, theophylline and theobromine in saliva using high performance liquid chromatography. *Annals of Clinical Biochemistry* 21, 120–124

Teale, J.D. (1978) Radioimmunoassay. In: *Scientific Foundations of Clinical Biochemistry*, vol.1 (Eds. Williams, D.L., Nunn, R.F. and Marks, V.), pp. 299–322. Heinemann Medical: London

Tune, L. (1984) Radioreceptor assays in clinical medicine: focus on serum anticholinergic drug concentration measurements. In: *Proceedings of the Second World Conference on Clinical Pharmacology and Therapeutics* (Eds. Lemberger, L. and Reidenberg, M.), pp. 836–850. American Society of Pharmacology and Experimental Therapeutics: Washington DC

White, L.O. and Reeves, D.S. (1981) Antibiotics: analytical techniques. In: *Therapeutic Drug Monitoring* (Eds. Richens, A. and Marks, V.), pp. 457–470. Churchill Livingstone: Edinburgh, New York

Widdop, B. (1985) *Therapeutic Drug Monitoring*. Churchill Livingstone: Edinburgh, New York

Appendix 3

Mechanisms of drug interactions

Neil Soni

The first anaesthetic agents, ether and nitrous oxide, were used originally as sole agents. Since then, as the armamentarium of drugs in anaesthesia has grown, so has the tendency to use multiple agents to produce a desired effect. Furthermore, in many instances the patients anaesthetized are already receiving quite a significant number of drugs. Consequently, not only are interactions anticipated, but also in the anaesthetic world a large number of the techniques employed are dependent on drug interactions to achieve the desired effect. In this Appendix the mechanism of drug interaction will be discussed with occasional reference to examples. A comprehensive review of all anaesthetic interactions is clearly impossible; it is the anaesthetist understanding the principal mechanisms which is important and which should enable interactions to be predicted and, if necessary, avoided.

To consider the actual size of the interaction problem in general medicine is itself a difficult undertaking. In some studies it has been suggested that hospital patients may receive more than eight prescribed drugs on average, and that will then be added to by further drugs for anaesthesia (Miller, 1973; May, Stewart and Cliff, 1974). In a trial assessment of pharmacies in the USA, 17 per cent of all prescriptions had potential for interactions to occur and one-third of these were judged highly significant. If these figures are extrapolated for the whole of the USA, it has been suggested that up to 80 million significant interactions would occur in one year just from general prescriptions (Medicom Database, 1983). Of course, in anaesthesia there are inevitably a lot of significant interactions, many of which are planned or anticipated. Indeed, the anaesthetic techniques may well depend on these interactions, not only for efficacy but also for safety. It is the unexpected or unpredicted interaction which poses the major threat.

It is important to determine what is meant by 'an interaction'. Essentially it is when the spheres of activity of two drugs overlap, so that the action of one drug will modify or affect the behaviour of another. This may occur in a variety of ways, and for the purpose of this chapter these interactions will be described as three groups – pharmaceutical occurring *in vitro*, pharmacokinetic and pharmacodynamic. The pharmacokinetic interaction refers generally to the way that the body deals with the drug and how this may be modified by other agents given concurrently, pharmacodynamic referring to the way the drug affects the body and again modification of this by interaction.

Pharmaceutical interactions

These may be divided into two groups: chemical and physical (Table A3.1).

Chemical

These are generally the reactions occurring before the drug is given to the patient. Almost every anaesthetist will have experienced the phenomenon of injecting a second drug into a giving set and seeing a precipitate form instantaneously. In situations such as that with thiopentone and vecuronium this precipitate will actually block the entire giving set, producing a potentially embarrassing moment. Obviously a drug interaction has occurred and this may well alter the efficacy of the agent being injected as well as the ability to inject any drug at all. However, there may well be an interaction taking place in other situations without a visible change in the tubing at all, and it is necessary for the anaesthetist to be aware of the variety of interactions which may occur not only in the operating theatre but also in the intensive care environment while drugs are being administered. Anaesthetic agents inevitably have to be stored prior to use and may in many instances, undergo deterioration whilst in storage. Frequently they are stored in a powder or a solid form, as in this state decomposition tends to occur more slowly. Exposure to light, changes in temperature, the addition of water or a mixing agent, may all tend to increase the rate of deterioration of the drug. The concentration of the solution formed may also be important, and as a general rule the rate of decomposition tends to increase with the concentration (Trissel, 1983).

The *acid–base* status and the pK_a of the drug often affect the solubility of the agent, and in most situations it is the ionized form of weak acids or bases which is more soluble. Consequently, changes in pH on mixing with other solutions may alter the overall pH and change the degree of ionization of the drug, and this may result in precipitation (Eggert, *et al.*, 1982). With regard to changes in pH, the degree of buffering which occurs is important. The solution with the greater buffering capability will tend to determine the final pH; consequently it is the less buffered drug which tends to precipitate out. Obviously the relative concentrations and volumes of each agent are important determinants of the degree of buffering available. An example of this is the administration of thiopentone in Hartmann's solution. If the thiopentone is mixed into a large volume of Hartmann's solution, there will be a significant change in pH as regards the thiopentone and precipitation may result. If, however, the thiopentone is given into an administration line in a bolus form the relative change in pH will be less as the concentration of thiopentone will be high relative to that of Hartmann's and precipitation is less likely to occur. If atracurium is administered into tubing containing thiopentone, its activity will be reduced by alkaline degeneration (Table A3.2).

A further phenomenon occurring in the mixture of drugs is the formation of *insoluble salts*, which may occur when drugs which interact are inadvertently mixed. In the cardiac arrest situation the addition of soluble calcium salts to infusion lines containing bicarbonate solution may well result in the formation of calcium carbonate, an insoluble salt, and this will of course result in fairly significant precipitation. This interaction is applicable in a wide variety of

Table A3.1 Pharmaceutical mechanisms

	Mechanism	Result
Chemical		
Acid–base	Alters pH + changes solubility	Precipitation occurs
Salt formation	Reaction may form insoluble salt	Precipitation occurs
Oxidation/reduction	—	Alters pharmacology
Hydrolysis	Addition of water + pH change	Alters pharmacology
Epimerization/racemization	Steric alteration of molecule	Alters pharmacology
Physical		
Osmolality	Damage to blood; solution supersaturation	Altered red blood cells; precipitate
Solvent system polarity	Solvent + aqueous changes Solubility	Precipitate
Sorption	Drug lipophilicity	Alters concentration of administered drug
Adsorption	Drug adherence	
Emulsion cracking	Cations; pH may alter globule size	Forms large globules; phase separation

circumstances, but is of particular relevance to parenteral nutrition; one must always be aware of the nature of anything to be added to parenteral nutrition solutions, to minimize the formation of insoluble salts.

Oxidation reactions are relatively common, reduction reactions less so. These may be spontaneous or catalysed by a variety of agents, including several heavy metals. Auto-oxidation of catecholamines occurs with light as well as with heavy metals (Newton, Fung and Williams, 1981). The products of oxidation reactions may be active or inactive, and in some instances may be toxic. Furthermore, although there may be visual changes in the solution, this may not occur until almost all the drug involved has been oxidized. This may significantly alter the action of the drug being administered. A variety of protective devices may be employed to prevent this form of reaction; for example, dark glass to protect the drug from light, the addition of antioxidants such as metabisulphite, or cation sequestering agents such as citrate.

Hydrolysis is a further form of chemical reaction which may occur, and this is frequently pH dependent. The addition of drugs such as suxamethonium to sodium thiopentone tends to change the pH in the direction of the thiopentone, and this may result in rapid hydrolysis of the suxamethonium (Grogono, 1974). Other groups of agents in which hydrolysis is an important potential reaction are the lactams, esters, amides and imines, which include the benzodiazepine group.

Epimerization or *racemization* of molecules in solutions also occurs. This will involve the alteration in the steric configuration of the molecule; an example is the change of adrenaline from an L to a D form, which occurs with a pH change in solution. The Maillard reaction is a further instance of a chemical interaction, in this case between the aldehyde carbonyl group of aldoses in dextrose solutions, and the amino groups in amino acid solution. This results in a colour change of the solution and precludes the storage of combined parenteral nutrition mixtures (Ellis, 1959). Although this reaction is minimal at room temperature, it becomes significant if the mixture is heat treated.

Some of the drugs commonly employed during anaesthesia are exposed to light for the first time during their use, and this may affect their stability. Photodegradation is dependent on the intensity and wavelength of the light involved (Lachman, Swartz and Cooper, 1960). This may catalyse oxidation or hydrolysis, and examples of drugs affected include sodium nitroprusside and the catecholamine group. The rate of deterioration of drug may vary considerably but, as with sodium nitroprusside, is significant enough to be of relevance in anaesthetic practice.

Whilst it is difficult to categorize the reaction involved, it seems reasonable to mention the interaction occurring between trichloroethylene and soda lime which results in dichloroacetylene formation. This particularly hazardous reaction takes place in the anaesthetic apparatus prior to administration to the patient and therefore anaesthetists should be aware of potential toxic reactions occurring *in vitro*, especially when employing newly introduced agents.

Physical

The other major group of pharmaceutical interactions may be described as the physical phenomena which may occur during the administration of drugs. The *osmolality* of the infusion fluid provides an example of an interaction which may occur on administration. The concurrent administration of blood with either 5% dextrose or mannitol may result in significant damage to the blood being given.

Solvent system polarity – the solubility of a drug in aqueous solution – is important in a variety of anaesthetic agents. If the solubility is poor it may be necessary for the drug to be dissolved in a specific solvent. Subsequent addition of the drug in solvent to an aqueous solution may reduce the solubility of the drug in that mixture and consequently the drug may precipitate out. An example of this occurs with diazepam, but once again it should be emphasized that the relative volumes and concentration of both the drugs and the solution to which it is being administered are of relevance in determining the degree of precipitation which occurs.

A further group of mechanisms which have been of considerable interest over the past few years are the interactions between certain drugs and the administration sets through which they are given. The reaction of paraldehyde with plastic syringes is probably the most obvious example of a major reaction. Other factors of considerable interest are those involving sorption, adsorption and solvent loss. *Sorption* is best described in relation to nitroglycerin and refers to the lipophilicity and polarity of the solution and its subsequent tendency to bind to different types of plastic or polyvinylchloride. The time that the drug is exposed to the surface and the area involved are also determinants of the quantity of drug removed from solution. This may result in significant changes in the concentration of the drug being administered and, consequently, changes in therapeutic effect. *Adsorption* is different, referring to the tendency of a drug to adhere to the surface of the container (whether glass or plastic), and considerable work has to be done with insulin in this regard. The amount of insulin removed is difficult to predict, but it has been suggested that the addition of a binding agent will reduce the amount of insulin adsorbed (Hirsch, Fratkin and Wood, 1977). *Solvent loss* through the plastic of containers may also occur, with a consequential change in drug concentration, but this is of doubtful clinical significance in anaesthetic practice.

Salting out is a phenomenon which occurs when electrolytes are added to supersaturated solutions such as mannitol. Another physical interaction which should be briefly described is the *emulsion cracking* which occurs when calcium salts are added to emulsions such as Intralipid. In emulsions the fat globules are held dispersed by the physical arrangement of the molecules and by electrostatic forces. Each globule carries a charge on its surface, known as the zeta potential, which repels other similarly charged globules. Ionization changes due to a reduction in pH or the addition of cations will reduce the zeta potential. The reduction in the electrostatic force will enable coalescence of the globules. This is termed 'aggregation' and results in an increase in size of the individual component globules of the emulsion. If the aggregates become large enough, flocculation is said to occur and this leads to phase separation. Whilst aggregates may not be visible to the naked eye, they may be associated with pathological problems relating to embolic phenomena. In clinical practice dextrose may, by alteration in pH, reduce zeta potential and increase

Table A3.2   Thiopentone administration: some of the drugs which interact *in vitro*

Alcuronium	Papaveretum
Pancuronium	Pethidine
Vecuronium	Ketamine
Tubocurare	Pentazocine
Atracurium	Metoclopramide
Suxamethonium	Droperidol
Midazolam	Glyceryl trinitrate

aggregation. Care must therefore be taken in determining which solutions are compatible with Intralipid infusion (Davis, 1982).

Pharmacokinetic interactions

'Pharmacokinetics' refers to the way in which the body deals with drugs, and this section discusses the way that it may be modified by a variety of interactions. This may occur during administration, distribution, biotransformation or elimination of the drug and some of the mechanisms involved are discussed below.

Administration

Drugs may be administered by a variety of routes. The oral route is not of great importance in anaesthetic practice other than for premedication, but is of considerable importance in the emergency department and this is an area in which anaesthetists are often involved. Furthermore, the oral absorption of drugs illustrates certain points as regards interactions and therefore is an important area to cover. When a drug is ingested and passes into the stomach, the rate at which it is subsequently absorbed depends on a variety of factors. The pK_a of the drug will determine the degree of ionization occurring in the stomach, which normally has a very low pH. Un-ionized drug may be able to be absorbed through the stomach lining, whilst ionized drug cannot be absorbed passively. Drugs such as H_2 antagonists or antacids will influence the stomach pH and change the amount of absorption taking place. Most drugs, however, are absorbed in the more alkaline small intestine. Drugs changing the speed of gastric emptying will alter the rate of delivery of other drugs to the site of absorption and influence uptake. Metoclopramide stimulates gastric emptying and increases the speed of uptake of many agents orally administered (Welling, 1984). The absorption of drugs may be influenced further by other agents present in the gastrointestinal tract at the same time. This mechanism may be utilized in at least two ways: first, chelating agents such as desferrioxamine may be used to chelate ferrous sulphate in the stomach; secondly, in less specific instances, activated charcoal has been used to help bind drugs in the intestine and thereby reduce absorption (Greensher *et al.*,

Table A3.3   Factors affecting oral absorption

Mechanism	Comment
Vomiting	Ipecacuanha, apomorphine
pH change	Alters ionization. May change gastric absorption (e.g. antacids, H_2 antagonists)
Enteric coating	Protects from acid dissolution. May alter if gastric pH high (e.g. antacids, H_2 antagonists – aspirin absorption)
Gastric motility	Rapid emptying may increase absorption Slow emptying may delay uptake
Malabsorption	Drug-induced by: 1. binding to fatty acids and bile acids causing steatorrhoea 2. interference with intestinal micellar phase + action on microvilli
Adsorption	Non-specific binding to drugs – charcoal. May also bind secreted drug and decrease enterohepatic cycling
Chelation	Specific and non-specific chelating agents
Splanchnic perfusion	Many drugs alter regional perfusion of the gut

1979). The more important mechanisms are summarized in Table A3.3.

To the anaesthetist the subcutaneous and intramuscular routes of administration are of considerably more importance. This of course includes local anaesthetic solutions. When a drug is given either intramuscularly or subcutaneously its uptake and distribution depend on a variety of factors. Whilst lipid solubility is important, the aqueous solubility of the drug is also significant because the drug must remain in solution at tissue pH long enough to be absorbed. Drugs prepared in solvents may, following administration, precipitate out in the tissue; this is due to the change in the solubility of the drug as it is mixed with interstitial fluid, a mechanism described in the section on pharmaceutical interactions. Examples of this include diazepam and phenytoin. This particular interaction has actually been utilized in clinical practice, and some drugs may be deliberately mixed in an oil solvent prior to injection in order to provide slow release of the active agent.

Distribution

After the administration of the drug it then has to be distributed, and this usually occurs via the blood stream. Even agents given for local effect, such as most of the local anaesthetic agents, will eventually be distributed systemically. The factors which may influence the distribution of the drug from the site of disposition operate in the same areas in which drug interactions may occur. Inhalational agents form a significant proportion of anaesthetic drug practice, and their uptake and distribution are largely determined by two factors: minute ventilation and cardiac output (Eger, 1982). It is the minute ventilation of the lungs that influences the rate of rise of alveolar concentration, which correlates well with the induction of anaesthesia, and it may be significantly reduced by a large number of anaesthetic agents. Premedication with narcotics, the use of induction agents and the inhalational agents themselves generally tend to decrease the minute ventilation and thereby slow induction. Conversely, the use of carbon dioxide has been advocated for increasing the speed of induction with inhalational agents. However, this technique has inherent risks if agents such as halothane are used.

Cardiac output and regional variations in perfusion will also influence the rate of rise of alveolar concentration of gases. Therefore, cardiac depression – which is an intrinsic side effect of many anaesthetic drugs – will tend to speed the rate of rise of the alveolar concentration, whilst other drugs which tend to increase cardiac output should slow the change in alveolar concentration. However, it is not only cardiac output which is important but also the regional distribution of that output which influences the speed of induction. Consequently, a reduced cardiac output not only speeds the rate of rise of alveolar concentration, but, by virtue of the physiological reflexes which come into play, also tends to increase the distribution of that output to the central nervous system – which will also enhance induction.

It can therefore be seen that a good many drugs used in anaesthetic practice will influence either the minute ventilation or the cardiac output, or both. Similarly, many drugs, whilst not having significant effects on the overall output, may well alter the regional perfusion, and this in turn may limit the perfusion through areas to which drugs have been administered. In this respect α-agonists, whilst possibly improving or altering cardiac output, may actually reduce muscle blood flow and skin perfusion, and thereby dramatically alter the rate at which intramuscularly or subcutaneously administered drugs are absorbed.

Local perfusion is of particular importance, especially when a local anaesthetic agent is administered to produce a nerve block. In clinical practice the concurrent administration of adrenaline may be used to reduce blood flow through the site of injection and reduce the rate of distribution of the local anaesthetic agent, and thereby not only prolong the duration of effect but also maintain a higher local concentration of anaesthetic solution for a longer period. The lipid solubility and pH of the drug and the tissue may also be important. Carbonated local anaesthetic solutions are said to improve the block obtained because the carbon dioxide tends to move across membranes readily and thereby reduces intracellular pH, increases the ionization of the local anaesthetic solution and enhances the anaesthetic effect (Bromage, 1965). Conversely, the addition of hyaluronidase to anaesthetic solutions tends to enhance the spread of the solution through the tissues. This has the dual effect of increasing absorption, with the potential for higher blood concentrations and toxicity, and also of reducing the duration of action of the drug. It does, however, increase the likelihood of the anaesthetic solution reaching its site of action.

In the lungs the actual uptake of drugs may also be modified by a variety of interactions, dependent on the physical nature of the gases involved. The second gas effect is an interaction by which there is an acceleration in the rate of rise of alveolar concentration when a gas is given concurrently with nitrous oxide. This is a result of both the second gas effect and the concentrating effect (Stoelting and Eger, 1979).

Protein binding

This particular mode of interaction is extensively and well described in the literature. Essentially, the majority of drugs on entering the circulation become bound to blood constituents. These include albumin, globulin, lipoproteins and cellular components such as erythrocytes. Quantitatively, albumin is the most important of these, and it is the effects of displacement of drugs from albumin-binding sites where interaction has been well documented. At normal body pH albumin tends to be negatively charged over all, but in fact consists of a complex molecule with a very large number of binding sites which may be of either polarity. Binding may be electrostatic, hydrogen binding or hydrophobic in nature, the hydrophobic binding occurring within the confines of the molecule. Binding usually obeys the laws of mass action, and the association and dissociation of drug is usually in the order of a few milliseconds. Many drugs will tend to bind at more than one site but each site will have its own dissociation constant which characterizes the various factors involved (Koch-Weser and Sellers, 1976). Obviously other influences such as temperature, pH and albumin concentration will all be important in determining drug binding.

It is the binding of drugs to albumin and to other sites which determines the distribution of a drug. This will tend to influence the quantity of free drug which is readily available and also the redistribution of drug if it becomes displaced from the albumin molecule. Binding may be competitive or non-competitive. The former implies competition for the same site; the latter occurs when the binding of the drug tends to alter the molecular configuration of the site, thereby blocking the binding of other drugs. The mode of interaction in either case is the displacement of a drug with an inherent increase in the concentration of free drug.

If a drug is highly albumin bound, a small degree of displacement will tend to increase the quantity of free drug very significantly and may produce pharmacological effects. These depend on whether the displaced drug remains free or whether it then binds to tissue or becomes rapidly distributed or eliminated. Hence not all displaced drug will necessarily remain free for long. If the quantity of free drug does tend to increase then the amount available for biotransformation and elimination will also increase, and in most situations this will tend to return the concentration of free drug to its original state. The end-result will be a reduction of the total available drug in the circulation, with somewhat less bound to albumin but with essentially the same concentration of free drug.

The drugs which are most likely to be affected can be predicted. These will be agents which are highly albumin bound, with a small volume of distribution and with a low therapeutic index. This mechanism has been well described in the literature, but in anaesthetic practice it is difficult to find evidence of interactions which have particularly significant clinical implications. Displacement of neuromuscular blocking drugs (Ghonheim, 1971) or reduced solubility of halothane by displacement from binding sites, thereby increasing the free drug (Laasberg and Hedley-Whyte, 1970), could have anaesthetic implications although these are probably not of great clinical relevance. A much quoted example is the prolongation of action of thiopentone by concomitant administration of sulphafurazole, which competes for binding sites. However, whilst this is of interest as regards the nature of the interaction, its significance in clinical practice is dubious (Csögör and Kerek, 1970).

Biotransformation

Following distribution, drugs are often altered prior to elimination. The biotransformation which occurs may change the pharmacological properties of the agent or merely convert it to a form which is more readily excreted. An example of biotransformation altering pharmacological effect is the interaction which occurs when protamine is given to reverse heparin. The basic protamine attaches and interacts with acidic heparin, forming a salt which lacks anticoagulant properties, and this occurs in the circulating blood volume. This simple acid/base interaction significantly reduces the activity of the drug although it does not actually produce a transformation of the chemical structure. In a similar way some chelating agents may be used to bind to active molecules in the circulation and inhibit their actions. However, the more significant interactions which are to be discussed are concerned with the physiological systems which normally biotransform drugs. These tend to involve enzyme systems in a variety of sites, both in major organs such as lungs and the liver and in individual situations such as at the neuromusclar junction. The kinetics of any drug dealt with by an enzyme system will be modified to some degree by any other agent which tends to affect the efficacy of the enzyme pathway. At the neuromuscular junction the effects of suxamethonium may be modified by agents which alter the availability of pseudocholinesterase. Whilst the problems associated with the use of anticholinesterase drugs such as ecothiopate are well known, the current use of many cytotoxic agents such as nitrogen mustard, cyclophosphamide and chlorambucil which may well reduce the clinical availability of pseudocholinesterase, is less well recognized as creating potential problems in anaesthetic practice. Conversely, tetrahydroaminacrine has been used to prolong the action of suxamethonium by the same mechanism.

The main organ systems concerned with biotransformation are the liver, the kidney and the lung, although almost all cells will have active metabolic sites which may alter drugs. The lung is a relatively active organ of biotransformation, with significant metabolism of agents such as prostaglandins. At the present time the clinical interactions occurring in the lung through metabolic systems are relatively few and poorly delineated. However, this is a site to be aware of in the future if there is further development of prostaglandin-like agents or prostaglandin inhibitors. The liver is the site probably best understood, and in this situation two different areas will be discussed: the delivery of the drug to the liver, and the metabolism of the drug through the hepatocellular systems.

A large variety of drugs affect hepatic blood flow. Consequently, the delivery of drugs to the liver for biotransformation may be reduced. A drug with a high intrinsic clearance may be of considerable importance in terms of its half-life. The intrinsic clearance is an index of the ability of, in this case, the liver to remove drug from the hepatic blood flow. Consequently, if flow exceeds intrinsic clearance, the quantity of drug removed is dependent on the intrinsic clearance; if flow is less than intrinsic clearance, it is the flow which will determine the quantity of drug removed. Therefore, drugs with high intrinsic clearances will be flow dependent; the best example in anaesthetic practice is probably lignocaine (Nies, Shand and Wilkinson, 1976). The pharmacological agents which tend to increase hepatic blood flow include glucagon, phenobarbitone and isoprenaline, whilst drugs which tend to reduce flow include propranolol, noradrenaline and most general anaesthetics. The general anaesthetics will have this effect if they tend to reduce cardiac output or modify regional blood flow. The effect of a significant reduction in hepatic blood flow will be to increase the half-life of lignocaine, and if infusions are being administered there will be a resultant increase in the plasma concentration (Heller and Friedman, 1984).

Whilst delivery of the drug is of course important, the main determinants of biotransformation are the metabolic pathways available in the liver cells. There are several enzyme systems of importance in the liver and these can be divided arbitrarily in terms of the microsomal fraction and the soluble fraction. The microsomal fraction contains the hydroxylation system involved in nitro reduction and azo reduction, the UDP-glucuronyl transferase and the microsomal oxidizing system. The soluble fraction contains the alcohol and aldehyde dehydrogenase, esterases, and *n*-acetyl transferase. Also within the cell located in the mitochondria are the monoamine oxidases (Birkett and Pond, 1975).

When two drugs are presented to the same enzyme system, they may interact in a competitive or non-competitive manner. Competition will occur up to the point at which the system becomes saturated. Non-competitive interaction implies either that one drug will be metabolized to the total exclusion of another or that the metabolism of one drug alters the enzyme system in such a way that the second drug cannot be metabolized. Furthermore, groups of agents may tend to induce or to inhibit the enzyme systems themselves. The microsomal hydroxylation system consists of three components – cytochrome P450, NADPH–cytochrome P450 reductase and phosphatidylcholine – and forms a large unit with a broad specificity. It may be induced by two different classes of drugs, the barbiturates included in the first group and the polycyclic hydrocarbons in the second. Induction by the barbiturates may enhance the metabolism of a range of drugs which may be quite different from the drugs which are preferentially metabolized if polycyclic hydrocarbons are used to induce the enzyme system. This may imply two slightly different enzyme systems or, alternatively, a very large molecule with different receptor sites within it. Following induction of the enzyme a susceptible drug will be metabolized more efficiently and this may result in a shorter half-life and consequently reduced serum levels, with a reduction in clinical efficacy. Conversely, if the inducing agent is withdrawn, there will be a regression of the enzyme system to its original state, with a reduction in the relative efficiency with which drugs are dealt with, and this will return the half-life and serum level of the drug to the preinduction level. If the drug dosage administered has been altered to compensate for the reduced half-life and serum levels, cessation of the inducing agent may result in higher levels with that dosage of drug and consequently toxicity may result. The drugs predominantly affected by such metabolisms are the sulphonylureas, the anticoagulants and diphenylhydantoin. These reactions may not be of great relevance to the anaesthetist, but they are important biological mechanisms.

It is reasonable in this context to comment on the time span over which induction may occur. Phenobarbitone may induce enzymes and result in a change in the rate of metabolism of other drugs within two days, but further increasing effects on metabolism will be seen over several weeks (Kristensen, Hansen and Skovsted, 1969). Similarly, removal of the inducing agent will result in regression of the enzyme system's efficacy over the ensuing two or more weeks (Kristensen, 1976). A further important interaction relating to induction is that which occurs when induction of an enzyme system may result in the production of toxic metabolites, as may be the case with halothane, and this has been discussed in Appendix 1.

The other two enzyme systems are the UDP-transferase which catalyses the glucuronidation of drugs and the microsomal ethanol-oxidizing system. Patients with chronic alcohol ingestion will tend to have well-induced liver function, but acute alcohol intake can result in saturation of the enzyme systems and thereby inhibition of further drug metabolism. This concept has been utilized in poisoning situations, where saturation of the enzyme system with ethanol may be used to prevent the formation of toxic metabolites from agents such as methanol or ethylene glycol. A further aspect of the inhibition of this enzyme system can be seen with antibiotics such as metronidazole which effectively block the conversion of acetaldehyde and result in accumulation and toxic manifestations of this metabolite (Thompson, 1980).

As a great many of the anaesthetic drugs used in everyday practice are metabolized to some extent in the liver, one might expect to see regular drug interactions occurring. Whilst this almost certainly does happen to a fairly large extent, the clinical significance of most of these reactions is not great. Nevertheless, it is as well to be aware of the mechanisms involved.

Elimination

Sooner or later most drugs or their metabolites have to be eliminated from the body, and this can occur at many sites. The lungs are of particular importance with the inhalational agents, whilst the liver, kidney and gastrointestinal tract are important with most of the parenterally administered drugs. The potential interactions occurring with a drug are very similar to those described above in the section on absorption and distribution of drugs. The minute ventilation and cardiac output are, in this situation, important determinants of the rate of fall of the alveolar concentration. Drugs which affect either of these factors will influence the rate of elimination of gaseous agents. The mechanism involved is the reverse of that occurring with uptake. At the end of anaesthesia the rapid transit of nitrous oxide (due to its solubility) into the alveolar space may result in effective dilution of the oxygen present there and cause diffusion hypoxia.

Renal excretion of drugs is particularly important in relation to highly ionized agents such as the muscle relaxants. The water solubility of drugs is in part determined by the ionization of the drug and this may well alter during the passage along the renal tubule. In the tubule, because water is avidly reabsorbed, there will be a concentration effect on the drug left inside, and this will produce a concentration gradient from the tubule into the interstitium. Changes in pH producing an increase in the un-ionized form of the drug, and hence an increase in lipid solubility, will allow its passage down the concentration gradient and out of the tubule, resulting in reabsorption (Kristensen, 1976). This effect may be clinically manipulated to increase the excretion of some drugs, especially in an overdose situation. If a patient has toxic levels of an acidic drug such as phenobarbitone or salicylate, increasing the urinary pH will maintain its relatively high ionization and will not allow reabsorption, thereby increasing excretion. Conversely, basic drugs may be eliminated in an acid urine. A further method of excretion via the kidney is that of drug secretion into the tubule. This is an active process and it may be blocked by drugs such as probenecid. It has been used to reduce the elimination of penicillin and thereby maintain drug concentrations in the serum. There are, of course, many other interactions of a far less specific nature. Renal toxicity may also adversely affect tubular function and result in impaired secretion of other agents. In the intensive care setting, with patients who are already at risk, the aminoglycosides may well produce an element of renal dysfunction which may alter the excretion of anaesthetic agents such as muscle relaxants. Obviously, drugs which significantly alter either the glomerular filtration rate or the regional perfusion of the kidney will also have potential for effects on drug excretion. A curious mechanism of interaction can occur mediated through the tubular response to thiazide. In this case, with the relative depletion of sodium due to the diuresis, lithium administered concurrently will in fact have a reduced renal clearance, and consequently its half-life may be prolonged. As this agent has a low therapeutic index this is a particularly hazardous interaction which may result in the patient coming under an anaesthetist's care in the intensive care environment (Petersen *et al.*, 1974).

Pharmacodynamics

The term 'pharmacodynamics' refers to the effects of a drug on a subject. Whilst most drugs may be given for a specific purpose, they more often than not have a wide range of side effects on different systems. In anaesthesia it is common practice to use groups of agents, each with specific actions, to provide an overall combined effect. In general terms, the end-result can be described in terms of an interaction of the pharmacodynamics of the drugs involved. The term 'balanced anaesthesia', coined in 1926 by J.S. Lundy of the Mayo Clinic, refers to just this type of interaction to produce a better form of anaesthesia.

The variety of actual and potential drug interactions in terms of pharmacodynamics is limitless. They can, for the purpose of discussion, be classified into three main areas: the interaction which may occur at a single receptor site; those occurring at a variety of receptor sites, and the general non-specific interactions mediated through unspecified sites of action. In general terms the interactions of drugs must be considered not only in the light of their specific actions but also in respect of the physiological reflex responses to their action which might be expected under normal conditions.

Considering the situation of the single receptor site, a sequence of events occurs resulting in receptor activation and consequent effect. The formation of a neurotransmitter agent, its release, movement across a synaptic cleft, binding and activation of a receptor, and its dissociation and elimination are all potential sites of interaction. Consideration of the uptake and storage of neurotransmitter agents will enable illustration of a mode of interaction. Any drug which tends to increase or reduce the amount of neurotransmitter stored will, by nature of the amount of transmitter available for release, alter the effects of any other drug which tends to release that transmitter. A slightly different illustration of effects on the release of neurotransmitter may be seen at the neuromuscular junction. In this instance the action of aminoglycosides may reduce prejunctional release of acetylcholine (Torda, 1980); in the normal patient this may have little significance in terms of neuromuscular function, but in the patient in whom a neuromuscular block with curariform drugs is present it may well produce significant clinical effect. Conversely, in this situation drugs of the aminopyridine group may increase the release of acetylcholine, an effect which has been used in clinical practice to reverse curariform drugs at the neuromuscular junction (Booij, 1980).

At the receptor itself stimulation by the neurotransmitter will result in a specific effect. Drugs may increase or decrease this effect when attached to the receptor. The form of interaction may be of a competitive or non-competitive nature. If competitive antagonism is present, whilst the maximum effect which the drug can produce will remain unchanged, the quantity of drug required to produce that effect will be greatly increased. However, if non-competitive antagonism occurs the implication is that the drug will alter the receptor in such a way as to prevent full agonist activity of the other agonist agent. Consequently, the maximum effect of a drug will be reduced independent of its concentration. An example of this can be seen at the adrenergic neuron where phentolamine, a competitive blocker, will tend to increase the concentration of agonist required to produce a maximum effect, whereas phenoxybenzamine a non-competitive blocker, will reduce the maximum effect achievable regardless of the concentration of agonist present. A further interaction may occur when both drugs have similar binding to receptors and interact in such a way that their effects are additive and may actually increase the total number of receptors which may be occupied at any one time. This may be due to the different geometry of the drugs, allowing greater access to the receptors and, therefore, synergism.

Following receptor activation, dissociation generally occurs and association will not recur if the drug or agonist is removed from the environment rapidly. Consequently, other agents which tend to reduce the elimination of the drug or agonist from the receptor vicinity will tend to alter the degree of receptor occupancy; this is another mode of interaction utilized in clinical practice. Using the model of the adrenergic neuron (Fig. A3.1), the drugs acting at each particular site have been demonstrated, and, as a drug at one site can interact with any other drug at any other site, the potential for major interactions occurring even within a single receptor system is immense. Awareness of these possible interactions can be used clinically either positively or to prevent disastrous consequences in anaesthetic practice.

The receptors, however, are generally parts of much larger systems; for example, the parasympathetic and the sympathetic nervous system. Physiological agonists often have a very specific action at a specific site, whereas pharmacological equivalents often have much more general effects

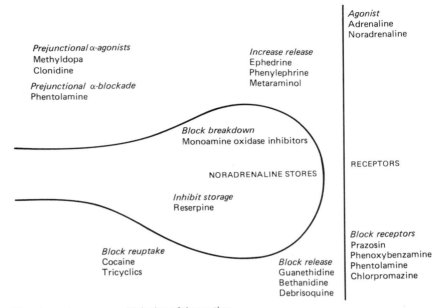

Fig. A3.1 Pharmacology of the adrenergic nerve terminal.

over a wide range of sites. Furthermore, whilst the physiological agonist may interact with a single receptor type, pharmacological agents very often affect more than only one receptor type – as is easily demonstrated by agents such as dopamine which will affect not only dopaminergic receptors but also α- and β-receptors. Another aspect of drug effect in this context is the fact that the sympathetic and parasympathetic nervous systems are in balance. The action of a drug to alter the tone of one system may result in an alteration of tone in the other. Consequently, in the presence of blockade of the sympathetic system, a drug whose side effect is a degree of agonist activity on the parasympathetic system may have a far greater pharmacological effect than would normally be predicted.

One particular illustration of interaction at different sites which is used in everyday anaesthetic practice is the use of reversal agents. Neostigmine is a non-specific cholinesterase inhibitor, which will tend to increase the concentration of acetylcholine in most areas of the body other than behind the blood–brain barrier. Muscarinic receptors will therefore also be stimulated and atropine is used routinely to block these unwanted side effects. This is an example of an interaction of drugs employed within the same receptor system to try to increase the specificity of action which is achieved. When using drugs which may affect a wide range of receptors it is essential for possible interactions occurring with other drugs within the same receptor system to be borne in mind.

Non-specific interactions

The largest single group of interactions occurring in anaesthetic practice are the non-specific interactions between drugs. There are a multiplicity of these, which may be mediated through a wide range of postulated mechanisms.

The concept of minimal alveolar concentration (MAC) as a means of evaluating the potency of an anaesthetic agent and being able to compare it with other drugs is a way of looking at the end-point of some types of interaction. The specific mechanism by which general anaesthesia is achieved is still not fully delineated. However, it is readily accepted that various pharmacological agents will reduce the MAC of certain inhalational agents such as halothane. It may therefore be assumed that at some point the primary drug, halothane, and the secondary agent are interacting at some physical or chemical site to enhance the overall effect. Analeptic agents, which may tend to reverse some of the anaesthetic agents, presumably act through similar pathways to achieve their effect, but again this is not known. Whilst it is conceptually easy to understand how a drug which has a sedative or narcotic action may influence MAC, it is more difficult to accept that the use of agents such as verapamil with halothane may significantly alter the MAC even though it appears to have no sedative or narcotic effects in its own right (Maze and Mason, 1983). Further information on the mechanism of general anaesthesia may in the future shed light on the mechanism by which these various drugs can interact to produce this overall effect.

The cardiovascular system is a fertile ground for non-specific interaction. Largely controlled by sympathetic and parasympathetic activity, many of the interactions can be predicted from a knowledge of the receptors involved and the reflex activity associated with activation or blockade of these receptors. It may be stated that a large number of anaesthetic drugs cause alterations in the cardiovascular system by means of depression of cardiac and smooth muscle contractility. This may in part be mediated through alterations in calcium flux into excitable cells (Altura and Altura, 1981). Indeed, the movement of calcium into and around the cell may have a significant influence on both neurotransmitter release and intrinsic muscle activity as well as cellular metabolic functions. In the future intracellular metabolism may be more readily identifiable as a site of major drug interaction. Already the effects of calcium antagonists on myocardial contractility and smooth muscle tone provide a plethora of interactions with anaesthetic agents. As has previously been stated, because the anaesthetic agents may have significant effects on calcium flux, there may well be an additive effect when calcium antagonists are also used. The role of calcium antagonists is rapidly expanding, and it is certain that in the future the mechanisms surrounding calcium channel opening and blocking will be important in terms of drug interaction and will be of clinical relevance to the anaesthetist.

Cardiac excitability is also of some importance. Halothane sensitizes the myocardium to catecholamines (Cullen and Miller, 1979) and by doing so will increase the tendency for hazardous interaction with catecholamines given concurrently. (The nature of this increase in excitability is not fully understood.) On the other hand, a wide variety of drugs tend to reduce cardiac excitability and this is in fact the function of a large group of antiarrhythmic

Table A3.4 Drugs altering electrolyte concentration

Electrolyte disturbance	Drug
Hypokalaemia	Diuretics, corticosteroids, glucose, insulin, laxatives, liquorice, topical silver nitrate, polymyxin, thiopentone
Hyperkalaemia	Potassium-sparing diuretics, suxamethonium
Hyponatraemia	Diuretics, sulphonylurea, vincristine, cyclophosphamide
Hypernatraemia	Osmotic diuretic, sodium bicarbonate, hypertonic saline
Hypomagnesaemia	Diuretics, laxatives
Hypermagnesaemia	Magnesium sulphate

agents. These have effects on the conduction system as well as on intrinsic myocardial contractility, and therefore have potential for interactions with drugs with similar effects (Adams, Mote and Pruett, 1982). Digoxin is particularly pertinent in this context and may well interact with many antiarrhythmic agents. It is of interest that halothane, which, as previously mentioned, tends to increase the excitability of the myocardium, has been reported as reducing the cardiotoxicity of digitalis-like drugs (Morrow, 1970). Again, the mechanism behind these interactions is difficult to delineate. The cardiovascular system is the site of the most threatening interactions for anaesthetists. Some agents in common use, such as fentanyl, are often used for relative cardiovascular stability. However, it has been noted that even with this drug a negative inotropic effect may be seen when it is used in combination with another stable agent, diazepam (Reves *et al.*, 1984). In this situation clinical observation has been confirmed by studies in laboratory preparations. It is important to note that the combination of two innocuous agents may result in haemodynamic changes which would not normally be anticipated.

A further area to consider is interactions which may be mediated by alterations in electrolyte balance. A large group of drugs influence electrolyte concentration in the body (Table A3.4), and the pharmacological effects of other agents may then be altered by the depletion of sodium, potassium, calcium or magnesium ions. Furthermore, intravascular depletion caused by diuretic therapy may predispose the patient to cardiovascular collapse in the presence of potent anaesthesic agents.

Hypokalaemia is relatively common in patients admitted to hospital for anaesthesia. The serum potassium is a relatively poor indicator of total potassium stores, but it is a quick and easy investigation to carry out and is one of the few ways of assessing the potassium balance. The two areas of significant interaction are the cardiovascular system and the neuromuscular junction. In most situations involving electrolyte depletion it is the acute changes in electrolyte concentration which play an important role in significant interactions rather than chronic depletion. Hypokalaemia tends to increase cardiac excitability due to increased automaticity, accelerated conductivity and delayed repolarization. This tends to reduce the threshold for arrhythmias and potentiates interaction with any drugs which increase arrhythmia susceptibility. These of course include anticholinergics, catecholamines and halothane (Vitez, 1983). The neuromuscular junction and skeletal muscle may also be affected. There is some debate as to the actual effect of low potassium on neuromuscular transmission. At the neuromuscular junction hypokalaemia tends to increase the end-plate transmembrane potential. However, this hyperpolarization may increase the action potential which occurs once the threshold is reached; therefore, although activation is less likely, when it does occur the amount of acetylcholine released may be increased (Miller, 1976). Hypokalaemia may result in profound muscle weakness and this may influence the use of neuromuscular blocking drugs indirectly.

Hyperkalaemia tends to reduce cardiac automaticity, conductivity and contractility, as well as producing a partial depolarization of the postjunctional skeletal muscle membrane. This impairs the response to stimulation. Patients with renal failure or on potassium-sparing diuretics may present with raised serum potassium and in this situation drugs such as suxamethonium may cause a further rise in the potassium level.

Similarly, hyponatraemia has anaesthetic interactions with potentiation of both local and inhalational agents, as well as haemodynamic effects associated with alterations in volume status. Calcium and magnesium changes caused by drug therapy may also have implications for anaesthetic agents. Magnesium in particular has effects on both neuromuscular transmission and peripheral vasodilatation. Magnesium sulphate infusions which are used in obstetric practice may have significant interactions with anaesthetic agents. These interactions may relate either to the cardiovascular effects due to peripheral vasodilatation or to the impairment of neuromuscular transmission in the presence of high magnesium levels.

These general interactions are by no means a comprehensive review of the pharmacodynamic interactions which are potentially available. The actual mechanism of action of many of the drugs used in anaesthesia is still unknown. As the physical alteration of membranes, the actual mechanisms of channel function and the intracellular actions of anaesthetic drugs become known, the mechanisms of interaction in these areas may become as familiar as those involving receptor function. However, they do serve to illustrate the diffuse areas in which they may occur.

Conclusion

This Appendix has attempted to categorize the mechanisms of drug interaction in anaesthesia along classic pharmacological lines. In doing so it is obvious that anaesthesia comprises a vast array of potential interactions, and it may be pertinent at this stage to look at the practical aspects of anaesthesia with relation to the potential interactions.

When an anaesthetist makes a preanaesthetic assessment not only the clinical status of the patient needs to be determined but also the polypharmacy to which the patient may be subjected. This may well influence the type of anaesthetic administered. A thorough working knowledge of the anaesthetic agents being used should include an awareness of their spheres of activity and where these may overlap with other drugs administered concomitantly.

Despite the advancement of anaesthesia as a science there is still considerable art involved in its successful practice. In this instance the science may be considered in terms of knowledge of the pharmacology of the drugs utilized, and thereby some comprehension of the mechanisms of interaction which may occur with their use. The art is to observe and learn from drug interactions in daily practice, and thereby to be able to select those which are clinically useful whilst avoiding those which are potentially dangerous.

References

Adams, R.J., Mote, S.P. and Pruett, J.K. (1982) Cardiovascular depressant effects of anesthetic agents and potential drug interaction. *Journal of the Medical Association of Georgia* **71**, 801

Altura, B.M. and Altura, B.T. (1981) General anesthetics and magnesium ions as calcium antagonists on vascular smooth muscle. In: *New Perspectives on Calcium Antagonists* (Ed. Weiss, E.B.), p. 131. Williams & Wilkins: Baltimore, MD

Birkett, D.J. and Pond, S.M. (1975) Medical drug interactions − a critical review. *Medical Journal of Australia* **1**, 687

Booij, L.H.D.J. (1980) Antagonism of ORG.NC45 neuromuscular blockade by neostigmine, pyridostigmine and 4-aminopyridine. *Anesthesia and Analgesia* **59**, 1

Bromage, P.R. (1965) A comparison of the hydrochloride and carbon dioxide salts of lidocaine and prilocaine in epidural analgesia. *Acta Anaesthesiologica Scandinavica* suppl. 16, 55

Csögör, S.I. and Kerek, S.F. (1970) Enhancement of thiopentone anaesthesia by sulphafurazole. *British Journal of Anaesthesia* **42**, 988

Cullen, B.F. and Miller, M.G. (1979) Drug interactions and anesthesia. *Anesthesia and Analgesia* **58**, 413

Davis, S.S. (1982) The stability of fat emulsions for intravenous administration. In: *Advances in Clinical Nutrition*, Second International Symposium on Nutrition, Bermuda (Ed. Johnston, I.D.A.), p. 213. MTP Press: Lancaster

Eger, E.I. (1982) Uptake, distribution and elimination of inhaled anaesthetics. In: *Scientific Foundations of Anaesthesia*, 3rd edn. (Eds. Scurr, C. and Feldman, S.A.), p. 467. Heinemann Medical: London

Eggert, L.D., Rusho, W.J., Mackay, M.W. *et al.* (1982) Calcium and phosphorus compatibility in parenteral nutrition solutions for neonates. *American Journal of Hospital Pharmacy* **39**, 49

Ellis, G.P. (1959) The Maillard reaction. *Advances in Carbohydrate Chemistry* **14**, 63

Ghonheim, N.M. (1971) Drug interactions. *Canadian Anaesthetists' Society Journal* **18**, 353

Greensher, J., Mofenson, H.C., Piccioni, A.L. and Fallon, P. (1979) Activated charcoal updated. *Journal of the American College of Emergency Physicians* **8**, 261

Grogono, A.W. (1974) Drug interactions in anaesthesia. *British Journal of Anaesthesia* **46**, 613

Heller, C.A. and Friedman, P.A. (1984) How cardiovascular drugs interact. *Journal of Cardiovascular Medicine* April, 285

Hirsch, J.I., Fratkin, M.J. and Wood, J.H. (1977) Clinical significance of insulin adsorption. *American Journal of Hospital Pharmacy* **34**, 583

Koch-Weser, J. and Sellers, E.M. (1976) Binding of drugs to serum albumin. *New England Journal of Medicine* **294**, 311 and 526

Kristensen, M.B. (1976) Drug interaction and clinical pharmacokinetics. *Clinical Pharmacokinetics* **1**, 351

Kristensen, M.B., Hansen, J.M. and Skovsted, L. (1969) The influence of phenobarbital on the half life of diphenylhydantoin. *Acta Medica Scandinavica* **185**, 347

Laasberg, L.H. and Hedley-Whyte, J. (1970) Halothane solubility in blood and solutions of plasma proteins. *Anesthesiology* **32**, 351

Lachman, L., Swartz, C.J. and Cooper, J. (1960) A comprehensive pharmaceutical testing laboratory. III. A light stability cabinet for evaluating the photosensitivity of pharmaceuticals. *Journal of the American Pharmaceutical Association* (Sci. Ed.) **49**, 213

May, F.E., Stewart, R.B. and Cliff, L.E. (1974) Drug use in the hospital: evaluation of determinants. *Clinical Pharmacology and Therapeutics* **16**, 834

Maze, M. and Mason, D.M. (1983) Verapamil decreases the MAC for halothane in dogs. *Anesthesia and Analgesia* **62**, 274

Medicom Database (1983) Evaluating drug interactions by computer. *American Pharmacy* **NS23**, 376

Miller, R.R. (1973) Drug surveillance utilizing epidemiological methods. A report from the Boston Collaborative Drug Surveillance Program. *American Journal of Hospital Pharmacy* **30**, 584

Miller, R.D. (1976) Antagonism of neuromuscular blockade. *Anesthesiology* **44**, 318

Morrow, D.H. (1970) Anaesthesia and digitalis toxicity. Effects of barbiturates and halothane on digoxin toxicity. *Anesthesia and Analgesia* **49**, 305

Newton, D.W., Fung, E.Y.Y. and Williams, D.A. (1981) Stability of five catecholamines and terbutaline sulfate in 5% dextrose injection in the absence and presence of aminophylline. *American Journal of Hospital Pharmacy* **38**, 1314

Nies, A.S., Shand, D.G. and Wilkinson, G.R. (1976) Altered hepatic blood flow and drug disposition. *Clinical Pharmacokinetics* **1**, 135

Petersen, V., Hvidt, S., Thansen, S. and Schou, M. (1974) Effect of prolonged thiazide treatment on renal lithium clearance. *British Medical Journal* **3**, 143

Reves, J.G., Kissin, I., Fournier, S.E. and Smith, L.R. (1984) Additive negative inotropic effect of a combination of diazepam and fentanyl. *Anesthesia and Analgesia* **63**, 97

Stoelting, R.K. and Eger, E.I. (1979) An additional explanation of the second gas effect. A concentrating effect. *Anesthesiology* **30**, 273

Thompson, W.L. (1980) Poisoning: the twentieth-century black death. In: *Critical Care. State of the Art* (Eds. Shoemaker, W.C. and Thompson, W.L.). Society of Critical Care Medicine: Fullerton, CA

Torda, T. (1980) The nature of gentamicin induced neuromuscular block. *British Journal of Anaesthesia* **52**, 325

Trissell, L.A. (1983) *Handbook on Injectable Drugs*, 3rd edn. American Society of Hospital Pharmacists: Bethesda, MD

Vitez, T.S. (1983) Electrolytes and the anesthetist. In: *American Society of Anesthesiologists Annual Meeting, 1983*, p. 128. American Society of Anesthesiologists

Welling, P.G. (1984) Interactions affecting drug absorption. *Clinical Pharmacokinetics* **9**, 404

Appendix 4
Steady state pharmacology

David J.R. Duthie and Walter S. Nimmo

'Steady state pharmacology' describes the equilibrium in which the rate of drug administration is equal to the rate of drug elimination from the body. Plasma and tissue concentrations are constant, avoiding the fluctuating plasma concentrations associated with conventional methods of drug administration. The drug must be delivered continuously, using some apparatus or delivery system to control its rate of adminstration. Its prescription is characterized by rate of delivery and duration rather than dose and dosing interval.

Advantages of steady state pharmacology

The most obvious advantage of rate-controlled preparations is that the duration of drug action is prolonged. This reduces dosing frequency and improves compliance. Conventional dosing produces fluctuating plasma drug concentrations. Rate-controlled preparations enhance safety by avoiding the initial toxic effects of large drug doses which are often given inappropriately to prolong drug action (Stanski and Watkins, 1982). They improve efficacy by avoiding subtherapeutic concentration at the end of a dosing interval. Parenteral systems avoid both first-pass metabolism and the variability in oral drug absorption related to meals, disease and altered gastrointestinal transit time (Rawlins and Bateman, 1985).

Abrupt withdrawal of medicines acting on the central nervous or cardiovascular systems may exacerbate symptoms (George, 1985). Severe effects, including sudden death, may follow withdrawal of β–adrenoceptor antagonists (Shand and Wood, 1978). Angina (Bala Subramanian *et al.*, 1983) and increased systemic vascular resistance (Casson, Jones and Parsons, 1984) have been shown after withdrawal of calcium antagonists. Parenteral rate-controlled preparations, such as transdermal nitroglycerin and clonidine, and intraocular pilocarpine allow therapy to continue without interruption when a patient is fasted before surgery or is unable to eat immediately afterwards.

At steady state, concentration-dependent drug effects are more recognizable than with continually fluctuating drug concentrations. Desired effects may be selected and toxic effects prevented by altering the rate of administration and changing the steady state concentration (Goldman, 1982; Urquhart, 1982). Therapeutic drug monitoring is simplified. The sample need no longer be taken at an exact time after dosing and results are still valid at the time of reporting and not of historical interest. The steady state concentration of a drug reflects well the amount of drug in the body and is a better indication of a drug's potency than the dose required (Koch-Weser, 1972).

Rate-controlled administration may allow the reintroduction of discarded drugs or simplify the adminstration of others with inconvenient dosing regimes. Clonides and pilocarpine are enjoying increased usage in rate-controlled preparations (Heilmann, 1985; Lawson, 1985). By increasing the choice of alternative drugs, those with long elimination half-lives may be superseded.

Disadvantages

One must ensure that steady state pharmacology demonstrates therapeutic advantages and not merely improved pharmacokinetic profiles. The advantages of rate therapy are fewer when using drugs with long half-lives and large therapeutic indices (the ratio of maximum tolerated concentration to minimum effective concentration). Pharmacokinetic data of plasma drug concentrations following bolus doses and short infusions may be unable to predict a drug's suitability for controlled delivery to steady state. Biological half-life may differ from plasma half-life in that drugs can persist at tissue receptors long after plasma concentrations have begun to fall.

The time taken to reach steady state may restrict the applications of rate-controlled therapy. With a constant rate of administration, it takes four to five elimination half-lives of a drug before 95 per cent steady state is reached. Whilst this is of no importance in prolonged therapy, such as maintenance antihypertensive therapy, it poses great problems when trying to achieve steady state within the relatively short time of a general anaesthetic.

Steady state concentration is dependent on the rate of both drug delivery and elimination.

$$\text{Rate of drug delivery} = \text{clearance} \times \text{drug concentration at steady state}$$

Whilst the rate of drug delivery may often be controlled, the rate of drug elimination cannot. Between-patient pharmacokinetic variation in clearance may make it impossible to predict an individual's resulting steady state plasma concentration. Pharmacodynamic variations in response to the plasma concentration obtained introduce further uncertainty to the response to a given rate of drug delivery. For example, an interpatient coefficient of variation of 39 per cent has been reported in the minimum effective analgesic concentration of pethidine in surgical patients (Austin, Stapleton and Mather, 1980).

Administering a drug at a constant rate to achieve steady state assumes that elimination is unchanging. There are many profound physiological changes during anaesthesia and in the days after surgery, but few data exist on whether or not they are sufficient to change drug clearance. Critically ill patients may exhibit impaired renal and hepatic function and marked changes in the distribution of fluid in the tissues and intravascular compartments. These may affect drug disposition in an unpredictable way.

The expense and trouble in achieving steady state plasma concentrations will be invalidated if active metabolites are produced or if tolerance to the drug's effects develops. A metabolite of morphine, morphine-6-glucuronide, has been shown to have greater analgesic activity than its parent compound in animals (Shimomura *et al.*, 1971). After distribution of a bolus dose, plasma concentrations of morphine-6-glucuronide can exceed those of morphine itself (Svensson *et al.*, 1982). Tolerance to morphine by infusion has been demonstrated within 4 hours in rats (Cox, Ginsburg and Osman, 1968) and it has been suggested that this may also occur within 24 hours in humans infused with methadone (Porter *et al.*, 1983) or morphine (Marshall *et al.*, 1985).

In patients with chronic pain, the longer the duration of opioid treatment, the less frequent is the need to increase the dose of opioid and the smaller is the increment in dose needed (Kanner and Foley, 1981). Tolerance to opioid drugs in patients with chronic pain may also represent advancing disease (Twycross and Wald, 1976). Tolerance due to enzyme induction found with barbiturates and central nervous system depressants develops insidiously over some days or weeks.

Drugs suitable for steady state pharmacology

A suitable drug and a reliable delivery system are necessary before attempting to achieve steady state concentrations with a drug. Little therapeutic gain is achieved by formulating a drug with a long intrinsic duration of action into a rate-controlled preparation (Prescott, 1984). Vitamins, haematinics, thyroxine, reserpine, barbiturate hypnotics, phenobarbitone, chlorpromazine, amitryptyline and diazepam have all been marketed inappropriately as slow release preparations. Rate-controlled antibiotic therapy has yet to demonstrate improved efficacy, and it increases aminoglycoside nephrotoxicity and ototoxicity (Schentag, 1985).

Drugs for which rate-controlled administration is suitable include those which have:

1. Plasma-concentration-dependent effects and toxicity.
2. Low therapeutic index.
3. Short elimination half-lives.
4. Necessity of continuous administration for optimum therapeutic effect.

The actions of drugs whose effects bear a relation to their plasma concentration may be ranked according to the concentrations at which they occur. For example, Guedel's stages of anaesthesia relate clinical signs to increasing partial pressures of ether in the alveoli and, by inference, in the central nervous system (Guedel, 1951). Hyoscine will inhibit motion sickness at concentrations lower than those associated with dry mouth, tachycardia, drowsiness, cycloplegia, amnesia and hallucinations (Shaw and Urquhart, 1980). The analgesic effect of morphine was improved and the adverse effects were reduced in one study of morphine infusion after cholecystectomy (Rutter, Murphy and Dudley, 1980).

Table A4.1   Drugs whose actions are related to their rates of administration

Acetazolamide	ACTH	Angiotensin II
Bleomycin	Carbamazepine	Chlordiazepoxide
Cytosine arabinoside	Diphenhydramine	Fentanyl
	Dopamine	
Frusemide	Glucagon	Heparin
Hydrochlorothiazide	Hyoscine	Insulin
Morphine	Nitroglycerin	Noradrenaline
Oestradiol	Phenacetin	Pilocarpine
Sodium nitroprusside	Vasopressin	Volatile anaesthetic agents

(Data from Urquhart, 1982)

Rate-controlled therapy may make it possible to select specifically the desired effects of a drug (Table A4.1). This assumes greater importance with drugs where the difference between maximum tolerated and minimum effective concentrations is small. Delivering the drug at a rate whose resulting steady state concentration is between therapeutic and toxic values will avoid the fluctuating plasma concentrations produced by pulsed dosing which result in alternating toxicity and ineffective therapy.

Drugs with short elimination half-lives may require inconveniently frequent dosing to maintain their effect. The cardiovascular drugs dopamine, isoprenaline, nitroprusside and nitroglycerin must be given by infusion to limit the potentially disastrous adverse effects of rapidly fluctuating plasma concentrations. The rate of infusion of these drugs is titrated continuously against effect; so steady state concentrations may never be reached.

Cancer chemotherapeutic agents must be present at particular phases of the division cycle of their target cells to exert their effect (Carlson and Sikic, 1983). These drugs, however, have concentration-dependent toxic effects. Maintaining appropriate steady state plasma concentrations of these drugs prolongs drug action and ensures that target cells are affected at susceptible stages of their division cycle, whilst maintaining plasma concentrations below toxic values. Enhanced efficacy with reduced toxicity has been claimed during studies using infusions of doxorubicin (Legha et al., 1982), bleomycin (Sikic et al., 1978) and fluorouracil (Seifert et al., 1975).

Methods of achieving steady state concentrations

Therapeutic systems, whether for intravenous, topical or oral use, all contain the following elements (Urquhart, 1982).

1. Drug reservoir.
2. Energy source.
3. Rate controller, to limit the rate of drug administration.
4. Delivery portal, through which the drug passes to the patient.
5. Platform, which constitutes the contained or supporting materials of the therapeutic system.

A constant delivery rate is necessary to maintain constant plasma concentrations of a drug subject to first-order elimination. The time taken to reach steady state is a function of the half-life of the drug. Five half-lives must

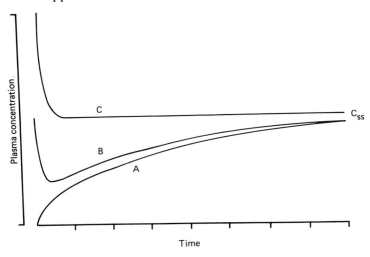

Fig. A4.1   Drug plasma concentrations produced by three infusion regimens. A: constant rate infusion alone $I = C_{ss}.Cl$. B: bolus of C_{ss}. V_1 followed by infusion I. C: bolus of C_{ss}. V_β followed by infusion I.
I = infusion rate; C_{ss} = steady state plasma concentration; Cl = clearance; V_β = apparent volume of distribution of a drug relating plasma concentration to amount of drug during slow elimination phase; V_1 = volume of central compartment.

elapse before steady state is reached (Fig. A4.1A), which is likely to be far too long to wait for a response. To reduce this delay, the therapeutic system may deliver the drug initially at a faster rate. For example, transdermal therapeutic systems containing hyoscine (TTS-hyoscine) contain hyoscine 140 μg in its adherent layer on the epidermal side of the rate-controlling microporous membrane. This serves as a priming dose before the constant delivery of hyoscine 0.5 mg over three days (Clissold and Heel, 1985). Intravenous infusion pumps under microprocessor control may be programmed to deliver sequentially infusions at different rates or concentrations to load the body compartments before maintaining a constant rate of infusion.

Two sequential infusions complicate the infusion regimen, but reduce the overshoot in plasma concentration (Fig. A4.2). The two infusion rates are calculated from the clearance, elimination half-life and desired drug plasma concentration. Shorter initial infusions reach steady state more quickly, but with a greater overshoot (Wagner, 1974).

Initial overshoot may be prevented using a bolus dose, maintenance infusion and an exponentially declining infusion (Krüger-Thiemer, 1968). This method has been developed in theory to produce an ideal lignocaine infusion regimen (Vaughan and Tucker, 1976) (Fig. A4.3).

Calculation of the component parts of the regimen is complex and involves many of a drug's pharmacokinetic parameters. Microprocessor-controlled infusion pumps are required to deliver the regimen using a solution of uniform concentration.

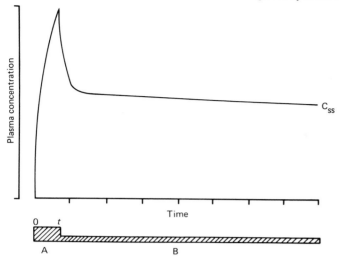

Fig. A4.2   Drug plasma concentrations produced by two sequential infusions. From time 0 to time t, A: initial fast infusion $I_1 = I_2/(1-e^{-\beta t})$ given that B: the second maintenance infusion, $I_2 = C_{ss}.Cl$ drug clearance and the elimination half-life are the only variables required to calculate the rate of both infusions. The shorter the time, t, of the initial infusion, the more rapidly is steady state achieved but with a greater overshoot. β = slow elimination phase hybrid rate constant.

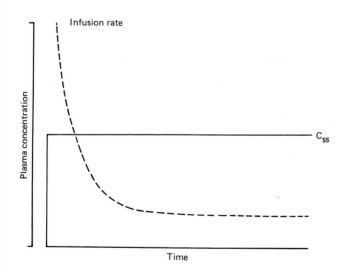

Fig. A4.3   Drug plasma concentrations produced by a bolus dose, a maintenance infusion and an exponentially declining infusion given simultaneously.
bolus dose: $C_{ss}V_1$; maintenance infusion: $C_{ss}Cl$; exponentially declining infusion: $X^0 (\alpha-k_{21}) (\beta-k_{21})^2.k_{21}.C^{-k_{21}\cdot t}$
where X^0 = dose given, α = fast hybrid rate constant and k_{21} = model rate constant between peripheral and central compartments.

Intravenous infusions to steady state

An initial bolus dose sufficient to load the central compartment offers little advantage over a simple infusion. The loading dose is distributed rapidly through peripheral compartments and the plasma concentration falls before climbing slowly to steady state (see Fig. A4.1b). A bolus dose sufficient to load every compartment prevents concentrations ever falling below steady state concentration (see Fig. A4.1c). The initial high concentrations produced are likely to cause toxic effects (Mitenko and Ogilvie, 1972).

Using the same principles, an alternative means of delivery with simple apparatus (shown in Fig. A4.4) has proved effective in achieving rapidly steady state concentrations of both lignocaine (Riddell *et al.*, 1984) and methohexitone (McMurray *et al.*, 1984). The maintenance solution is connected to a mixing vial which contains a more concentrated solution. The tubing from the mixing vial to the patient contains the loading dose. When the infusion pump is turned on, the patient receives a constant rate of infusion of a solution whose concentration declines exponentially from the original mixing vial solution to that of the maintenance solution.

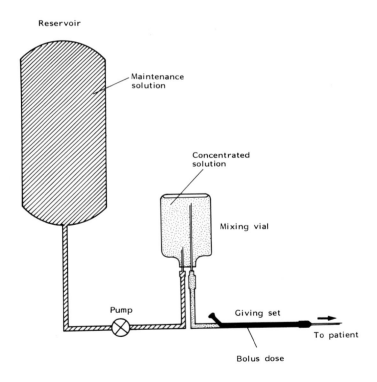

Fig. A4.4 Apparatus used to achieve steady state rapidly using three different solutions infused sequentially at a constant rate: (1) the bolus dose is injected into the giving set; (2) the concentrated solution is mixed in the vial with (3) the maintenance solution from the reservoir. (After Riddell *et al.*, 1984.)

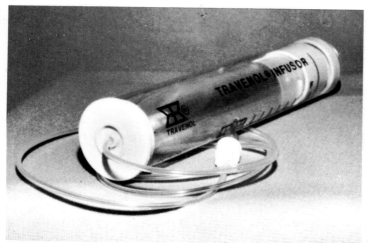

Fig. A4.5   The Baxter Travenol infusor.

Maintenance infusions may be delivered at a constant rate by syringe drivers or volumetric pumps. A lightweight disposable pump which requires no external power source had been introduced recently. The Baxter Travenol infusor (Fig. A4.5) delivers drugs dissolved in dextrose 5% solution at a constant rate of 2 ml per hour for 24 hours (Nimmo and Todd, 1985).

Examples of drugs delivered to steady state

Inhaled anaesthetic agents

The time taken to approach steady state with nitrous oxide and the modern halogenated volatile anaesthetic agents is short. The alveolar concentration of the poorly soluble nitrous oxide, delivered at high concentrations, nears the inspired gas concentration within 10 minutes, and the alveolar concentration of halothane is half the inspired concentration of 1% after 20 minutes (Eger, 1968).

Complete equilibrium with the fat- and vessel-poor tissues will not be reached, and some loss of anaesthetic agent will occur through leaks in the anaesthetic system and the surgical wound. Except for nitrous oxide and, in prolonged anaesthesia, the modern halogenated volatile anaesthetic agents, inhaled anaesthetic agents continue to be taken up throughout an anaesthetic. However, once the vessel-rich group of tissues is saturated, alveolar tension, which relates to that of the brain, approaches the inspired tension and the uptake of the anaesthetic agent is diminished appreciably. The patient remains at a near constant depth of anaesthesia until the inspired concentration of the anaesthetic agent is changed.

Minimum alveolar concentrations (MAC) published for inhaled anaesthetic agents each represent the mean of an assumed normal distribution of ED_{50} within the population. As far as variation within the population allows, the depth of anaesthesia desired can be selected by delivering an inspired concentration of an agent, which is a multiple or fraction of its MAC value.

Steady state will be approached more quickly using a relatively insoluble anaesthetic agent delivered at high concentration with increased ventilation of the lungs.

Intravenous anaesthetic agents

Infusions of intravenous anaesthetic agents have been used as part of the technique of total intravenous anaesthesia, to sedate patients whose lungs are ventilated artificially and to protect the brain after head injury or an episode of hypoxia.

The minimum infusion rate (MIR) has been used to compare potencies of drugs administered intravenously to produce anaesthesia but these do not necessarily reflect true potencies or steady state (Sear and Prys-Roberts, 1979).

The half-lives of barbiturates, etomidate and propofol are too long for the minimum infusion rate alone to be used to reach steady state plasma concentrations during an anaesthetic. Some success has been obtained using a three-stage infusion of methohexitone to attain steady state rapidly (McMurray et al., 1984).

Opioid analgesic drugs

The changing analgesic requirements of a patient during surgery have led to the development of interactive rate control of analgesic infusions. Microprocessor-controlled infusion pumps, programmed with the pharmacokinetic data for drugs such as alfentanil and fentanyl, are used to adjust drug input continuously to achieve the desired steady state concentrations for predicted surgical stimulation (Schüttler, Stoeckel and Schwilden, 1985).

Pain after surgery may last for days and is controlled poorly when treated with intramuscular opioids given 'on demand' (Hug, 1980). Analgesia may be improved by infusing opioids to steady state. The minimum effective analgesic plasma concentration required to relieve pain after surgery was determined for pethidine (Austin, Stapleton and Mather, 1980), and pain was controlled well when pethidine was infused to steady state by a series of three declining infusion rates begun after hysterectomy. Despite the two loading infusions, four out of ten patients reported severe pain in the first 3 hours when pethidine concentrations were below the minimum effective analgesic concentration (Stapleton, Austin and Mather, 1979). When constant rate infusions of fentanyl were begun 2 hours before surgery and supplemented by a further bolus dose during anaesthesia before skin incision, 44 patients attained steady state concentrations before surgery ended. They remained at steady state with effective analgesia until the infusions were discontinued at 24 hours (Duthie and Nimmo, 1985).

Tolerance to opioid infusions, as reported for methadone (Porter et al., 1983) and morphine (Marshall et al., 1985), may limit the usefulness of this regimen.

Neuromuscular-blocking agents

The introduction of the short acting, competitive neuromuscular-blocking agents has been followed by attempts to achieve unchanging neuromuscular blockade using continuous intravenous infusions (Flynn *et al.*, 1983; Mirakhur and Ferres, 1984). Monitoring drug effect by twitch height of evoked muscle contraction, the dose of drug needed to produce comparable effects was similar when given as an infusion or by intermittent dosing.

Repeat bolus doses of vecuronium had to be given every 12 minutes to maintain the twitch height below 25 per cent of control height; so the administration of vecuronium is simplified considerably by infusing at a rate necessary to achieve steady state effect (Noeldge, Hinsken and Buzello, 1984).

Hyoscine

Hyoscine is a competitive inhibitor of the muscarinic ACh receptors and an effective antiemetic. Its effects have been ranked according to measured urinary excretion rates, and increasing excretion rates are related to bradycardia, antiemetic effects, dry mouth, drowsiness and, lastly, tachycardia (Shaw and Urquhart, 1980). A transdermal preparation delivering 0.5 mg hyoscine at a constant rate over 3 days has been shown to provide effective prophylaxis against motion sickness at steady state with a reduced incidence of toxic side effects (Price *et al.*, 1981) and may be useful for perioperative nausea.

Insulin

Patients in severe diabetic ketoacidosis (pH $\leq$ 7.1) who received soluble insulin by a constant rate intravenous infusion required less insulin and suffered less hypoglycaemia than a comparable group who received insulin by 2-hourly intravenous and intramuscluar injections. The dose of the injections was related to plasma blood sugar concentrations, whereas the infusions were at a constant rate of 8 units of insulin per hour. Bicarbonate was withheld from the infusion group. The fall of plasma glucose and 3-hydroxybutyrate concentrations and the rise of arterial pH were similar in both groups.

During the first 6 hours of therapy the injection group received an average of 5.4 times the dose of insulin given to the infusion group and a third of the injection group experienced hypoglycaemia. None of the infusion group became hypoglycaemic (Lutterman, Adriaansen and van't Laar, 1979).

Heparin

Therapeutic effects with reduced toxicity can be achieved by infusing heparin to steady state. In patients treated with intravenous heparin there were no differences in mortality or recurrent thromboembolic complications between a group receiving heparin by continuous infusion and two groups receiving 4-hourly injections with or without laboratory control. The incidence of major haemorrhagic complications was seven times higher in both injection groups than in the infusion group. A smaller dose of heparin was required in the infusion group to maintain the partial thromboplastin time in the therapeutic range, but this difference just failed to achieve statistical significance (Salzman *et al.*, 1975).

Oxygen

Oxygen is given often to overcome hypoxaemia immediately after anaesthesia. An accurate assessment of pulmonary gas exchange in spontaneously breathing patients is possible only when using fixed performance oxygen delivery systems whose function is independent of patient factors. Low flow (anaesthetic circuits) and high flow (Ventimasks) systems will deliver a constant inspired oxygen concentration throughout the breathing cycle. The resultant arterial oxygen tension is obtained at steady state, which is not possible with variable performance oxygen delivery systems.

Conclusions

Administering a drug to steady state avoids the fluctuating plasma concentrations obtained with conventional divided dosing. There is the potential to select therapeutic effects whilst avoiding both toxic effects and subtherapeutic plasma drug concentrations. The benefits of steady state pharmacology are more obvious when using drugs with short elimination half-lives and narrow therapeutic indices. With more widespread application, rate-controlled drug administration may help improve the use of such drugs. Modern technology will facilitate rate-controlled drug administration.

References

Austin, K.L., Stapleton, J.V. and Mather, L.E. (1980) Relationship between blood meperidine concentrations and analgesic response: a preliminary report. *Anaesthesiology* **53**, 460–466

Bala Subramanian, V., Bowles, M.J., Khurmi, N.S., Davies, E.B., O'Hara, M.J. and Raftery, A.B. (1983) Calcium antagonist withdrawal syndrome: objective demonstration with frequency modulated ambulatory ST-segment monitoring. *British Medical Journal* **286**, 520–521

Carlson, R.W. and Sikic, B.I (1983) Continous infusion or bolus injection in cancer chemotherapy. *Annals of Internal Medicine* **99**, 823–833

Casson, W.R., Jones, R.M. and Parsons, R.S. (1984) Nifedipine and cardiopulmonary bypass. Post-bypass management after continuation or withdrawal of therapy. *Anaesthesia* **39**, 1197–1201

Clissold, S.P. and Heel, R.C. (1985) Transdermal hyoscine (scopolamine). A preliminary review of its pharacodynamic properties and therapeutic efficacy. *Drugs* **29**, 189–207

Cox, B.M., Ginsburg, M, and Osman, O.H. (1968) Acute tolerance to narcotic analgesic drugs. *British Journal of Pharmacology* **33**, 245–256

Duthie, D.J.R. and Nimmo, W.S. (1985) The pharmacokinetics of fentanyl by constant rate i.v. infusion for pain relief after surgery. *Anesthesiology* **63**, A282

Eger, E.I. (1968) Applications of a mathematical model of gas uptake. In: *Uptake and Distribution of Anaesthetic Agents* (Eds. Papper, E.M. and Kitz, R.J.), pp. 88–103. Mcgraw-Hill: New York

Flynn, P.J., Hughes, R., Walton, B. and Jothilingham, S. (1983) Use of atracurium infusions for general surgical procedures including cardiac surgery with induced hypothermia. *British Journal of Anaesthesia* 55, 135S–138S

George, C.F. (1985) Hazards of the abrupt withdrawal of drugs. *Prescribers' Journal* 25, 31–39

Goldman, P. (1982) Rate controlled drug delivery. *New England Journal of Medicine* 307, 286–290

Guedel, A.E. (1951) *Inhalation Anaesthesia: a fundamental guide*, 2nd ed., Macmillan: London

Heilmann, K. (1985) Long-term follow-up of controlled-release pilocarpine therapy. In: *Rate Control in Drug Therapy* (Eds. Prescott, L.F. and Nimmo, W.S.), pp. 265–275. Churchill Livingstone: Edinburgh

Hug, C.C. (1980) Improving analgesic therapy. *Anesthesiology* 53, 441–443

Kanner, R.M. and Foley, K.M. (1981) Patterns of narcotic drug use in a cancer pain clinic. *Annals of the New York Academy of Sciences* 362, 161–172

Koch-Weser, J., (1972) Drug therapy, Serum drug concentrations as therapeutic guides. *New England Journal of Medicine* 287, 227–231

Krüger-Thiemer, E. (1968) Continuous intravenous infusion and multicompartment accumulation. *European Journal of Pharmacology* 4, 317–324

Lawson, A.A.H. (1985) Clinical studies and pharmacological studies with transdermal clonidine. In: *Rate Control in Drug Therapy* (Eds. Prescott, L.F. and Nimmo, W.S.), pp. 215–219, Churchill Livingstone. Edinburgh

Legha, S.S., Benjamin, R.S., MacKay, B., *et al.* (1982) Reduction of doxorubicin cardiotoxicity by prolonged continuous intravenous infusion. *Annals of Internal Medicine* 96, 133–139

Lutterman, J.A., Adriaansen, A.A.J. and van't Laar, A. (1979) Treatment of severe diabetic ketoacidosis. A comparative study of two methods. *Diabetologia* 17, 17–21

Marshall, H., Porteous, C., McMillan, I., Macpherson, S.G. and Nimmo, W.S. (1985) Relief of pain by infusion of morphine after operation: does tolerance develop? *British Medical Journal* 291, 19–21

McMurray, T. J., Riddell, J.G., Dundee, J.W. and McAllister, C.B. (1984) A new simple method for rapidly achieving and maintaining constant methohexitone concentrations. *British Journal of Anaesthesia* 56, 429P

Mirakhur, R.K. and Ferres, C.J, (1984) Muscle relaxation with an infusion of vecuronium. *European Journal of Anaesthesiology* 1, 353–359

Mitenko, P.A. and Ogilvie, R.I. (1972) Rapidly achieved plasma concentration plateaus, with observations on theophylline kinetics. *Clinical Pharmacology and Therapeutics* 13, 329–335

Nimmo, W.S. and Todd, J.G. (1985) Fentanyl by constant rate i.v. infusion for postoperative analgesia. *British Journal of Anaesthesia* 57, 250–254

Noeldge, G., Hinsken, H. and Buzello, W. (1984) Comparison between the continuous infusion of vecuronium and the intermittent administration of pancuronium and vecuronium. *British Journal of Anaesthesia* 56, 473–477

Porter, E.J.B., McQuay, H.J., Bullingham, R.E.S., Weir, L., Allen, M.C. and Moore, R.A. (1983) Comparison of effects of intraoperative and postoperative methadone: acute tolerance to the postoperative dose? *British Journal of Anaesthesia* 55, 325–332

Prescott, L.F. (1984) Historical review and perspective of rate control in drug therapy. In: *Rate Control in Drug Therapy* (Eds. Prescott, L.F. and Nimmo, W.S.), pp. 1–10. Churchill Livingstone: Edinburgh

Price, N.M., Schmitt, L.G., McGuire, J., Shaw, J.E. and Trobough, G. (1981) Transdermal scopolamine in the prevention of motion sickness at sea. *Clinical Pharmacology and Therapeutics* 29, 414–419

Rawlins, M.D. and Bateman, D.N. (1985) The contribution of absorption to variation in response to drugs. In: *Rate Control in Drug Therapy* (Eds. Prescott, L.F. and

Nimmo, W.S.), pp. 11–18. Churchill Livingstone: Edinburgh

Riddell, J.G., McAllister, C.B., Wilkinson, G.R., Wood, A.J.J. and Roden, D.M. (1984) A new method for constant plasma drug concentrations: application to lidocaine. *Annals of Internal Medicine* **100**, 25–28

Rutter, P.C., Murphy, F. and Dudley, H.A.F. (1980) Morphine: controlled trial of different methods of administration for postoperative pain relief. *British Medical Journal* **281**, 12–13

Salzman, E.W., Daykin, D., Shapiro, R.M. and Rosenberg, R. (1975) Management of heparin therapy. *New England Journal of Medicine* **292**, 1046–1050

Schentag, J.J. (1985) Rate-controlled antibiotic therapy. In: *Rate Control in Drug Therapy* (Eds. Prescott, L.F. and Nimmo, W.S.), pp. 282–288. Churchill Livingstone: Edinburgh

Schüttler, J., Stoeckel, H. and Schwilden, H. (1985) Clinical experience with interactive rate control of intravenous anaesthesia. In: *Rate Control in Drug Therapy* (Eds. Prescott, L.F. and Nimmo, W.S.), pp. 232–236. Churchill Livingstone: Edinburgh

Sear, J.W. and Prys-Roberts, C. (1979) Dose-related haemodynamic effects of continuous infusions of Althesin in man. *British Journal of Anaesthesia* **51**, 867–874

Seifert, P., Baker, L.H., Reed, M.L. and Vaitkevicius, V.K. (1975) Comparison of continously infused 5-fluorouracil with bolus injections in treatment of patients with colorectal adenocarcinoma. *Cancer* **36**, 123–128

Shand, D.G. and Wood, A.J.J. (1978) Propranolol withdrawal syndrome—why? *Circulation* **58**, 202–203

Shaw, J.E. and Urquhart, J. (1980) Programmed, systemic drug delivery by the transdermal route. *Trends in Pharmacological Sciences* **1**, 208–211

Shimomura, K., Kamato, O., Ueki, S. *et al.* (1971) Analgesia effects of morphine glucuronides. *Tohoku Journal of Experimental Medicine* **105**, 45–52

Sikic, B.I., Collins, J.M., Mimaugh, E.G. and Gram, T.E. (1978) Improved therapeutic index of bleomycin when administered by continuous infusion in mice. *Cancer Treatment Reports* **62**, 2011–2017

Stanski, D.R. and Watkins, W.D. (1982) *Drug Disposition in Anaesthesia*, p. 91. Grune & Stratton: New York

Stapleton, J.V., Austin, K.L. and Mather, L.E. (1979) A pharmacokinetic approach to postoperative pain: continuous infusion of pethidine. *Anaesthesia and Intensive Care* **7**, 25–32

Svensson, J.O., Rane, A., Sawe, J. and Sjoquist, F. (1982) Determination of morphine, morphine-3-glucuronide and (tentatively) morphine-6-glucuronide in plasma and urine using ion-pair high performance liquid chromatography. *Journal of Chromatography* **230**, 427–432

Twycross, R.G. and Wald, S.J. (1976) Long term use of diamorphine in advanced cancer. In: *Advances in Pain Research and Therapy*, vol. II (Eds. Bonica, J.J. and Albe-Fessard, D.G.), pp. 653–661. Raven Press: New York

Urquhart, J. (1982) Rate controlled drug dosage. *Drugs* **23**, 207–226

Vaughan, D.P. and Tucker, G.T. (1976) General derivation of the ideal intravenous drug input required to achieve and maintain a constant plasma drug concentration. Theoretical application to lignocaine therapy. *European Journal of Clinical Pharmacology* **10**, 433–440

Wagner, J.G. (1974) A safe method for rapidly achieving plasma concentration plateaus. *Clinical Pharmacology and Therapeutics* **16**, 691–700

Index